Healthy Heart Sourcebook for Women

Heart Diseases & Disorders
Sourcebook, 2nd Edition

Household Safety Sourcebook

Immune System Disorders Sourcebook

Infant & Toddler Health Sourcebook

Infectious Diseases Sourcebook

Injury & Trauma Sourcebook

Kidney & Urinary Tract Diseases &
Disorders Sourcebook

Learning Disabilities Sourcebook,
2nd Edition

Leukemia Sourcebook

Liver Disorders Sourcebook

Lung Disorders Sourcebook

Medical Tests Sourcebook, 2nd Edition

Men's Health Concerns Sourcebook,
2nd Edition

Mental Health Disorders Sourcebook,
2nd Edition

Mental Retardation Sourcebook

Movement Disorders Sourcebook

Obesity Sourcebook

Osteoporosis Sourcebook

Pain Sourcebook, 2nd Edition

Pediatric Cancer Sourcebook

Physical & Mental Issues in Aging
Sourcebook

Podiatry Sourcebook

Pregnancy & Birth Sourcebook,
2nd Edition

Prostate Cancer

Public Health Sourcebook

Reconstructive & Cosmetic Surgery
Sourcebook

Rehabilitation Sourcebook

Respiratory Diseases & Disorders
Sourcebook

Sexually Transmitted Diseases
Sourcebook, 2nd Edition

Skin Diso

Sleep Disc

Sports Inju

Stress-Rela

Stroke Sou

Substance Abuse Sourcebook

Surgery Sourcebook

Transplantation Sourcebook

Traveler's Health Sourcebook

Vegetarian Sourcebook

Women's Health Concerns Sourcebook,
2nd Edition

Workplace Health & Safety Sourcebook

Worldwide Health Sourcebook

Teen Health Series

Cancer Information for Teens

Diet Information for Teens

Drug Information for Teens

Fitness Information for Teens

Mental Health Information
for Teens

Sexual Health Information
for Teens

Skin Health Information
for Teens

Sports Injuries Information
for Teens

Genetic Disorders
SOURCEBOOK

Third Edition

Health Reference Series

Third Edition

Genetic Disorders
SOURCEBOOK

Basic Consumer Health Information about Hereditary Diseases and Disorders, Including Facts about the Human Genome, Genetic Inheritance Patterns, Disorders Associated with Specific Genes, Such as Sickle Cell Disease, Hemophilia, and Cystic Fibrosis, Chromosome Disorders, Such as Down Syndrome, Fragile X Syndrome, and Turner Syndrome, and Complex Diseases and Disorders Resulting from the Interaction of Environmental and Genetic Factors, Such as Allergies, Cancer, and Obesity

Along with Facts about Genetic Testing, Suggestions for Parents of Children with Special Needs, Reports on Current Research Initiatives, a Glossary of Genetic Terminology, and Resources for Additional Help and Information

Edited by
Karen Bellenir

Omnigraphics

615 Griswold Street • Detroit, MI 48226

Bibliographic Note

Because this page cannot legibly accommodate all the copyright notices, the Bibliographic Note portion of the Preface constitutes an extension of the copyright notice.

Edited by Karen Bellenir

Health Reference Series

Karen Bellenir, Managing Editor
David A. Cooke, M.D., Medical Consultant
Elizabeth Barbour, Permissions Associate
Dawn Matthews, Verification Assistant
Laura Pleva Nielsen, Index Editor
EdIndex, Services for Publishers, Indexers

* * *

Omnigraphics, Inc.

Matthew P. Barbour, Senior Vice President
Kay Gill, Vice President—Directories
Kevin Hayes, Operations Manager
Leif Gruenberg, Development Manager
David P. Bianco, Marketing Director

* * *

Peter E. Ruffner, Publisher

Frederick G. Ruffner, Jr., Chairman

Copyright © 2004 Omnigraphics, Inc.

ISBN 0-7808-0742-1

Library of Congress Cataloging-in-Publication Data

Genetic disorders sourcebook : basic consumer health information about hereditary diseases and disorders, including facts about the human genome, genetic inheritance patterns, disorders associated with specific genes, such as sickle cell disease, hemophilia, and cystic fibrosis, chromosome disorders, such as Down syndrome, fragile x syndrome, and Turner syndrome, and complex diseases and disorders resulting from the interaction of environmental and genetic factors, such as allergies, cancer, and obesity; along with facts about genetic testing, suggestions for parents of children with special needs, reports on current research initiatives, a glossary of genetic terminology, and resources for additional help and information--3rd ed. / Karen Bellenir.
    p. cm.
  Includes bibliographical references and index.
  ISBN 0-7808-0742-1 (hardcover : alk. paper)
  1. Human chromosome abnormalities--Popular works. I. Bellenir, Karen.
  RB155.5.G455 2004
  616'.042--dc22

                                                                  2004020841

Table of Contents

Visit www.healthreferenceseries.com to view *A Contents Guide to the Health Reference Series*, a listing of more than 10,000 topics and the volumes in which they are covered.

Preface xi

Part I: Understanding Inheritance

Chapter 1—Genes and How They Work 3

Chapter 2—The Human Genome 15

Chapter 3—What Are Genetic Disorders? 37

Chapter 4—How Are Genetic Disorders Inherited? 47

Part II: Disorders Associated with Specific Genes

Chapter 5—Albinism 57

Chapter 6—Alpha-1 Antitrypsin Deficiency 67

Chapter 7—Bleeding Disorders 77

   Section 7.1—Hemophilia A (Factor
         VIII Deficiency) 78

   Section 7.2—Hemophilia B (Factor
         IX Deficiency) 83

   Section 7.3—Factor I Deficiency
         (Afibrinogenemia) 85

   Section 7.4—von Willebrand Disease 87

Chapter 8—Blood Disorders 91

    Section 8.1—Fanconi Anemia 92

    Section 8.2—Hemochromatosis 96

    Section 8.3—Sickle Cell Anemia 101

    Section 8.4—Thalassemia 107

Chapter 9—Color Blindness 111

Chapter 10—Connective Tissue Disorders 115

    Section 10.1—Questions and Answers
               about Heritable Disorders
               of Connective Tissue 116

    Section 10.2—Ehlers-Danlos Syndrome 120

    Section 10.3—Marfan Syndrome 122

Chapter 11—Cystic Fibrosis 129

Chapter 12—Glycogen Storage Disease 135

Chapter 13—Growth Disorders 139

    Section 13.1—What Is a Growth Disorder? ... 140

    Section 13.2—Achondroplasia 144

    Section 13.3—Other Less Common Types
               of Dwarfism 147

Chapter 14—Hereditary Deafness 155

Chapter 15—Huntington Disease 159

Chapter 16—Inborn Errors of Metabolism 171

    Section 16.1—Biotinidase Deficiency 172

    Section 16.2—Galactosemia 173

    Section 16.3—Maple Syrup Urine Disease 175

    Section 16.4—Phenylketonuria (PKU) 177

    Section 16.5—Tyrosinemia 182

    Section 16.6—Urea Cycle Disorders 184

Chapter 17—Leukodystrophies 189

Chapter 18—Lipid Storage Diseases 199

    Section 18.1—Batten Disease 200

    Section 18.2—Fabry Disease 206

    Section 18.3—Gaucher Disease 210

    Section 18.4—Mucolipidoses 214

Section 18.5—Mucopolysaccharidoses 216

Section 18.6—Niemann-Pick Disease 226

Section 18.7—Sandhoff Disease 234

Section 18.8—Tay-Sachs Disease 236

Chapter 19—Neurofibromatoses 243

Chapter 20—Neuromuscular Disorders 249

Section 20.1—Barth Syndrome 250

Section 20.2—Charcot-Marie-Tooth
Disease 251

Section 20.3—Mitochondrial Myopathies 257

Section 20.4—Muscular Dystrophies 258

Section 20.5—Spinal Muscular Atrophy 273

Chapter 21—Rett Syndrome 285

Chapter 22—Tuberous Sclerosis 289

Chapter 23—Wilson Disease 295

Part III: Chromosome Disorders

Chapter 24—Chromosome Abnormalities 299

Chapter 25—Angelman Syndrome 303

Chapter 26—Cri du Chat Syndrome 311

Chapter 27—DiGeorge Syndrome 319

Chapter 28—Down Syndrome 325

Section 28.1—Basic Facts about Down
Syndrome 326

Section 28.2—Understanding the
Different Types of Down
Syndrome 329

Section 28.3—How Is Down Syndrome
Diagnosed in a Newborn? 331

Section 28.4—Health Issues in Down
Syndrome 332

Section 28.5—Early Intervention and
Down Syndrome 333

Chapter 29—Edwards Syndrome 339

Chapter 30—Fragile X Syndrome 343

Chapter 31—Klinefelter Syndrome... 359

Chapter 32—Patau Syndrome 369

Chapter 33—Prader-Willi Syndrome 373

Chapter 34—Triple X Syndrome 377

Chapter 35—Turner Syndrome 379

Chapter 36—Williams Syndrome.. 387

Part IV: Complex Disorders with a Genetic Component

Chapter 37—The Interplay of Genes and the Environment.... 393

Chapter 38—Cancer Genetics 395

        Section 38.1—Cancer Genetics Overview 396

        Section 38.2—Heredity and Breast Cancer ... 407

        Section 38.3—Heredity and Colon Cancer 409

        Section 38.4—Heredity and Skin Cancer 411

        Section 38.5—Heredity and Prostate
                  Cancer 414

Chapter 39—Genital and Urinary Tract Defects 417

Chapter 40—Diabetes and Genetics 425

Chapter 41—Genetic Factors in Obesity 433

Chapter 42—Multiple Genetic and Environmental
          Factors Influence Heart Disorders 437

        Section 42.1—Congenital Cardiovascular
                  Defects 438

        Section 42.2—Familial Dilated
                  Cardiomyopathy 450

        Section 42.3—Genetics Linked with
                  Sudden Cardiac Death 456

Chapter 43—Genetics and High Blood Pressure 459

Chapter 44—Hereditary Factors in Allergy and Asthma 463

        Section 44.1—Genetic Risk for Allergy
                  and Asthma.............................. 464

Section 44.2—Scientists Identify Genes
that Regulate Allergic
Response to Diesel Fumes 466

Chapter 45—Heredity and Parkinson Disease 469

Chapter 46—Genes and the Development of
Alzheimer's Disease 471

Chapter 47—Mental Illness: Evidence of a Genetic
Component 477

Section 47.1—Family History of
Mental Illness 478

Section 47.2—Hunting for Genes
Associated with Mental
Illnesses 481

Chapter 48—Addiction and Genetics... 485

Section 48.1—The Genetics of Alcoholism 486

Section 48.2—Gene Linked to Drug
Addiction 493

Section 48.3—Is There an Inherited
Vulnerability to Nicotine
Addiction? 495

Part V: Genetics and Family Matters

Chapter 49—Genetic Counseling 501

Chapter 50—Genetic Testing 507

Chapter 51—Evaluating Gene Tests 513

Chapter 52—Prenatal Testing.. 517

Chapter 53—Newborn Screening Tests.................................... 531

Chapter 54—A Guide for Parents of Children with
Chronic Conditions 535

Chapter 55—Special Education Services for Children
with Disabilities 549

Chapter 56—Genetics Privacy and Legislation 557

Chapter 57—Genetic Discrimination in Health Insurance 567

ix

Chapter 58—Planning for the Future for People with
    Special Needs 571

Part VI: Genetic Research

Chapter 59—The Human Genome Project 579

Chapter 60—Beyond Genes: Scientists Venture Deeper
    Into the Human Genome 583

Chapter 61—Recently Developed Medical Technologies 587

Chapter 62—Single Nucleotide Polymorphisms (SNPs).......... 595

Chapter 63—Novel Mechanism Preserves Y Chromosome
    Genes 599

Chapter 64—Gene Discovery Opens Door to Further
    Research in Inherited Neurological
    Disorders 603

Chapter 65—Researchers Identify Gene for Premature
    Aging Disorder 607

Chapter 66—Behavioral Genetics 613

Chapter 67—The Promise of Pharmacogenomics 623

Chapter 68—Gene Therapy 627

Part VII: Additional Help and Information

Chapter 69—Glossary of Genetic Terms 635

Chapter 70—Newborn Screening Programs in the
    United States 655

Chapter 71—Resources for Information about Genetics
    and Genetic Research 677

Chapter 72—Genetic Disorders: A Directory of
    Information and Support Resources 683

Index **713**

Preface

About This Book

All people share more than 99 percent of the same hereditary information. The remaining fraction of a percent is responsible for the differences that make each person unique. Some gene variations produce physical traits, such as eye, hair, and skin color. Other gene variations, called mutations, can alter the way the body's cells function and lead to medical consequences. All together, genetic alterations are directly responsible for an estimated 5,000 disorders. In addition, researchers are discovering that genes also play a role in the development of many other diseases by influencing how the body responds to environmental factors. The study of genetics is demonstrating how some of the most significant circumstances in a person's life can be affected by some of the smallest pieces in the genetic puzzle.

Genetic Disorders Sourcebook, Third Edition explains how human inheritance works and offers facts about disorders linked to mutations in specific genes, such as sickle cell disease, hemophilia, and cystic fibrosis, or to chromosome abnormalities, such as Down syndrome, fragile X syndrome, and Turner syndrome. A section on disorders that arise from the complex interaction of genetic and environmental factors describes the hereditary components of such disorders as allergies, Alzheimer's disease, cancer, diabetes, high blood pressure, and obesity. A section on genetics and family matters offers information for parents of children with disabilities, provides facts about genetic privacy and discrimination, and describes genetic counseling, prenatal testing, and newborn screening programs. Reports on current research initiatives describe the development of new medical technologies that hold the promise of transforming the future of medical care. A glossary of genetic terms and resource directories for additional help and information are also included.

How to Use This Book

This book is divided into parts and chapters. Parts focus on broad areas of interest. Chapters are devoted to single topics within a part.

Part I: Understanding Inheritance provides answers to basic questions about cells and cellular functioning, DNA (deoxyribonucleic acid), genes, chromosomes, and the human genome. It describes the processes that lead to genetic disorders and explains different types of inheritance patterns.

Part II: Disorders Associated with Specific Genes describes disorders linked to mutations that cause a gene to malfunction. Researchers estimate that humans have approximately 30,000 different genes, each of which consists of a unique sequence of DNA and comprises from several hundred to more than two million DNA bases. Genes accomplish their tasks by providing instructions that control the activities of every cell in the body. Genetic disorders result from malfunctions in this process. Examples include albinism, hemophilia, muscular dystrophy, phenylketonuria (PKU), and sickle cell anemia.

Part III: Chromosome Disorders describes disorders caused by changes in the number or form of the chromosomes, the structures that carry the genes. A typical human cell contains 46 chromosomes, one set of 23 chromosomes inherited from a biological mother and another set of 23 chromosomes inherited from a biological father. Changes in the number of chromosomes, such as inheriting three instead of two copies of a particular chromosome, or in the structure of chromosomes, such as a portion of a chromosome being deleted or repeated, lead to medical syndromes that can affect many areas of physical and mental development. These types of hereditary disorders are known as chromosomal abnormalities. Examples include Down syndrome, fragile x syndrome, and Turner syndrome.

Part IV: Complex Disorders with a Genetic Component describes disorders where genetic variations are linked to higher risks for certain diseases because they influence a person's susceptibility to hazards in his or her environment. According to the Centers for Disease Control and Prevention (CDC), researchers now believe that virtually all human diseases result from the interaction of genetic susceptibility factors and modifiable environmental factors, which are broadly defined to include infectious, chemical, physical, nutritional, and behavioral factors. Examples of diseases with identified genetic links include cancer, diabetes, high blood pressure, obesity, and Alzheimer's disease.

Part V: Genetics and Family Matters offers information about such topics as genetic counseling, prenatal testing, and newborn screening. It provides tips for parents of children with chronic conditions and disabilities and discusses ethical issues related to the use of genetic information.

Part VI: Genetic Research reports on recent developments, innovative medical technologies, and new discoveries that may impact the future course of medical care.

Part VII: Additional Help and Information provides a glossary of genetic terms, state contacts for newborn screening programs, a list of resources for information about genetics and genetic research, and a directory of information and support resources for specific genetic disorders.

Bibliographic Note

This volume contains documents and excerpts from publications issued by the following U.S. government agencies: Alzheimer's Disease Education and Referral Center; Centers for Disease Control and Prevention (CDC); Genetics Home Reference, a service of the National Library of Medicine; Human Genome Project; National Cancer Institute; National Center for Biotechnology Information; National Digestive Diseases Information Clearinghouse; National Dissemination Center for Children with Disabilities (NICHCY); National Human Genome Research Institute; National Institute of Allergy and Infectious Diseases; National Institute of Arthritis and Musculoskeletal and Skin Diseases; National Institute of Child Health and Human Development; National Institute of Diabetes and Digestive and Kidney Diseases; National Institute of Mental Health; National Institute of Neurological Disorders and Stroke; National Institute on Alcohol

Abuse and Alcoholism; National Institute on Drug Abuse; Oak Ridge National Laboratory; and the U.S. Food and Drug Administration (FDA).

In addition, this volume contains copyrighted documents from the following organizations: A.D.A.M., Inc.; Alpha-1 Association; American Association for the Advancement of Science; American Heart Association; American Liver Foundation; Angelman Syndrome Foundation; Cincinnati Children's Hospital Medical Center; Cri Du Chat Support Group of Australia, Inc.; Duke University Medical Center; Ehlers-Danlos National Foundation; Emory University School of Medicine, Department of Human Genetics; Families of Spinal Muscular Atrophy; Fanconi Amenia Research Fund, Inc.; Harvard Medical School Center for Hereditary Deafness; HeartCenterOnline, Inc.; International Albinism Center at the University of Minnesota; Johns Hopkins Department of Orthopaedic Surgery; Late Onset Tay-Sachs Foundation; Lippincott Williams and Wilkins; Maple Syrup Urine Disease Family Support Group; March of Dimes Birth Defects Foundation; MedicineNet, Inc.; Muscular Dystrophy Association; National Association for Down Syndrome; National Down Syndrome Society; National Gaucher Foundation; National Hemophilia Foundation; National Newborn Screening and Genetics Resource Center; National Niemann-Pick Disease Foundation; National Organization of Rare Disorders (NORD); National Tay-Sachs and Allied Diseases Association, Inc.; National Urea Cycle Disorders Foundation; Nemours Center for Children's Health Media, a division of The Nemours Foundation; Prader-Willi Syndrome Association; University of Illinois Eye Center; University of Michigan Health System; University of Texas Health Science Center at Houston; and Williams Syndrome Association.

Full citation information is provided on the first page of each chapter. Every effort has been made to secure all necessary rights to reprint the copyrighted material. If any omissions have been made, please contact Omnigraphics to make corrections for future editions.

Acknowledgements

In addition to the organizations and agencies listed above, special thanks go to many others who have worked hard to help bring this book to fruition, especially editorial assistants Elizabeth Bellenir, Sandra Lawton, and Dawn Matthews, permissions associate Liz Barbour, and indexer Edward J. Prucha.

About the Health Reference Series

The *Health Reference Series* is designed to provide basic medical information for patients, families, caregivers, and the general public. Each volume takes a particular topic and provides comprehensive coverage. This is especially important for people who may be dealing with a newly diagnosed disease or a chronic disorder in themselves or in a family member. People looking for preventive guidance, information about disease warning signs, medical statistics, and risk factors for health problems will also find answers to their questions in the *Health Reference Series*. The *Series*, however, is not intended to serve as a tool for diagnosing illness, in prescribing treatments, or as a substitute for the physician/patient relationship. All people concerned about medical symptoms or the possibility of disease are encouraged to seek professional care from an appropriate health care provider.

Locating Information within the Health Reference Series

The *Health Reference Series* contains a wealth of information about a wide variety of medical topics. Ensuring easy access to all the fact sheets, research reports, in-depth discussions, and other material contained within the individual books of the series remains one of our highest priorities. As the *Series* continues to grow in size and scope, however, locating the precise information needed by a reader may become more challenging.

A *Contents Guide to the Health Reference Series* was developed to direct readers to the specific volumes that address their concerns. It presents an extensive list of diseases, treatments, and other topics of general interest compiled from the Tables of Contents and major index headings. To access *A Contents Guide to the Health Reference Series*, visit www.healthreferenceseries.com.

Medical Consultant

Medical consultation services are provided to the *Health Reference Series* editors by David A. Cooke, M.D. Dr. Cooke is a graduate of Brandeis University, and he received his M.D. degree from the University of Michigan. He completed residency training at the University of Wisconsin Hospital and Clinics. He is board-certified in Internal Medicine. Dr. Cooke currently works as part of the University of Michigan Health System and practices in Brighton, MI. In his free time, he enjoys writing, science fiction, and spending time with his family.

Our Advisory Board

We would like to thank the following board members for providing guidance to the development of this series:

Dr. Lynda Baker,
Associate Professor of Library and Information Science,
Wayne State University, Detroit, MI

Nancy Bulgarelli,
William Beaumont Hospital Library, Royal Oak, MI

Karen Imarisio,
Bloomfield Township Public Library, Bloomfield Township, MI

Karen Morgan,
Mardigian Library, University of Michigan-Dearborn, Dearborn, MI

Rosemary Orlando,
St. Clair Shores Public Library, St. Clair Shores, MI

Health Reference Series *Update Policy*

The inaugural book in the *Health Reference Series* was the first edition of *Cancer Sourcebook* published in 1989. Since then, the *Series* has been enthusiastically received by librarians and in the medical community. In order to maintain the standard of providing high-quality health information for the layperson the editorial staff at Omnigraphics felt it was necessary to implement a policy of updating volumes when warranted.

Medical researchers have been making tremendous strides, and it is the purpose of the *Health Reference Series* to stay current with the most recent advances. Each decision to update a volume is made on an individual basis. Some of the considerations include how much new information is available and the feedback we receive from people who use the books. If there is a topic you would like to see added to the update list, or an area of medical concern you feel has not been adequately addressed, please write to:

Editor
Health Reference Series
Omnigraphics, Inc.
615 Griswold Street
Detroit, MI 48226
E-mail: editorial@omnigraphics.com

Part One

Understanding Inheritance

Chapter 1

Genes and How They Work

What is a cell?

Cells are the basic building blocks of all living things. The human body is composed of trillions of cells. They provide structure for the body, take in nutrients from food, convert those nutrients into energy, and carry out specialized functions. Cells also contain the body's hereditary material and can make copies of themselves.

Cells have many parts, each with a different function. Some of these parts, called organelles, are specialized structures that perform certain tasks within the cell. Human cells contain the following major parts, listed in alphabetical order:

- **Cytoplasm:** The cytoplasm is fluid inside the cell that surrounds the organelles.

- **Endoplasmic reticulum (ER):** This organelle helps process molecules created by the cell and transport them to their specific destinations either inside or outside the cell.

- **Golgi apparatus:** The Golgi apparatus packages molecules processed by the endoplasmic reticulum to be transported out of the cell.

"The Basics: Genes and How They Work," from *Genetics Home Reference: A Guide to Understanding Genetic Conditions,* a service of the U.S. National Library of Medicine, January 2003, updated March 2004; available online at http://ghr.nlm.nih.gov.

- **Lysosomes and peroxisomes:** These organelles are the recycling center of the cell. They digest foreign bacteria that invade the cell, rid the cell of toxic substances, and recycle worn-out cell components.

- **Mitochondria:** Mitochondria are complex organelles that convert energy from food into a form that the cell can use. They have their own genetic material, separate from the DNA in the nucleus, and can make copies of themselves.

- **Nucleus:** The nucleus serves as the cell's command center, sending directions to the cell to grow, mature, divide, or die. It also houses DNA (deoxyribonucleic acid), the cell's hereditary material. The nucleus is surrounded by a membrane called the nuclear envelope, which protects the DNA and separates the nucleus from the rest of the cell.

- **Plasma membrane:** The plasma membrane is the outer lining of the cell. It separates the cell from its environment and allows materials to enter and leave the cell.

- **Ribosomes:** Ribosomes are organelles that process the cell's genetic instructions to create proteins. These organelles can float freely in the cytoplasm or be connected to the endoplasmic reticulum.

What is DNA?

DNA, or deoxyribonucleic acid, is the hereditary material in humans and almost all other organisms. Nearly every cell in a person's body has the same DNA. Most DNA is located in the cell nucleus (where it is called nuclear DNA), but a small amount of DNA can also be found in the mitochondria (where it is called mitochondrial DNA or mtDNA).

The information in DNA is stored as a code made up of four chemical bases: adenine (A), guanine (G), cytosine (C), and thymine (T). Human DNA consists of about 3 billion bases, and more than 99 percent of those bases are the same in all people. The order, or sequence, of these bases determines the information available for building and maintaining an organism, similar to the way in which letters of the alphabet appear in a certain order to form words and sentences.

DNA bases pair up with each other, A with T and C with G, to form units called base pairs. Each base is also attached to a sugar molecule and a phosphate molecule. Together, a base, sugar, and phosphate are called a nucleotide. Nucleotides are arranged in two long strands that form a spiral called a double helix. The structure of the double helix is somewhat like a ladder, with the base pairs forming the ladder's rungs and the sugar and phosphate molecules forming the vertical side pieces of the ladder.

An important property of DNA is that it can replicate, or make copies of itself. Each strand of DNA in the double helix can serve as a pattern for duplicating the sequence of bases. This is critical when cells divide because each new cell needs to have an exact copy of the DNA present in the old cell.

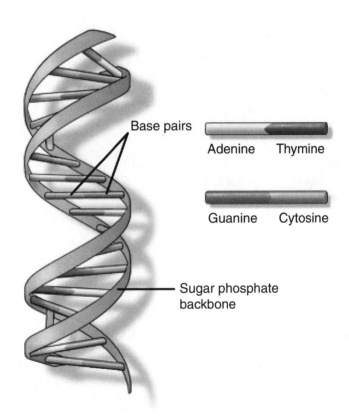

Figure 1.1. *DNA is a double helix formed by base pairs attached to a sugar-phosphate backbone (Source: U.S. National Library of Medicine).*

What is a gene?

A gene is the basic physical and functional unit of heredity. Genes, which are made up of DNA, act as instructions to make molecules called proteins. In humans, genes vary in size from a few hundred DNA bases to more than 2 million bases. The Human Genome Project has estimated that humans have between 30,000 and 40,000 genes.

Every person has two copies of each gene, one inherited from each parent. Most genes are the same in all people, but a small number of genes (less than 1 percent of the total) are slightly different between people. Alleles are forms of the same gene with small differences in their sequence of DNA bases. These small differences contribute to each person's unique physical features.

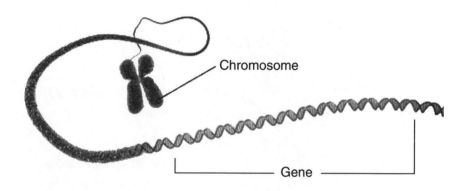

Figure 1.2. *Genes are made up of DNA. Each chromosome contains many genes (Source: U.S. National Library of Medicine).*

What is a chromosome?

In the nucleus of each cell, the DNA molecule is packaged into thread-like structures called chromosomes. Each chromosome is made up of DNA tightly coiled many times around proteins called histones that support its structure.

Chromosomes are not visible in the cell's nucleus—not even under a microscope—when the cell is not dividing. However, the DNA that makes up chromosomes becomes more tightly packed during cell division and is then visible under a microscope. Most of what research-ers know about chromosomes was learned by observing chromosomes during cell division.

Each chromosome has a constriction point called the centromere, which divides the chromosome into two sections, or "arms." The short arm of the chromosome is labeled the "p arm." The long arm of the chromosome is labeled the "q arm." The location of the centromere on each chromosome gives the chromosome its characteristic shape, and can be used to help describe the location of specific genes.

How many chromosomes do people have?

In humans, each cell normally contains 23 pairs of chromosomes, for a total of 46. Twenty-two of these pairs, called autosomes, look the same in both males and females. The 23rd pair, the sex chromosomes,

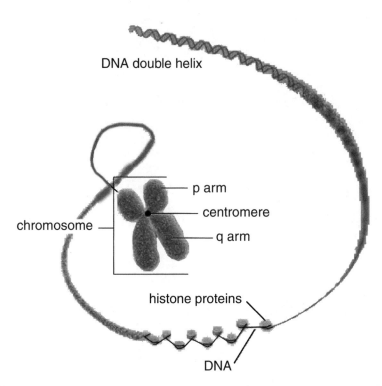

Figure 1.3. *DNA and histone proteins are packaged into structures called chromosomes (Source: U.S. National Library of Medicine).*

7

differ between males and females. Females have two copies of the X chromosome, while males have one X and one Y chromosome.

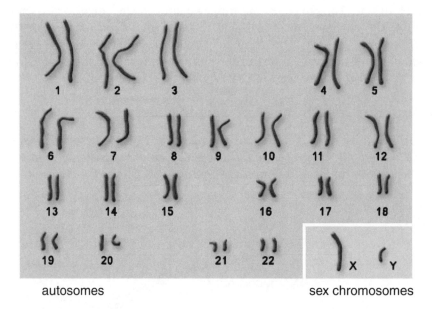

autosomes   sex chromosomes

Figure 1.4. The 22 autosomes are numbered by size. The other two chromosomes, X and Y, are the sex chromosomes (Source: U.S. National Library of Medicine).

How do geneticists indicate the location of a gene?

Geneticists use a standardized way of describing the location of a particular gene on a chromosome. A gene's location is often written as a position:

17q12

It can also be written as a range, if less is known about the exact location:

17q12-q21

These combinations of numbers and letters provide a gene's "address" on a chromosome. The address is made up of several parts:

- The chromosome on which the gene can be found. The first number or letter used to describe a gene's location represents the chromosome. Chromosomes 1 through 22 (the autosomes) are designated by their chromosome number. The sex chromosomes are designated by X or Y.

- The arm of the chromosome. Each chromosome is divided into two sections, or arms, based on the location of a narrowing (constriction) called the centromere. By convention, the shorter arm is called p, and the longer arm is called q. The chromosome arm is the second part of the gene's address. For example, 5q is the long arm of chromosome 5, and Xp is the short arm of the X chromosome.

- The position of the gene on the p or q arm. The position of a gene is based on a standard pattern of light and dark bands that appear when the chromosome is stained in a certain way. The position is usually designated by two digits (representing a region and a band), which are sometimes followed by a decimal point and one or more additional digits (representing sub-bands within a light or dark area). The number indicating gene position increases with distance from the centromere. For example: 14q21 represents the long arm of chromosome 14 at position 21. 14q21 is closer to the centromere than 14q22.

Sometimes, the abbreviations "cen" or "ter" are also used to describe a gene's location. "Cen" indicates that the gene is very close to the centromere. For example, 16pcen refers to the short arm of chromosome 16 near the centromere. "Ter" stands for terminus, which indicates that the gene is very close to the end of the p or q arm. For example, 14qter refers to tip of the long arm of chromosome 14.

What are proteins and what do they do?

Proteins are large, complex molecules that play many critical roles in the body. They do most of the work in cells and are required for the structure, function, and regulation of the body's tissues and organs.

Proteins are made up of hundreds or thousands of smaller units called amino acids, which are attached to one another in long chains. There are 20 different types of amino acids that can be combined to make a protein. The sequence of amino acids determines each protein's unique 3-dimensional structure and its specific function.

9

Proteins can be described according to their large range of functions in the body. See Table 1.1.

Table 1.1. Proteins and Their Functions in the Body

Function	Description	Examples
Antibody	Antibodies bind to specific foreign particles, such as viruses and bacteria, to help protect the body.	Immunoglobulin G (IgG)
Enzyme	Enzymes carry out almost all of the thousands of chemical reactions that take place in cells. They also assist with the formation of new molecules by reading the genetic information stored in DNA.	RNA polymerase
Messenger	Messenger proteins, such as some types of hormones, transmit signals to coordinate biological processes between different cells, tissues, and organs.	Growth hormone
Structural component	These proteins provide structure and support for cells. On a larger scale, they also allow the body to move.	Microtubules, microfilaments, intermediate filaments
Transport/ storage molecule	These proteins bind and carry atoms and small molecules within cells and throughout the body.	Ferritin

How does a gene make a protein?

Most genes contain the information needed to make functional molecules called proteins. (A few genes produce other molecules that help the cell assemble proteins.) The journey from gene to protein is complex and tightly controlled within each cell. It consists of two major steps: transcription and translation. Together, transcription and translation are known as gene expression.

During the process of transcription, the information stored in a gene's DNA is transferred to a similar molecule called RNA (ribonucleic acid) in the cell nucleus. Both RNA and DNA are made up of a chain of nucleotide bases, but they have slightly different chemical properties. The type of RNA that contains the information for making a protein is called messenger RNA (mRNA) because it carries the information, or message, from the DNA out of the nucleus into the cytoplasm.

Translation, the second step in getting from a gene to a protein, takes place in the cytoplasm. The mRNA interacts with a specialized complex called a ribosome, which reads the sequence of mRNA bases. Each sequence of three bases, called a codon, usually codes for one particular amino acid. (Amino acids are the building blocks of proteins.) A type of RNA called transfer RNA (tRNA) assembles the protein, one amino acid at a time. Protein assembly continues until the ribosome encounters a stop codon (a sequence of three bases that does not code for an amino acid).

The flow of information from DNA to RNA to proteins is one of the fundamental principles of molecular biology. It is so important that it is sometimes called the central dogma.

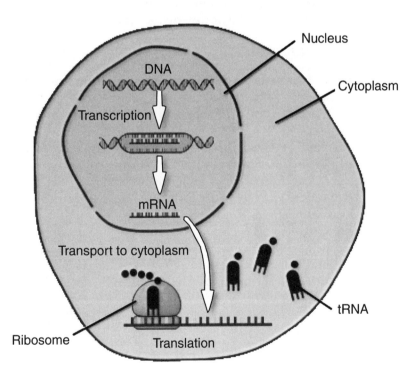

Figure 1.5. Through the processes of transcription and translation, information from genes is used to make proteins (Source: U.S. National Library of Medicine).

11

Can genes be turned on and off in cells?

Yes. Each cell expresses, or turns on, only a fraction of its genes. The rest of the genes are repressed, or turned off. The process of turning genes on and off is known as gene regulation. Gene regulation makes a brain cell look and act different from a liver cell or a muscle cell. It also allows cells to react quickly to changes in their environments and is an important part of normal development. Although we know that the regulation of genes is critical for life, this complex process is not yet fully understood.

Gene regulation can occur at any point during gene expression, but most commonly occurs at the level of transcription (when the information in a gene's DNA is transferred to mRNA). Signals from the environment or from other cells activate proteins called transcription factors. These proteins bind to regulatory regions of a gene and increase or decrease the level of transcription. By controlling the level of transcription, this process can determine the amount of protein product that is made by a gene at any given time.

How do cells divide?

There are two types of cell division: mitosis and meiosis. Most of the time when people refer to cell division, they mean mitosis, the process of making new body cells. Meiosis is the type of cell division that creates egg and sperm cells.

Mitosis is a fundamental process for life. During mitosis, a cell duplicates all of its contents, including its chromosomes, and splits to form two identical daughter cells. Because this process is so critical, the steps of mitosis are carefully controlled by a number of genes. When mitosis is not regulated correctly, health problems such as cancer can result.

The other type of cell division, meiosis, ensures that humans have the same number of chromosomes in each generation. It is a two-step process that reduces the chromosome number by half—from 46 to 23—to form sperm and egg cells. When the sperm and egg cells unite at conception, each contributes 23 chromosomes so the resulting embryo will have the usual 46. Meiosis also allows genetic variation through a process of DNA shuffling while the cells are dividing.

How do genes control the growth and division of cells?

A variety of genes are involved in the control of cell growth and division. The cell cycle is the cell's way of replicating itself in an organized,

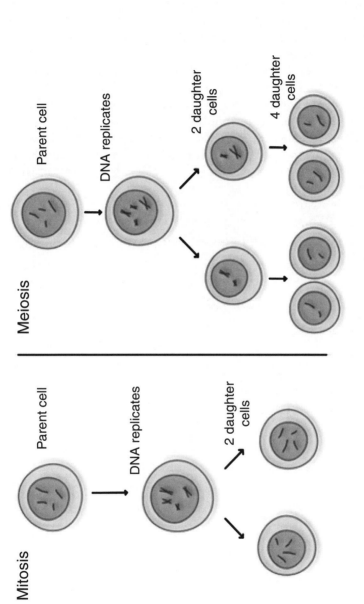

Figure 1.6. *Mitosis and meiosis, the two types of cell division (Source: U.S. National Library of Medicine).*

step-by-step fashion. Tight regulation of this process ensures that a dividing cell's DNA is copied properly, any errors in the DNA are repaired, and each daughter cell receives a full set of chromosomes. The cycle has checkpoints (also called restriction points), which allow certain genes to check for mistakes and halt the cycle for repairs if something goes wrong.

If a cell has an error in its DNA that cannot be repaired, it may undergo programmed cell death (apoptosis). Apoptosis is a common process throughout life that helps the body get rid of cells it doesn't need. Cells that undergo apoptosis break apart and are recycled by a type of white blood cell called a macrophage. Apoptosis protects the body by removing genetically damaged cells that could lead to cancer, and it plays an important role in the development of the embryo and the maintenance of adult tissues.

Cancer results from a disruption of the normal regulation of the cell cycle. When the cycle proceeds without control, cells can divide without order and accumulate genetic defects that can lead to a cancerous tumor.

Chapter 2

The Human Genome

What Is a Genome?

A genome is an organism's complete set of DNA, including all of its genes. Each genome contains all of the information need to build and maintain that organism. In humans, a copy of the entire genome—more than 3 billion DNA base pairs—is contained in all cells that have a nucleus. Genes code for proteins that attach to the genome at the appropriate positions and switch on a series of reactions called gene expression.

Brief History

In 1909, Danish botanist Wilhelm Johanssen coined the word gene for the hereditary unit found on a chromosome. Nearly 50 years earlier, Gregor Mendel had characterized hereditary units as factors—observable differences that were passed from parent to offspring. Today we know that a single gene consists of a unique sequence of DNA that provides the complete instructions to make a functional

---

This chapter contains excerpts from "What is a Genome?" *A Science Primer: A Basic Introduction to the Science Underlying NCBI Resources*, from the National Center for Biotechnology Information (NCBI), revised March 2004. The full text of this document can be found online through the NCBI website at http://www.ncbi.nih.gov. The first paragraph is excerpted from "The Human Genome Project and Genomic Research," *Genetics Home Reference: Your Guide to Understanding Genetic Conditions*, a service of the U.S. National Library of Medicine, March 2003.

product, called a protein. Genes instruct each cell type—such as skin, brain, and liver—to make discrete sets of proteins at just the right times, and it is through this specificity that unique organisms arise.

The Physical Structure of the Human Genome

Nuclear DNA

Inside each of our cells lies a nucleus, a membrane-bounded region that provides a sanctuary for genetic information. The nucleus contains long strands of DNA that encode this genetic information. A DNA chain is made up of four chemical bases: adenine (A) and guanine (G), which are called purines, and cytosine (C) and thymine (T), referred to as pyrimidines. Each base has a slightly different composition, or combination of oxygen, carbon, nitrogen, and hydrogen. In a DNA chain, every base is attached to a sugar molecule (deoxyribose) and a phosphate molecule, resulting in a nucleic acid or nucleotide. Individual nucleotides are linked through the phosphate group, and it is the precise order, or sequence, of nucleotides that determines the product made from that gene.

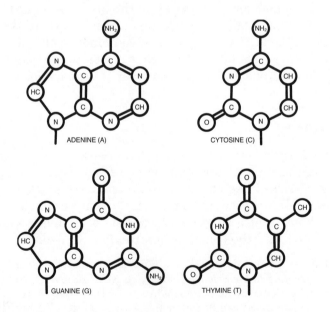

Figure 2.1. *Each DNA base is made up of the sugar 2'-deoxyribose linked to a phosphate group and one of the four bases depicted above: adenine (top left), cytosine (top right), guanine (bottom left), and thymine (bottom right).*

16

The DNA that constitutes a gene is a double-stranded molecule consisting of two chains running in opposite directions. The chemical nature of the bases in double-stranded DNA creates a slight twisting force that gives DNA its characteristic gently coiled structure, known as the double helix. The two strands are connected to each other by chemical pairing of each base on one strand to a specific partner on the other strand. Adenine (A) pairs with thymine (T), and guanine (G) pairs with cytosine (C). Thus, A-T and G-C base pairs are said to be complementary. This complementary base pairing is what makes DNA a suitable molecule for carrying our genetic information—one strand of DNA can act as a template to direct the synthesis of a complementary strand. In this way, the information in a DNA sequence is readily copied and passed on to the next generation of cells.

5' to 3' Direction: A DNA chain, also called a strand, has a sense of direction, in which one end is chemically different than the other. The so-called 5' end terminates in a 5' phosphate group (-PO4); the 3' end terminates in a 3' hydroxyl group (-OH). This is important because DNA strands are always synthesized in the 5' to 3' direction.

Organelle DNA

Not all genetic information is found in nuclear DNA. Both plants and animals have an organelle—a "little organ" within the cell—called the mitochondrion (plural, mitochondria). Each mitochondrion has its own set of genes. Plants also have a second organelle, the chloroplast, which also has its own DNA. Cells often have multiple mitochondria, particularly cells requiring lots of energy, such as active muscle cells. This is because mitochondria are responsible for converting the energy stored in macromolecules into a form usable by the cell, namely, the adenosine triphosphate (ATP) molecule. Thus, they are often referred to as the power generators of the cell.

Unlike nuclear DNA (the DNA found within the nucleus of a cell), half of which comes from our mother and half from our father, mitochondrial DNA is only inherited from our mother. This is because mitochondria are only found in the female gametes or eggs of sexually reproducing animals, not in the male gamete, or sperm. Mitochondrial DNA also does not recombine; there is no shuffling of genes from one generation to the other, as there is with nuclear genes.

Why don't sperm have mitochondria? Large numbers of mitochondria are found in the tail of sperm, providing them with an engine that generates the energy needed for swimming toward the egg. However, when the sperm enters the egg during fertilization, the tail falls off, taking away the father's mitochondria.

Why Is There a Separate Mitochondrial Genome?

The energy-conversion process that takes place in the mitochondria takes place aerobically, in the presence of oxygen. Other energy conversion processes in the cell take place anaerobically, or without oxygen. The independent aerobic function of these organelles is thought to have evolved from bacteria that lived inside of other simple organisms in a mutually beneficial, or symbiotic, relationship, providing them with aerobic capacity. Through the process of evolution, these tiny organisms became incorporated into the cell, and their genetic systems and cellular functions became integrated to form a single functioning cellular unit. Because mitochondria have their own DNA, RNA, and ribosomes, this scenario is quite possible. This theory is also supported by the existence of a eukaryotic organism, called the amoeba, which lacks mitochondria. Therefore, amoeba must always have a symbiotic relationship with an aerobic bacterium.

Why Study Mitochondria?

There are many diseases caused by mutations in mitochondrial DNA (mtDNA). Because the mitochondria produce energy in cells, symptoms of mitochondrial diseases often involve degeneration or functional failure of tissue. For example, mtDNA mutations have been identified in some forms of diabetes, deafness, and certain inherited heart diseases. In addition, mutations in mtDNA are able to accumulate throughout an individual's lifetime. This is different from mutations in nuclear DNA, which has sophisticated repair mechanisms to limit the accumulation of mutations. Mitochondrial DNA mutations can also concentrate in the mitochondria of specific tissues. A variety of deadly diseases are attributable to a large number of accumulated mutations in mitochondria. There is even a theory, the Mitochondrial Theory of Aging, that suggests that accumulation of mutations in mitochondria contributes to, or drives, the aging process. These defects are associated with Parkinson's and Alzheimer's disease, although it is not known whether the defects actually cause or are a direct result of the diseases. However, evidence suggests that the mutations contribute to the progression of both diseases.

In addition to the critical cellular energy-related functions, mitochondrial genes are useful to evolutionary biologists because of their maternal inheritance and high rate of mutation. By studying patterns of mutations, scientists are able to reconstruct patterns of migration and evolution within and between species. For example, mtDNA analysis has been used to trace the migration of people from Asia across the Bering Strait to North and South America. It has also been used to identify an ancient maternal lineage from which modern man evolved.

Ribonucleic Acids

Just like DNA, ribonucleic acid (RNA) is a chain, or polymer, of nucleotides with the same 5' to 3' direction of its strands. However, the ribose sugar component of RNA is slightly different chemically than that of DNA. RNA has a 2' oxygen atom that is not present in DNA. Other fundamental structural differences exist. For example, uracil takes the place of the thymine nucleotide found in DNA, and RNA is, for the most part, a single-stranded molecule. DNA directs the synthesis of a variety of RNA molecules, each with a unique role in cellular function. For example, all genes that code for proteins are first made into an RNA strand in the nucleus called a messenger RNA (mRNA). The mRNA carries the information encoded in DNA out of the nucleus to the protein assembly machinery, called the ribosome, in the cytoplasm. The ribosome complex uses mRNA as a template to synthesize the exact protein coded for by the gene.

Other Forms of RNA: In addition to mRNA, DNA codes for other forms of RNA, including ribosomal RNAs (rRNAs), transfer RNAs (tRNAs), and small nuclear RNAs (snRNAs). rRNAs and tRNAs participate in protein assembly whereas snRNAs aid in a process called splicing—the process of editing of mRNA before it can be used as a template for protein synthesis.

Proteins

Although DNA is the carrier of genetic information in a cell, proteins do the bulk of the work. Proteins are long chains containing as many as 20 different kinds of amino acids. Each cell contains thousands of different proteins:

- **enzymes** that make new molecules and catalyze nearly all chemical processes in cells

- **structural components** that give cells their shape and help them move

- **hormones** that transmit signals throughout the body; antibodies that recognize foreign molecules

- **transport molecules** that carry oxygen

The genetic code carried by DNA is what specifies the order and number of amino acids and, therefore, the shape and function of the protein.

The Central Dogma—a fundamental principle of molecular biology—states that genetic information flows from DNA to RNA to protein. Ultimately, however, the genetic code resides in DNA because only DNA is passed from generation to generation. Yet, in the process of making a protein, the encoded information must be faithfully transmitted first to RNA then to protein. Transferring the code from DNA to RNA is a fairly straightforward process called transcription. Deciphering the code in the resulting mRNA is a little more complex. It first requires that the mRNA leave the nucleus and associate with a large complex of specialized RNAs and proteins that, collectively, are called the ribosome. Here the mRNA is translated into protein by decoding the mRNA sequence in blocks of three RNA bases, called codons, where each codon specifies a particular amino acid. In this way, the ribosomal complex builds a protein one amino acid at a time, with the order of amino acids determined precisely by the order of the codons in the mRNA.

A given amino acid can have more than one codon. These redundant codons usually differ at the third position. For example, the amino acid serine is encoded by UCU, UCC, UCA, and/or UCG. This redundancy is key to accommodating mutations that occur naturally as DNA is replicated and new cells are produced. By allowing some of the random changes in DNA to have no effect on the ultimate protein sequence, a sort of genetic safety net is created. Some codons do not code for an amino acid at all but instruct the ribosome when to stop adding new amino acids.

The First Codon: In 1961, Marshall Nirenberg and Heinrich Matthaei correlated the first codon (UUU) with the amino acid phenylalanine. After that, it was not long before the genetic code for all 20 amino acids was deciphered.

Table 2.1. RNA triplet codons and their corresponding amino acids. (A translation chart of the 64 RNA codons)

	U	C	A	G
U	UUU Phenylalanine	UCU Serine	UAU Tyrosine	UGU Cysteine
	UUC Phenylalanine	UCC Serine	UAC Tyrosine	UGC Cysteine
	UUA Leucine	UCA Serine	UAA Stop	UGA Stop
	UUG Leucine	UCG Serine	UAG Stop	UGG Tryptophan
C	CUU Leucine	CCU Proline	CAU Histidine	CGU Arginine
	CUC Leucine	CCC Proline	CAC Histidine	CGC Arginine
	CUA Leucine	CCA Proline	CAA Glutamine	CGA Arginine
	CUG Leucine	CCG Proline	CAG Glutamine	CGG Arginine
A	AUU Isoleucine	ACU Threonine	AAU Asparagine	AGU Serine
	AUC Isoleucine	ACC Threonine	AAC Asparagine	AGC Serine
	AUA Isoleucine	ACA Threonine	AAA Lysine	AGA Arginine
	AUG Methionine	ACG Threonine	AAG Lysine	AGG Arginine
G	GUU Valine	GCU Alanine	GAU Aspartate	GGU Glycine
	GUC Valine	GCC Alanine	GAC Aspartate	GGC Glycine
	GUA Valine	GCA Alanine	GAA Glutamate	GGA Glycine
	GUG Valine	GCG Alanine	GAG Glutamate	GGG Glycine

The Core Gene Sequence: Introns and Exons

Genes make up about one percent of the total DNA in our genome. In the human genome, the coding portions of a gene, called exons, are interrupted by intervening sequences, called introns. In addition, a eukaryotic gene does not code for a protein in one continuous stretch of DNA. Both exons and introns are transcribed into mRNA, but before it is transported to the ribosome, the primary mRNA transcript is edited. This editing process removes the introns, joins the exons together, and adds unique features to each end of the transcript to make a mature mRNA. One might then ask what the purpose of an intron is if it is spliced out after it is transcribed. It is still unclear what all the functions of introns are, but scientists believe that some serve as the site for recombination, the process by which progeny derive a combination of genes different from that of either parent, resulting in novel genes with new combinations of exons, the key to evolution.

21

From Genes to Proteins: Start to Finish

We just discussed that the journey from DNA to mRNA to protein requires that a cell identify where a gene begins and ends. This must be done both during the transcription and the translation process.

Transcription

Transcription, the synthesis of an RNA copy from a sequence of DNA, is carried out by an enzyme called RNA polymerase. This molecule has the job of recognizing the DNA sequence where transcription is initiated, called the promoter site. In general, there are two promoter sequences upstream from the beginning of every gene. The location and base sequence of each promoter site vary for prokaryotes (bacteria) and eukaryotes (higher organisms), but they are both recognized by RNA polymerase, which can then grab hold of the sequence and drive the production of an mRNA.

Eukaryotic cells have three different RNA polymerases, each recognizing three classes of genes. RNA polymerase II is responsible for synthesis of mRNAs from protein-coding genes. This polymerase requires a sequence resembling TATAA, commonly referred to as the TATA box, which is found 25–30 nucleotides upstream of the beginning of the gene, referred to as the initiator sequence.

Transcription terminates when the polymerase stumbles upon a termination, or stop signal. In eukaryotes, this process is not fully understood. Prokaryotes, however, tend to have a short region composed of G's and C's that is able to fold in on itself and form complementary base pairs, creating a stem in the new mRNA. This stem then causes the polymerase to trip and release the nascent, or newly formed, mRNA.

Translation

The beginning of translation, the process in which the genetic code carried by mRNA directs the synthesis of proteins from amino acids, differs slightly for prokaryotes and eukaryotes, although both processes always initiate at a codon for methionine. For prokaryotes, the ribosome recognizes and attaches at the sequence AGGAGGU on the mRNA, called the Shine-Dalgarno sequence, that appears just upstream from the methionine (AUG) codon. Curiously, eukaryotes lack this recognition sequence and simply initiate translation at the amino acid methionine, usually coded for by the bases AUG, but sometimes GUG. Translation is terminated for both prokaryotes and eukaryotes when the ribosome reaches one of the three stop codons.

Structural Genes, Junk DNA, and Regulatory Sequences

Structural Genes: Sequences that code for proteins are called structural genes. Although it is true that proteins are the major components of structural elements in a cell, proteins are also the real workhorses of the cell. They perform such functions as transporting nutrients into the cell; synthesizing new DNA, RNA, and protein molecules; and transmitting chemical signals from outside to inside the cell, as well as throughout the cell—both critical to the process of making proteins.

Junk DNA: Over 98 percent of the genome is of unknown function. Although often referred to as junk DNA, scientists are beginning to uncover the function of many of these intergenic sequences—the DNA found between genes.

Regulatory Sequences: A class of sequences called regulatory sequences makes up a numerically insignificant fraction of the genome but provides critical functions. For example, certain sequences indicate the beginning and end of genes, sites for initiating replication and recombination, or provide landing sites for proteins that turn genes on and off. Like structural genes, regulatory sequences are inherited; however, they are not commonly referred to as genes.

Other DNA Regions: Forty to forty-five percent of our genome is made up of short sequences that are repeated, sometimes hundreds of times. There are numerous forms of this repetitive DNA, and a few have known functions, such as stabilizing the chromosome structure or inactivating one of the two X chromosomes in developing females, a process called X-inactivation. The most highly repeated sequences found so far in mammals are called satellite DNA because their unusual composition allows them to be easily separated from other DNA. These sequences are associated with chromosome structure and are found at the centromeres (or centers) and telomeres (ends) of chromosomes. Although they do not play a role in the coding of proteins, they do play a significant role in chromosome structure, duplication, and cell division. The highly variable nature of these sequences makes them an excellent marker by which individuals can be identified based on their unique pattern of their satellite DNA.

Another class of non-coding DNA is the pseudogene, so named because it is believed to be a remnant of a real gene that has suffered mutations and is no longer functional. Pseudogenes may have arisen through the duplication of a functional gene, followed by inactivation of one of the copies. Comparing the presence or absence of pseudogenes is one method used by evolutionary geneticists to group species and to determine relatedness. Thus, these sequences are thought to carry a record of our evolutionary history.

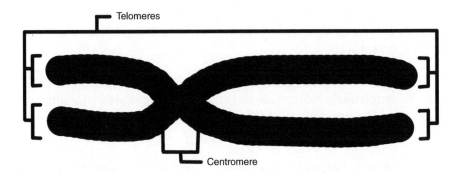

Figure 2.2. A chromosome. A chromosome is composed of a very long molecule of DNA and associated proteins that carry hereditary information. The centromere, shown at the center of this chromosome, is a specialized structure that appears during cell division and ensures the correct distribution of duplicated chromosomes to daughter cells. Telomeres are the structures that seal the end of a chromosome. Telomeres play a critical role in chromosome replication and maintenance by counteracting the tendency of the chromosome to otherwise shorten with each round of replication.

How Many Genes Do Humans Have?

In February 2001, two largely independent draft versions of the human genome were published. Both studies estimated that there are 30,000 to 40,000 genes in the human genome, roughly one-third the number of previous estimates. More recently scientists estimated that there are less than 30,000 human genes. However, we still have to make guesses at the actual number of genes, because not all of the human genome sequence is annotated and not all of the known sequence has been assigned a particular position in the genome.

So, how do scientists estimate the number of genes in a genome? For the most part, they look for tell-tale signs of genes in a DNA sequence. These include: open reading frames, stretches of DNA, usually greater than 100 bases, that are not interrupted by a stop codon such as TAA, TAG or TGA; start codons such as ATG; specific sequences found at splice junctions, a location in the DNA sequence where RNA removes the non-coding areas to form a continuous gene transcript for translation into a protein; and gene regulatory sequences. This process is dependent on computer programs that search for these patterns in various sequence databases and then make predictions about the existence of a gene.

From One Gene–One Protein to a More Global Perspective

Only a small percentage of the 3 billion bases in the human genome becomes an expressed gene product. However, of the approximately one percent of our genome that is expressed, 40 percent is alternatively spliced to produce multiple proteins from a single gene. Alternative splicing refers to the cutting and pasting of the primary mRNA transcript into various combinations of mature mRNA. Therefore the one gene–one protein theory, originally framed as "one gene–one enzyme," does not precisely hold.

With so much DNA in the genome, why restrict transcription to a tiny portion, and why make that tiny portion work overtime to produce many alternate transcripts? This process may have evolved as a way to limit the deleterious effects of mutations. Genetic mutations occur randomly, and the effect of a small number of mutations on a single gene may be minimal. However, an individual having many genes each with small changes could weaken the individual, and thus the species. On the other hand, if a single mutation affects several alternate transcripts at once, it is more likely that the effect will be devastating—the individual may not survive to contribute to the next generation. Thus, alternate transcripts from a single gene could reduce the chances that a mutated gene is transmitted.

Gene Switching: Turning Genes On and Off

The estimated number of genes for humans, less than 30,000, is not so different from the 25,300 known genes of *Arabidopsis thaliana*, commonly called mustard grass. Yet, we appear, at least at first glance, to be a far more complex organism. A person may wonder how this increased complexity is achieved. One answer lies in the regulatory system that turns genes on and off. This system also precisely controls the amount of a gene product that is produced and can further modify the product after it is made. This exquisite control requires multiple regulatory input points. One very efficient point occurs at transcription, such that an mRNA is produced only when a gene product is needed. Cells also regulate gene expression by post-transcriptional modification; by allowing only a subset of the mRNAs to go on to translation; or by restricting translation of specific mRNAs to only when the product is needed. At other levels, cells regulate gene expression through DNA folding, chemical modification of the nucleotide bases, and intricate feedback mechanisms in which some of the gene's own protein product directs the cell to cease further protein production.

Controlling Transcription

Promoters and Regulatory Sequences: Transcription is the process whereby RNA is made from DNA. It is initiated when an enzyme, RNA polymerase, binds to a site on the DNA called a promoter sequence. In most cases, the polymerase is aided by a group of proteins called transcription factors that perform specialized functions, such as DNA sequence recognition and regulation of the polymerase's enzyme activity. Other regulatory sequences include activators, repressors, and enhancers. These sequences can be *cis*-acting (affecting genes that are adjacent to the sequence) or *trans*-acting (affecting expression of the gene from a distant site), even on another chromosome.

The Globin Genes—An Example of Transcriptional Regulation: An example of transcriptional control occurs in the family of genes responsible for the production of globin. Globin is the protein that complexes with the iron-containing heme molecule to make hemoglobin. Hemoglobin transports oxygen to our tissues via red blood cells. In the adult, red blood cells do not contain DNA for making new globin; they are ready-made with all of the hemoglobin they will need.

During the first few weeks of life, embryonic globin is expressed in the yolk sac of the egg. By week five of gestation, globin is expressed in early liver cells. By birth, red blood cells are being produced, and globin is expressed in the bone marrow. Yet, the globin found in the yolk is not produced from the same gene as is the globin found in the liver or bone marrow stem cells. In fact, at each stage of development, different globin genes are turned on and off through a process of transcriptional regulation called switching.

To further complicate matters, globin is made from two different protein chains: an alpha-like chain coded for on chromosome 16; and a beta-like chain coded for on chromosome 11. Each chromosome has the embryonic, fetal, and adult form lined up on the chromosome in a sequential order for developmental expression. The developmentally regulated transcription of globin is controlled by a number of *cis*-acting DNA sequences, and although there remains a lot to be learned about the interaction of these sequences, one known control sequence is an enhancer called the locus control region (LCR). The LCR sits far upstream on the sequence and controls the alpha genes on chromosome 16. It may also interact with other factors to determine which alpha gene is turned on.

Thalassemias are a group of diseases characterized by the absence or decreased production of normal globin, and thus hemoglobin, leading to decreased oxygen in the system. There are alpha and beta thalassemias, defined by the defective gene, and there are variations of each of these, depending on whether the embryonic, fetal, or adult forms are affected and/or expressed. Although there is no known cure for the thalassemias, there are medical treatments that have been developed based on our current understanding of both gene regulation and cell differentiation. Treatments include blood transfusions, iron chelators, and bone marrow transplants. With continuing research in the areas of gene regulation and cell differentiation, new and more effective treatments may soon be on the horizon, such as the advent of gene transfer therapies.

The Influence of DNA Structure and Binding Domains: Sequences that are important in regulating transcription do not necessarily code for transcription factors or other proteins. Transcription can also be regulated by subtle variations in DNA structure and by chemical changes in the bases to which transcription factors bind. As stated previously, the chemical properties of the four DNA bases differ slightly, providing each base with unique opportunities to chemically react with other molecules. One chemical modification of DNA, called methylation, involves the addition of a methyl group (-CH3). Methylation frequently occurs at cytosine residues that are preceded by guanine bases, oftentimes in the vicinity of promoter sequences. The methylation status of DNA often correlates with its functional activity, where inactive genes tend to be more heavily methylated. This is because the methyl group serves to inhibit transcription by attracting a protein that binds specifically to methylated DNA, thereby interfering with polymerase binding. Methylation also plays an important role in genomic imprinting, which occurs when both maternal and paternal alleles are present but only one allele is expressed while the other remains inactive. Another way to think of genomic imprinting is as "parent of origin differences" in the expression of inherited traits.

Considerable intrigue surrounds the effects of DNA methylation, and many researchers are working to unlock the mystery behind this concept.

Controlling Translation

Translation is the process whereby the genetic code carried by an mRNA directs the synthesis of proteins. Translational regulation occurs through the binding of specific molecules, called repressor proteins, to a sequence found on an RNA molecule. Repressor proteins prevent a gene from being expressed. As we have just discussed, the default state for a gene is that of being expressed via the recognition of its promoter by RNA polymerase. Close to the promoter region is another *cis*-acting site called the operator, the target for the repressor protein. When the repressor protein binds to the operator, RNA polymerase is prevented from initiating transcription, and gene expression is turned off.

Translational control plays a significant role in the process of embryonic development and cell differentiation. Upon fertilization, an egg cell begins to multiply to produce a ball of cells that are all the same. At some point, however, these cells begin to differentiate, or change into specific cell types. Some will become blood cells or kidney cells, whereas others may become nerve or brain cells. When all of the cells formed are alike, the same genes are turned on. However, once differentiation begins, various genes in different cells must become active to meet the needs of that cell type. In some organisms, the egg houses store immature mRNAs that become translationally active only after fertilization. Fertilization then serves to trigger mechanisms that initiate the efficient translation of mRNA into proteins. Similar mechanisms serve to activate mRNAs at other stages of development and differentiation, such as when specific protein products are needed.

Mechanisms of Genetic Variation and Heredity

Does Everyone Have the Same Genes?

When you look at the human species, you see evidence of a process called genetic variation, that is, there are immediately recognizable differences in human traits, such as hair and eye color, skin pigment, and height. Then there are the not so obvious genetic variations, such as blood type. These expressed, or phenotypic, traits are attributable to genotypic variation in a person's DNA sequence. When two individuals display different phenotypes of the same trait, they are said to have two different alleles for the same gene. This means that the gene's sequence is slightly different in the two individuals, and the gene is said to be polymorphic, "poly" meaning many and "morph" meaning shape or form. Therefore, although people generally have the same genes, the genes do not have exactly the same DNA sequence. These polymorphic sites influence gene expression and also serve as markers for genomic research efforts.

Genetic Variation

Most genetic variation occurs during the phases of the cell cycle when DNA is duplicated. Mutations in the new DNA strand can manifest as base substitutions, such as when a single base gets replaced with another; deletions, where one or more bases are left out; or insertions, where one or more bases are added. Mutations can either be synonymous, in which the variation still results in a codon for the same amino acid or non-synonymous, in which the variation results in a codon for a different amino acid. Mutations can also cause a frame shift, which occurs when the variation bumps the reference point for reading the genetic code down a base or two and results in loss of part, or sometimes all, of that gene product. DNA mutations can also be introduced by toxic chemicals and, particularly in skin cells, exposure to ultraviolet radiation.

Mutations that occur in somatic cells—any cell in the body except gametes and their precursors—will not be passed on to the next generation. This does not mean, however, that somatic cell mutations, sometimes called acquired mutations, are benign. For example, as your skin cells prepare to divide and produce new skin cells, errors may be inadvertently introduced when the DNA is duplicated, resulting in a daughter cell that contains the error. Although most defective cells die quickly, some can persist and may even become cancerous if the mutation affects the ability to regulate cell growth.

Mutations and the Next Generation

There are two places where mutations can be introduced and carried into the next generation. In the first stages of development, a sperm cell and egg cell fuse. They then begin to divide, giving rise to cells that differentiate into tissue-specific cell types. One early type of differentiated cell is the germ line cell, which may ultimately develop into mature gametes. If a mutation occurs in the developing germ line cell, it may persist until that individual reaches reproductive age. Now the mutation has the potential to be passed on to the next generation.

Mitosis and Meiosis: The manner in which a cell replicates differs with the various classes of life forms, as well as with the end purpose of the cell replication. Cells that compose tissues in multicellular organisms typically replicate by organized duplication and spatial separation of their cellular genetic material, a process called mitosis. Meiosis is the mode of cell replication for the formation of sperm and egg cells in plants, animals, and many other multicellular life forms. Meiosis differs significantly from mitosis in that the cellular progeny have their complement of genetic material reduced to half that of the parent cell.

Mutations may also be introduced during meiosis, the mode of cell replication for the formation of sperm and egg cells. In this case, the germ line cell is healthy, and the mutation is introduced during the actual process of gamete replication. Once again, the sperm or egg will contain the mutation, and during the reproductive process, this mutation may then be passed on to the offspring.

One should bear in mind that not all mutations are bad. Mutations also provide a species with the opportunity to adapt to new environments, as well as to protect a species from new pathogens. Mutations are what lie behind the popular saying of "survival of the fittest," the basic theory of evolution proposed by Charles Darwin in 1859. This theory proposes that as new environments arise, individuals carrying certain mutations that enable an evolutionary advantage will survive to pass this mutation on to its offspring. It does not suggest that a mutation is derived from the environment, but that survival in that environment is enhanced by a particular mutation. Some genes, and even some organisms, have evolved to tolerate mutations better than others. For example, some viral genes are known to have high mutation rates. Mutations serve the virus well by enabling adaptive traits, such as changes in the outer protein coat so that it can escape detection and thereby destruction by the host's immune system. Viruses also produce certain enzymes that are necessary for infection of a host cell. A mutation within such an enzyme may result in a new form that still allows the virus to infect its host but that is no longer blocked by an anti-viral drug. This will allow the virus to propagate freely in its environment.

Mendel's Laws—How We Inherit Our Genes

In 1866, Gregor Mendel studied the transmission of seven different pea traits by carefully test-crossing many distinct varieties of peas. Studying garden peas might seem trivial to those of us who live in a modern world of cloned sheep and gene transfer, but Mendel's simple approach led to fundamental insights into genetic inheritance, known today as Mendel's Laws. Mendel did not actually know or understand the cellular mechanisms that produced the results he observed. Nonetheless, he correctly surmised the behavior of traits and the mathematical predictions of their transmission, the independent segregation of alleles during gamete production, and the independent assortment of genes. Perhaps as amazing as Mendel's discoveries was the fact that his work was largely ignored by the scientific community for over 30 years.

Mendel's Principles of Genetic Inheritance

Law of Segregation: Each of the two inherited factors (alleles) possessed by the parent will segregate and pass into separate gametes (eggs or sperm) during meiosis, which will each carry only one of the factors.

Law of Independent Assortment: In the gametes, alleles of one gene separate independently of those of another gene, and thus all possible combinations of alleles are equally probable.

Law of Dominance: Each trait is determined by two factors (alleles), inherited one from each parent. These factors each exhibit a characteristic dominant, co-dominant, or recessive expression, and those that are dominant will mask the expression of those that are recessive.

How Does Inheritance Work?

Our discussion here is restricted to sexually reproducing organisms where each gene in an individual is represented by two copies, called alleles—one on each chromosome pair. There may be more than two alleles, or variants, for a given gene in a population, but only two alleles can be found in an individual. Therefore, the probability that a particular allele will be inherited is 50:50, that is, alleles randomly and independently segregate into daughter cells, although there are some exceptions to this rule.

The term diploid describes a state in which a cell has two sets of homologous chromosomes, or two chromosomes that are the same. The maturation of germ line stem cells into gametes requires the diploid number of each chromosome be reduced by half. Hence, gametes are said to be haploid—having only a single set of homologous chromosomes. This reduction is accomplished through a process called meiosis, where one chromosome in a diploid pair is sent to each daughter gamete.

Human gametes, therefore, contain 23 chromosomes, half the number of somatic cells—all the other cells of the body.

Because the chromosome in one pair separates independently of all other chromosomes, each new gamete has the potential for a totally new combination of chromosomes. In humans, the independent segregation of the 23 chromosomes can lead to as many as 16 to 17 million different combinations in one individual's gametes. Only one of these gametes will combine with one of the nearly 17 million possible combinations from the other parent, generating a staggering potential for individual variation. Yet, this is just the beginning. Even more variation is possible when you consider the recombination between sections of chromosomes during meiosis as well as the random mutation that can occur during DNA replication. With such a range of possibilities, it is amazing that siblings look so much alike.

Expression of Inherited Genes

Gene expression, as reflected in an organism's phenotype, is based on conditions specific for each copy of a gene. As we just discussed, for every human gene there are two copies, and for every gene there can be several variants or alleles. If both alleles are the same, the gene is said to be homozygous. If the alleles are different, they are said to be heterozygous. For some alleles, their influence on phenotype takes precedence over all other alleles. For others, expression depends on whether the gene appears in the homozygous or heterozygous state. Still other phenotypic traits are a combination of several alleles from several different genes. Determining the allelic condition used to be accomplished solely through the analysis of pedigrees, much the way Mendel carried out his experiments on peas. However, this method can leave many questions unanswered, particularly for traits that are a result of the interaction between several different genes. Today, molecular genetic techniques exist that can assist researchers in tracking the transmission of traits by pinpointing the location of individual genes, identifying allelic variants, and identifying those traits that are caused by multiple genes.

The Nature of Alleles: A dominant allele is an allele that is almost always expressed, even if only one copy is present. Dominant alleles express their phenotype even when paired with a different allele, that is, when heterozygous. In this case, the phenotype appears the same in both the heterozygous and homozygous states. Just how the dominant allele overshadows the other allele depends on the gene, but in some cases the dominant gene produces a gene product that the other allele does not. Well-known dominant alleles occur in the human genes for Huntington disease, a form of dwarfism called achondroplasia, and polydactylism (extra fingers and toes).

On the other hand, a recessive allele will be expressed only if there are two identical copies of that allele, or for a male, if one copy is present on the X chromosome. The phenotype of a recessive allele is only seen when both alleles are the same. When an individual has one dominant allele and one recessive allele, the trait is not expressed because it is overshadowed by the dominant allele. The individual is said to be a carrier for that trait. Examples of recessive disorders in humans include sickle cell anemia, Tay-Sachs disease, and phenylketonuria (PKU).

A particularly important category of genetic linkage has to do with the X and Y sex chromosomes. These chromosomes not only carry the genes that determine male and female traits, but also those for some other characteristics as well. Genes that are carried by either sex chromosome are said to be sex linked. Men normally have an X and a Y combination of sex chromosomes, whereas women have two X's. Because only men inherit Y chromosomes, they are the only ones to inherit Y-linked traits. Both men and women can have X-linked traits because both inherit X chromosomes.

X-linked traits not related to feminine body characteristics are primarily expressed in the phenotype of men. This is because men have only one X chromosome. Subsequently, genes on that chromosome that do not code for gender are expressed in the male phenotype, even if they are recessive. In women, a recessive allele on one X chromosome is often masked in their phenotype by a dominant normal allele on the other. This explains why women are frequently carriers of X-linked traits but more rarely have them expressed in their own phenotypes. In humans, at least 320 genes are X-linked. These include the genes for hemophilia, red–green color blindness, and congenital night blindness. There are at least a dozen Y-linked genes, in addition to those that code for masculine physical traits.

It is now known that one of the X chromosomes in the cells of human females is completely, or mostly, inactivated early in embryonic life. This is a normal self-preservation action to prevent a potentially harmful double dose of genes. Recent research points to the *Xist* gene on the X chromosome as being responsible for a sequence of events that silences one of the X chromosomes in women. The inactivated X chromosomes become highly compacted structures known as Barr bodies. The presence of Barr bodies has been used at international sport competitions as a test to determine whether an athlete is a male or a female.

Exceptions to Mendel's Laws

There are many examples of inheritance that appear to be exceptions to Mendel's laws. Usually, they turn out to represent complex interactions among various allelic conditions. For example, co-dominant alleles both contribute to a phenotype. Neither is dominant over the other. Control of the human blood group system provides a good example of co-dominant alleles.

Pleiotropism, or pleiotropy, refers to the phenomenon in which a single gene is responsible for producing multiple, distinct, and apparently unrelated phenotypic traits, that is, an individual can exhibit many different phenotypic outcomes. This is because the gene product is active in many places in the body. An example is Marfan's syndrome, where there is a defect in the gene coding for a connective tissue protein. Individuals with Marfan's syndrome exhibit abnormalities in their eyes, skeletal system, and cardiovascular system.

Some genes mask the expression of other genes just as a fully dominant allele masks the expression of its recessive counterpart. A gene that masks the phenotypic effect of another gene is called an epistatic gene; the gene it subordinates is the hypostatic gene. The gene for albinism in humans is an epistatic gene. It is not part of the interacting skin-color genes. Rather, its dominant allele is necessary for the development of any skin pigment, and its recessive homozygous state results in the albino condition, regardless of how many other pigment genes may be present. Because of the effects of an epistatic gene, some individuals who inherit the dominant, disease-causing gene show only partial symptoms of the disease. Some, in fact, may show no expression of the disease-causing gene, a condition referred to as nonpenetrance. The individual in whom such a nonpenetrant mutant gene exists will be phenotypically normal but still capable of passing the deleterious gene on to offspring, who may exhibit the full-blown disease.

Then we have traits that are multigenic, that is, they result from the expression of several different genes. This is true for human eye color, in which at least three different genes are responsible for determining eye color. A brown/blue gene and a central brown gene are both found on chromosome 15, whereas a green/blue gene is found on chromosome 19. The interaction between these genes is not well understood. It is speculated that there may be other genes that control other factors, such as the amount of pigment deposited in the iris. This multigenic system explains why two blue-eyed individuals can have a brown-eyed child.

Speaking of eye color, have you ever seen someone with one green eye and one brown eye? In this case, somatic mosaicism may be the culprit. This is probably easier to describe than explain. In multicellular organisms, every cell in the adult is ultimately derived from the single-cell fertilized egg. Therefore, every cell in the adult normally carries the same genetic information. However, what would happen if a mutation occurred in only one cell at the two-cell stage of development? Then the adult would be composed of two types of cells: cells with the mutation and cells without. If a mutation affecting melanin production occurred in one of the cells in the cell lineage of one eye but not the other, then the eyes would have different genetic potential for melanin synthesis. This could produce eyes of two different colors.

Penetrance refers to the degree to which a particular allele is expressed in a population phenotype. If every individual carrying a dominant mutant gene demonstrates the mutant phenotype, the gene is said to show complete penetrance.

The Four Basic Blood Types: There are four basic blood types, and they are O, A, B, and AB. We know that our blood type is determined by the alleles that we inherit from our parents. For the blood type gene, there are three basic blood type alleles: A, B, and O. We all have two alleles, one inherited from each parent. The possible combinations of the three alleles are OO, AO, BO, AB, AA, and BB. Blood types A and B are co-dominant alleles, whereas O is recessive. A co-dominant allele is apparent even if only one is present; a recessive allele is apparent only if two recessive alleles are present. Because blood type O is recessive, it is not apparent if the person inherits an A or B allele along with it. So, the possible allele combinations result in a particular blood type in this way:

OO = blood type O
AO = blood type A
BO = blood type B
AB = blood type AB
AA = blood type A
BB = blood type B

You can see that a person with blood type B may have a B and an O allele, or they may have two B alleles. If both parents are blood type B and both have a B and a recessive O, then their children will either be BB, BO, or OO. If the child is BB or BO, they have blood type B. If the child is OO, he or she will have blood type O.

35

Chapter 3

What Are Genetic Disorders?

What does it mean if a disorder seems to run in my family?

A particular disorder might be described as running in a family if more than one person in the family has the condition. Some disorders that affect multiple family members are caused by gene mutations, which can be inherited (passed down from parent to child). Other conditions that appear to run in families are not inherited. Instead, environmental factors such as dietary habits or a combination of genetic and environmental factors are responsible for these disorders.

It is not always easy to determine whether a condition in a family is inherited. A genetics professional can use a person's family history (a record of health information about a person's immediate and extended family) to help determine whether a disorder has a genetic component.

What is a gene mutation and how do mutations occur?

A gene mutation is a permanent change in the DNA sequence that makes up a gene. Mutations range in size from one DNA base to a large segment of a chromosome.

Gene mutations occur in two ways: they can be inherited from a parent or acquired during a person's lifetime. Mutations that are

"Genetic Disorders," from *Genetics Home Reference: Your Guide to Understanding Genetic Conditions,* a service of the U.S. National Library of Medicine, updated March 9, 2004; available online at http://ghr.nlm.nih.gov.

passed from parent to child are called hereditary mutations or germline mutations (because they are present in the egg and sperm cells, which are also called germ cells). This type of mutation is present throughout a person's life in virtually every cell in the body.

Acquired (or sporadic) mutations, on the other hand, occur in the DNA of individual cells at some time during a person's life. These

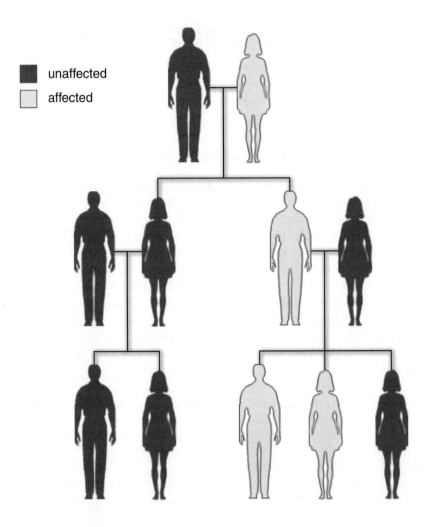

Figure 3.1. Condition Affecting Members of a Family: Some disorders are seen in more than one generation of a family.

changes can be caused by environmental factors such as ultraviolet radiation from the sun, or can occur if a mistake is made as DNA copies itself during cell division. Acquired mutations in somatic cells (cells other than sperm and egg cells) cannot be passed on to the next generation. If a mutation occurs in an egg or sperm cell during a person's life, however, there is a chance that the person's children will inherit the mutation.

How can gene mutations cause disorders?

To function correctly, each cell depends on thousands of proteins to do their jobs in the right places at the right times. Sometimes, gene mutations prevent one or more of these proteins from working properly. By changing a gene's instructions for making a protein, a mutation can cause the protein to malfunction or to be missing entirely. When a mutation alters a protein that plays a critical role in the body, a medical condition can result. A condition caused by mutations in one or more genes is called a genetic disorder.

It is important to note that genes themselves do not cause disease— genetic disorders are caused by mutations that make a gene function improperly. For example, when people say that someone has the cystic fibrosis gene, they are usually referring to a mutated version of the *CFTR* gene, which causes the disease. All people, including those without cystic fibrosis, have a version of the *CFTR* gene.

Do all gene mutations cause disorders?

No. Only a small percentage of mutations cause genetic disorders— most have no impact on health. For example, some mutations alter a gene's DNA base sequence but don't change the function of the protein made by the gene.

Often, gene mutations that could cause a genetic disorder are repaired by certain enzymes before the gene is expressed (makes a protein). Each cell has a number of pathways through which enzymes recognize and repair mistakes in DNA. Because DNA can be damaged or mutated in many ways, the process of DNA repair is an important way in which the body protects itself from disease.

A very small percentage of all mutations actually have a positive effect. These mutations lead to new versions of proteins that help an organism and its future generations better adapt to changes in their environment. For example, a beneficial mutation could result in a protein that protects the organism from a new strain of bacteria.

What kinds of gene mutations are possible?

The DNA sequence of a gene can be altered in a number of ways. Gene mutations have varying effects on health, depending on where they occur and whether they alter the function of essential proteins. The types of mutations include:

- **Missense mutation:** This type of mutation is a change in one DNA base pair that results in the substitution of one amino acid for another in the protein made by a gene.

- **Nonsense mutation:** A nonsense mutation is also a change in one DNA base pair. Instead of substituting one amino acid for another, however, the altered DNA sequence prematurely signals the cell to stop building a protein. This type of mutation results in a shortened protein that may function improperly or not at all.

- **Insertion:** An insertion changes the number of DNA bases in a gene by adding a piece of DNA. As a result, the protein made by the gene may not function properly.

- **Deletion:** A deletion changes the number of DNA bases in a gene by removing a piece of DNA. The deleted DNA may alter the function of the resulting protein.

- **Duplication:** A duplication consists of a piece of DNA that is abnormally copied one or more times. This type of mutation may alter the function of the resulting protein.

- **Frameshift mutation:** This type of mutation occurs when the addition or loss of DNA bases changes a gene's reading frame. A reading frame consists of groups of three bases that each code for one amino acid. A frameshift mutation shifts the grouping of these bases and changes the code for amino acids. The resulting protein is usually nonfunctional. Insertions, deletions, and duplications can all be frameshift mutations.

- **Repeat expansion:** Nucleotide repeats are short DNA sequences that are repeated a number of times in a row. For example, a trinucleotide repeat is made up of three-base-pair sequences, and a tetranucleotide repeat is made up of four-base-pair sequences. A repeat expansion is a mutation that increases the number of times that the short DNA sequence is repeated. This type of mutation can cause the resulting protein to function improperly.

What are the different ways in which a genetic condition can be inherited?

Some genetic conditions are caused by mutations in a single gene. These conditions are usually inherited in one of several straightforward patterns, depending on the gene involved. See Table 3.1.

Many other disorders are caused by a combination of the effects of multiple genes or by interactions between genes and the environment. Such disorders are more difficult to analyze because their genetic causes are often unclear, and they do not follow the patterns of inheritance described above. Examples of conditions caused by multiple genes or gene/environment interactions include heart disease, diabetes, schizophrenia, and certain types of cancer.

If a genetic disorder runs in my family, what are the chances that my children will have the condition?

When a genetic disorder is diagnosed in a family, family members often want to know the likelihood that they or their children will develop the condition. This can be difficult to predict in some cases because many factors influence a person's chances. One important factor is how the condition is inherited. For example:

- A person affected by an autosomal dominant disorder has a 50-percent chance of passing the mutated gene to each child. There is also a 50-percent chance that a child will not inherit the mutated gene.

- For an autosomal recessive disorder, two unaffected people who each carry one copy of the mutated gene (carriers) have a 25-percent chance with each pregnancy of having a child affected by the disorder. There is a 75-percent chance with each pregnancy that a child will be unaffected.

- The chance of passing on an X-linked dominant condition differs between men and women because men have one X and one Y chromosome, while women have two X chromosomes. A man passes on his Y chromosome to all of his sons and his X chromosome to all of his daughters. Therefore, the sons of a man with an X-linked dominant disorder will not be affected, and his daughters will all inherit the condition. A woman passes on one or the other of her X chromosomes to each child. Therefore, a woman with an X-linked dominant disorder has a 50-percent chance of having an affected daughter or son with each pregnancy.

Table 3.1. Inheritance Patterns

Inheritance Pattern	Description	Examples
Autosomal dominant	Only one mutated copy of the gene is needed for a person to be affected by an autosomal dominant disorder. Each affected person usually has one affected parent.	Huntington disease, neurofibromatosis 1
Autosomal recessive	Two copies of the gene must be mutated for a person to be affected by an autosomal recessive disorder. An affected person usually has unaffected parents who each carry a single copy of the mutated gene (and are referred to as carriers).	cystic fibrosis, sickle cell anemia
X-linked dominant	X-linked dominant disorders are caused by mutations in genes on the X chromosome. Only a few disorders have this inheritance pattern. Females are more frequently affected than males, and the chance of passing on an X-linked dominant disorder differs between men and women.	X-linked hypophosphatemia
X-linked recessive	X-linked recessive disorders are also caused by mutations in genes on the X chromosome. Males are more frequently affected than females, and the chance of passing on the disorder differs between men and women.	hemophilia A, Duchenne muscular dystrophy
Mitochondrial	This type of inheritance, also known as maternal inheritance, applies to genes in mitochondrial DNA. (Mitochondria, which are structures in each cell that convert molecules into energy, each contain a small amount of DNA.) Because only egg cells contribute mitochondria to the developing embryo, only females can pass on mitochondrial conditions to their children.	Leber's hereditary optic neuropathy (LHON)

- Because of the difference in sex chromosomes, the probability of passing on an X-linked recessive disorder also differs between men and women. The sons of a man with an X-linked recessive disorder will not be affected, and his daughters will carry one copy of the mutated gene. With each pregnancy, a woman who carries an X-linked recessive disorder has a 50-percent chance of having sons who are affected and a 50-percent chance of having daughters who carry one copy of the mutated gene.

It is important to note that the chance of passing on a genetic condition applies equally to each pregnancy. For example, if a couple has a child with an autosomal recessive disorder, the chance of having another child with the disorder is still 25 percent (or one in four). Having one child with a disorder does not protect future children from inheriting the condition. Conversely, having a child without the condition does not mean that future children will definitely be affected.

Although the chances of inheriting a genetic condition appear straightforward, in some cases factors such as a person's family history and the results of genetic testing can modify those chances. In addition, some people with a disease-causing mutation never develop any health problems or may experience only mild symptoms of the disorder. If a disease that runs in a family does not have a clear-cut inheritance pattern, predicting the likelihood that a person will develop the condition can be particularly difficult.

Because estimating the chance of developing or passing on a genetic disorder can be complex, genetics professionals can help people understand these chances and make informed decisions about their health.

Can changes in chromosomes cause disorders?

Yes. Changes that affect entire chromosomes or large segments of chromosomes can cause problems with growth, development, and function of the body's systems. These changes can affect many genes along the chromosome and alter the proteins made by those genes. Conditions caused by a change in the number or structure of chromosomes are known as chromosomal disorders. Many chromosomal disorders are not inherited.

Human cells normally contain 23 pairs of chromosomes, for a total of 46 in each cell. A change in the number of chromosomes leads to a chromosomal disorder. A gain or loss of chromosomes from the normal 46 is called aneuploidy. Down syndrome is an example of a condition caused by aneuploidy—people with Down syndrome have an extra copy of chromosome 21, for a total of 47 chromosomes in each cell.

Chromosomal disorders can also be caused by changes in chromosome structure. These changes are caused by the breakage and reunion of chromosome segments when an egg or sperm cell is formed. Pieces of DNA can be rearranged within one chromosome, or transferred between two or more chromosomes. The effects of structural changes depend on their size and location. Some disorders caused by changes in chromosome structure can be passed from parent to child.

Why are some genetic conditions more common in particular ethnic groups?

Some genetic disorders are more likely to occur among people who trace their ancestry to a particular geographic area. People in an ethnic group often share certain versions of their genes, which have been passed down from common ancestors. If one of these shared genes contains a disease-causing mutation, a particular genetic disorder may be more frequently seen in the group.

Examples of genetic conditions that are more common in particular ethnic groups are sickle cell anemia, which is more common in people of African, African American, or Mediterranean heritage; and Tay-Sachs disease, which is more likely to occur among people of Ashkenazi (eastern and central European) Jewish or French Canadian ancestry. It is important to note, however, that these disorders can occur in any ethnic group.

How are genetic conditions named?

Genetic conditions are not named in one standard way (unlike genes, which are given an official name and symbol by a formal committee). Doctors who treat families with a particular disorder are often the first to propose a name for the condition. Expert working groups may later revise the name to improve its usefulness. Naming is important because it allows accurate and effective communication about particular conditions, which will ultimately help researchers find new approaches to treatment.

Disorder names are often derived from one or a combination of sources:

- The basic genetic or biochemical defect that causes the condition (for example, alpha-1 antitrypsin deficiency);

- One or more major signs or symptoms of the disorder (for example, sickle cell anemia);

- The parts of the body affected by the condition (for example, retinoblastoma);

- The name of a physician or researcher, often the first person to describe the disorder (for example, Marfan syndrome, which was named after Dr. Antoine Bernard-Jean Marfan);

- A geographic area (for example, familial Mediterranean fever, which occurs mainly in populations bordering the Mediterranean Sea); or

- The name of a patient or family with the condition (for example, amyotrophic lateral sclerosis, which is also called Lou Gehrig disease after a famous baseball player who had the condition).

Disorders named after a specific person or place are called eponyms. There is debate as to whether the possessive form (for example, Alzheimer's disease) or the nonpossessive form (Alzheimer disease) of eponyms is preferred. As a rule, medical geneticists use the nonpossessive form, and this form may become the standard for doctors in all fields of medicine.

The HUGO Gene Nomenclature Committee (HGNC) designates an official name and symbol (an abbreviation of the name) for each known human gene. Some official gene names include additional information in parentheses, such as related genetic conditions, subtypes of a condition, or inheritance pattern. The HGNC is a non-profit organization funded by the U.K. Medical Research Council and the U.S. National Institutes of Health. The Committee has named more than 13,000 of the estimated 30,000 to 40,000 genes in the human genome.

During the research process, genes often acquire several alternate names and symbols. Different researchers investigating the same gene may each give the gene a different name, which can cause confusion. The HGNC assigns a unique name and symbol to each human gene, which allows effective organization of genes in large databanks, aiding the advancement of research.

Chapter 4

How Are Genetic Disorders Inherited?

Long before the advent of genetic testing or even complete understanding of DNA and RNA, astute observers noticed that genetic
traits, including many disorders, were passed from one generation to
another in somewhat predictable patterns. These came to be known
as autosomal dominant, autosomal recessive, X-linked recessive and X-
linked dominant patterns of inheritance. To understand heredity, you
have to know a little about human chromosomes and how they work.

Chromosomes come in pairs in the cell's nucleus. Humans have 46
chromosomes in each cell nucleus, which are actually 23 pairs of chromosomes. For 22 of these pairs, numbered chromosome 1 through
chromosome 22, the chromosomes are the same; that is, they carry
genes for the same traits. One chromosome comes from a person's
mother, the other from his father. The 23rd pair is an exception and
determines gender. The 23rd chromosomal pair differs according to
whether you're a male or a female. Males have an X and a Y chromosome, while females have two Xs for this 23rd pair of chromosomes.
Every female gets one X chromosome from her mother and one X from
her father. Every male gets an X chromosome from his mother and a
Y from his father.

Excertped from "Facts About Genetic Disorders," with permission from the
Muscular Dystrophy Association, www.mdausa.org. © 2000 The Muscular Dys-
trophy Association. For additional information, call the Muscular Dystrophy
Association National Headquarters toll-free at (800) 572-1717. To find an
MDA office in your area, look in your local telephone book, or click on "Clinics
and Services" on the MDA website.

Y chromosomes are unique to males and, in fact, determine maleness. If a man passes to his child an X chromosome from this 23rd pair, it will be a girl; if he donates a Y, it will be a boy.

Autosomal dominant conditions require only one mutation to show themselves.

When specialists use the term autosomal dominant, they mean that the genetic mutation is on an autosome, one of the chromosomes that's not an X or a Y. They also mean that the condition caused by the mutation can occur even if only one of the two paired autosomes carries the mutation. It's a way of saying that the mutated gene is dominant over the normal gene.

In autosomal dominant disorders, the chance of having an affected child is 50 percent with each conception.

Autosomal recessive conditions require two mutations to show themselves. When they use the term autosomal recessive, they mean that the disorder is again located on chromosomes that aren't Xs or Ys. However, when a disorder is recessive, it takes two mutated genes to cause a visible disorder in a person.

The word "recessive" comes from the idea that, when only one gene mutation exists, it may remain undetected ("recede" into the background) for several generations in a family—until someone has a child with another person who also has a mutation in that same autosomal gene. Then, the two recessive genes can come together in a child and produce the signs and symptoms of a genetic disorder.

You can think of recessive genes as "weaker" than "dominant" genes, in that it takes two of them to cause a problem.

People with one gene mutation for disorders that require two to produce the disorder are said to be carriers of the disorder. Carriers are usually protected from showing symptoms of a genetic disease by the presence of a normal corresponding gene on the other chromosome of each chromosome pair.

Sometimes, biochemical or other electrical testing or certain conditions (for example, vigorous exercise or fasting) will reveal subtle cellular abnormalities in carriers of various genetic conditions.

In autosomal recessive disorders, the chance of having an affected child is 25 percent with each conception.

Another important inheritance pattern is the *X-linked pattern*. X-linked disorders affect males and females differently. X-linked disorders come from mutations in genes on the X chromosome.

X-linked disorders affect males more severely than they do females. The reason is that females have two X chromosomes, while males have only one. If there's a mutation in an X-chromosome gene, the female has a second, "backup," X chromosome that almost always carries a normal version of the gene and can usually compensate for the mutated gene. The male, on the other hand, has no such backup; he has a Y chromosome paired with his sole X. In reality, females sometimes have disease symptoms in X-linked conditions despite the presence of a backup X chromosome. In some X-linked disorders, females routinely show symptoms of the disease, although they're rarely as serious (or lethal) as those in the males.

Some experts prefer the term X-linked recessive for the type of X-linked disorder in which females rarely show symptoms and X-linked dominant for the type in which females routinely show at least some disease symptoms.

Females with mild or no disease symptoms who have one mutated gene on an X chromosome and a normal version of the gene on the other X chromosome are called carriers of an X-linked disorder.

In X-linked recessive disorders, when the mother is a carrier, the chance of having an affected child is 50 percent for each male child. If the father has the mutation and is able to have children, boys won't be affected, because they receive only a Y chromosome from him. Girls receive his X chromosome and will be carriers.

Can inheritance diagrams predict what my family will look like?

No. Many of us have seen diagrams like those of autosomal dominant, autosomal recessive and X-linked recessive inheritance during our school years or perhaps in medical offices. Unfortunately, these diagrams very often lead to misunderstandings.

The diagrams are mathematical calculations of the odds that one gene or the other in a pair of genes will be passed on to a child during any particular conception.

These are the same kinds of calculations one would make if asked to predict the chances of a coin landing as heads or tails. With each coin toss (assuming the coin isn't weighted and the conditions are otherwise impartial), the chances that the coin will land in one position or the other are 50 percent.

In reality, if you were to toss a coin six times, you might come up with any number of combinations: All your tosses might be heads, or five could be heads with one tails, or four might be tails with two heads.

In fact, every coin toss was a new set of odds: 50 percent heads, 50 percent tails. The second coin toss wasn't the least bit influenced by the first, nor the third by the first two, nor the sixth by the previous five.

So it is with the conception of children. If the odds of passing on a certain gene (say a gene on the X chromosome that carries a mutation versus a gene on the other X chromosome that doesn't) are 50 percent for each conception, they remain 50 percent no matter how many children you have.

Don't be misled by an orderly diagram that shows one out of two children getting each gene so that a family of four children has two children with and two children without the gene in question.

Like the coin toss where six tosses turned up six heads, you could have six children who all inherit the gene.

What happens in actual families?

In real life, it's impossible to predict which genes will be passed on to which children at each conception. This kind of prediction would be the same as trying to predict the outcome of any particular coin toss. Even though the overall odds are 50 percent heads and 50 percent tails, you can get six heads in a row.

How can a disease be genetic if no one else in the family has it?

This is a question often asked by people who have received a diagnosis of a genetic disorder or who have had a child with such a diagnosis. "But, doctor," they often say, "There's no history of anything like this in our family, so how can it be genetic?" This is a very understandable source of confusion.

Very often, a genetic (or hereditary) disorder occurs in a family where no one else has been known to have it.

One way for this to happen is the mechanism of recessive inheritance. In recessive disorders, it takes two mutated genes to cause disease symptoms. A single genetic mutation may have been present and passed down in a family for generations but only now has a child inherited a second mutation from the other side of the family and so developed the disease.

A similar mechanism occurs with X-linked disorders. The family may have carried a mutation on the X chromosome in females for generations, but until someone gives birth to a male child with this mutation, the genetic disorder remains only a potential, not an actual, disease. Females rarely have significant symptoms in X-linked disorders.

Another way for a child to develop a dominant or X-linked disease that's never been seen in the family follows this scenario: One or more of the father's sperm cells or one or more of the mother's egg cells develops a mutation. Such a mutation would never be detected by standard medical tests or even by DNA tests, which generally sample the blood cells. However, if this particular sperm or egg is used to conceive a child, he or she will be born with the mutation. This scenario isn't rare.

Until recently, when parents who didn't have a genetic disorder and tested as "noncarriers" gave birth to a child with a genetic disorder, they were reassured that the mutation was a one-time event in a single sperm or egg cell and that it would be almost impossible for it to happen again.

Unfortunately, especially in the case of Duchenne dystrophy, this proved to be false reassurance. We now know that sometimes more than one egg cell can be affected by a mutation that isn't in the mother's blood cells and doesn't show up on standard carrier tests. Such mothers can give birth to more children with Duchenne dystrophy because subsequent egg cells with the Duchenne mutation can be used to conceive a child.

In a sense, these mothers actually are carriers—but carriers only in some of their cells. They can be thought of as "partial" carriers. Another term is mosaic carrier. It's very hard to estimate the precise risk of passing on the disorder in these cases.

It's very likely that this kind of situation occurs in other neuromuscular genetic disorders, although most haven't been as well studied as Duchenne dystrophy. For example, more than one sperm or egg cell could pass on a dominant mutation to more than one of a parent's children. Or, in a recessive disorder like spinal muscular atrophy, a child could inherit one mutation from a parent who's a full carrier, and then acquire a second genetic mutation from the other parent, a mosaic carrier. Standard carrier testing wouldn't pick up any problem in the latter parent.

In practical terms, the most important message of recent research is that a genetic test that looks only at blood cells and shows that a parent is not a carrier can't be completely relied upon with regard to the risk of having another affected child. The mutation may be present in cells that weren't tested, and if those include some of the sperm or egg cells, there's a risk that more than one affected child could be born.

A geneticist or genetic counselor can help you make informed decisions regarding childbearing if you've already had a child with a genetic disorder. The recurrence risk is different in different disorders.

Are there genes outside the cell's nucleus?

Yes. There's actually another small set of genes that we all possess, inside our cells but outside the cell nucleus. The cell nucleus is where most of our genes reside on the 23 pairs of chromosomes already discussed.

The additional genes, which make up less than one percent of a cell's DNA, are the mitochondrial genes, and they exist on circular chromosomes inside mitochondria, the "energy factories" of cells. (The singular for mitochondria is mitochondrion.)

What are genes doing inside the mitochondria?

There are about 37 genes, mostly involved in energy production, inside the mitochondria. Scientists believe that mitochondria were once independent organisms resembling today's bacteria, and that when they became part of human and animal cells, they kept their own genes. These genes, arranged on circular chromosomes, carry the recipes for 13 proteins needed for mitochondrial functions. They also code for 24 specialized RNA molecules that are needed to assist in the production of other mitochondrial proteins. For reasons that will become clear, it's important to know that mitochondria also use proteins made by genes in the cell's nucleus. These proteins are "imported" into the mitochondria.

Can disease-causing mutations occur in mitochondrial genes?

Yes. Disease-causing mutations can occur in the mitochondrial genes. The disorders are often, as one would predict, associated with energy deficits in cells with high energy requirements, such as nerve and muscle cells. The disorders as a whole are called mitochondrial disorders. Mitochondrial disorders affecting muscle are known as mitochondrial myopathies.

How are mitochondrial mutations inherited?

Mitochondrial DNA inheritance comes only through the mother and is therefore completely different from nuclear (from the nucleus) DNA inheritance. The rules for recessive, dominant and X-linked inheritance don't apply at all. An embryo receives its mitochondria from the mother's egg cell, not the father's sperm cell, at conception. (Research suggests that sperm mitochondria are eliminated by the egg cell.)

Mutations can exist in some of the mitochondria in a person's cells and never cause much, if any, trouble. (In fact, one theory of aging says that it's caused by an accumulation of mutations in mitochondrial DNA.) The normal mitochondria are usually enough to produce the needed energy for the body. But once a person has a certain percentage of mutated mitochondria (perhaps 30 percent or so), the energy deficits become crucial and a mitochondrial disorder can result.

Mothers can pass on mitochondrial mutations to their children, but fathers can't, so mitochondrial DNA inheritance follows a pattern called maternal inheritance. The severity of the child's disorder depends on how many normal versus abnormal mitochondria the child receives from the mother.

Mitochondrial DNA mutations can also occur during development of an embryo. Not all mitochondrial mutations are inherited. Some occur as an embryo is developing in the womb. Researchers have found that embryonic mitochondrial mutations generally occur after sperm or egg cells have formed in the affected embryo, so, as far as has been observed, these mutations are not passed on to the next generation.

Does DNA from the cell's nucleus affect the mitochondria?

Yes. DNA from the nucleus also affects mitochondrial function, so some mitochondrial disorders are inherited according to the same rules as are other genetic disorders.

Most mitochondrial proteins aren't made in the mitochondria but come from genes in the cell's nucleus. These nuclear proteins are later imported into the mitochondria, where they too help with energy production.

As you may have guessed, mutations can also occur in these nuclear genes that affect mitochondria. So, that's another way to get a "mitochondrial disorder" —but one that's not caused by mutated mitochondrial DNA. Nuclear DNA that affects mitochondrial function is inherited according to the autosomal and X-linked patterns.

For family planning, it's important to know exactly what kind of DNA mutation exists in a family with a mitochondrial disorder— whether it's a mitochondrial DNA mutation or a nuclear DNA mutation. As you can see, these have very different patterns of inheritance and implications for the family.

Part Two

Disorders Associated with Specific Genes

Chapter 5

Albinism

What is albinism?

The word "albinism" refers to a group of inherited conditions. People with albinism have little or no pigment in the eyes, skin, and hair (or in some cases in the eyes alone). They have inherited from their parents an altered copy of a gene that does not work correctly. The altered gene does not allow the body to make the usual amounts of a pigment called melanin.

Approximately one in 17,000 people have one of the types of albinism. About 18,000 people in the United States are affected. Albinism affects people from all races. The parents of most children with albinism have normal hair and eye color for their ethnic background and do not have a family history of albinism.

What is melanin pigment?

Melanin is a dark compound that is called a photoprotective pigment. The major role of melanin pigment in the skin is to absorb the ultraviolet (UV) light that comes from the sun so that the skin is not damaged. Sun exposure normally produces a tan which is an increase in melanin pigment in the skin. Many people with albinism do not

Text in this chapter is excerpted and reprinted with permission from "Facts About Albinism," by Richard A. King, M.D., Ph.D., C. Gail Summers, M.D., James W. Haefemeyer, M.D., M.S., and Bonnie S. LeRoy, M.S. Copyright © 2000 The International Albinism Center at the University of Minnesota. To view the complete text of this booklet, or for additional information, visit http://www.cbc.umn.edu/iac/.

have melanin pigment in their skin and do not tan with exposure to the sun. As a result, their skin is sensitive to the sun light and they develop a sun burn. In people with albinism, all other parts of the skin are normal even if there is no melanin in the skin.

Melanin pigment is important in other areas of the body, such as the eye and the brain, but it is not known what the melanin pigment does in these areas. Melanin pigment is normally present in the retina. The area of the retina called the fovea does not develop correctly if melanin pigment is not present in the retina during development. The nerve connections between the retina and the brain are also altered if melanin pigment is not present in the retina during development.

The iris normally has melanin pigment, and this makes the iris opaque to light (no light goes through an opaque iris). Iris pigment in albinism is reduced, and the iris is translucent to light, but the iris develops and functions normally in albinism.

Table 5.1. Genes Involved in Pigmentation

Gene	Location
Tyrosinase	Chromosome 11
P	Chromosome 15
Dopachrome tautomerase (TRP2)	Chromosome 13
DHICA oxidase (TRP1)	Chromosome 9
Hermansky-Pudlak syndrome (HPS)	Chromosome 10
Ocular albinism (OA1)	Chromosome X

What are the problems with albinism?

The eye needs melanin pigment to develop normal vision. People with albinism have impairment of vision because the eye does not have a normal amount of melanin pigment during development. The skin needs pigment for protection from sun damage, and people with albinism often sunburn easily. In tropical areas, many people with albinism who do not protect their skin get skin cancers.

There are several less common types of albinism which involve other problems also, such as mild problems with blood clotting, or problems with hearing.

Albinism may cause social problems, because people with albinism look different from their families, peers, and other members of their ethnic group.

Growth and development of a child with albinism should be normal and intellectual development is normal. Developmental milestones should be achieved at the expected age. General health of a child and an adult with albinism is normal, and the reduction in melanin pigment in the skin, hair and the eyes should have no effect on the brain, the cardiovascular system, the lungs, the gastrointestinal tract, the genitourinary system, the musculoskeletal system, or the immune system. Life span is normal.

What eye problems result from albinism?

People with albinism, whether it involves the eyes alone or involves the skin and the hair, often have several eye problems. Ophthalmologists and optometrists can help people with albinism compensate for their eye problems, but they cannot cure them.

Visual acuity: People with albinism are not "blind," but their vision (also called visual acuity) is not normal, and cannot be corrected completely with glasses. Extreme farsightedness or nearsightedness, and astigmatism are common, Correction with glasses can improve acuity in many people with albinism. Corrected visual acuity ranges from 20/20 (can see at 20 feet what should be seen at 20 feet; this is considered normal) to 20/400 (see at 20 feet what should be seen at 400 feet; this is considered legally blind). Normal or near-normal vision is unusual, however, even when glasses are worn.

For help with visual acuity, eye doctors experienced in low vision can prescribe a variety of devices. No one device can serve the needs of all persons in all situations, since different occupations and hobbies require the use of vision in different ways. Young children may simply need glasses, and older children can sometimes benefit from bifocal glasses. Low vision clinics may prescribe telescopic lenses mounted on glasses, sometimes called bioptics, for close-up work as well as for distant vision. Recently smaller and lighter telescopes have been developed; however, ordinary glasses or bifocals with a strong reading correction may serve well for many people with albinism.

Nystagmus: Nystagmus is an involuntary movement of the eyes back and forth. Attempted treatments to control nystagmus have included biofeedback, contact lenses, and surgery. The most promising may be eye muscle surgery that reduces the movement of the eyes; however, vision may not improve in all cases due to other associated eye abnormalities. People with albinism may find ways of reducing nystagmus while reading, such as placing a finger by the eye, or tilting the head at an angle where nystagmus is dampened.

Strabismus: Strabismus means that the eyes do not fixate and track together. Strabismus is common in albinism and is related to the altered development of the optic nerves. It is usually not severe and the tends to alternate between involving the right and the left eye. Despite this condition, people with albinism do have some depth perception, although it is not as sharp as when both eyes can work together.

Ophthalmologists may prefer to treat infants with strabismus starting at about six months age, before the function of their eyes has developed fully. They may recommend that parents patch one eye to promote the use of the non-preferred eye. In other cases, the alignment of the eyes may improve with the wearing of glasses. Correction of strabismus by surgery or by injection of medicine into the muscles around the eyes does not completely correct the problem. Although these treatments may improve the alignment of the eyes and enhance psycho-social development and interpersonal interactions, they cannot correct the improper routing of the nerves to the brain. Depth perception is not improved with eye muscle surgery.

Photophobia: Sensitivity to light is called photophobia. The iris allows "stray" light to enter the eye and cause sensitivity. For photophobia, eye doctors can prescribe dark glasses that shield the eyes from bright light, or photochromic lenses that darken on exposure to brighter light. There is no proof that dark glasses will improve vision, even when used at a very early age, but they may improve comfort. Children and adults with albinism who do not like tinted lenses may benefit more from wearing a cap or a visor when outdoors in the sun.

Iris color: It is a common, but false, notion that people with albinism must have red eyes. In fact the color of the iris varies from a dull gray to blue to brown. (A brown iris is common in ethnic groups with darker pigmentation.) Under certain lighting conditions, there is a reddish or violet hue reflected through the iris because it has very little pigment. This reddish reflection comes from the retina, which is the surface lining the inside of the eye. This reddish reflection is similar to that which occurs when a flash photograph is taken of a person looking directly at the camera making the eyes appear red. With some types of albinism the red color can reflect back through the iris as well as through the pupil.

Foveal hypoplasia: One major abnormality of the eye in albinism involves lack of development of the fovea; this condition is known as foveal hypoplasia. The fovea is a small but important area of the retina in the inside of the eye. The retina contains the nerve cells that detect the light entering the eye and transmit the signal for the light to the brain. The fovea is the area of the retina that allows sharp vision, which is required for activities such as reading. This area of the retina does not develop in albinism. It is not known why the fovea does not develop normally with albinism, but it is related to the lack of melanin pigment in the retina during development of the eye. The developing eye seems to need melanin for organizing the fovea.

Nerve signals: Another major abnormality of the eye in albinism involves the development of the nerves that connect the retina to the brain. People with albinism have an unusual pattern for sending nerve signals from the eye to the brain. This unusual pattern for nerve signals probably prevents the eyes from working well together and causes reduced depth perception.

How do we classify albinism?

Two main categories of albinism are: "oculocutaneous albinism" (AHK-you-low-CU-tain-ee-us), called OCA, and "ocular albinism" (AHK-you-lahr), called OA. OCA means that melanin pigment is missing in the skin, the hair, and the eyes. OA means that the melanin pigment is missing mainly in the eyes, and the skin and hair appear normal. OCA is more common than OA.

Oculocutaneous albinism (OCA): For many years, the term "albinism" referred only to people who had white hair, white skin, and blue eyes. Individuals who had OCA and pigmented hair and eyes were identified, particularly in African and African-American populations, and terms such as *incomplete albinism, partial albinism*, or *imperfect albinism* were used for this, but these terms are inappropriate and are no longer used.

In the 1980s the classification of OCA was expanded using very careful skin, hair, and eye examinations. The reason for this was the knowledge that there were more than 50 gene loci that controlled pigmentation in the mouse, and it was suggested that careful analysis of skin, hair, and eye pigmentation of individuals with OCA could help identify the human equivalent of each of these genes. A number of types of OCA were identified, including platinum OCA, minimal pigment OCA, yellow OCA, temperature-sensitive OCA, autosomal recessive ocular albinism, and brown OCA. In the 1990s, we were able to identify the genes involved in most types of OCA, and found that the classifications based on hair, skin, and eye color are not accurate and that it is better to classify OCA types based on the specific gene involved. We have now identified five genes that are associated with the development of OCA and one gene that is involved in OA.

Table 5.2. Genes Associated with Albinism.

Gene	Type of Albinism
Tyrosinase gene	OCA1 (OCA1A and OCA1B)
P gene	OCA2
TRP1 gene	OCA3
HPS gene	Hermansky-Pudlak Syndrome
CHS gene	Chediak Higashi Syndrome
OA1 gene	X-linked ocular albinism

OCA1 (tyrosinase related oculocutaneous albinism): One of the two most common types of albinism is tyrosinase related OCA, produced by loss of function of the tyrosinase enzyme in the melanocyte. This results from inherited mutations of the tyrosinase gene. Classical OCA, with a total absence of melanin in the skin, hair, and eyes over the lifetime of the affected individual is the most obvious type of OCA1, but there is a wide range of pigmentation associated with tyrosinase gene mutations. The range in phenotypes extends from total absence to near normal cutaneous pigmentation, but the ocular features are always present and help identify an individual as having albinism.

An important distinguishing characteristic of OCA1 is the presence of marked hypopigmentation at birth. Most individuals affected with a type of OCA1 have white hair, milky white skin, and blue eyes at birth. The irides can be very light blue and translucent so that the whole iris appears pink or red in ambient or bright light. During the first and second decade of life, the irides usually become a darker blue and may remain translucent or become lightly pigmented with reduced translucency. The skin remains white or appears to have more color with time. Sun exposure produces erythema and a burn if the skin is has little pigment and is unprotected, but may tan well if cutaneous pigment has developed. Pigmented lesions (nevi, freckles, lentigines) develop in the skin of individuals who have developed pigmented hair and skin.

OCA1A (classic tyrosinase-negative OCA): Individuals with OCA1A or the classic tyrosinase-negative OCA are unable to make melanin in their skin, hair, or eyes, because they have no active tyrosinase enzyme. They are born with white hair and skin and blue eyes, and there is no change as they mature into teenagers and adults. They never develop melanin in these tissues. The phenotype is the same in all ethnic groups around the world and at all ages. With time, the hair may develop a dense rather than a translucent white or a slight yellow tint but this usually from the denaturing of the hair protein with the use of different shampoos. The irides are translucent and appear pink early in life and often turn a gray-blue color with time. No pigmented lesions develop in the skin, although amelanotic nevi can be present.

Visual acuity for OCA1A is usually in the legally-blind range, 20/200 to 20/400, although near vision may be better if the print is held close to the eyes. Vision usually does not improve with age. Photophobia and nystagmus cause more problems with OCA1A than with other types. Vision often does not correct well with glasses, but low vision aids help.

OCA1B: OCA1B is produced by mutations of the tyrosinase gene that result in enzyme with some residual or "leaky" activity. The variation in the pigmentation in individuals with OCA1B is wide from very little cutaneous pigment to nearly normal skin and hair pigment. Mutations coding for enzyme with differing amounts of residual activity are the primary cause of this variation, and a moderate amount of residual activity can lead to near normal cutaneous pigmentation and the mistaken diagnosis of ocular albinism. Ethnic and family pigment patterns influence the pigmentation of an individual with OCA1B, and hair color can be light red or brown in some families where this is the predominant pigment pattern.

OCA2 (P-gene related oculocutaneous albinism: The common features of OCA2 include the presence of hair pigment at birth and iris pigment at birth or early in life. Localized skin pigment (nevi, freckles, and lentigines) can develop, often in sun exposed regions of the skin, but tanning is usually absent. Both OCA1B and OCA2 have a broad range of pigmentation that, in part, reflects the genetic background of the affected individual. There may be some accumulation of pigment in the hair with age but this is much less pronounced as that found in OCA1B, and many individuals with OCA2 have the same hair color throughout life. OCA2 is the most common type of OCA in the world, primarily because of the high frequency in equatorial Africa.

Brown OCA: Brown OCA is a type of albinism that is recognized in the African and the African-American populations, but not in other populations to date. In African and African-American individuals with Brown OCA, the hair and skin color are light brown, and the irides are gray to tan at birth. With time there is little change in skin color, but the hair may turn darker and the irides may accumulate more tan pigment. Affected individuals are recognized as having albinism because they have all of the ocular features of albinism. The iris has punctate and radial translucency, and moderate retinal pigment is present. The skin may darken with sun exposure. Visual acuity ranges from 20/60 to 20/150.

OCA3 (TRP1-related OCA): A type of OCA known as 'Rufous' or 'Red OCA' in the South African population results from mutations of the gene for TRP1. Individuals with OCA who have red hair and reddish-brown pigmented skin have been reported in Africa and in New Guinea, but clinical descriptions are incomplete, and similar individuals in the U.S. population have not been identified and reported.

Hermansky-Pudlak syndrome (HPS): The Hermansky-Pudlak syndrome includes OCA, an abnormality of platelets that usually leads to mild bleeding, and the accumulation of a material called ceroid in tissues throughout the body. HPS is a pigmenting type of OCA. Skin and eye pigment develop in many affected individuals, but the amount of pigment that forms is quite variable. Some affected individuals have marked hypopigmentation of their skin and hair similar to that of OCA1A, others have white skin and yellow or blond hair similar to OCA1B or OCA2, and still others have only moderate hypopigmentation suggesting that they may have OA rather than OCA. The variation can be seen within families.

The most important medical problems in HPS are usually related to the lung and the gastrointestinal tract changes. The bleeding problem in HPS is related to a deficiency of granules in the platelets that store material needed for normal platelet function.

Chediak-Higashi syndrome (CHS): The Chediak-Higashi syndrome is a rare syndrome that includes an increased susceptibility to bacterial infections, hypopigmentation, and the presence of giant granules in white blood cells. The skin, hair, and eye pigment is reduced or diluted in CHS, but the affected individuals often do not have obvious albinism and the hypopigmentation may only be noted when compared to other family members. Hair color is light brown to blond, and the hair has a metallic silver-gray sheen. The skin is creamy white to slate gray. Iris pigment is present, and nystagmus and photophobia may be present or absent.

OA1 X-linked ocular albinism: Ocular albinism involves the eyes only. X-linked ocular albinism occurs primarily in males. Skin color is usually normal or slightly lighter than the skin of other family members. Eye color may be in the normal range, but examination of the back of the eye (retina) through the pupil shows that there is no pigment in the retina. Females who carry the gene for X-linked ocular albinism may show a mixture of pigmented and non-pigmented areas in their retinas. Visual acuity in X-linked albinism is in the range of 20/50 to 20/400.

How can you determine the type of albinism present?

It is usually possible to determine the type of albinism present with a careful history of pigment development and an examination of the skin, hair, and eyes. The only type of albinism that has white hair at birth is OCA1. Individuals with other types of OCA will have some hair pigment at birth, although it may be very slight in amount. It can be difficult to tell if the hair is completely white or very lightly pigmented in a very young child, and changes in pigment over time will usually help clarify the OCA type present.

The most accurate test for determining the specific type of albinism is a gene test. A small sample of blood is obtained from the affected individual and the parents. By a complex process, a genetic laboratory can "sequence" the code of the DNA (the chemical that carries the 'genetic code' of each gene) to identify the changes (mutations) in the gene that cause albinism in the family. The test is useful only for families that contain individuals with albinism. It cannot be performed practically as a screening test for the general population. None of the tests available are capable of detecting all of the mutations of the genes that cause albinism, and responsible mutations cannot be detected in a small number of individuals and families with albinism.

The test can be used to determine if a fetus has albinism. For this purpose a sample would be obtained by amniocentesis, a procedure which involves using a needle to draw fluid from the uterus, at 16 to 18 weeks gestation. Those considering such testing should be aware that given proper support children with albinism can function well and have normal life spans.

Where can I get more information about albinism?

The International Albinism Center is a center for research about albinism and health care for albinism. Contact:

The International Albinism Center
University of Minnesota
P.O. Box 485 Mayo, 420 Delaware Street S.E.
Minneapolis, Minnesota 55455
Phone: 612-624-0144
Website: http://www.cbc.umn.edu/iac/facts.htm

About the Authors

Richard A. King, M.D., Ph.D., Professor of Medicine and in the Institute of Human Genetics at the University of Minnesota, has conducted research on albinism for more than fifteen years, and coordinates the International Albinism Center.

C. Gail Summers, M.D., Professor of Ophthalmology at the University of Minnesota, is involved in research on vision and albinism, and is co-director of the International Albinism Center.

James W. Haefemeyer, M.D., M.S., is a family practice physician in Minneapolis, Minnesota, who has albinism and is a NOAH (National Organization for Albinism and Hypopigmentation) Scientific Advisor.

Bonnie S. LeRoy, M.S., is an Associate Professor in the Department of Cell Biology, Genetics and Development and Director of the Graduate Program in Genetics Counseling at the University of Minnesota.

Chapter 6

Alpha-1 Antitrypsin Deficiency

General Information

What is alpha-1-antitrypsin?

Alpha-1-antitrypsin (alpha-1) is a protein that is produced mostly by the liver. Its primary function is to protect the lungs from neutrophil elastase. Neutrophil elastase is an enzyme that normally serves a useful purpose in lung tissue—it digests damaged or aging cells and bacteria in order to provide for healing. However, once it is done digesting those proteins, it does not stop, and attacks the lung tissue. Alpha-1-antitrypsin, in sufficient amounts, will trap and destroy the neutrophil elastase before it has a chance to begin damaging the delicate lung tissue.

Alpha-1-antitrypsin is an acute-phase reactive protein, which simply means that the production of alpha-1 can increase to three or four times the normal amount to protect tissues. This occurs in times of infection, pregnancy, or other situations that subject the body to an increase in neutrophil elastase. If you have a severe deficiency of alpha-1, your serum levels will not show a meaningful increase of alpha-1 in response to infections or other biological stress.

Reprinted with permission from the Alpha-1 Association, http://www.alpha1 .org. © 2004 Alpha-1 Association. All rights reserved. This material was reviewed for accuracy by medical advisor, Jack Lieberman, M.D.

How does alpha-1-antitrypsin deficiency affect you?

Alpha-1 is mostly manufactured in the liver. In alpha-1 deficient persons, the amount of alpha-1 produced may be close to normal, however, the liver does not secrete a normal amount into the bloodstream. If there is insufficient alpha-1-antitrypsin circulating, the destructive action of the damaging enzyme is largely unchecked and lung tissue is destroyed. In addition, what little alpha-1-antitrypsin circulating is defective and cannot effectively "trap" the elastase before it destroys healthy lung tissue. Persons with alpha-1 often have emphysema as a primary disease. In addition, they may have asthma, chronic bronchitis, and become susceptible to lung infections, and any of these conditions can cause further damage if not treated promptly.

Another disease that some alpha patients have is cirrhosis of the liver. This affects very young alpha-1 children, as well as 12%–15% of adult alpha patients. There is no cure, and for those who suffer progressive damage, a liver transplant is currently the only option available for survival.

Very rarely, alphas may also have a disease known as panniculitis. This is a skin affectation that occurs in children and adults alike.

What gives you alpha-1-antitrypsin deficiency?

Alpha-1-antitrypsin deficiency is an inherited disorder, and it occurs when both parents pass on an abnormal gene (*PiZ*) to their child. This results in a phenotype of *PiZZ* (Pi is protease inhibitor). People with normal amounts of alpha-1 have two normal genes (*PiMM*). If a person inherits one normal gene and one abnormal gene, they are carriers of the disease and are phenotyped *PiMZ*. Although there are many different alleles (or variants of the gene) that have been mapped, *PiZ* is the most common allele that can cause lung disease, and it usually results in the most severe cases.

What is emphysema?

Emphysema is a lung disease caused by the destruction of the delicate walls of small air sacs (alveoli). With this destruction, air sacs lose their elasticity and form larger, inefficient sacs that cannot properly exchange oxygen and carbon dioxide with the bloodstream. In addition, it becomes harder to breathe since each drawn breath inflates the lungs, but the lungs do not return to normal with the exhaled breath. This causes air to become trapped, leading to overinflation of the air sacs, which can cause additional damage. Emphysema caused by alpha-1 is a progressive disease—the destructive action continues until the lungs can no longer bring in oxygen to the bloodstream.

Alpha-1 emphysema, also called genetic emphysema, usually causes symptoms in people while they are in their 30s or 40s. While there is no cure for alpha-1, there are treatments available for the symptoms as well as a replacement therapy that may slow down or halt the destruction.

What is cirrhosis?

Cirrhosis is a chronic degenerative disease of the liver. It is often caused by alcohol abuse or as the result of infections such as hepatitis, and it has other causes as well. One risk factor for cirrhosis is having alpha-1-antitrypsin deficiency.

With cirrhosis, the liver deteriorates, the lobes become fibrous, and there is a great deal of fatty accumulation. This leads to problems with the liver's role in detoxifying drugs and alcohol, the absorption of vitamins is reduced, and there is an adverse effect on the gastrointestinal functions and the bilirubin and hormonal metabolic functions.

Some of the symptoms of cirrhosis include nausea, flatulence, weight loss, weakness, and abdominal pain.

What is panniculitis?

Panniculitis is an inflammation of fat just beneath the skin, causing the skin to harden and form lumps, patches, or lesions. It is likely that the damage is initiated by destructive action of unrestrained neutrophils. In some patients, damage from panniculitis may occur after an incident of trauma to the affected area. It occurs in children as well as adults, and has been linked to the ZZ and MZ phenotypes and possibly other alleles as well.

Lung Disease

How are lungs affected?

Alpha-1-antitrypsin protects the delicate tissues of the lungs by binding to neutrophil elastase, a protein released by white blood cells which digests bacteria and other foreign objects in the lungs. When a person who is deficient of alpha-1-antitrypsin inhales irritants, or contracts a lung infection, the neutrophil elastase released in the lungs continues digesting irritants unchecked, eventually destroying healthy lung tissue. The eventual result of the destruction of healthy lung tissue by neutrophil elastase is emphysema.

However, alpha-1-antitrypsin deficiency emphysema (also known as "genetic" or "inherited" emphysema) is different than emphysema caused by smoking ("acquired" emphysema). In emphysema caused by smoking the damage usually affects the upper portion of the lungs. In the alpha-1 patient, the lower regions of the lungs are first affected. With either cause, the lungs are hyperinflated due to air trapping caused by the destruction of the lung tissue, and the diaphragms are flattened due to the hyperinflation of the lungs.

Many people with alpha-1 also have chronic bronchitis. With this, the lung lining becomes swollen and congested with mucus, restricting air flow. The bronchi (air passages) often go into bronchospasms, which are contractions of the muscles which further reduce air flow. This often results in a chronic cough.

Asthma is common in patients with alpha-1. It is characterized by wheezing, coughing, and shortness of breath. Asthma is often precipitated by allergens, stress, exercise, and infections. In alpha-1 patients, symptoms of asthma can be managed with medications.

What are some lung risk factors associated with alpha-1?

Of utmost importance for people diagnosed with alpha-1-antitrypsin deficiency is immediate smoking cessation. No other single factor can improve an alpha's chance for survival. Inhaling smoke into the lungs summons massive amounts of neutrophil elastase to the lungs. Additionally, cigarette smoke renders the available alpha-1 antitrypsin useless.

Avoiding irritants such as chemicals, pollution, dust, and ozone, is also extremely important. Protecting yourself against lung infections, when possible, is highly advisable. Most physicians recommend pneumonia vaccines and annual flu shots.

In short, any type of irritant, bacteria, or virus that could make its way to the lungs should be avoided. Limiting these risks, and thus reducing the amount of neutrophil elastase needed in the lungs, can have a profound affect on limiting lung damage.

How is alpha-1 diagnosed in patients with lung problems?

Although alpha-1 is one of the most common genetic disorders in the world, it is often misdiagnosed. Many times patients are told they have asthma, bronchitis, symptoms related to stress, emphysema caused by smoking, or simply chronic obstructive pulmonary disease of unknown cause.

The most common indicators of alpha-1 include shortness of breath, a chronic cough, and abnormal liver test results. If you have any of these symptoms there is a simple blood test that can detect alpha-1-antitrypsin levels.

This test is also recommended if you have relatives, especially siblings, who have been diagnosed with alpha-1 or if there is a family history of early emphysema, with or without smoking.

What medical tests are used to monitor alpha-1 patients with lung disease?

Blood Tests: There is a simple blood test that measures the amount of alpha-1 circulating in your blood serum. If your levels are 45% or less than normal, additional testing may be performed in order to determine the phenotype. Some laboratories will test phenotypes on all samples, in order to detect heterozygous carriers of an abnormal alpha-1 variant.

Phenotypes: There are two types of units used to report alpha-1 levels: milligrams per 100 ml (mg%) and micromoles per liter (µM/L). The micromolar level is based on a highly purified laboratory standard for detecting alpha-1 levels. To avoid confusion with the commercial testing standard of mg% (which overestimated alpha-1 levels by 35–40%), use alpha-1 levels to determine phenotype. Both provide the same basic phenotype information to the alpha patient (see Table 6.1).

Table 6.1. Common alpha-1 phenotypes and the levels associated with them.

Phenotype	µM/L	mg%
MM	20–53	150–350
MZ	12–28	90–210
SS	13–27	100–210
SZ	10–16	75–120
ZZ	2.5–7	20–45
NULL	0	0

Alpha-1 levels of 11 µM/L (80 mg%) or less put you at greatest risk of developing alpha-1 related emphysema. Smokers with intermediate deficiency levels (80–160 mg%) are also at increased risk of lung disease.

The M gene refers to the normal gene. Over 75 alleles (gene variations) have been mapped, some of which can cause alpha-1. The S, Z and Null genes are the most common ones that cause alpha-1 deficiencies.

The Null gene is one that produces no detectable levels of alpha-1. Alphas with the Null-Null phenotype are at the greatest risk of developing emphysema, yet none have suffered liver damage as a result of their alpha-1.

What medications and treatments are available for alpha-1-related lung diseases?

Most physicians recommend medications for alpha-1 emphysema which are commonly used to treat asthma patients. There is no medicinal treatment for emphysema, and emphysema is incurable. However, many alphas also have an "asthma component" to their alpha-1. Keeping the airways open and free of inflammation, therefore, is an extremely important issue for alphas.

What surgeries are used to treat lung problems in alpha-1 patients?

Lung Volume Reduction: Lung volume reduction consists of cutting out damaged portions of the lung, thereby reducing its size by around 20%. It may seem strange to remove part of a lung when a patient has problems breathing, but the basis behind it makes sense. With emphysema, the alveoli in the lungs hyperinflate, become enlarged and less efficient in assisting with the exchange of blood gases. As a result, the over-expanded lung pushes against the healthier portions of lung, decreasing its effectiveness. It also pushes against the diaphragm, causing it to lose its natural shape and effectiveness.

When damaged, overinflated portions of the lungs are removed, more room is created for the diaphragm to move and for the normal parts of the lungs to inflate and deflate.

Alpha-1 patients have undergone this surgery with mixed results. Some have greatly improved their lung function, while others note little or no change. One of the problems alphas face with lung volume reduction is that their lung damage is often quite diffuse with no relatively good lung to expand and to have improved function in response to the surgery.

Lung Transplant: Patients with alpha-1 who have end-stage lung disease may be candidates for a lung transplant, if all other medical options have been exhausted. One or both lungs are removed and replaced with healthy lungs from a recently deceased human donor. There have been some transplants using lobes from living donors, that have met with some success, but this is a fairly new procedure and long-term results are not available.

Liver Disease

How are livers affected?

In 12–15% of alpha patients, the liver is affected, sometimes with lung damage as well. This can lead to cirrhosis of the liver, which is chronic, progressive and fatal. There are two primary theories that address liver disease in alpha patients.

The external attack theory: Due to the lack of alpha-1 circulating, the liver is subject to attacks by neutrophil elastase, other destructive enzymes, or bacteria.

The internal attack theory: In most cases of alpha-1, much of the alpha-1 synthesized in the liver is defective and therefore cannot be secreted (released) into the bloodstream. Only a small amount of alpha-1 is secreted. The remainder of the alpha-1 that accumulates in the liver cell membranes may cause the destruction of the liver. The possible method of destruction has not yet been determined.

What are some risks of developing liver disease?

For *PiZZ* alphas, the risks of developing liver disease vary depending on age, and other factors. Around 10% of newborns with ZZ genotypes have liver disease that leads to fatal childhood cirrhosis. The risk is slightly higher in adults. Overall, approximately 12%–15% of all ZZ genotypes develop liver disease.

1. The risk appears to be slightly higher in male ZZ's.
2. Liver disease can occur simultaneously with lung disease.
3. Other factors may increase the risk, such as excessive alcohol consumption and exposure to occupational toxins. It is theorized that genetic factors also play a role in development of liver disease.
4. In persons with null/null genotype (where no alpha-1-antitrypsin is produced at all) there have been no reported cases of liver disease.

What are the major blood test indicators that may signal liver disease?

Albumin and globulin are two classes of proteins that constitute the total protein in your blood. Abnormal ratios of these two proteins may indicate liver disease.

Bilirubin is the normal breakdown product from hemoglobin in red blood cells. Total bilirubin is composed of direct and indirect bilirubin. Liver disease may be indicated if total bilirubin and direct bilirubin are elevated, especially if there are also increased levels of the enzymes alkaline phosphate, serum glutamic oxaloacetic transaminase, lactate dehydrogenase, and GGTP.

What are the medications and treatments for alpha-1 liver disease?

There is currently no cure for liver damage caused by alpha-1. There are supportive measures used to treat conditions that develop as a result of liver damage. It is important to provide essential nutrients to the liver through a healthy diet and use of vitamin supplements. Phenobarbital or cholestyramine may be prescribed for severe jaundice or itching. Diuretics are used in the case of body fluid buildup.

Liver Transplant: The only treatment that offers a chance of survival for alpha children and adults with severe liver disease is a liver transplant. Upon the completion of the transplant, the genotype of the patient is changed, and the new liver begins synthesizing and secreting normal amounts of alpha-1. This has occurred as soon as two days post-transplant. Survival outcomes vary depending on many factors.

Panniculitis Treatment

Treatment for panniculitis associated with alpha-1 may include the use of dapsone, which may inhibit the damaging reactions of the neutrophils. For alphas with panniculitis, the use of augmentation therapy using human-derived alpha-1 (Prolastin®) seems to promote healing and prevent future damage. Many doctors are recommending long-term alpha-1 replacement for alpha-1 panniculitis patients.

Other Information

What is my prognosis for the future?

If diagnosed with alpha-1-antitrypsin deficiency, your prognosis will vary depending on the following factors. However, none of them can be reliable determinants on their own. It is believed that they interact to an unknown degree. It is also believed that there may be an unknown genetic factor that plays a role in whether an alpha-1 individual will have lung or liver damage or panniculitis.

How does the amount of alpha-1 in my blood affect disease risk?

If you have at least 15% of the normal amount of alpha-1 circulating in your bloodstream, it is thought that your lungs will be protected from the destructiveness of neutrophil elastase if you don't smoke. This is still under study by many researchers, and the results have been mixed.

What measures of lung function affect risk?

The higher your FEV1 (forced expiratory volume) is, the better. Persons with FEV1 results between 30% and 65% will generally have the fastest rate of decline.

How does smoking status affect disease risks?

If you smoke, you will lose lung function much faster than a non-smoker or an ex-smoker. It is estimated that smoking cuts an average of 15 years off the life of a person with alpha-1. Not only do the chemicals from tobacco products cause an increase in neutrophil elastase, but the smoke also reduces the effect of alpha-1 that is left in your lungs.

Why are lung infections a problem?

Each lung infection you get draws a large amount of neutrophil elastase to your lungs. Once there, they fight off the infection, then begin destroying delicate lung tissue, with very little alpha-1 to stop them. You lose lung function quickly in this manner. If you seek prompt medical treatment each time you suffer from respiratory illnesses, you can help protect your lungs.

Why is exposure to obnoxious lung irritants a problem?

Any chemical that can be inhaled into the lungs can act as an irritant. Breathing pollutants and exposure to substances such as asbestos can attract a great number of neutrophil elastase to your lungs, and as is the case with infection and smoking, you will lose valuable lung function much faster with additional exposure.

What other factors are linked to health risks for people with alpha-1?

There may be many other factors that play a role in the health of a person with alpha-1. Many people with alpha-1 live long, healthy lives with very little or no signs of liver or lung damage.

The chance of avoiding liver disease is fairly high for most alpha patients, as an average of less than 15% may develop liver damage. Avoiding or minimizing use or exposure of any substance that can damage your liver may be advised, particularly if you have some high liver enzyme levels.

The onset of alpha-1 related panniculitis is extremely rare. It is possible that other unknown genetic causes may increase an alpha's chances of contracting this skin disease.

Living with Alpha-1

There are many different ways alpha-1 affects people. Some have severe manifestations in the form of lung, liver or skin disease, while others have mild symptoms or live without obvious signs of disease into old age.

When you are diagnosed as having alpha-1-antitrypsin deficiency, you can expect to go through a grieving process. As a result you may be on a rollercoaster of emotions. There is no right or wrong way to express your feelings about having this disease. People handle it in many different ways. Some go on as if nothing happened, while others become heavily involved in as many aspects of alpha-1 as they can. Most alphas fall somewhere in between. It is important to deal with your emotions in the manner that works for you. Many people find that belonging to a support group is very helpful. Hearing from others who share your disease, and the subsequent problems that surface because of it, can help you deal with the many aspects of alpha-1: the financial, the medical, the societal and the personal.

Chapter 7

Bleeding Disorders

Chapter Contents

Section 7.1—Hemophilia A (Factor VIII Deficiency)................. 78
Section 7.2—Hemophilia B (Factor IX Deficiency).................... 83
Section 7.3—Factor I Deficiency (Afibrinogenemia).................. 85
Section 7.4—von Willebrand Disease 87

Section 7.1

Hemophilia A (Factor VIII Deficiency)

What Is It?

Hemophilia is a bleeding disorder caused by a deficiency in one of the blood clotting factors. Hemophilia A (often called classic hemophilia) accounts for about 80 percent of all hemophilia cases. It is a deficiency in clotting factor VIII.

Hemophilia A is a hereditary disorder in which the clotting ability of the blood is impaired and excessive bleeding results. Small wounds and punctures are usually not a problem, but uncontrolled internal bleeding can result in pain and swelling and permanent damage, especially to joints and muscles.

Severity of symptoms can vary, and severe forms become apparent early on. Prolonged bleeding is the hallmark of hemophilia A and typically occurs when an infant is circumcised. Additional bleeding manifestations make their appearance when the infant becomes mobile. Mild cases may go unnoticed until later in life when there is excessive bleeding and clotting problems in response to surgery or trauma. Internal bleeding may happen anywhere, and bleeding into joints is common.

The incidence of hemophilia A is one out of 10,000 live male births. About 17,000 Americans have hemophilia. Women may have it, but it's very rare. With treatment and management, the outcome is good. Most men with hemophilia are able to lead relatively normal lives.

Inheritance Pattern

Hemophilia A is caused by an inherited sex-linked recessive trait with the defective gene located on the X chromosome. Females are carriers of this trait. Fifty percent of the male offspring of female carriers have the disease and fifty percent of their female offspring are carriers. All female children of a male with hemophilia are carriers of the trait.

One third of all cases of hemophilia A occur when there is no family history of the disorder. In these cases, hemophilia develops as the result of a new or spontaneous gene mutation.

Genetic counseling may be advised for carriers. Female carriers can be identified by testing. A woman is definitely a hemophilia carrier if she is:

- The biological daughter of a man with hemophilia

- The biological mother of more than one son with hemophilia

- The biological mother of one hemophilic son and has at least one other blood relative with hemophilia

A woman may or may not be a hemophilia carrier if she is:

- The biological mother of one son with hemophilia

- The sister of a male with hemophilia

- An aunt, cousin, or niece of an affected male related through maternal ties

- The biological grandmother of one grandson with hemophilia

The only way a woman could ever have hemophilia is if her father has it and her mother carries the gene. Women who are carriers can also be symptomatic carriers, whereby they do experience factor deficiencies.

Symptoms and Diagnosis

Hemophilia is caused by several different gene abnormalities. The severity of the symptoms of hemophilia A depends on how a particular gene abnormality affects the activity of factor VIII. When the activity is less than one percent of normal, episodes of severe bleeding occur and recur for no apparent reason. Symptoms include:

- Bruising

- Spontaneous bleeding

- Bleeding into joints and associated pain and swelling

- Gastrointestinal tract and urinary tract hemorrhage

- Blood in the urine or stool

- Prolonged bleeding from cuts, tooth extraction, and surgery

People whose clotting activity is five percent of normal may have only mild hemophilia. They rarely have unprovoked bleeding episodes, but surgery or injury may cause uncontrolled bleeding, which can be fatal. Milder hemophilia may not be diagnosed at all, although some people whose clotting activity is 10 to 25 percent of normal may have prolonged bleeding after surgery, dental extractions, or a major injury.

Generally, the first bleeding episode occurs before 18 months of age, often after a minor injury. A child who has hemophilia bruises easily. Even an injection into a muscle can cause bleeding that results in a large bruise (hematoma). Recurring bleeding into the joints and muscles can ultimately lead to crippling deformities. Bleeding can swell the base of the tongue until it blocks the airway, making breathing difficult. A slight bump on the head can trigger substantial bleeding in the skull, causing brain damage and death.

A doctor may suspect hemophilia in a child whose bleeding is unusual. A laboratory analysis of blood samples can determine whether the child's clotting is abnormally slow. If it is, the doctor can confirm the diagnosis of hemophilia A and can determine the severity by testing the activity of factor VIII.

Treatments

Hemophilia is treated by infusing the missing clotting factor. The amount infused depends upon the severity of bleeding, the site of the bleeding, and the size of the patient. In the past, mild hemophilia A was typically treated with infusion of cryoprecipitate or desmopressin acetate (DDAVP), which causes release of factor VIII that is stored within the body on the lining of blood vessels. Today, experts recommend desmopressin injection or Stimate nasal spray.

Clotting factors are found in plasma and, to a greater extent, in plasma concentrates. Some plasma concentrates are intended for home use and can be self-administered, either on a regular basis to prevent bleeding or at the first sign of bleeding. More often, they are administered three times a day, but both the dose and frequency depend on the severity of the bleeding problem. The dose is adjusted according to the results of periodic blood tests. During a bleeding episode, more clotting factors are needed.

To prevent a bleeding crisis, people with hemophilia and their families can be taught to administer factor VIII concentrates at home at the first signs of bleeding. People with severe forms of the disease may need regular prophylactic infusions, which bring factor levels higher than one percent to prevent bleeds.

Depending on the severity of the disease, DDAVP or factor VIII concentrate may be given prior to dental extractions and surgery to prevent bleeding. Immunization with hepatitis B vaccine is necessary because of the increased risk of exposure to hepatitis due to frequent infusions of blood products.

Gene therapy and fetal tissue implant techniques are under study as possible treatments.

People who have hemophilia should avoid situations that might cause bleeding. They should be conscientious about dental care so they won't need to have teeth extracted. People who have hemophilia should also avoid certain drugs that can aggravate bleeding problems:

- Aspirin

- Heparin

- Warfarin

- Certain analgesics such as nonsteroidal anti-inflammatory drugs

Treatment should be coordinated by a healthcare practitioner who is expert in the field, such as a hematologist or hemophilia treatment center nurse.

The National Hemophilia Foundation's Medical and Scientific Advisory Council (MASAC) made recommendations for treatment of hemophilia in November of 1999. They include:

- Factor VIII products for patients who are HIV seronegative, including recombinant factor VIII, especially for young and newly diagnosed patients who have not received any blood or plasma-derived products.

- Immunoaffinity purified factor VIII concentrates for patients who are HIV seropositive.

- Cryoprecipitate is not recommended because of the risk of HIV and hepatitis infection. Despite greatly improved screening and purification for viral inactivation in blood products, cryoprecipitate can still contain viruses.

- Mild hemophilia A should be treated with desmopressin, in a DDAVP injection or Stimate nasal spray.

Complications

- Chronic joint deformities, caused by recurrent bleeding into the joint, may be managed by an orthopedic specialist.

- Intracerebral hemorrhage is another possible complication.

Some persons with hemophilia develop antibodies to transfused factor VIII. As a result, the transfusions are ineffective. If antibodies are detected in blood samples, the dosage of the plasma concentrates may be increased, or different types of clotting factors or drugs to reduce the antibody levels may be used.

In the past, the plasma concentrates carried the risk of transmitting blood-borne diseases such as hepatitis and AIDS. About 60 percent of persons with hemophilia who were treated with plasma concentrates in the early 1980s were infected with HIV. However, the risk of transmitting HIV infection through plasma concentrates has been virtually eliminated by today's use of screened and processed blood and a genetically engineered factor VIII (recombinant).

Section 7.2

Hemophilia B
(Factor IX Deficiency)

What Is It?

Hemophilia is a bleeding disorder caused by a deficiency in one of the blood clotting factors. Hemophilia B (also called "Christmas disease" after Stephen Christmas, a 20th-century British boy who was first diagnosed with it) is a deficiency in clotting factor IX.

Hemophilia A is seven times more common than hemophilia B. The incidence of hemophilia B is one out of 34,500 men.

Hemophilia B is a hereditary disorder in which the clotting ability of the blood is impaired and prolonged bleeding results. Small wounds and punctures are usually not a problem. But uncontrolled internal bleeding can result in pain and swelling and permanent damage, especially to joints and muscles.

The outcome is good with treatment and management. Most people with Hemophilia B are able to lead relatively normal lives.

Inheritance Pattern

Hemophilia B is caused by an inherited sex-linked recessive trait with the defective gene located on the X chromosome. Females are carriers of this trait. Fifty percent of the male offspring of female carriers will have the disease, and fifty percent of their female offspring will be carriers. All female children of a male with hemophilia will be carriers of the trait.

One fifth of all cases of hemophilia B occur when there is no family history of the disorder. In these cases, hemophilia develops as the result of a new or spontaneous gene mutation.

Genetic counseling may be advised for carriers. Female carriers can be identified by testing. A woman is definitely a hemophilia carrier if she is:

- The biological daughter of a man with hemophilia
- The biological mother of more than one son with hemophilia
- The biological mother of one hemophilic son and has at least one other blood relative with hemophilia

A woman may or may not be a hemophilia carrier if she is:

- The biological mother of one son with hemophilia
- The sister of a male with hemophilia
- An aunt, cousin, or niece of an affected male related through maternal ties
- The biological grandmother of one grandson with hemophilia

Symptoms and Diagnosis

Hemophilia is caused by several different gene abnormalities. Severity of Hemophilia B symptoms depends on how a particular gene abnormality affects the activity of factor IX. When the activity is less than one percent of normal, episodes of prolonged bleeding may occur for no apparent reason.

Severity of symptoms can vary, but severe forms become apparent early on. Prolonged bleeding is the disease's hallmark and typically manifests itself when an infant is circumcised. Additional bleeding manifestations make their appearance when the infant becomes mobile. Mild cases may go unnoticed until later in life, when they occur in response to surgery or trauma. Internal bleeding may occur anywhere and bleeding into joints is common.

Risk factors are a family history of bleeding and being male. The incidence of hemophilia B is one out of 34,500 men. Symptoms include:

- Nosebleeds
- Bruising
- Spontaneous bleeding
- Bleeding into joints and associated pain and swelling
- Gastrointestinal tract and urinary tract hemorrhage
- Blood in the urine or stool
- Prolonged bleeding from cuts, tooth extraction, and surgery
- Prolonged bleeding following circumcision

Treatments

Like hemophilia A, hemophilia B is typically treated by infusing the missing clotting factor. The amount infused depends upon the severity of bleeding, the site of the bleeding, and the size of the patient. Hepatitis B vaccine is recommended for individuals with hemophilia B because they are at increased risk of developing hepatitis due to exposure to blood products.

Gene therapy and fetal tissue implant techniques are under study as possible treatments.

Section 7.3

Factor I Deficiency (Afibrinogenemia)

What Is It?

Fibrinogen, also known as factor I, is needed for most types of platelet aggregation. It's the last step in the clotting process, the "glue" that holds the clot together. People who have a factor I deficiency have a combined bleeding and clotting disorder, meaning that both platelets and clotting are abnormal. Since its discovery in 1920, there have only been about 200 cases of this disorder.

Included under factor I deficiency are several rare coagulation disorders known as congenital fibrinogen defects. They include:

- afibrinogenemia

- hypofibrinogenemia

- dysfibrinogenemia

The first two are called quantitative abnormalities because they have to do with an absent or low quantity of fibrinogen. The third is called a qualitative abnormality because the fibrinogen does not work well.

Afibrinogenemia is the complete absence of fibrinogen. Hypofibrinogenemia is a low level of fibrinogen—less than 100 mg in 1 dL of blood. Both conditions are inherited in an autosomal fashion and can affect males and females.

The severity of the disorder is related to the amount of fibrinogen. Afibrinogenemia is usually discovered in newborns and can cause bleeding from the umbilical cord, genitourinary tract, or central nervous system. People with hypofibrinogenemia may have little, moderate, or severe bleeding.

Dysfibrinogenemias are due to variations in the factor I molecule. More than 70 different types of dysfibrinogenemia have been identified.

Inheritance Pattern

The disorder is not sex-linked as is hemophilia. It affects both males and females with equal frequency. It is autosomal recessive, which means if the clotting defect is inherited from a parent, the child will be a genetic carrier of the condition, but may or may not have symptoms.

Symptoms and Diagnosis

Few people who have any of these disorders suffer symptoms, although some are predisposed to form blood clots (thrombosis).

Treatments

Many people with hypofibrinogenemia or dysfibrinogenemia need no treatment. Those who require treatment may be given cryoprecipitate or fresh frozen plasma. Anticoagulants are sometimes prescribed to reduce the risk of thrombosis. The goal of treatment is to raise the patient's fibrinogen level to 100 mg/dL for minor bleeding and up to 200 mg/dL for surgery or severe bleeding. (One unit of fresh frozen plasma has about 450 mg of fibrinogen.)

Complications

Plasma levels of fibrinogen exceeding 1000 mg/dL have been reported to possibly increase the risk of thrombosis. In women, menstrual bleeding can be a severe problem and must be controlled.

Section 7.4

von Willebrand Disease

The most commonly inherited bleeding disorder is von Willebrand Disease (vWd) and it occurs in both males and females.

What is von Willebrand Factor?

von Willebrand Factor (vWF) is a clotting protein in the blood. It is produced in the cells that line the blood vessels and then is released into the blood stream.

Bleeding occurs when blood vessels are injured. Platelets, a type of blood cell, stick to the injured vessel and form a platelet plug. von Willebrand factor acts as a glue to help the platelets stick to the injury site. Simultaneously, other coagulation factors work together to form a clot, further sealing the area of damage.

How does someone get von Willebrand Disease?

von Willebrand Disease is known as an inherited or genetic disorder meaning it is passed down through families through information in the cells called genes.

What are the signs and symptoms of von Willebrand Disease?

von Willebrand Disease (vWD) can be a mild disorder associated with few, if any, symptoms. Sometimes people are not diagnosed until they have excessive bleeding following a serious injury, accident, invasive dental work, or surgery. In other cases, diagnosis of one family member may lead to a diagnosis in other family members as well.

Bleeding usually involves the mucous membranes, the delicate tissues that line such body passages as the nose, mouth, uterus, vagina, stomach and intestines. Some of the usual symptoms of vWD include frequent nosebleeds, easy bruising, heavy menstrual flow, and excessive bleeding following surgery, childbirth, or dental work.

How is it diagnosed?

vWD may be difficult disorder to diagnose. It is often hard to distinguish individuals with mild vWD from those without. Children whose symptoms are fairly mild may live for many years without a diagnosis or perhaps may never be diagnosed. It may also be hard to distinguish between vWD and other bleeding disorders.

Laboratory tests are an important part of diagnosis. Repeat testing is often necessary in order to get a clear answer.

The tests most frequently performed in people who might have vWD are:

- Bleeding time—measures how long it takes a cut on your child's arm to stop bleeding

- Factor VIII activity—measures how much factor VIII is present in your child's blood

- Ristocetin cofactor activity—tests how well vWF works

- vWF antigen—measures how much vWF protein is present in your child's blood whether or not it works properly

- Multimer analysis—examines the structure of vWF molecules

What are the different types of von Willebrand Disease?

Type I: The von Willebrand factor is deficient in quantity. This type is the most common form of the disease.

Type II: The von Willebrand factor is deficient and does not function normally.

Type IIA: vWF does not form proper multimers.

Type IIB: vWF multimers are too active and bind to platelets in the blood, resulting in removal of platelets and vWF from the blood.

Type IIM: vWF does not bind to platelets well.

Type IIN: vWF does not bind to factor VIII well.

Type III: There is an absence of von Willebrand factor in the blood. An associated low level of coagulation factor VIII also occurs. This type is the most severe form of the disease.

What treatment is available?

The treatment goal of von Willebrand Disease is to normalize the level of vWd factor and clotting factor VIII in the blood, allowing for routine blood clotting. Treatment is based on the type and severity of disease. If your child only has bruising or nosebleeds, medications may not be necessary. Serious bleeding issues may require more sophisticated treatment including:

- **Cryoprecipitate:** Cryoprecipitate is a fraction of human plasma, the liquid part of blood. It contains both factor VIII and von Willebrand factor. If cryoprecipitate is obtained from a well-screened unaffected family member or donor, it may be a viable treatment option. However, in general the Medical and Scientific Advisory council of the National Hemophilia Foundation no longer recommends this treatment method due to its associated risks.

- **Desmopressin (DDAVP):** DDAVP is a synthetic hormone used to stimulate the release of von Willebrand factor and factor VIII found in storage sites of cells that line the blood vessels. Desmopressin can be given by vein, subcutaneously, or in the form of a nasal spray. DDAVP does offer convenient treatment for some vWd patients, but unfortunately it does not work effectively in all von Willebrand patients. Tests can be performed to see whether your child adequately responds to this type of therapy.

- **Factor VIII Concentrates:** Alphanate and Humate P (factor VIII) coagulation products contain von Willebrand factor and are suitable for treating von Willebrand disease. These concentrates have been purified to reduce the risk of blood-borne viruses. However, not all types of factor VIII products are appropriate for treating von Willebrand disease, because not all factor VIII concentrates contain von Willebrand factor.

Chapter 8

Blood Disorders

Chapter Contents

Section 8.1—Fanconi Anemia 92
Section 8.2—Hemochromatosis 96
Section 8.3—Sickle Cell Anemia 101
Section 8.4—Thalassemia 107

Section 8.1

Fanconi Anemia

What Is Fanconi Anemia?

Fanconi anemia (FA) is one of the inherited anemias that leads to bone marrow failure (aplastic anemia). It is a recessive disorder: if both parents carry a defect (mutation) in the same FA gene, each of their children has a 25% chance of inheriting the defective gene from both parents. When this happens, the child will have FA.

There are at least eleven FA genes (A, B, C, D1 (BRCA2), D2, E, F, G, I, J, and L). These eleven account for almost all of the cases of Fanconi anemia. Mutations in FA-A, FA-C, and FA-G are the most common and account for approximately 85% of the FA patients worldwide. FA-D1, FA-D2, FA-E, FA-F, and FA-L account for 10%. FA-B, FA-I, and FA-J represent less than 5% of FA patients. Eight of the Fanconi anemia genes have been cloned.

FA occurs equally in males and females. It is found in all ethnic groups. Though considered primarily a blood disease, it can affect all systems of the body. Many patients eventually develop acute myelogenous leukemia (AML) and at a very early age. FA patients are extremely likely to develop head and neck, gynecological, and/or gastrointestinal squamous cell carcinomas, again at a much earlier age than in squamous cell carcinoma patients in the general population. Patients who have had a successful bone marrow transplant and, thus, are cured of the blood problem associated with FA still must have regular examinations to watch for signs of cancer.

Additional Information about Fanconi Anemia

Causes, Incidence, and Risk Factors

Fanconi's anemia is inherited in an autosomal recessive fashion, thus one copy of an abnormal gene is passed on by each parent. It occurs in all racial and ethnic groups. It is classically diagnosed between 2 and 15 years of age.

The disease is caused by a genetic defect that prevents cells from fixing damaged DNA or removing toxic, oxygen-free radicals that damage cells. Patients may be suspected of having the disease, if they have particular birth defects or develop decreased blood counts.

Symptoms

This set of physical abnormalities occur in 80% of the cases:

- Skin pigment change: darkened areas of the skin, cafe-au-lait spots, vitiligo
- Short stature
- Upper limb anomalies: missing, extra, or misshapen thumbs; underdeveloped or absent radius bone in the forearm; anomalies of the hands; abnormalities of the ulna
- Small testicles, genital changes
- Other skeletal anomalies: congenital hip abnormality, scoliosis, spinal or rib malformations, small head
- Eye/eyelid anomalies
- Kidney malformations
- Ear anomalies/deafness
- Hip, leg, and toe abnormalities
- Gastrointestinal/cardiopulmonary malformations

Other potential symptoms:

- Mental retardation
- Learning disability
- Low birth weight
- Failure to thrive
- An affected sibling

Signs and Tests

Common tests performed for evaluation of Fanconi's anemia include:

- CBC (complete blood count) initially demonstrates low platelets (thrombocytopenia), then low neutrophils (a type of white blood cell), and finally low hemoglobin (anemia), which develops over months to years.

- Bone marrow biopsy.

- Clastogenic stress-induced chromosomal breakage analysis on blood cells of patients and their siblings to diagnose the disease. Here, chemotherapy is added to a blood sample to check for abnormal damage to chromosomes.

- HLA (human leukocyte antigen) tissue typing on the patient and their family members to determine if any are matching bone marrow donors.

- Hand x-ray, and other imaging studies (x-ray, CT scan, MRI) to evaluate any anomalies.

- Hearing test.

- Developmental assessment.

- Ultrasound of the kidneys.

- Amniocentesis or chorionic villous sampling has been used for prenatal diagnosis.

Treatment

If the hematological changes are mild to moderate and the patient does not require transfusions, a period of observation is currently recommended with frequent blood count checks and yearly bone marrow examinations. Observations for the development of secondary malignancies are also performed. In the short term, growth factors (such as erythropoietin, G-CSF [granulocyte colony-stimulating factor], and GM-CSF [granulocyte-macrophage colony-stimulating factor]) can be used to improve blood counts. Other growth factors for platelet stimulation are currently under investigation.

Bone marrow transplantation can cure the blood count problems associated with Fanconi's anemia. A HLA matched sibling is the best donor source, although umbilical cord blood cells and unrelated bone marrow can also be used. This therapy is very effective, and although there are associated toxicities, there has been improvement in the care of Fanconi patients during the transplant. There is approximately a 70% success rate for those patients fortunate enough to have a donor.

Even though a successful bone marrow transplant can cure the bone marrow problems from Fanconi's anemia, patients are at risk for other cancers and must be regularly followed by a physician.

Prior to bone marrow transplantation, androgen therapy (oxymetholone, nandrolone decanoate) combined with low doses of steroids (hydrocortisone, prednisone) was the standard treatment, and this approach is currently used if the patient does not have an appropriate bone marrow donor. Typically, 50–75% of patients initially respond to androgen therapy, however, all patients will rapidly relapse when the drug is stopped. In most cases, these drugs eventually become ineffective.

Symptoms due to low blood counts, such as bleeding, infections, or symptomatic anemia (fatigue, shortness of breath, chest pain, dizziness), are treated with transfusions or antibiotics as needed. Patients with low neutrophil counts, who develop a fever, are usually treated with intravenous antibiotics.

Most patients visit a hematologist, an endocrinologist, and an ophthalmologist regularly. An orthopedist, gynecologist, or nephrologist may be seen as needed.

Expectations (Prognosis)

The reported survival of patients with Fanconi's anemia is highly varied, ranging from 2 to 25 years. The prognosis is especially poor if blood counts are low. Survival has likely been improved with the development and refinement of therapies, such as bone marrow transplantation.

Although bone marrow transplantation can restore blood counts, patients with Fanconi's anemia remain predisposed to a variety of cancers (leukemia, myelodysplastic syndrome, liver cancer, and others).

Women with Fanconi's anemia who become pregnant should be closely followed by a physician as they often require transfusions throughout pregnancy. Fertility is decreased in males, although a small number of Fanconi patients have fathered children.

Prevention

Fanconi's anemia is an inherited disorder, and little can be done to prevent the disease short of genetic counseling for families known to be affected as a result. However, some complications, such as pneumococcal pneumonia, hepatitis, and varicella infections, can be prevented by vaccination.

Additionally, patients should avoid known carcinogens and undergo regular cancer screening to detect malignancies early in their course, should they arise.

Section 8.2

Hemochromatosis

National Digestive Diseases Information Clearinghouse (NDDIC), National Institute of Diabetes and Digestive and Kidney Diseases (NIDDK), NIH Pub. No. 02-4620, August 2002. This text was reviewed by Bruce R. Bacon, M.D., Saint Louis University School of Medicine; and Anthony Tavill, M.D., Case Western Reserve University School of Medicine.

Hemochromatosis, the most common form of iron overload disease, is an inherited disorder that causes the body to absorb and store too much iron. The extra iron builds up in organs and damages them. Without treatment, the disease can cause these organs to fail.

Iron is an essential nutrient found in many foods. The greatest amount is found in red meat and iron-fortified bread and cereal. In the body, iron becomes part of hemoglobin, a molecule in the blood that transports oxygen from the lungs to all body tissues.

Healthy people usually absorb about 10 percent of the iron contained in the food they eat to meet the body needs. People with hemochromatosis absorb more than the body needs. The body has no natural way to rid itself of excess iron, so extra iron is stored in body tissues, especially the liver, heart, and pancreas.

Causes

Genetic or hereditary hemochromatosis is mainly associated with a defect in a gene called *HFE*, which helps regulate the amount of iron absorbed from food. There are two known important mutations in *HFE*, named C282Y and H63D. C282Y is the most important. When C282Y is inherited from both parents, iron is over absorbed from the diet and hemochromatosis can result. H63D usually causes little increase in iron absorption, but a person with H63D from one parent and C282Y from the other may rarely develop hemochromatosis.

The genetic defect of hemochromatosis is present at birth, but symptoms rarely appear before adulthood. A person who inherits the defective gene from both parents may develop hemochromatosis. A person who inherits the defective gene from only one parent is a carrier for the disease but usually does not develop it. However, carriers might have a slight increase in iron absorption.

Scientists hope that further study of *HFE* will reveal how the body normally metabolizes iron. They also want to learn how iron injures cells and whether it contributes to organ damage in other diseases, such as alcoholic liver disease, hepatitis C, porphyria cutanea tarda, heart disease, reproductive disorders, cancer, autoimmune hepatitis, diabetes, and joint disease.

Juvenile hemochromatosis and neonatal hemochromatosis are two forms of the disease that are not caused by an *HFE* defect. Their cause is unknown. The juvenile form leads to severe iron overload and liver and heart disease in adolescents and young adults between the ages of 15 and 30, and the neonatal form causes the same problems in newborn infants.

Risk Factors

Hereditary hemochromatosis is one of the most common genetic disorders in the United States. It most often affects Caucasians of Northern European descent, although other ethnic groups are also affected. About 5 people in 1,000 (0.5 percent) of the U.S. Caucasian population carry two copies of the hemochromatosis gene and are susceptible to developing the disease. One person in 8 to 12 is a carrier of the abnormal gene. Hemochromatosis is less common in African Americans, Asian Americans, Hispanic Americans, and American Indians.

Although both men and women can inherit the gene defect, men are about five times more likely to be diagnosed with the effects of hereditary hemochromatosis than women. Men also tend to develop problems from the excess iron at a younger age.

Symptoms

Joint pain is the most common complaint of people with hemochromatosis. Other common symptoms include fatigue, lack of energy, abdominal pain, loss of sex drive, and heart problems. Symptoms tend to occur in men between the ages of 30 and 50 and in women over age 50. However, many people have no symptoms when they are diagnosed.

If the disease is not detected early and treated, iron may accumulate in body tissues and may eventually lead to serious problems such as:

- arthritis

- liver disease, including an enlarged liver, cirrhosis, cancer, and liver failure

- damage to the pancreas, possibly causing diabetes

- heart abnormalities, such as irregular heart rhythms or congestive heart failure

- impotence

- early menopause

- abnormal pigmentation of the skin, making it look gray or bronze

- thyroid deficiency

- damage to the adrenal gland

Diagnosis

A thorough medical history, physical examination, and routine blood tests help rule out other conditions that could be causing the symptoms. This information often provides helpful clues, such as a family history of arthritis or unexplained liver disease.

Blood tests can determine whether the amount of iron stored in the body is too high. The transferrin saturation test determines how much iron is bound to the protein that carries iron in the blood. The serum ferritin test shows the level of iron in the liver. If either of these tests shows higher than normal levels of iron in the body, doctors can order a special blood test to detect the *HFE* mutation, which will help confirm the diagnosis. (If the mutation is not present, hereditary hemochromatosis is not the reason for the iron buildup, and the doctor will look for other causes.) A liver biopsy, in which a tiny piece of liver tissue is removed and examined under a microscope, may be needed. It will show how much iron has accumulated in the liver and whether the liver is damaged.

Hemochromatosis is often undiagnosed and untreated. It is considered rare and doctors may not think to test for it. The initial symptoms can be diverse and vague and can mimic the symptoms of many other diseases. Also, doctors may focus on the conditions caused by hemochromatosis—arthritis, liver disease, heart disease, or diabetes—rather than on the underlying iron overload. However, if the iron overload caused by hemochromatosis is diagnosed and treated before organ damage has occurred, a person can live a normal, healthy life.

Hemochromatosis is usually treated by a specialist in liver disorders (hepatologist), digestive disorders (gastroenterologist), or blood disorders (hematologist). Because of the other problems associated with hemochromatosis, several other specialists may be on the treatment team, such as an endocrinologist, cardiologist, or rheumatologist. Internists or family practitioners can also treat the disease.

Treatment

Treatment is simple, inexpensive, and safe. The first step is to rid the body of excess iron. The process is called phlebotomy, which means removing blood. Depending on how severe the iron overload is, a pint of blood will be taken once or twice a week for several months to a year, and occasionally longer. Blood ferritin levels will be tested periodically to monitor iron levels. The goal is to bring blood ferritin levels to the low end of normal and keep them there. Depending on the lab, that means 25 to 50 micrograms of ferritin per liter of serum. Depending on the amount of iron overload at diagnosis, reaching normal levels can take many phlebotomies.

Once iron levels return to normal, maintenance therapy, which involves giving a pint of blood every 2 to 4 months for life, begins. Some people may need it more often. An annual blood ferritin test will help determine how often blood should be removed.

The earlier hemochromatosis is diagnosed and treated in appropriate cases, the better. If treatment begins before any organs are damaged, associated conditions—such as liver disease, heart disease, arthritis, and diabetes—can be prevented. The outlook for people who already have these conditions at diagnosis depends on the degree of organ damage. For example, treating hemochromatosis can stop the progression of liver disease in its early stages, which means a normal life expectancy. However, if cirrhosis has developed, the person's risk of developing liver cancer increases, even if iron stores are reduced to normal levels. Appropriate regular follow-up with a specialist is necessary.

People who have complications of hemochromatosis may want to consider getting treatment from a specialized hemochromatosis center. These centers are located throughout the country.

People with hemochromatosis should not take iron supplements. Those who have liver damage should not drink alcoholic beverages because they may further damage the liver.

Although treatment cannot cure the conditions associated with established hemochromatosis, it will help most of them. The main exception is arthritis, which does not improve even after excess iron is removed.

Tests for Hemochromatosis

Screening for hemochromatosis (testing people who have no symptoms) is not a routine part of medical care or checkups. However, researchers and public health officials do have some suggestions:

- Brothers and sisters of people who have hemochromatosis should have their blood tested to see if they have the disease or are carriers.

- Parents, children, and other close relatives of people who have the disease should consider testing.

- Doctors should consider testing people who have joint disease, severe and continuing fatigue, heart disease, elevated liver enzymes, impotence, and diabetes, because these conditions may result from hemochromatosis.

Since the genetic defect is common and early detection and treatment are so effective, some researchers and education and advocacy groups have suggested that widespread screening for hemochromatosis would be cost-effective and should be conducted. However, a simple, inexpensive, and accurate test for routine screening does not yet exist, and the available options have limitations. For example, the genetic test provides a definitive diagnosis, but it is expensive. The blood test for transferrin saturation is widely available and relatively inexpensive, but it may have to be done twice with careful handling to confirm a diagnosis and to show that it is the consequence of iron overload.

Hope through Research

Current research in hemochromatosis is concentrated in four areas.

Genetics: Scientists are working to understand more about how the *HFE* gene normally regulates iron levels and why not everyone with an abnormal pair of genes develops the disease.

Pathogenesis: Scientists are studying how iron injures body cells. Iron is an essential nutrient, but above a certain level it can damage or even kill the cell.

Epidemiology: Research is under way to explain why the amounts of iron people normally store in their bodies differ. Research is also being conducted to determine how many people with the defective *HFE* gene go on to develop symptoms, as well as why some people develop symptoms and others do not.

Screening and testing: Scientists are working to determine at what age testing is most effective, which groups should be tested, and what the best tests for widespread screening are.

Section 8.3

Sickle Cell Anemia

What is sickle cell disease?

It is an inherited disease of red blood cells which can cause attacks of pain, damage to vital organs, risk of serious infections and can lead to early death. Sickle cell disease affects the main protein inside the red blood cells called hemoglobin. The disease occurs when a person inherits one sickle cell gene from each parent or a combination of one sickle cell gene plus one of several other abnormal hemoglobin genes.

Hemoglobin in the red blood cells carries oxygen from the lungs and takes it to every part of the body. The main hemoglobin in the red blood cells of people with sickle cell disease is not normal. Red blood cells containing mainly normal hemoglobin are round and flexible. In people with sickle cell disease, the abnormal hemoglobin forces the cells to lose their normally round and flexible shape, becoming distorted and rigid. Under a microscope, these abnormal cells may look like the C-shaped farm tool called a sickle.

Sickle cells tend to become trapped and to be destroyed in small blood vessels (veins and arteries), the spleen, the liver and other organs. This results in a shortage of red blood cells, or anemia. Anemia can cause an affected child to be pale, short of breath, easily tired and have slowed growth and physical development. Certain conditions, such as infections or enlargement of the spleen, may worsen the anemia by speeding up destruction of red blood cells. Infections also can reduce red blood cell production, leading to worsening of anemia.

There are several forms of sickle cell disease. The most common forms are referred to as SS (the child inherits two sickle cell genes), SC (the child inherits one sickle cell gene and one gene for another abnormal type of hemoglobin called C), and S beta thalassemia (the child inherits one sickle cell gene and one gene for a type of thalassemia, another inherited anemia). The effects of sickle cell disease vary greatly from one person to the next. Some affected people rarely are ill while others are frequently hospitalized.

What special problems do babies and young children with sickle cell disease have?

Infants and young children with sickle cell disease are especially vulnerable to severe bacterial infections, such as those that cause meningitis and blood infection. Infections are the leading cause of death in children with sickle cell disease. However, early diagnosis and treatment have dramatically reduced the risk of infections and death. For this reason, more than 40 states now screen newborns for sickle cell disease.

Newborn testing alerts physicians to begin treatment before dangerous infections occur. Studies show that daily treatment with the antibiotic penicillin, beginning by 2 months of age and continuing to at least 5 years, reduces the risk of the most serious infections by about 85 percent.

It is very important for babies and children with sickle cell disease to receive the regular childhood vaccinations. Two of these vaccinations, the Hib (*Haemophilus influenzae* b) vaccine and the pneumococcal vaccine (Prevar), which are recommended for all babies starting at 2 months of age, help protect against potentially life-threatening bacterial infections. Children with sickle cell disease also should receive another type of pneumococcal vaccine (23-valent pneumococcal vaccine), which protects against additional types of bacteria, starting at age 2. The meningococcal vaccine, which protects against meningitis, is recommended at age 5 for all children with sickle cells disease. Children with sickle cell disease also should have yearly flu (influenza) shots, beginning after 6 months of age, early during the flu season (usually September or October).

One of the most serious complications of sickle cell anemia is stroke, a bleed or blockage of blood within the blood vessels of the brain. About 10 percent of children with sickle cell anemia have a stroke, which can lead to lasting disabilities, by age 20. The risk is highest between the ages of 4 and 6 years. A 1998 study found that regular blood transfusions greatly reduce the risk of a first stroke in children with sickle cell anemia who have been identified as being at increased risk of stroke, based upon a special ultrasound examination of the brain. Regular transfusions also reduce the risk of another stroke in children who already have had a stroke. Unfortunately, regular transfusions pose some major risks—including a potentially fatal build-up of iron in the body, infections, and other problems—so this treatment is not routine. The decision to attempt this treatment should be made by a family and their doctors after a thorough discussion with a pediatric hematologist who is experienced with this treatment. Children who receive regular transfusions also must undergo a complicated and time-consuming treatment aimed at reducing iron levels in their body.

What causes the pain in sickle cell disease?

At times, sickle blood cells become stuck in tiny blood vessels that exist throughout the body. When they get stuck, the cells pile up and block the blood vessels. This cuts off the blood supply to nearby tissues so that cells cannot get through to bring oxygen to them. Without oxygen, the area becomes inflamed, injured, and often very painful.

This blockage of blood vessels is known as a sickle cell pain episode or crisis. Pain episodes may be very severe and need to be treated in the hospital with pain-killing drugs or, more often, they are milder and can be treated at home. If the blockage is long-lasting, it can destroy areas of tissue. Sickle cell pain occurs most frequently in bones.

Until recently, there was no effective treatment to prevent the sickling that causes a pain crisis other than transfusions. A 1995 study reported that treatment with a drug called hydroxyurea reduced the number of pain crises in severely affected adults by about 50 percent. In 1998, the Food and Drug Administration (FDA) approved use of this drug in patients over 18 years of age who have had at least three painful crises in the previous year. However, long-term use of hydroxyurea in affected children is not yet routinely recommended because it is not known whether it could have any adverse effects on growth and development. Studies to date in children indicate that hydroxyurea is effective and well tolerated, at least in the short-term. One small study also found that the drug helped prevent a second stroke in children who already have had one stroke. Researchers continue to study the long-term safety of the drug in children, and whether it may help to prevent organ damage in affected children.

Can a person catch sickle cell disease from someone who has it?

No. The disease is inherited and is not contagious. To inherit the disease, a child must receive two sickle cell genes, one from each parent who carries a sickle cell gene.

Do we all have the same chance of inheriting sickle cell disease?

No. In the United States, most cases of sickle cell disease occur among African Americans, and Hispanics of Caribbean ancestry. About one in every 400 African Americans has sickle cell disease. It also affects people of Arabian, Greek, Maltese, Italian, Sardinian, Turkish, and Indian ancestry.

Is sickle cell trait the same thing as sickle cell disease?

No. A person who inherits the sickle cell gene from one parent and the normal type of that gene from the other parent is said to have sickle cell trait. A simple blood test can distinguish sickle cell trait from sickle cell disease. One in 12 African Americans in this country has sickle cell trait. They generally are as healthy as noncarriers, rarely having any health problems related to the trait. Sickle cell trait cannot change to become sickle cell disease. However, when two people with sickle cell trait have a child, their child may inherit two sickle cell genes and have the disorder.

What are the chances that parents with sickle cell trait will pass it on to their children?

There is a 50/50 (50 percent) chance that a child born to parents who both carry a sickle cell gene will have the trait, like the parents. There is a 25 percent chance that the child will have sickle cell disease. There also is a 25 percent chance that the child will have neither the trait nor the disease.

Each successive pregnancy has the same set of chances. If only one parent has the trait and the other has no abnormal hemoglobin gene, there is no chance that their children will have sickle cell disease. However, there is a 50/50 chance of each child having the trait.

Can a woman with sickle cell disease have a safe pregnancy?

Yes. However, affected women are at increased risk of complications that can affect their health and that of their babies. During pregnancy, the disease may become more severe and painful crises may occur more frequently. A pregnant woman with sickle cell disease is at increased risk of preterm labor, and of having a low-birthweight baby. However, with early prenatal care and careful monitoring throughout pregnancy, women with sickle cell disease can have a healthy pregnancy and delivery. If the baby's father has sickle cell trait, the baby has a 50 percent chance of having the disease. If he does not, the baby will have only the trait.

Is there a test for sickle cell disease or trait?

Yes. Readily available blood tests such as hemoglobin electrophoresis will identify people who have either sickle cell trait or a form of the disease, as well as a number of other less common inherited hemoglobin abnormalities. There also are prenatal tests to determine whether the baby will have sickle cell disease, carry the trait or be unaffected. If both parents have the sickle cell trait, in three out of four cases, the prenatal test will reveal that the fetus will not have sickle cell disease.

Where is sickle cell testing and treatment available?

Couples who are planning to have a baby can get carrier testing at medical centers and sickle cell treatment facilities. A genetic counselor at the nearest medical center can refer a couple for testing and discuss the risks to their offspring. Other sources of testing and counseling, as well as treatment of those with sickle cell disease, include the pediatric department or hematology (blood) division of your local hospital. Couples also can check with their doctor or the Sickle Cell Disease Association of America for resources in their area. As mentioned previously, many states test newborns for sickle cell disease as part of their newborn screening program.

Is there a cure for sickle cell disease?

About 100 children with sickle cell disease have been cured through a bone marrow transplant, using donated bone marrow from an immunologically matched sibling. However, a cure using this approach carries a high risk: About 10 percent of children who underwent bone marrow transplants for severe sickle cell disease have died. Other approaches are being tested, such as transplants using cells from umbilical cord blood. Studies on gene therapy for sickle cell disease may someday offer a cure at less risk. Currently, researchers are studying a number of new drug treatments, in addition to hydroxyurea, for reducing the severity and frequency of complications of the disease. These include treatment with an antifungal drug called clotrimazole, which may help prevent red blood cells from sickling. Recent studies also suggest that inhaling the gas nitric oxide also may help prevent sickling. There also has been much progress in medical care that limits damage to the organs from sickling. This care has greatly improved survival and the quality of life for many affected individuals.

Is the March of Dimes supporting research on sickle cell disease?

The March of Dimes has been a major supporter of sickle cell disease research. Grantees currently are seeking to develop new treatments to prevent pain episodes and organ damage. They also are seeking to identify genetic and environmental factors that influence the severity of symptoms, in order to improve prognosis and treatment of affected children.

References

Adams, R.J., et al. Prevention of a first stroke by transfusions in children with sickle cell anemia and abnormal results on transcranial Doppler ultrasonography. *New England Journal of Medicine,* volume 339, number 1, July 2, 1998, pages 5–11.

Steinberg, M.H. Management of sickle cell disease. *New England Journal of Medicine,* volume 340, number 13, April 1, 1999, pages 1021–1030.

Wethers, D.L. Sickle cell disease in childhood: Part 1. Laboratory diagnosis, pathophysiology and health maintenance. *American Family Physician,* volume 62, number 5, September 1, 2000, pages 1013–1020.

Section 8.4

Thalassemia

"Learning about Thalassemia," National Human Genome
Research Institute (NHGRI), http://www.genome.gov, updated
February 2004.

What Do We Know about Heredity and Thalassemia?

Thalassemia is actually a group of inherited diseases of the blood
that affect a person's ability to produce hemoglobin, resulting in anemia. Hemoglobin is a protein in red blood cells that carries oxygen
and nutrients to cells in the body. About 100,000 babies worldwide
are born with severe forms of thalassemia each year. Thalassemia
occurs most frequently in people of Italian, Greek, Middle Eastern,
Southern Asian, and African Ancestry.

The two main types of thalassemia are called alpha and beta, depending on which part of an oxygen-carrying protein in the red blood
cells is lacking. Both types of thalassemia are inherited in the same
manner. The disease is passed to children by parents who carry the
mutated thalassemia gene. A child who inherits one mutated gene is
a carrier, which is sometimes called thalassemia trait. Most carriers
lead completely normal, healthy lives.

A child who inherits two thalassemia trait genes—one from each
parent—will have the disease. A child of two carriers has a 25 percent chance of receiving two trait genes and developing the disease,
and a 50 percent chance of being a thalassemia trait carrier.

Most individuals with alpha thalassemia have milder forms of
the disease, with varying degrees of anemia. The most severe form
of alpha thalassemia, which affects mainly individuals of South-
east Asian, Chinese, and Filipino ancestry, results in fetal or newborn death.

A child who inherits two copies of the mutated gene for beta thalassemia will have beta thalassemia disease. The child can have a mild
form of the disease, known as thalassemia intermedia, which causes
milder anemia that rarely requires transfusions.

Thalassemia Major: A Serious Disorder

The more severe form of the disease is thalassemia major, also called Cooley's anemia. It is a serious disease that requires regular blood transfusions and extensive medical care.

Those with thalassemia major usually show symptoms within the first two years of life. They become pale and listless and have poor appetites. They grow slowly and often develop jaundice. Without treatment, the spleen, liver and heart soon become greatly enlarged. Bones become thin and brittle. Heart failure and infection are the leading causes of death among children with untreated thalassemia major.

The use of frequent blood transfusions and antibiotics has improved the outlook for children with thalassemia major. Frequent transfusions keep their hemoglobin levels near normal and prevent many of the complications of the disease. But repeated blood transfusions lead to iron overload—a buildup of iron in the body—that can damage the heart, liver and other organs. Drugs known as iron chelators can help rid the body of excess iron, preventing or delaying problems related to iron overload.

Thalassemia has been cured using bone marrow transplants. However, this treatment is possible only for a small minority of patients who have a suitable bone marrow donor. The transplant procedure itself is still risky and can result in death.

Gene Therapy Offers Hope for a Cure

Scientists are working to develop a gene therapy that may offer a cure for thalassemia. Such a treatment might involve inserting a normal beta globin gene (the gene that is abnormal in this disease) into the patient's stem cells, the immature bone marrow cells that are the precursors of all other cells in the blood.

Another form of gene therapy could involve using drugs or other methods to reactivate the patient's genes that produce fetal hemoglobin—the form of hemoglobin found in fetuses and newborns. Scientists hope that spurring production of fetal hemoglobin will compensate for the patient's deficiency of adult hemoglobin.

Is There a Test for Thalassemia?

Blood tests and family genetic studies can show whether an individual has thalassemia or is a carrier. If both parents are carriers, they may want to consult with a genetic counselor for help in deciding whether to conceive or whether to have a fetus tested for thalassemia.

Prenatal testing can be done around the 11th week of pregnancy using chorionic villi sampling (CVS). This involves removing a tiny piece of the placenta. Or the fetus can be tested with amniocentesis around the 16th week of pregnancy. In this procedure, a needle is used to take a sample of the fluid surrounding the baby for testing.

Assisted reproductive therapy is also an option for carriers who don't want to risk giving birth to a child with thalassemia. A new technique, pre-implantation genetic diagnosis (PGD), used in conjunction with in vitro fertilization, may enable parents who have thalassemia or carry the trait to give birth to healthy babies. Embryos created in-vitro are tested for the thalassemia gene before being implanted into the mother, allowing only healthy embryos to be selected.

Chapter 9

Color Blindness

Color blindness is used in colloquial terms to refer to the difficulty in telling colors apart but a more correct term would be color vision defect. Color blindness is a misnomer because only a small percentage of people are unable to see any color.

Color vision is important in many everyday tasks, such a driving a car (does that traffic light mean "stop" or "go"?). Persons with color vision defects may be at a disadvantage in school or at work. In fact, lack of normal color vision may limit career opportunities. For example, normal color vision is vital in such jobs as color printing and color photography. Abnormal color vision can even be dangerous in certain situations, such as in rail and water navigation. For this reason, persons with color vision defects are excluded by law from certain occupations.

What causes color vision defects?

Color vision depends on the absorption of light by visual pigments contained within specialized cells in the eye called photoreceptors. There are two types of photoreceptors: rods and cones. Rods, which provide vision in dim light, have no ability to distinguish between colors. Cones are responsible for color vision. There are three different

This chapter contains the document, "Color Blindness" from the "Eye Facts" series of documents. Reprinted with permission from the website of the University of Illinois Eye Center, http://www.uic.edu/com/eye. © 2004 University of Illinois Board of Trustees. All rights reserved.

types of come pigment in the normal eye. Color vision occurs within the visual part of the brain compares electrical signals from the different types of cones.

Defects in color vision are either inherited or acquired. Inherited defects result mainly from missing or incorrect visual pigments. There are different types of inherited defects, with different levels of severity. Color vision defects sometimes can be acquired, as a result of eye disease or normal aging or as a side effect of certain medications. In acquired defects, other parts of the eye besides cones and cone pigments may be affected.

What are the types of inherited color vision defects?

There are three groups of inherited color vision defects: monochromacy, dichromacy, and anomalous trichromacy. The last two groups are subdivided into red-green and blue-yellow types of defects. Inherited red-green color vision defects are more common in males (1 to 8 percent depending on race) than in females (about 0.4 percent). Inherited blue-yellow defects are rare in either sex.

Monochromacy: Rod monochromats, or complete achromats, are truly "color blind" since they cannot distinguish any hues (for example, blue, green, yellow and red). They see only different degrees of lightness. For them, the world appears to be shades of gray, black and white. They also have poor visual acuity, aversion to bright light, and nystagmus (an involuntary, rapid movement of the eyes).

To have rod monochromacy, someone must inherit a gene for the disorder from both parents. This condition occurs in approximately one in 30,000 of the population.

Dichromacy is a less severe form of color defect than monochromacy. Dichromats can tell some hues apart. Dichromacy is divided into three types: protanopia, deuteranopia, and tritanopia.

Protanopia and deuteranopia are red-green defects. Persons with red-green defects have difficulty distinguishing between reds, greens, and yellows but can discriminate between blues and yellows. Protanopes often can name red and green correctly because green looks lighter to them than red.

Males have red-green defects if they inherit a defective gene from their mother. Affected males pass the defective gene to all of their daughters but none of their sons. Females who inherit only one defective gene are carriers of that gene. Females who inherit the gene for red-green defect from both parents are affected.

Hereditary tritanopia is a blue-yellow defect. Persons with blue-yellow defects cannot see the difference between blues and yellows but can distinguish between reds and greens. Tritanopia is somewhat rare (affecting between one and 15,000 and one in 50,000) and occurs equally in both sexes. Tritanopes usually have fewer problems in performing everyday tasks than do those with red-green dichromacy.

Anomalous Trichromacy: The ability of anomalous trichromats to distinguish between hues is better than dichromats but still not normal. Red-green anomalous trichromacy is subdivided into protanomaly and deuteranomaly. Both types are inherited in the same way as for red-green dichromacy. The severity can range from mild to extreme. Some persons with the mildest forms may not even realize their color vision is abnormal.

A third type of anomalous trichromacy is tritanomaly. This condition is more often acquired than inherited.

How are color vision defects diagnosed?

Specialized color vision tests can easily detect color vision defects. Pseudoisochromatic plate tests are commonly used to screen for inherited color vision defects. In this group of tests, a pattern of colored dots forms a number or letter against a background of other colored dots. Persons with normal color vision can discern these patterns, but those with color defects cannot. A sample of this test can be found online at http://www.uic.edu/com/eye/LearningAboutVision/EyeFacts/ColorBlindness.htm.

Arrangement tests are a second type of color vision test. They are used to measure the severity of inherited color vision defects or to test for acquired color defects. The person being tested must arrange color chips in order of similarity.

Can color vision defects be cured?

No cure exists for inherited color vision defects since they are caused by missing or incorrect visual pigments. Acquired color vision defects can be corrected sometimes if the underlying cause can be treated.

Special aids have been developed to help persons with color vision defects distinguish some of the colors that cause them trouble. These devices include specially tinted contact lenses and eyeglasses. However, these aids do not provide normal color vision and therefore should be used with caution.

Chapter 10

Connective Tissue Disorders

Chapter Contents

Section 10.1—Questions and Answers about
             Heritable Disorders of Connective Tissue......... 116
Section 10.2—Ehlers-Danlos Syndrome 120
Section 10.3—Marfan Syndrome 122

115

Section 10.1

Questions and Answers about Heritable Disorders of Connective Tissue

National Institute of Arthritis and Musculoskeletal and Skin Diseases
(NIAMS), NIH Pub. No. 01-4790, July 2001.

This chapter describes a family of more than 200 disorders that affect connective tissues. These disorders result from alterations (mutations) in genes responsible for building tissues. Alterations in these genes may change the structure and development of skin, bones, joints, heart, blood vessels, lungs, eyes, and ears. Some mutations also change how these tissues work.

All of these diseases are directly related to mutations in genes, and thus are called "heritable." Some other connective tissue problems are not directly linked to mutations in tissue-building genes, although some people may be genetically predisposed to becoming affected. The disorders discussed in this chapter are called heritable (genetic) disorders of connective tissue (HDCTs). Many, but not all, of them are rare.

Some Common Heritable Connective Tissue Disorders

Physicians and scientists have identified more than 200 heritable connective tissue disorders. Some of the more common ones are listed below. Some of these are really groups of disorders and may be known by other names.

Ehlers-Danlos syndrome: The problems present in Ehlers-Danlos syndrome (EDS), a group of approximately ten disorders, include changes in the physical properties of skin, joints, blood vessels, and other tissues such as ligaments and tendons. People with EDS have some degree of joint looseness, fragile small blood vessels, and abnormal scar formation and wound healing. Soft, velvety skin stretches excessively but returns to normal after being pulled. Some forms of EDS can present problems with the spine, including curved spine; the eyes; and weak internal organs, including the uterus, intestines, and large blood vessels. Mutations in several different genes are responsible for different symptoms in the several types of EDS. In most cases, the genetic defect involves collagen, the major protein-building material of bone.

Epidermolysis bullosa: The characteristic feature of epidermolysis bullosa (EB) is blistering in the skin. Some forms of the disease may involve the gastrointestinal tract, the pulmonary system, muscle, or the bladder. Most forms are evident at birth. This disorder can be both disabling and disfiguring, and some forms may lead to early death. The disease results when skin layers separate after minor trauma. Defects of several proteins within the skin are at fault.

Marfan syndrome: People with Marfan syndrome tend to have excessively long bones and are commonly thin, with long, "spider-like" fingers. Other problems include skeletal malformations, abnormal position of the lens of the eye, and enlargement at the beginning part of the aorta, the major vessel carrying blood away from the heart. If left untreated, an enlarged aorta can lead to hemorrhage and even death. This disorder results from mutations in the gene that makes fibrillin-1, a protein important to connective tissue.

Osteogenesis imperfecta: People with osteogenesis imperfecta (OI) have bones that fracture easily, low muscle mass, and joint and ligament laxity. There are four major types of OI ranging in severity from mild to lethal. The appearance of people with OI varies considerably. Individuals may also have a blue or gray tint to the sclera (whites of the eyes), thin skin, growth deficiencies, and fragile teeth. They may develop scoliosis, respiratory problems, and hearing loss. Also known as "brittle bone disease," this disorder arises from mutations in the two genes that make type I collagen, a protein important to bones and skin. These mutations cause the body to make either too little or poor-quality type I collagen.

Questions and Answers about HDCTs

What is connective tissue?

Connective tissue is the material between the cells of the body that gives tissues form and strength. This "cellular glue" is also involved in delivering nutrients to the tissue, and in the special functioning of certain tissues. Connective tissue is made up of dozens of proteins, including collagens, proteoglycans, and glycoproteins. The combination of these proteins can vary between tissues. The genes that encode these proteins can harbor defects or mutations, which can affect the functioning of certain properties of connective tissue in selected tissues. This can lead to a HDCT.

Who gets HDCTs?

Scientists estimate that as many as 1 million people in the United States may have a heritable disorder of connective tissue. Generally, these conditions affect people of all ethnic groups and ages, and both genders are commonly affected. Many of these disorders are rare. Some may not be evident at birth, but only declare themselves after a certain age or after exposure to a particular environmental stress.

Does anything increase the chances of having a genetic disease?

Several factors increase the likelihood that a person will inherit an alteration in a gene. If you are concerned about your risk, you should talk to your health care provider or a genetic counselor.

The following factors may increase the chance of getting or passing on a genetic disease:

- Parents who have a genetic disease

- A family history of a genetic disease

- Parents who are closely related or part of a distinct ethnic or geographic community

- Parents who do not show disease symptoms, but "carry" a disease gene in their genetic makeup (this can be discovered through genetic testing).

What are the symptoms of a HDCT?

Each disorder has different symptoms. For instance, some diseases, such as Marfan syndrome, osteogenesis imperfecta, and certain chondrodysplasias (disorders of long-bone development) cause bone growth problems. People with bone growth disorders may have brittle bones or bones that are too long or too short. In some of these disorders, joint looseness or joints that are too tight can cause problems.

The skin can be affected as well. Ehlers-Danlos syndrome results in stretchy or loose skin, while in the disease cutis laxa, deficient elastic fibers cause the skin to hang in folds. Epidermolysis bullosa results in blistered skin. Pseudoxanthoma elasticum causes skin, eye, and heart problems, and closed-off or blocked blood vessels. Marfan syndrome and some forms of Ehlers-Danlos syndrome lead to weak blood vessels. Some disorders cause people to be unusually tall (Marfan syndrome) or short (chondrodysplasias, osteogenesis imperfecta), or to have head and facial structure malformations (Apert syndrome, Pfeiffer syndrome).

It is critical for affected individuals and their family members to work closely with their health care teams. Symptoms of HDCTs are extremely variable, and some disorders can pose severe health risks even when affected individuals have no symptoms.

How do doctors diagnose HDCTs?

Diagnosis always rests first on a combination of family history, medical history, and physical examination. Because many of these conditions are uncommon, the family physician may suspect a diagnosis but be uncertain about how to confirm it. At this point, referral to experienced clinicians, often medical geneticists, can be extremely valuable either to confirm or to exclude the suspected diagnosis. Laboratory tests are available to confirm the diagnosis for many HDCTs, but not for all.

Once a diagnosis is made, laboratory studies may be available to provide some or all of the following:

- Prenatal testing to identify an affected fetus to assist in family planning.

- Newborn screening to spot a condition that may become evident later in life.

- Carrier testing to identify adults who, without symptoms, carry a genetic mutation for a disease.

- Predictive testing to spot people at risk for developing a genetic connective tissue disease later in life. These tests are helpful for diseases that run in the family.

What treatments are available?

Each disorder requires a specific program for management and treatment. In most instances, regular monitoring is important to assess, for example, diameter of the aorta in people with Marfan syndrome, extent of scoliosis (spine curvature) in people with OI or some forms of EDS, and whether there is protrusion of the spine into the base of the skull in people with OI. For some conditions, specific metabolic treatment is useful (for example, vitamin B_6 in people with homocystinuria, a metabolic disorder resulting from a liver enzyme deficiency). In others, systemic treatment with drugs like beta blockers is appropriate. Maintaining general health is also important for people with all HDCTs, as is staying in touch with specialists who will be aware of emerging new treatments.

Section 10.2

Ehlers-Danlos Syndrome

What Is Ehlers-Danlos Syndrome?

Individuals with EDS have a defect in their connective tissue, the tissue which provides support to many body parts such as the skin, muscles and ligaments. The fragile skin and unstable joints found in EDS are the result of faulty collagen. Collagen is a protein which acts as a "glue" in the body, adding strength and elasticity to connective tissue.

Ehlers-Danlos syndrome (EDS) is a heterogeneous group of heritable connective tissue disorders, characterized by articular (joint) hypermobility, skin extensibility, and tissue fragility. There are six major types of EDS. The different types of EDS are classified according to their manifestations of signs and symptoms. Each type of EDS is a distinct disorder that "runs true" in a family. This means that an individual with vascular type EDS will not have a child with classical type EDS.

Symptoms

Clinical manifestations of EDS are most often skin and joint related and may include:

- **Skin:** Soft velvet-like skin; variable skin hyper-extensibility; fragile skin that tears or bruises easily (bruising may be severe); severe scarring; slow and poor wound healing; development of molluscoid pseudo tumors (fleshy lesions associated with scars over pressure areas).

- **Joints:** Joint hypermobility; loose/unstable joints which are prone to frequent dislocations and/or subluxations; joint pain; hyperextensible joints (they move beyond the joint's normal range); early onset of osteoarthritis.

- **Miscellaneous/Less Common:** Chronic, early onset, debilitating musculoskeletal pain (usually associated with the hypermobility type); arterial/intestinal/uterine fragility or rupture (usually associated with the vascular type); scoliosis at birth and scleral fragility (associated with the kyphoscoliosis type); poor muscle tone (associated with the arthrochalasia type); mitral valve prolapse; and gum disease.

Prevalence

At this time, research statistics of EDS show the prevalence as one in 5,000 to one in 10,000. It is known to affect both males and females of all racial and ethnic backgrounds.

Hereditary Patterns

The two known inheritance patterns for EDS include autosomal dominant and autosomal recessive. Regardless of the inheritance pattern, we have no choice in which genes we pass on to our children.

Prognosis

The prognosis of EDS depends on the specific type. Life expectancy can be shortened with the vascular type of EDS due to the possibility of organ and vessel rupture. Life expectancy is usually not affected in the other types.

Section 10.3

Marfan Syndrome

"Questions and Answers about Marfan Syndrome," National Institute of Arthritis and Musculoskeletal and Skin Diseases (NIAMS), NIH Pub. No. 02-5000, October 2001.

What is Marfan syndrome?

Marfan syndrome is a heritable condition that affects the connective tissue. The primary purpose of connective tissue is to hold the body together and provide a framework for growth and development. In Marfan syndrome, the connective tissue is defective and does not act as it should. Because connective tissue is found throughout the body, Marfan syndrome can affect many body systems, including the skeleton, eyes, heart and blood vessels, nervous system, skin, and lungs.

Marfan syndrome affects men, women, and children, and has been found among people of all races and ethnic backgrounds. It is estimated that at least one in 5,000 people in the United States have the disorder.

What are the characteristics of Marfan syndrome?

Marfan syndrome affects different people in different ways. Some people have only mild symptoms, while others are more severely affected. In most cases, the symptoms progress as the person ages. The body systems most often affected by Marfan syndrome are:

- **Skeleton:** People with Marfan syndrome are typically very tall, slender, and loose jointed. Since Marfan syndrome affects the long bones of the skeleton, arms, legs, fingers, and toes may be disproportionately long in relation to the rest of the body. A person with Marfan syndrome often has a long, narrow face, and the roof of the mouth may be arched, causing the teeth to be crowded. Other skeletal abnormalities include a sternum (breastbone) that is either protruding or indented, curvature of the spine (scoliosis), and flat feet.

- **Eyes:** More than half of all people with Marfan syndrome experience dislocation of one or both lenses of the eye. The lens may be slightly higher or lower than normal and may be shifted off to one side. The dislocation may be minimal, or it may be pronounced and obvious. Retinal detachment is a possible serious complication of this disorder. Many people with Marfan syndrome are also nearsighted (myopic), and some can develop early glaucoma (high pressure within the eye) or cataracts (the eye's lens loses its clearness).

- **Heart and blood vessels** (cardiovascular system): Most people with Marfan syndrome have abnormalities associated with the heart and blood vessels. Because of faulty connective tissue, the wall of the aorta (the large artery that carries blood from the heart to the rest of the body) may be weakened and stretch, a process called aortic dilatation. Aortic dilatation increases the risk that the aorta will tear (aortic dissection) or rupture, causing serious heart problems or sometimes sudden death. Sometimes, defects in heart valves can also cause problems. In some cases, certain valves may leak, creating a "heart murmur," which a doctor can hear with a stethoscope. Small leaks may not result in any symptoms, but larger ones may cause shortness of breath, fatigue, and palpitations (a very fast or irregular heart rate).

- **Nervous system:** The brain and spinal cord are surrounded by fluid contained by a membrane called the dura, which is composed of connective tissue. As people with Marfan syndrome get older, the dura often weakens and stretches, then begins to weigh on the vertebrae in the lower spine and wear away the bone surrounding the spinal cord. This is called dural ectasia. These changes may cause only mild discomfort or may lead to radiated pain in the abdomen or to pain, numbness, or weakness of the legs.

- **Skin:** Many people with Marfan syndrome develop stretch marks on their skin, even without any weight change. These stretch marks can occur at any age and pose no health risk. However, people with Marfan syndrome are also at increased risk for developing an abdominal or inguinal hernia where a bulge develops that contains part of the intestines.

- **Lungs:** Although connective tissue abnormalities make the tiny air sacs within the lungs less elastic, people with Marfan syndrome generally do not experience noticeable problems with their lungs. If, however, these tiny air sacs become stretched or swollen, the risk of lung collapse may increase. Rarely, people with Marfan syndrome may have sleep-related breathing disorders such as snoring or sleep apnea (a sleep disorder characterized by brief periods when breathing stops).

What causes Marfan syndrome?

Marfan syndrome is caused by a defect (mutation) in the gene that determines the structure of fibrillin, a protein that is an important part of connective tissue. A person with Marfan syndrome is born with the disorder, even though it may not be diagnosed until later in life. Although everyone with Marfan syndrome has a defect in the same gene, the mutation is specific to each family and not everyone experiences the same characteristics to the same degree. This is called variable expression, meaning that the defective gene expresses itself in different ways in different people. Scientists do not yet understand why variable expression occurs in people with Marfan syndrome.

The defective gene can be inherited: The child of a person who has Marfan syndrome has a 50 percent chance of inheriting the disease. Sometimes a new gene defect occurs during the formation of sperm or egg cells, but two unaffected parents have only a one in 10,000 chance of having a child with Marfan syndrome. Possibly 25 percent of cases are due to a spontaneous mutation at the time of conception.

How is Marfan syndrome diagnosed?

There is no specific laboratory test, such as a blood test or skin biopsy, to diagnose Marfan syndrome. The doctor and/or geneticist (a doctor with special knowledge about inherited diseases) relies on observation and a complete medical history, including:

- information about any family members who may have the disorder or who had an early, unexplained heart-related death

- a thorough physical examination, including an evaluation of the skeletal frame for the ratio of arm/leg size to trunk size

- an eye examination, including a "slit lamp" evaluation

- heart tests such as an echocardiogram (a test that uses ultrasound waves to examine the heart and aorta).

The doctor may diagnose Marfan syndrome if the patient has a family history of the disease and there are specific problems in at least two of the body systems known to be affected. For a patient with no family history of the disease, at least three body systems must be affected before a diagnosis is made. Moreover, two of the systems must show clear signs that are relatively specific for Marfan syndrome.

In some cases, a genetic analysis may be useful, but such analyses are often time consuming and may not provide any additional helpful information. Family members of a person diagnosed with Marfan syndrome should not assume they are not affected if there is no knowledge that the disorder existed in previous generations of the family. After a clinical diagnosis of a family member, a genetic study might identify the specific mutation for which a test can be performed to determine if other family members are affected.

What types of doctors treat Marfan syndrome?

Because a number of body systems may be affected, a person with Marfan syndrome should be cared for by several different types of doctors. A general practitioner or pediatrician may oversee routine health care and refer the patient to specialists such as a cardiologist (a doctor who specializes in heart disorders), an orthopaedist (a doctor who specializes in bones), or an ophthalmologist (a doctor who specializes in eye disorders) as needed. Some people with Marfan syndrome are also treated by a geneticist.

What treatment options are available?

There is no cure for Marfan syndrome. To develop one, scientists may have to identify and change the specific gene responsible for the disorder before birth. However, a range of treatment options can minimize and sometimes prevent complications. The appropriate specialists will develop an individualized treatment program; the approach the doctor uses depends on which systems have been affected.

- **Skeletal:** Annual evaluations are important to detect any changes in the spine or sternum. This is particularly important in times of rapid growth, such as adolescence. A serious deformity can not only be disfiguring but can also prevent the heart and lungs from functioning properly. In some cases, an orthopedic brace or surgery may be recommended to limit damage and disfigurement.

- **Eyes:** Early, regular eye examinations are key to catching and correcting any vision problems associated with Marfan syndrome. In most cases, eyeglasses or contact lenses can correct the problem, although surgery may be necessary in some cases.

- **Heart and blood vessels:** Regular checkups and echocardiograms help the doctor evaluate the size of the aorta and the way the heart is working. The earlier a potential problem is identified and treated, the lower the risk of life-threatening complications. Those with heart problems are encouraged to wear a medical alert bracelet and to go to the emergency room if they experience chest, back, or abdominal pain. Some heart valve problems can be managed with drugs such as beta-blockers, which may help decrease stress on the aorta. In other cases, surgery to replace a valve or repair the aorta may be necessary. Surgery should be performed before the aorta reaches a size that puts it at high risk for tear or rupture. Following heart surgery, extreme care must be followed to prevent endocarditis (inflammation of the lining of the heart cavity and valves). Dentists should be alerted to this risk; they are likely to recommend that the patient be prescribed protective medicines before they perform dental work.

- **Nervous system:** If dural ectasia (swelling of the covering of the spinal cord) develops, medication may help minimize any associated pain.

- **Lungs:** It is especially important that people with Marfan syndrome not smoke, as they are already at increased risk for lung damage. Any problems with breathing during sleep should be assessed by a doctor.

Pregnancy poses a particular concern due to the stress on the body, particularly the heart. A pregnancy should be undertaken only under conditions specified by obstetricians and other specialists familiar with Marfan syndrome and be followed as a high-risk condition.

While eating a balanced diet is important for maintaining a healthy lifestyle, no vitamin or dietary supplement has been shown to help slow, cure, or prevent Marfan syndrome.

What are some of the emotional and psychological effects of Marfan syndrome?

Being diagnosed and learning to live with a genetic disorder can cause social, emotional, and financial stress. It often requires a great deal of adjustment in outlook and lifestyle. A person who is an adult when Marfan syndrome is diagnosed may feel angry or afraid. There may also be concerns about passing the disorder to future generations or about its physical, emotional, and financial implications.

The parents and siblings of a child diagnosed with Marfan syndrome may feel sadness, anger, and guilt. It is important for parents to know that nothing that they did caused the fibrillin gene to mutate. Parents may be concerned about the genetic implications for siblings or have questions about the risk to future children. Some children with Marfan syndrome are advised to restrict their activities. This may require a lifestyle adjustment that may be hard for a child to understand or accept.

For both children and adults, appropriate medical care, accurate information, and social support are key to living with the disease. Genetic counseling may also be helpful in understanding the disease and its potential impact on future generations.

What is the outlook for a person with Marfan syndrome?

While Marfan syndrome is a lifelong disorder, the outlook has improved in recent years. Early diagnosis and advances in medical technology have improved the quality of life for people with Marfan syndrome and lengthened their lifespan. In addition, early identification of risk factors (such as aortic dilation) allows doctors to intervene and prevent or delay complications. Advances being made by researchers provide hope for the future. With early diagnosis and appropriate management, the life expectancy for someone with Marfan syndrome is similar to that of the average person.

What research is being conducted to help people with Marfan syndrome?

Scientists are approaching research on Marfan syndrome from a variety of perspectives. One approach is to better understand what happens once the genetic defect or mutation occurs. How does it change the way connective tissue develops and functions in the body? Why are people with Marfan syndrome affected differently? Scientists are searching for the answers to these questions both by studying the genes themselves and by studying large family groups affected by the disease. Newly developed mouse models that carry mutations in the fibrillin gene may help scientists better understand the disorder. Animal studies that are preliminary to gene therapy are also under way.

Other scientists are focusing on ways to treat some of the complications that arise in people with Marfan syndrome. Clinical studies are being conducted to evaluate the usefulness of certain medications in preventing or reducing problems with the aorta. Researchers are also working to develop new surgical procedures to help improve the cardiac health of people with Marfan syndrome.

Chapter 11

Cystic Fibrosis

Cystic fibrosis (CF) is a genetic disorder that particularly affects the lungs and digestive system and makes a child more vulnerable to repeated lung infections. Now, thanks to high-tech medical advances in drug therapy and genetics, children born with CF can look forward to longer and more comfortable lives. In the last 10 years, research into all aspects of CF has helped doctors to understand the illness better and to develop new therapies. In the future, ongoing research may help find a cure.

What Is Cystic Fibrosis?

Currently affecting more than 30,000 children and young adults in the United States, cystic fibrosis makes children sick by disrupting the normal function of epithelial cells—cells that make up the sweat glands in the skin and that also line passageways inside the lungs, liver, pancreas, and digestive and reproductive systems.

In CF, the inherited CF gene directs the body's epithelial cells to produce a defective form of a protein called CFTR (or cystic fibrosis transmembrane conductance regulator) found in cells that line the lungs, digestive tract, sweat glands, and genitourinary system. When

This information was provided by KidsHealth, one of the largest resources online for medically reviewed health information written for parents, kids, and teens. For more articles like this one, visit www.KidsHealth.org, or www.TeensHealth.org. © 2004 The Nemours Center for Children's Health Media, a division of The Nemours Foundation.

the CFTR protein is defective, epithelial cells can't regulate the way chloride (part of the salt called sodium chloride) passes across cell membranes. This disrupts the essential balance of salt and water that is needed to maintain a normal thin coating of fluid and mucus inside the lungs, pancreas, and passageways in other organs. The mucus becomes thick, sticky, and hard to move.

Normally, mucus in the lungs traps germs, which are then cleared out of the lungs. But in CF, the thick, sticky mucus and the germs it has trapped remain in the lungs, and the lungs become infected.

In the pancreas, thick mucus blocks the channels that would normally carry important enzymes to the intestines to digest foods. When this happens, the child's body can't process or absorb nutrients properly, especially fats. The child has problems gaining weight, even with a normal diet and a good appetite.

A Family's Risk for CF

Humans have 23 pairs of chromosomes made of the inherited genetic chemical called DNA. The CF gene is found on chromosome number 7. It takes two copies of a CF gene—one inherited from each parent—for a child to show symptoms of CF. Persons born with only one CF gene (inherited from only one parent) and one normal gene are CF carriers. CF carriers do not show CF symptoms themselves, but can pass the problem CF gene to their children. Scientists estimate that about 12 million Americans are currently CF carriers. If two CF carriers have a child, there is a one in four chance that the child will have CF.

There are more than 1,200 different mutations of the CF gene that can lead to cystic fibrosis (some mutations cause milder symptoms than others). About 70% of people with CF have the disease because they inherited the mutant gene *Delta F508* from both of their parents. This can be detected by genetic testing, which can be done in children, both before and after birth, and in adults who are thinking about starting or enlarging their families.

Of all ethnic groups, Caucasians have the highest inherited risk for CF, and Asian Americans have the lowest. In the United States today, about one of every 3,600 Caucasian children is born with CF. This compares with one of every 17,000 African Americans and only one of every 90,000 Asian Americans. Although the chances of inherited risk may vary, CF has been described in every geographic area of the world among every ethnic population.

Scientists don't know exactly why the CF gene evolved in humans, but they have some evidence to show that it helped to protect earlier generations from the bacteria that cause cholera, a severe intestinal infection.

How CF Affects Children

The diagnosis of CF is usually made before an affected child is 3 years old. However, about 15% of those with CF are diagnosed later in life (even adulthood). Symptoms usually center around the lungs and digestive organs and can be more or less severe.

A few children with CF begin having symptoms at birth. Some are born with a condition called meconium ileus. Although all newborns have meconium—the thick, dark, putty-like substance that usually passes from the rectum in the first few days of a baby's life—in CF, the meconium can be too thick and sticky to pass and can completely block the intestines.

More commonly, though, babies born with CF don't gain weight as expected. They fail to thrive in spite of a normal diet and a good appetite. In these children, mucus blocks the passageways of the pancreas and prevents pancreatic digestive juices from entering the child's intestines. Without these digestive juices, the intestines can't absorb fats and proteins completely, so nutrients pass out of the body unused rather than helping the child's body grow. Poor fat absorption makes the child's stools appear oily and bulky and increases the child's risk for deficiencies of the fat-soluble vitamins (vitamins A, D, E, and K). Unabsorbed fats may also cause excessive intestinal gas, an abnormally swollen belly, and abdominal pain or discomfort.

Because CF also affects epithelial cells in the skin's sweat glands, children with CF may have a salty "frosting" on their skin or taste "salty" when their parents kiss them. They may also lose abnormally large amounts of body salt when they sweat on hot days.

Cystic fibrosis is the most common cause of pancreatic insufficiency in children, but a condition called Shwachman-Diamond syndrome (SDS) is the second most common cause. SDS is a genetic condition that causes a reduced ability to digest food because digestive enzymes don't work properly. Some of the symptoms of SDS are similar to those of CF, so it may be confused with cystic fibrosis. However, in children with SDS, the sweat test is normal.

Because CF produces thick mucus within the respiratory tract, a child with CF may suffer from nasal congestion, sinus problems, wheezing, and asthma-like symptoms. As CF symptoms progress,

131

the child may develop a chronic cough that produces globs of thick, heavy, discolored mucus. They may also suffer from repeated lung infections.

As chronic infections reduce lung function, the person's ability to breathe often decreases. A person with CF may eventually begin to feel short of breath, even when resting. Despite aggressive medical therapy, lung disease develops in nearly all patients with CF and is a common cause of disability and shortened life span.

Identifying a Child with CF

By performing genetic tests during pregnancy, parents can now learn whether their unborn children may have CF. But even when genetic tests confirm CF, there's still no way to predict beforehand whether a specific child's CF symptoms will be severe or mild. Genetic testing can also be done on a child after birth, and can be performed on parents, siblings, and other relatives who are considering having a family.

After birth, the standard diagnostic test for CF is called the sweat test—an accurate, safe, and painless way to diagnose CF. In the sweat test, a small electric current is used to carry the chemical pilocarpine into the skin of the child's forearm. This stimulates sweat glands in the area to produce sweat. Over a period of 30 to 60 minutes, sweat is collected on filter paper or gauze and tested for chloride.

To diagnose CF, two sweat tests are generally performed in a lab accredited by the Cystic Fibrosis Foundation. A child must have a sweat chloride result of greater than 60 on two separate sweat tests to make the diagnosis of CF.

Several other tests serve as standard parts of the routine care used to monitor a child's CF:

- chest X-rays

- blood tests to evaluate nutritional status

- bacterial studies that confirm the growth of *Pseudomonas aeruginosa*, *Staphylococcus aureus*, or *Haemophilus influenza* bacteria in a child's lungs (these bacteria are common in CF but may not affect healthy people exposed to CF)

- pulmonary function tests (PFTs) to measure the effects of CF on a child's breathing (PFTs are done as soon as the child is old enough to be able to cooperate in the testing procedure; infant PFTs are currently being studied.)

Treating a Child with CF

When kids are first diagnosed with CF, they may or may not have to spend some time in the hospital, depending on their condition. If they do, they'll have diagnostic tests, especially baseline measurements of their breathing (lung function) and a nutritional assessment. Before they leave, their doctors will make sure that their lungs are clear and that they've started a diet with digestive enzymes and vitamins that will help them to gain weight normally. Afterward, they'll probably see their doctor for follow-up visits at least once every one to three months.

The basic daily care program of a child with CF varies from child to child, but usually includes pulmonary therapy (treatments to maintain lung function) and nutritional therapy (a high-calorie, high-fat diet with vitamin supplements). Children with CF can also take oral doses of pancreatic enzymes to help them digest food better. They may also occasionally need oral or inhaled antibiotics to treat lung infections and mucolytic medication (a mucus-thinning drug) to keep mucus fluid and flowing.

One of the newest treatments for CF that's still being researched is an inhaled spray containing normal copies of the CF gene. These normal genes deliver the correct copy of the CF gene into the lungs of CF patients. Since 1993, more than 100 CF patients have been treated with CF gene therapy, and test trials are underway in at least nine different medical centers throughout the country and other centers around the world. Another new therapy, called protein repair therapy, aims at repairing the defective CFTR protein. Numerous medications, including a spice called curcumin, are also being tested at clinical centers across the country.

Caring for a child with CF can be tough at times, but parents need not feel alone. Their child's doctor or family doctor can usually refer them to a local support group linked to the Cystic Fibrosis Foundation.

—Reviewed by: Raj Padman, MD, May 2004

Chapter 12

Glycogen Storage Disease

What is glycogen storage disease?

Glucose is a large energy source for the body. It is stored by the body in the form of glycogen and later released into the body with the help of enzymes.

Glycogen storage disease (GSD) is a group of inherited (born with) disorders where an abnormal amount or type of glycogen settles in the liver and causes failure of the liver's ability to break down glycogen to supply glucose to the rest of the body. This happens when one or more of the many enzymes (proteins produced by the body) needed to convert sugar (glucose) into its storage form (glycogen) are missing.

Many sugars (including glucose) are present in foods and are used by the body as a source of energy. After a meal, blood glucose levels rise. The body stores the extra glucose that is not needed right away as glycogen in the liver and muscles. Later, as the blood glucose levels in the body begin to dip, the body uses this stored energy.

These sugars, stored in the form of glycogen, need to be processed by enzymes in the body before they can carry out their functions. If the enzymes needed to process them are missing, these sugars can accumulate, causing problems.

There are at least 10 different types of GSDs, which are put into groups, based on the enzyme that is missing. The most common forms of GSD are Types I, II, III and IV. Glycogen storage diseases affect approximately one in about 20,000 people.

What are the causes?

When glucose is changed into glycogen, a different enzyme is required at each step. If one of these enzymes is defective (not normal) and fails to complete its step, the process stops. These enzyme defects cause glycogen storage diseases.

GSD is inherited and occurs because of an inherited defective gene from both parents. If both parents carry the defective gene, there is:

- A 25% chance that their child will develop the disorder
- A 50% chance that their child will receive one defective gene from one of the parents, which means the child will not show symptoms of the disorder but is a "carrier"
- A 25% chance their child will receive both normal genes, one from each parent, and will have a GSD

What are the signs and symptoms?

Symptoms vary based on the enzyme that is missing. They usually result from the buildup of glycogen or from an inability to produce glucose when needed. Because GSD occurs mainly in muscles and the liver, those areas show the most obvious symptoms.

Symptoms may include:

- Growth failure
- Muscle cramps
- Low blood sugar
- A greatly enlarged liver
- A swollen belly

The age when symptoms begin and how severe they are depends on the type of GSD. Children with GSD I rarely develop cirrhosis (liver disease), but they are at an increased risk for developing liver tumors.

In some ways, GSD III is a milder version of GSD I. It also is a very rare cause of liver failure, but it may cause fibrosis (early scarring of the liver, which may be caused by a healing response to injury, infection or inflammation). GSD II is a muscle disease and does not affect the liver.

Glycogen storage disease IV causes cirrhosis; it may also cause heart or muscle dysfunction. Often, infants born with GSD IV are diagnosed with enlarged livers and failure to thrive within their first year of life; they develop cirrhosis of the liver by age 3–5.

How is it diagnosed?

The four major symptoms of GSD I, III and IV are:

- Low blood sugar
- Enlarged liver
- Growth problems
- Abnormal blood test results

An exam of a sample of liver tissue is done to tell if a certain enzyme is missing. A diagnosis can be confirmed by a biopsy of the affected organ(s) that shows the amount of glycogen and enzyme activity.

What is the treatment?

Treatment depends on the type of glycogen storage disease. Some GSD types cannot be treated; others are fairly easy to control by treating the symptoms.

For the types of GSD that can be treated, patients must carefully follow a special diet.

Frequent high carbohydrate meals during the day. For some children, eating several small meals rich in sugars and starches every day helps prevent blood sugar levels from dropping.

Cornstarch. For some young children over the age of 2, giving uncooked cornstarch every four to six hours—including during overnight hours—also can relieve the problem.

Continuous nighttime feeding. In order to maintain the blood glucose level, a tube is inserted into the stomach each evening to send a solution with a high concentration of glucose. This helps control the blood sugar level. Younger children will have to use this tube each evening, but doctors feel that this may not be necessary once they get older. In the daytime the tube is removed, but the patient must eat foods rich in sugars and starches about every three hours. This treatment can be successful in reversing most symptoms.

Drug treatment. GSD tends to cause uric acid (a waste product) to accumulate, which can cause gout (painful inflammation of the joints) and kidney stones. Medication is often necessary to prevent this.

In some types of this disease, children must limit their amount of exercise to reduce muscle cramps.

What is the long-term prognosis?

Some GSD types cannot be treated, while others are fairly easy to control by treating the symptoms. Patients with treatable GSD do very well if the blood glucose level is maintained within the normal range. Maintaining a healthy blood glucose level can reverse all of the signs of this disease, allowing the child to lead a long, relatively normal life.

In the more severe cases of GSD, infection and other complications are likely to occur. These include liver, heart and respiratory failure. If liver failure occurs, receiving a liver transplant is the only option. Transplants have been effective in reversing the symptoms of GSD.

Chapter 13

Growth Disorders

Chapter Contents

Section 13.1—What Is a Growth Disorder?.............................. 140
Section 13.2—Achondroplasia 144
Section 13.3—Other Less Common Types of Dwarfism........... 147

Section 13.1

What Is a Growth Disorder?

This information was provided by KidsHealth, one of the largest resources online for medically reviewed health information written for parents, kids, and teens. For more articles like this one, visit www.KidsHealth.org, or www.TeensHealth.org. © 2001 The Nemours Center for Children's Health Media, a division of The Nemours Foundation.

Lately it seems as though your child is looking up to her classmates—literally. Whereas the other kids in her class have been getting taller and developing into young adults, your child's growth seems to be lagging behind. Her classmates now tower over her. Is something wrong?

What Is a Growth Disorder?

A growth disorder is any type of problem in infants, kids, or teens that prevents them from meeting realistic expectations of growth. Disorders may include failure to thrive in infancy, failure to gain height and weight in young children, and short stature or delayed sexual development in teens.

Common Growth Disorders and Their Causes

This section will discuss a sampling of normal variant growth patterns, such as familial short stature and constitutional growth delay, and growth disorders, such as growth hormone deficiency and Turner syndrome.

Although it's common for newborns to lose a little weight in the first few days, some infants continue to show slower than expected weight gain and growth, a condition known as failure to thrive. Usually caused by inadequate nutrition or a feeding problem, failure to thrive is most common in children younger than age 3. Failure to thrive may also be a symptom of another problem, such as an infection or a digestive problem. Child neglect or abuse may also be associated with failure to thrive.

Shorter parents tend to have shorter children, a condition known as familial (or genetic) short stature. This term applies to short children who do not have any symptoms of diseases that affect growth. Children with familial short stature still have growth spurts and enter puberty at normal ages, but they usually will only reach a height similar to that of their parents.

Constitutional growth delay describes children who are small for their ages but who are growing at a normal rate. They usually have a delayed "bone age," which means that their skeletal maturation is younger than their age in years. (A child's bone age is measured by taking an x-ray of a child's hand and wrist and comparing it to standard x-ray findings seen in children of the same age.)

These children do not have any signs or symptoms of diseases that affect growth. They tend to reach puberty later than their peers do, with delay in the onset of sexual development and the pubertal growth spurt. But because they continue to grow until an older age, they tend to catch up to their peers when they reach adult height. One or both parents or other close relatives of these children often experienced a similar "late-bloomer" growth pattern.

Children diagnosed with familial short stature or constitutional growth delay often face social problems because they are short or don't enter puberty when their classmates do. "Most importantly, children and their families need to be reassured that their child does not have a disease or medical condition that poses a threat to their health or requires treatment," says Steven Dowshen, MD, a pediatric endocrinologist. However, these kids may need extra help coping with teasing by their peers or reassurance that they will grow and develop eventually.

Other Causes of Growth Disorders

Diseases of the kidneys, heart, gastrointestinal tract, lungs, or other body systems may lead to growth disorders. Other symptoms in children with these illnesses usually give clues as to the disease causing the growth delay. However, poor growth may be the first sign of a problem in some of these conditions.

Endocrine diseases (diseases involving hormones, the chemical messengers of the body) involve a deficiency or excess of hormones and can be responsible for growth failure during childhood and adolescence. Growth hormone deficiency is a disorder that involves the pituitary gland (the small gland at the base of the brain that secretes several hormones, including growth hormone). A damaged or malfunctioning pituitary gland may not produce enough hormones for normal growth. Hypothyroidism is a condition in which the thyroid gland fails to make enough thyroid hormone, which is essential for normal bone growth.

Turner syndrome, one of the most common growth problems, occurs in girls and is a genetic syndrome in which there is a missing or abnormal X chromosome. In addition to short stature, girls with Turner syndrome usually don't undergo normal sexual development because their ovaries (sex organs that produce eggs and female hormones) fail to mature and function normally.

How Is a Growth Disorder Diagnosed?

The number of tests needed to detect a growth disorder depends on the findings at each step of evaluation. A short child who is healthy and growing at a normal rate may just be observed throughout childhood, but a child who has stopped growing or is growing more slowly than expected will often need additional testing.

Your child's doctor or endocrinologist will look for signs of the many possible causes of short stature and growth failure. Blood tests may be performed to look for hormone and chromosome abnormalities as well as to rule out other diseases associated with growth failure. A bone age x-ray is frequently done, and special scans (such as an MRI) can check the pituitary gland for abnormalities.

To measure the ability of the child's pituitary gland to produce growth hormone, the doctor (usually a pediatric endocrinologist) may perform a growth hormone stimulation test. This involves giving the child certain medications that cause the pituitary gland to secrete growth hormone and then drawing several small blood samples to check growth hormone levels over a period of time after the medications are given.

Treatment

Although the treatment of a growth problem is usually not an urgent situation, earlier diagnosis and treatment of some conditions may help kids achieve a more typical adult height.

If an underlying medical condition is identified, specific treatment may result in improved growth. Growth failure due to hypothyroidism, for example, is usually simply treated by giving the child thyroid hormone replacement therapy in pill form.

Growth hormone injections for children with growth hormone deficiency, Turner syndrome, and chronic kidney failure may help them reach a more normal height. "Human growth hormone is generally considered safe and effective," Dr. Dowshen says, although full treatment may take many years and not all children will have a good response. The treatment can be quite costly (approximately $20,000 to $30,000 per year), although most health insurance plans will cover the costs.

Helping Your Child

You can boost your child's self-esteem by providing positive reinforcement and emphasizing other characteristics, like her intelligence, personality, and talents. Dr. Dowshen recommends de-emphasizing the focus on height as a measure of social acceptance. Your child should be taught that her value doesn't come from height but from her other qualities.

Kids who are very self-conscious about their size may need some additional help in coping. "In some cases, evaluation and treatment by a mental health professional may be indicated," Dr. Dowshen says.

If You Suspect a Problem

If you are concerned about your child's growth, take her to her doctor. Depending on the findings of the examination, the doctor may refer your child to a pediatric endocrinologist, who can help diagnose and treat specific growth disorders.

It's also important to be on the lookout for the social and emotional problems that kids with growth disorders face. It's not easy being the shortest kid in the class and it's never any fun being teased. Helping your child build self-esteem and emphasizing her abilities—regardless of how tall she grows—might be just what the doctor ordered.

Section 13.2

Achondroplasia

"Patient Guide to Achondroplasia," reprinted with permission from the Johns Hopkins University School of Medicine Department of Orthopaedic Surgery. © 2000. All rights reserved.

What is achondroplasia?

"Dysplasia" means abnormal development. "Achondroplasia" refers to the abnormal development of cartilage ("chondro"). Because the skeleton develops by the ossification of cartilage, this leads to an abnormal development of the bones, most commonly causing them to be much shorter than normal.

Achondroplasia is the most common of all skeletal dysplasias. This condition leads to patients attaining a full grown height under four feet. The greatest shortening occurs in the humerus (the bone between the shoulder and the elbow) and the femur (the bone between the hip and the knee). There may also be underdevelopment of the face.

What causes achondroplasia?

Achondroplasia is a genetic disease. This means that a gene that directs a specific process in the body does not work properly. In this particular condition, a protein in the body called the "fibroblast growth factor receptor" begins to function abnormally. The result is that the growth of bones, which normally occurs in the cartilage of the growth plate, is slowed. This leads to shorter bones, abnormally shaped bones, and shorter stature.

The genetic defect can be passed from a parent to his or her child. In the case of achondroplasia, however, it more commonly is the result of a spontaneous mutation (a sudden genetic defect) that occurs in the developing embryo.

What are the signs and symptoms of achondroplasia?

Patients with achondroplasia have a short stature, a long trunk, and shortened limbs, which are noticeable at birth. Adults usually reach a height of between 42 and 56 inches. The head is large and the forehead is prominent. Portions of the face can be underdeveloped as well.

At birth, the legs appear straight, but as a child begins to walk, he or she develops a knock-knee or bowed-leg deformity. The hands and the feet appear large, but the fingers and toes are short and stubby. Straightening of the arm at the elbow may be restricted, but usually does not keep a patient with achondroplasia from doing any specific activities.

In addition, the child may develop an excessive curve of the lower back and a waddling walking pattern.

What are the different types of achondroplasia?

There are several recognized developmental disorders that mimic achondroplasia. First, in a condition called pseudo-achondroplasia, the face of the child appears normal, but he or she may have irregular growth plates in the hips and knees. In another condition called hypochondroplasia, the child is less severely affected. He or she usually develops a height over 54 inches and does not ever get spinal stenosis (see below).

What is the treatment of achondroplasia?

Unfortunately, there is no treatment that can cure this condition. Surgery is sometimes needed to correct specific skeletal deformities. For example, in patients with severe knock-knee or bowed legs, the pediatric orthopaedic surgeon can perform an osteotomy in which he or she cuts the bones of the leg and allows them to heal in a more correct anatomical position. For significant spinal kyphosis a spinal fusion sometimes is performed (permanently connecting otherwise separate vertebrae).

The most serious complication of achondroplasia is the narrowing of the spinal canal called "spinal stenosis." The canal houses the spinal cord and such narrowing can lead to a compression of the cord and severe neurological problems. Surgical decompression of the cord is needed to relieve the pressure on it. This is done by opening the canal at the affected levels in a procedure called a "laminectomy."

Should my child see a doctor regularly?

Yes. It is important to follow a doctor to make sure that spinal stenosis does not develop. The physician evaluates the strength of the extremities and bladder control. Weakness and loss of bladder control are both signs of developing spinal stenosis.

How will the child do in the long run with achondroplasia?

The prognosis depends on the severity of the disease. Patients who have two copies of the deficient gene (that is, one from each parent, also known as "homozygous") generally die a few weeks to months after birth. Those with one copy (that is, from only one parent, also known as "heterozygous") have a normal life span and intelligence. They are usually independent in their daily life activities. Many of these patients, in fact, have gone on to do great things in life.

For further information, please contact:

- The Human Growth Foundation (HGF): http://www.hgfound.org

- Little People of America (LPA): http://www.lpaonline.org

- Kathryn and Alan C. Greenberg Center for Skeletal Dysplasias: http://www.med.jhu.edu/Greenberg.Center/Greenberg.Center

Section 13.3

Other Less Common Types of Dwarfism

Information in this section is excerpted with permission from several Rare Disease Reports produced by the National Organization for Rare Disorders (NORD), P.O. Box 1968, Danbury, CT 06813-1968, (800) 999-NORD (6673). © 2000–2004 NORD. All rights reserved. Full-text reports for these and many other disorders, which include information on symptoms, causes, treatments, and clinical trials, can be purchased individually or by subscription on the NORD website at http://www.rarediseases.org.

Bloom Syndrome

Bloom syndrome is a rare genetic disorder characterized by short stature; increased sensitivity to light (photosensitivity); multiple small dilated blood vessels on the face (facial telangiectasia), often resembling a butterfly in shape; immune deficiency leading to increased susceptibility to infections; and, perhaps most importantly, a markedly increased susceptibility to cancer of any organ, but especially to leukemia and lymphoma. Some clinicians classify Bloom syndrome as a chromosomal breakage syndrome; that is, a disorder associated with a high frequency of chromosomal breaks and rearrangements. It is suspected that there is a link between the frequency of chromosomal breaks and the increased propensity toward malignancies.

Bloom syndrome is inherited as an autosomal recessive genetic trait. It is often included among the Jewish genetic diseases.

Cockayne Syndrome

Cockayne syndrome (CS) is a rare form of dwarfism. It is an inherited disorder whose diagnosis depends on the presence of three signs (1) growth retardation; that is, short stature, (2) abnormal sensitivity to light (photosensitivity), and (3) prematurely aged appearance (progeria). In the classical form of Cockayne syndrome (CS type I) the symptoms are progressive and typically become apparent after the age of one year. An early onset or congenital form of Cockayne syndrome (CS type II) is apparent at birth (congenital). There is a third form, known as Cockayne syndrome Type III (CS type III), that

147

presents later in the child's development and is generally a milder form of the disease. A fourth form, now recognized as xeroderma pigmentosa-Cockayne syndrome (XP-CS), combines features of both of these disorders.

Diastrophic Dysplasia

Diastrophic dysplasia, which is also known as diastrophic dwarfism, is a rare disorder that is present at birth (congenital). The range and severity of associated symptoms and physical findings may vary greatly from case to case. However, the disorder is often characterized by short stature and unusually short arms and legs (short-limbed dwarfism); abnormal development of bones (skeletal dysplasia) and joints (joint dysplasia) in many areas of the body; progressive abnormal curvature of the spine (scoliosis and/or kyphosis); abnormal tissue changes of the outer, visible portions of the ears (pinnae); and/or, in some cases, malformations of the head and facial (craniofacial) area.

In most infants with diastrophic dysplasia, the first bone within the body of each hand (first metacarpals) may be unusually small and "oval shaped," causing the thumbs to deviate away (abduction) from the body ("hitchhiker thumbs"). Other fingers may also be abnormally short (brachydactyly) and joints between certain bones of the fingers (proximal interphalangeal joints) may become fused (symphalangism), causing limited flexion and restricted movement of the finger joints. Affected infants also typically have severe foot deformities (talipes or "clubfeet") due to abnormal deviation and fusion of certain bones within the body of each foot (metatarsals). In addition, many children with the disorder experience limited extension, partial (subluxation) or complete dislocation, and/or permanent flexion and immobilization (contractures) of certain joints.

In most infants with diastrophic dysplasia, there is also incomplete closure of bones of the spinal column (spina bifida occulta) within the neck area and the upper portion of the back (lower cervical and upper thoracic vertebrae). In addition, during the first year of life, some affected children may begin to develop progressive abnormal sideways curvature of the spine (scoliosis). During adolescence, individuals with the disorder may also develop abnormal front-to-back curvature of the spine (kyphosis), particularly affecting vertebrae within the neck area (cervical vertebrae). In severe cases, progressive kyphosis may lead to difficulties breathing (respiratory distress). Some individuals may also be prone to experiencing partial dislocation (subluxation) of joints between the central areas (bodies) of cervical vertebrae, potentially resulting in spinal cord injury. Such injury may cause muscle weakness (paresis) or paralysis and/or life-threatening complications.

In addition, most newborns with diastrophic dysplasia have or develop abnormal fluid-filled sacs (cysts) within the outer, visible portions of the ears (pinnae). Within the first weeks of life, the pinnae become swollen and inflamed and unusually firm, thick, and abnormal in shape. Over time, the abnormal areas of tissue (lesions) may accumulate deposits of calcium salts (calcification) and eventually develop into bone (ossification). Some affected infants may also have abnormalities of the head and facial (craniofacial) area including incomplete closure of the roof of the mouth (cleft palate) and/or abnormal smallness of the jaws (micrognathia). In addition, in some affected infants, abnormalities of supportive connective tissue (cartilage) within the windpipe (trachea), voice box (larynx), and certain air passages in the lungs (bronchi) may result in collapse of these airways, causing life-threatening complications such as respiratory obstruction and difficulties breathing. In some individuals with the disorder, additional symptoms and physical findings may also be present. Diastrophic dysplasia is inherited as an autosomal recessive trait.

Dyggve-Melchior-Clausen Syndrome

Dyggve-Melchior-Clausen syndrome is a rare autosomal recessive disorder. Major symptoms may include short stature, mental retardation, bulging of the chest sternum, flattening of the vertebrae and upper border of the pelvis (iliac crest), shortening of the bones in the middle portion of the hand (metacarpals) and changes in the long bones. Patients with the Smith-McCort dwarfism form of this disorder do not have mental retardation.

Ellis-van Creveld Syndrome

Ellis-van Creveld syndrome is a rare genetic disorder characterized by short limb dwarfism, additional fingers and/or toes (polydactyly), abnormal development of fingernails and, in over half of the cases, congenital heart defects. This disorder is inherited through an autosomal recessive trait.

Growth Hormone Deficiency

Growth hormone is manufactured in the pituitary gland. If it is missing or reduced in quantity during infancy or childhood, it results in growth retardation, short stature and other maturation delays.

Growth hormone deficiency (GHD) causes an absence or delay of lengthening and widening of the skeletal bones inappropriate to the chronological age of the child. A sufficient quantity of growth hormone is required during childhood to maintain growth and normalize sexual maturity. In some cases the onset of the disorder occurs prenatally (before birth), and in others the condition occurs months or years later. Laboratory testing is necessary before a diagnosis of growth hormone deficiency is made because growth and maturity delays can be caused by a wide variety of other factors, including normal genetic influences.

Hallermann-Streiff Syndrome

Hallermann-Streiff syndrome is a rare genetic disorder that is primarily characterized by distinctive malformations of the skull and facial (craniofacial) region; sparse hair (hypotrichosis); eye (ocular) abnormalities; dental defects; degenerative skin changes (atrophy), particularly in the scalp and nasal regions; and/or short stature (that is, dwarfism). Characteristic craniofacial features include a short, broad head (brachycephaly) with an unusually prominent forehead and/or sides of the skull (frontal and/or parietal bossing); a small, underdeveloped lower jaw (hypoplastic mandible); a narrow, highly arched roof of the mouth (palate); and a thin, pinched, tapering nose. Many affected individuals also have clouding of the lenses of the eyes at birth (congenital cataracts); unusually small eyes (microphthalmia); and/or other ocular abnormalities. Dental defects may include the presence of certain teeth at birth (natal teeth) and absence (hypodontia or partial adontia), malformation, and/or improper alignment of teeth. In almost all cases, Hallermann-Streiff syndrome has appeared to occur randomly for unknown reasons (sporadically) and may be the result of a new change to genetic material (mutation).

Hypochondroplasia

Hypochondroplasia is a genetic disorder characterized by small stature and disproportionately short arms, legs, hands, and feet (short-limbed dwarfism). Short stature often is not recognized until early to mid childhood or, in some cases, as late as adulthood. In those with the disorder, bowing of the legs typically develops during early childhood but often improves spontaneously with age. Some affected individuals may also have an abnormally large head (macrocephaly), a relatively prominent forehead, and/or other physical abnormalities associated with the disorder. In addition, in about 10 percent of cases, mild mental retardation may be present.

In some cases, hypochondroplasia appears to occur randomly for unknown reasons (sporadically) with no apparent family history. In other instances, the disorder is familial with autosomal dominant inheritance.

Kniest Syndrome

Kniest syndrome is a type of dwarfism that is characterized by unusually short arms and legs, a round face with hollow or depressed areas, swelling and stiffness of the joints, and a stiff drawing up (contractures) of the fingers. Cleft palate, abnormal curvature of the spine (scoliosis), and vision and/or hearing problems may also occur. Intellect is usually normal in people with this syndrome.

Laron Syndrome

Laron syndrome (LTD1), a rare genetic disorder, is caused by the body's inability to use the growth hormone (GH) that it produces. The problem lies not in the production of growth hormone but rather in a defective GH-receptor. This defect prevents the proper binding of the GH molecule leaving high levels of unbound growth hormone in the plasma.

LTD1 is characterized by short stature, delayed bone age and, less frequently, blue eyes and hip degeneration as well as high levels of circulating growth hormone.

A second form of the disorder known as Laron syndrome type II (LTD2) shows typical clinical features of the Laron syndrome but is due to a defect in the biochemical processing of growth hormone after the hormone has been bound on the cell surface.

Metatropic Dysplasia I

Metatropic dysplasia I is a rare genetic disorder characterized by extremely small stature, with short arms and legs. Other characteristics of this disorder are a narrow thorax, short ribs, and kyphoscoliosis (backward and sideways curvature of the spinal column) which develops into short trunk dwarfism.

McKusick Type Metaphyseal Chondrodysplasia

McKusick type metaphyseal chondrodysplasia is a rare progressive inherited disorder characterized by unusually fine, sparse hair and short stature with abnormally short arms and legs (short-limbed dwarfism). Portions of the long bones of the arms and legs develop abnormally with unusual cartilage formations and subsequent abnormal bone formation at the large (bulbous) end portions (metaphyses) of these long bones (metaphyseal chondrodysplasia). In addition, most individuals with McKusick type metaphyseal chondrodysplasia may exhibit impairment of specialized cells (T-cells) that play an important role in helping the body's immune system to fight infection (cellular immunodeficiency). Affected individuals may also have abnormally low levels of certain white blood cells (neutropenia and lymphopenia); low levels of circulating red blood cells (anemia); and/or increased susceptibility to certain infections, such as chickenpox. In some cases, affected infants may also exhibit improper intestinal absorption of certain necessary nutrients (malabsorption) and/or dental abnormalities such as unusually small teeth (microdontia). Some individuals with the disorder may also have additional physical abnormalities. The range and severity of symptoms vary widely from case to case. McKusick type metaphyseal chondrodysplasia is inherited as an autosomal recessive genetic trait.

Multiple Epiphyseal Dysplasia

Multiple epiphyseal dysplasia (MED) is a rare inherited spectrum of disorders characterized by malformation (dysplasia) of the "growing portion" or head of the long bones (epiphyses). Affected individuals may have an abnormally short thighbone (femur), unusually short hands and fingers, mild short stature, a waddling gait, and/or pain in the hips and knees. In some cases, painful swelling and inflammation of certain joints (arthritis) may be present as early as five years of age. Most cases of multiple epiphyseal dysplasia are inherited as autosomal dominant traits; rare cases are inherited as autosomal recessive traits.

Pseudoachondroplastic Dysplasia

Pseudoachondroplastic dysplasia is a rare inherited disorder characterized by skeletal malformations resulting in short legs and mild to moderate short stature (short-limbed dwarfism). Affected individuals may have short, stubby fingers (brachydactyly), abnormally bowed legs (genu varum), and/or a malformation in which the knees are abnormally close together and the ankles are unusually far apart (genu valgum). In addition, affected individuals may have spinal abnormalities including abnormally increased curvature of the bones of the lower spine (lumbar lordosis) and front-to-back curvature of the spine (kyphosis). Cases of pseudoachondroplastic dysplasia are due to mutations of the *COMP* gene. Most cases of pseudoachondroplastic dysplasia are inherited as an autosomal dominant trait. However, a recessive form of the disorder may also exist.

Schwartz-Jampel Syndrome

Schwartz-Jampel syndrome (SJS) is a rare genetic disorder characterized by abnormalities of the skeletal muscles, including muscle weakness and stiffness (myotonic myopathy); abnormal bone development (bone dysplasia); permanent bending or extension of certain joints in a fixed position (joint contractures); and/or growth delays resulting in abnormally short stature (dwarfism). Affected individuals may also have small, fixed facial features and various abnormalities of the eyes, some of which may cause impaired vision. The range and severity of symptoms may vary from case to case. Two types of the disorder have been identified that may be differentiated by age of onset and other factors. Schwartz-Jampel syndrome type 1, which is considered the classical form of the disorder, may become apparent during early to late infancy or childhood. Schwartz-Jampel syndrome type 2, a more rare form of the disorder, is typically recognized at birth (congenital). Most researchers now believe that SJS type 2 is actually the same disorder as Stuve-Wiedemann syndrome and not a form of Schwartz-Jampel syndrome.

Schwartz-Jampel syndrome is thought to be inherited as an autosomal recessive trait. However, some cases reported in the medical literature suggest an autosomal dominant inheritance pattern.

Spondyloepiphyseal Dysplasia, Congenital

Congenital spondyloepiphyseal dysplasia is a rare genetic disorder characterized by growth deficiency before birth (prenatally), spinal malformations, and/or abnormalities affecting the eyes. As affected individuals age, growth deficiency eventually results in short stature (dwarfism) due, in part, to a disproportionately short neck and trunk, and a hip deformity in which the thigh bone is angled toward the center of the body (coxa vara). In most cases, affected individuals may have diminished muscle tone (hypotonia), abnormal front-to-back and side-to-side curvature of the spine (kyphoscoliosis), abnormal inward curvature of the spine (lumbar lordosis), and/or unusual protrusion of the breast bone (sternum), a condition known as pectus carinatum.

Affected individuals also have abnormalities affecting the eyes including nearsightedness (myopia) and, in approximately 50 percent of cases, detachment of the nerve-rich membrane lining the eye (retina). Congenital spondyloepiphyseal dysplasia is inherited as an autosomal dominant trait.

Spondyloepiphyseal Dysplasia Tarda

Spondyloepiphyseal dysplasia tarda (SEDT) is a rare, hereditary, skeletal disorder that affects males only. Physical characteristics include moderate short-stature (dwarfism), moderate to severe spinal deformities, barrel-chest, disproportionately short trunk, and premature osteoarthritis.

An extremely rare form of SEDT, the Toledo type, differs from typical SEDT by its autosomal recessive mode of genetic transmission and by the presence of a metabolic abnormality in the urine.

Weill-Marchesani Syndrome

Weill-Marchesani syndrome is a rare, genetic disorder characterized by short stature; an unusually short, broad head (brachycephaly) and other facial abnormalities; hand defects, including unusually short fingers (brachydactyly); and distinctive eye (ocular) abnormalities. These typically include unusually small, round lenses of the eyes (spherophakia) that may be prone to dislocating (ectopia lentis) as well as other ocular defects. Due to such abnormalities, affected individuals may have varying degrees of visual impairment, ranging from nearsightedness (myopia) to blindness. Researchers suggest that Weill-Marchesani syndrome may have autosomal recessive or autosomal dominant inheritance.

Chapter 14

Hereditary Deafness

Hearing is a complex process, so it should be no surprise that the causes of hearing loss are also complex. Hearing loss can occur because of damage to the ear, especially the inner ear. For example, infants may be born with hearing loss caused by a viral infection that was acquired during pregnancy. At other times the cause is genetic and therefore due to changes in the genes involved in the hearing process. Sometimes, hearing loss is due to a combination of genetic and environmental factors. There is, for example, a genetic change that makes some people more likely to develop hearing loss after taking certain antibiotic medications.

Understanding the genetic causes of deafness has important benefits. This knowledge not only allows doctors to inform families about their chances of having children with hearing loss, but it can also influence the way a person's deafness is treated. Whether a person's hearing loss is going to worsen can sometimes be predicted if the specific cause is known. Also, deafness may be only one of a group of medical problems that a person may have. For example, some people with hearing loss also have problems that affect other parts of the body, such as the heart, kidneys, or eyes. Knowing the genetic cause in these cases allows a doctor to be aware that there might be problems in other systems as well.

Excerpted with permission from, *Understanding the Genetics of Deafness: A Guide for Patients and Families,* a booklet by the Harvard Medical School Center for Hereditary Deafness. © 2004. All rights reserved. The complete text of this booklet is available at http://hearing.harvard.edu.

It might seem reasonable to suspect a genetic cause of deafness only if the hearing loss runs in the family. But it is common for children to have genetic deafness even though neither one of their parents are affected. This deafness can also be passed on to future generations. Genetic tests can, therefore, be helpful even if there is only one person in the family with hearing loss.

How is hearing loss detected and diagnosed?

It is important to detect hearing loss as early as possible so that a child can develop appropriate communication and learning skills. For this reason, many states now give a simple, painless hearing test to all newborn babies to determine if they can hear sound. Without this newborn screening, hearing losses might not be noticed by parents, teachers or doctors until the child begins to have difficulties speaking and learning, sometimes as late as age 2 or 3 years. Therefore, it is important to have this test done at a very early age. Babies who do not pass this screening test are referred to an audiologist for more in-depth testing.

An audiologist will first determine the severity and type of hearing loss. The severity of hearing loss is measured by observing how loud a sound needs to be for the child to hear it. This is often referred to as the hearing threshold level. The different types of hearing loss are classified according to what part of the hearing system is affected. Sound is picked up by the outer ear and then passes through the ear canal to the middle ear. Problems in these places cause conductive hearing loss. After passing through the middle ear, the sound then travels to a part of the inner ear called the cochlea, where it is changed to a signal that can be sent down the hearing nerve to the brain. Problems here cause sensorineural hearing loss.

Next, an effort is made to find the cause of the hearing loss. The pediatrician, family practitioner or audiologist involved in the care of the infant or child with a newly diagnosed hearing loss will often refer them to an otolaryngologist for further evaluation of the cause of the hearing loss. Some kinds of hearing loss occur when the hearing system is damaged by things like loud noise, head injury, medications, or infections. Sometimes, knowledge of these causes can help to treat the hearing loss or stop it from getting worse.

Another possibility is that the hearing loss is genetic. This means that it is carried down through a family. This is why recording a detailed family history is very important. There are two main forms of genetic deafness: syndromic, in which there can be other medical problems in addition to the hearing loss, and nonsyndromic, where the only obvious medical problem is the loss of hearing. Although most hereditary hearing loss is nonsyndromic, there are also many syndromes that have deafness as a feature. A list of common deafness syndromes is given in Table 14.1. Identification of these syndromes is particularly important in helping to predict whether other medical problems might occur. Deciding whether a hearing loss is syndromic or nonsyndromic is not always easy because some problems can be subtle or only detected by special tests. For example, a special eye exam is required to diagnose Usher syndrome and an electrocardiogram is needed to identify Jervell and Lange-Nielsen syndrome (see Table 14.1). As a result, a doctor may ask for the help of other specialists such as a cardiologist, ophthalmologist, or clinical geneticist.

Table 14.1. Common Forms of Syndromic Deafness

Syndrome	Main Features (Besides Deafness)
Alport	Kidney problems
Branchio-oto-renal	Neck cysts and kidney problems
Jervell and Lange-Nielsen	Heart problems
Neurofibromatosis type 2	Tumors of the hearing and balance nerve
Pendred	Thyroid enlargement
Stickler	Unusual facial features, eye problems, arthritis
Usher syndrome	Progressive blindness
Waardenburg syndrome	Skin pigment changes

Although a family history can help find a genetic cause, the absence of a family history of deafness does not mean that the deafness is not genetic. In fact, genetic deafness may appear for the first time in a child whose parents are not deaf and may not have any family history of deafness. It is, therefore, important to combine information from physical exams, clinical tests, a family history, and genetic tests to identify the cause of hearing loss. This can help in the treatment and management of the deafness, and to predict the possibility of passing on the deafness to future generations.

How is hearing loss inherited?

It is estimated that about half of all childhood deafness is due to hereditary causes. These hereditary causes involve genes in the hearing process that are inherited or passed down in a family.

There are also cases in which a genetic mutation is seen for the first time in a person whose parents do not carry the mutation. This type of mutation is called a spontaneous mutation and is usually caused because of a DNA change in a gene in the parent's sperm or egg cells. This is one way that genetic inheritance of a trait can suddenly begin within a family when ancestors were not affected. In this case it would have been impossible to predict that the child would be affected, but the chance of future generations having deafness can be determined.

Although there are many forms of hearing loss that are caused by mutations in single genes, other types are believed to require mutations in two or more genes for a person to be affected. Also, mutations in some genes do not appear to cause hearing loss directly. Instead, they put a person at risk for deafness due to environmental factors, such as exposure to loud noise or antibiotics. The continued study of people with hearing loss is needed to understand these situations and the sometimes complex connections between genetics and hearing loss.

Chapter 15

Huntington Disease

Introduction

In 1872, the American physician George Huntington wrote about an illness that he called "an heirloom from generations away back in the dim past." He was not the first to describe the disorder, which has been traced back to the middle ages at least. One of its earliest names was chorea, which, as in choreography, is the Greek word for dance. The term chorea describes how people affected with the disorder writhe, twist, and turn in a constant, uncontrollable dance-like motion. Later, other descriptive names evolved. Hereditary chorea emphasizes how the disease is passed from parent to child. Chronic progressive chorea stresses how symptoms of the disease worsen over time. Today, physicians commonly use the simple term Huntington disease (HD) to describe this highly complex disorder that causes untold suffering for thousands of families.

In the United States alone, about 30,000 people have HD; estimates of its prevalence are about one in every 10,000 persons. At least 150,000 others have a 50 percent risk of developing the disease and thousands more of their relatives live with the possibility that they, too, might develop HD.

Text in this chapter is excerpted from "Huntington's Disease—Hope through Research," National Institute of Neurological Disorders and Stroke (NINDS), 2001. The full text of this document is available online at http://www.ninds.nih.gov/health_and_medical/pubs/huntington_disease-htr.htm.

What Causes Huntington Disease?

HD results from genetically programmed degeneration of nerve cells, called neurons, in certain areas of the brain. This degeneration causes uncontrolled movements, loss of intellectual faculties, and emotional disturbance. Specifically affected are cells of the basal ganglia, structures deep within the brain that have many important functions, including coordinating movement. Within the basal ganglia, HD especially targets neurons of the striatum, particularly those in the caudate nuclei and the pallidum. Also affected is the brain's outer surface, or cortex, which controls thought, perception, and memory.

How Is HD Inherited?

HD is found in every country of the world. It is a familial disease, passed from parent to child through a mutation, or misspelling, in the normal gene.

The genetic defect responsible for HD is a small sequence of DNA on chromosome 4 in which several base pairs are repeated many, many times. The normal gene has three DNA bases, composed of the sequence CAG. In people with HD, the sequence abnormally repeats itself dozens of times. Over time—and with each successive generation—the number of CAG repeats may expand further.

Each parent has two copies of every chromosome but gives only one copy to each child. Each child of an HD parent has a 50/50 chance of inheriting the HD gene. If a child does not inherit the HD gene, he or she will not develop the disease and cannot pass it to subsequent generations. A person who inherits the HD gene, and survives long enough, will sooner or later develop the disease. In some families, all the children may inherit the HD gene; in others, none do. Whether one child inherits the gene has no bearing on whether others will or will not share the same fate.

A small number of cases of HD are sporadic, that is, they occur even though there is no family history of the disorder. These cases are thought to be caused by a new genetic mutation—an alteration in the gene that occurs during sperm development and that brings the number of CAG repeats into the range that causes disease.

What Are the Major Effects of the Disease?

Early signs of the disease vary greatly from person to person. A common observation is that the earlier the symptoms appear, the faster the disease progresses.

Family members may first notice that the individual experiences mood swings or becomes uncharacteristically irritable, apathetic, passive, depressed, or angry. These symptoms may lessen as the disease progresses or, in some individuals, may continue and include hostile outbursts or deep bouts of depression.

HD may affect the individual's judgment, memory, and other cognitive functions. Early signs might include having trouble driving, learning new things, remembering a fact, answering a question, or making a decision. Some may even display changes in handwriting. As the disease progresses, concentration on intellectual tasks becomes increasingly difficult.

In some individuals, the disease may begin with uncontrolled movements in the fingers, feet, face, or trunk. These movements—which are signs of chorea—often intensify when the person is anxious. HD can also begin with mild clumsiness or problems with balance. Some people develop choreic movements later, after the disease has progressed. They may stumble or appear uncoordinated. Chorea often creates serious problems with walking, increasing the likelihood of falls.

The disease can reach the point where speech is slurred and vital functions, such as swallowing, eating, speaking, and especially walking, continue to decline. Some individuals cannot recognize other family members. Many, however, remain aware of their environment and are able to express emotions.

Some physicians have employed a recently developed Unified HD Rating Scale, or UHDRS, to assess the clinical features, stages, and course of HD. In general, the duration of the illness ranges from 10 to 30 years. The most common causes of death are infection (most often pneumonia), injuries related to a fall, or other complications.

At What Age Does HD Appear?

The rate of disease progression and the age at onset vary from person to person. Adult-onset HD, with its disabling, uncontrolled movements, most often begins in middle age. There are, however, other variations of HD distinguished not just by age at onset but by a distinct array of symptoms. For example, some persons develop the disease as adults, but without chorea. They may appear rigid and move very little, or not at all, a condition called akinesia.

Some individuals develop symptoms of HD when they are very young—before age 20. The terms early-onset or juvenile HD are often used to describe HD that appears in a young person. A common sign of HD in a younger individual is a rapid decline in school performance. Symptoms can also include subtle changes in handwriting and slight problems with movement, such as slowness, rigidity, tremor, and rapid muscular twitching, called myoclonus. Several of these symptoms are similar to those seen in Parkinson's disease, and they differ from the chorea seen in individuals who develop the disease as adults. These young individuals are said to have akinetic-rigid HD or the Westphal variant of HD. People with juvenile HD may also have seizures and mental disabilities. The earlier the onset, the faster the disease seems to progress. The disease progresses most rapidly in individuals with juvenile or early-onset HD, and death often follows within 10 years.

Individuals with juvenile HD usually inherit the disease from their fathers. These individuals also tend to have the largest number of CAG repeats. The reason for this may be found in the process of sperm production. Unlike eggs, sperm are produced in the millions. Because DNA is copied millions of times during this process, there is an increased possibility for genetic mistakes to occur. To verify the link between the number of CAG repeats in the HD gene and the age at onset of symptoms, scientists studied a boy who developed HD symptoms at the age of two, one of the youngest and most severe cases ever recorded. They found that he had the largest number of CAG repeats of anyone studied so far—nearly 100. The boy's case was central to the identification of the HD gene and at the same time helped confirm that juveniles with HD have the longest segments of CAG repeats, the only proven correlation between repeat length and age at onset.

A few individuals develop HD after age 55. Diagnosis in these people can be very difficult. The symptoms of HD may be masked by other health problems, or the person may not display the severity of symptoms seen in individuals with HD of earlier onset. These individuals may also show symptoms of depression rather than anger or irritability, or they may retain sharp control over their intellectual functions, such as memory, reasoning, and problem-solving.

There is also a related disorder called senile chorea. Some elderly individuals display the symptoms of HD, especially choreic movements, but do not become demented, have a normal gene, and lack a family history of the disorder. Some scientists believe that a different gene mutation may account for this small number of cases, bu this has not been proven.

How Is HD Diagnosed?

The discovery of the HD gene in 1993 resulted in a direct genetic test to make or confirm a diagnosis of HD in an individual who is exhibiting HD-like symptoms. Using a blood sample, the genetic test

162

analyzes DNA for the HD mutation by counting the number of repeats in the HD gene region. Individuals who do not have HD usually have 28 or fewer CAG repeats. Individuals with HD usually have 40 or more repeats. A small percentage of individuals, however, have a number of repeats that fall within a borderline region (see Table 15.1).

Table 15.1. CAG Repeats and Risk for Developing Huntington Disease

Number of CAG Repeats	Outcome
less than or equal to 28	Normal range; individual will not develop HD
29–34	Individual will not develop HD but the next generation is at risk
35–39	Some, but not all, individuals in this range will develop HD; next generation is also at risk
greater than or equal to 40	Individual will develop HD

What Is Presymptomatic Testing?

Presymptomatic testing is used for people who have a family history of HD but have no symptoms themselves. If either parent had HD, the person's chance would be 50/50. In the past, no laboratory test could positively identify people carrying the HD gene—or those fated to develop HD—before the onset of symptoms. That situation changed in 1983, when a team of scientists supported by the National Institute of Neurological Disorders and Stroke (NINDS) located the first genetic marker for HD—the initial step in developing a laboratory test for the disease.

A marker is a piece of DNA that lies near a gene and is usually inherited with it. Discovery of the first HD marker allowed scientists to locate the HD gene on chromosome 4. The marker discovery quickly led to the development of a presymptomatic test for some individuals, but this test required blood or tissue samples from both affected and unaffected family members in order to identify markers unique to that particular family. For this reason, adopted individuals, orphans, and people who had few living family members were unable to use the test.

Discovery of the HD gene has led to a less expensive, scientifically simpler, and far more accurate presymptomatic test that is applicable to the majority of at-risk people. The new test uses CAG repeat length to detect the presence of the HD mutation in blood.

There are many complicating factors that reflect the complexity of diagnosing HD. In a small number of individuals with HD—one to three percent—no family history of HD can be found. Some individuals may not be aware of their genetic legacy, or a family member may conceal a genetic disorder from fear of social stigma. A parent may not want to worry children, scare them, or deter them from marrying. In other cases, a family member may die of another cause before he or she begins to show signs of HD. Sometimes, the cause of death for a relative may not be known, or the family is not aware of a relative's death. Adopted children may not know their genetic heritage, or early symptoms in an individual may be too slight to attract attention.

How Does a Person Decide Whether to be Tested?

The anxiety that comes from living with a 50 percent risk for HD can be overwhelming. How does a young person make important choices about long-term education, marriage, and children? How do older parents of adult children cope with their fears about children and grandchildren? How do people come to terms with the ambiguity and uncertainty of living at risk?

Some individuals choose to undergo the test out of a desire for greater certainty about their genetic status. They believe the test will enable them to make more informed decisions about the future. Others choose not to take the test. They are able to make peace with the uncertainty of being at risk, preferring to forego the emotional consequences of a positive result, as well as possible losses of insurance and employment. There is no right or wrong decision, as each choice is highly individual.

Whatever the results of genetic testing, the at-risk individual and family members can expect powerful and complex emotional responses. The health and happiness of spouses, brothers and sisters, children, parents, and grandparents are affected by a positive test result, as are an individual's friends, work associates, neighbors, and others. Because receiving test results may prove to be devastating, testing guidelines call for continued counseling even after the test is complete and the results are known.

Is There a Treatment for HD?

Physicians may prescribe a number of medications to help control emotional and movement problems associated with HD. It is important to remember however, that while medicines may help keep these clinical symptoms under control, there is no treatment to stop or reverse the course of the disease.

Antipsychotic drugs, such as haloperidol, or other drugs, such as clonazepam, may help to alleviate choreic movements and may also be used to help control hallucinations, delusions, and violent outbursts. Antipsychotic drugs, however, are not prescribed for another form of muscle contraction associated with HD, called dystonia, and may in fact worsen the condition, causing stiffness and rigidity. These medications may also have severe side effects, including sedation, and for that reason should be used in the lowest possible doses.

For depression, physicians may prescribe fluoxetine, sertraline, nortriptyline, or other compounds. Tranquilizers can help control anxiety and lithium may be prescribed to combat pathological excitement and severe mood swings. Medications may also be needed to treat the severe obsessive-compulsive rituals of some individuals with HD.

Most drugs used to treat the symptoms of HD have side effects such as fatigue, restlessness, or hyperexcitability. Sometimes it may be difficult to tell if a particular symptom, such as apathy or incontinence, is a sign of the disease or a reaction to medication.

What Kind of Care Does the Individual with HD Need?

Although a psychologist or psychiatrist, a genetic counselor, and other specialists may be needed at different stages of the illness, usually the first step in diagnosis and in finding treatment is to see a neurologist. While the family doctor may be able to diagnose HD, and may continue to monitor the individual's status, it is better to consult with a neurologist about management of the varied symptoms.

Problems may arise when individuals try to express complex thoughts in words they can no longer pronounce intelligibly. It can be helpful to repeat words back to the person with HD so that he or she knows that some thoughts are understood. Sometimes people mistakenly assume that if individuals do not talk, they also do not understand. Never isolate individuals by not talking, and try to keep their environment as normal as possible. Speech therapy may improve the individual's ability to communicate.

It is extremely important for the person with HD to maintain physical fitness as much as his or her condition and the course of the disease allows. Individuals who exercise and keep active tend to do better than those who do not. A daily regimen of exercise can help the person feel better physically and mentally. Although their coordination may be poor, individuals should continue walking, with assistance if necessary. Those who want to walk independently should be allowed to do so as long as possible, and careful attention should be given to keeping their environment free of hard, sharp objects. This will help ensure maximal independence while minimizing the risk of injury from a fall. Individuals can also wear special padding during walks to help protect against injury from falls. Some people have found that small weights around the ankles can help stability. Wearing sturdy shoes that fit well can help too, especially shoes without laces that can be slipped on or off easily.

Impaired coordination may make it difficult for people with HD to feed themselves and to swallow. As the disease progresses, persons with HD may even choke. In helping individuals to eat, caregivers should allow plenty of time for meals. Food can be cut into small pieces, softened, or pureed to ease swallowing and prevent choking. While some foods may require the addition of thickeners, other foods may need to be thinned. Dairy products, in particular, tend to increase the secretion of mucus, which in turn increases the risk of choking. Some individuals may benefit from swallowing therapy, which is especially helpful if started before serious problems arise. Suction cups for plates, special tableware designed for people with disabilities, and plastic cups with tops can help prevent spilling. The individual's physician can offer additional advice about diet and about how to handle swallowing difficulties or gastrointestinal problems that might arise, such as incontinence or constipation.

Caregivers should pay attention to proper nutrition so that the individual with HD takes in enough calories to maintain his or her body weight. Sometimes people with HD, who may burn as many as 5,000 calories a day without gaining weight, require five meals a day to take in the necessary number of calories. Physicians may recommend vitamins or other nutritional supplements. In a long-term care institution, staff will need to assist with meals in order to ensure that the individual's special caloric and nutritional requirements are met. Some individuals and their families choose to use a feeding tube; others choose not to.

Individuals with HD are at special risk for dehydration and therefore require large quantities of fluids, especially during hot weather. Bendable straws can make drinking easier for the person. In some cases, water may have to be thickened with commercial additives to give it the consistency of syrup or honey.

What Research Is Being Done?

Although HD attracted considerable attention from scientists in the early 20th century, there was little sustained research on the disease until the late 1960s when the Committee to Combat Huntington Disease and the Huntington Chorea Foundation, later called the Hereditary Disease Foundation, first began to fund research and to campaign for federal funding. In 1977, Congress established the Commission for the Control of Huntington Disease and Its Consequences, which made a series of important recommendations. Since then, Congress has provided consistent support for federal research, primarily through the National Institute of Neurological Disorders and Stroke, the government's lead agency for biomedical research on disorders of the brain and nervous system. The effort to combat HD proceeds along the following lines of inquiry, each providing important information about the disease:

- **Basic neurobiology:** Now that the HD gene has been located, investigators in the field of neurobiology—which encompasses the anatomy, physiology, and biochemistry of the nervous system—are continuing to study the HD gene with an eye toward understanding how it causes disease in the human body.

- **Clinical research:** Neurologists, psychologists, psychiatrists, and other investigators are improving our understanding of the symptoms and progression of the disease in patients while attempting to develop new therapeutics.

- **Imaging:** Scientific investigations using PET and other technologies are enabling scientists to see what the defective gene does to various structures in the brain and how it affects the body's chemistry and metabolism.

- **Animal models:** Laboratory animals, such as mice, are being bred in the hope of duplicating the clinical features of HD and can soon be expected to help scientists learn more about the symptoms and progression of the disease.

- **Fetal tissue research:** Investigators are implanting fetal tissue in rodents and nonhuman primates with the hope that success in this area will lead to understanding, restoring, or replacing functions typically lost by neuronal degeneration in individuals with HD.

These areas of research are slowly converging and, in the process, are yielding important clues about the gene's relentless destruction of mind and body. The NINDS supports much of this exciting work.

Clinical Studies

Scientists are pursuing clinical studies that may one day lead to the development of new drugs or other treatments to halt the disease's progression. Examples of NINDS-supported investigations, using both asymptomatic and symptomatic individuals, include:

- **Genetic studies on age of onset, inheritance patterns, and markers found within families:** These studies may shed additional light on how HD is passed from generation to generation.

- **Studies of cognition, intelligence, and movement:** Studies of abnormal eye movements, both horizontal and vertical, and tests of patients' skills in a number of learning, memory, neuropsychological, and motor tasks may serve to identify when the various symptoms of HD appear and to characterize their range and severity.

- **Clinical trials of drugs:** Testing of various drugs may lead to new treatments and at the same time improve our understanding of the disease process in HD. Classes of drugs being tested include those that control symptoms, slow the rate of progression of HD, and block effects of excitotoxins, and those that might correct or replace other metabolic defects contributing to the development and progression of HD.

Imaging

NINDS-supported scientists are using positron emission tomography (PET) to learn how the gene affects the chemical systems of the body. PET visualizes metabolic or chemical abnormalities in the body, and investigators hope to ascertain if PET scans can reveal any abnormalities that signal HD. Investigators conducting HD research are also using PET to characterize neurons that have died and chemicals that are depleted in parts of the brain affected by HD.

Like PET, a form of magnetic resonance imaging (MRI) called functional MRI can measure increases or decreases in certain brain chemicals thought to play a key role in HD. Functional MRI studies are also helping investigators understand how HD kills neurons in different regions of the brain.

Imaging technologies allow investigators to view changes in the volume and structures of the brain and to pinpoint when these changes occur in HD. Scientists know that in brains affected by HD, the basal ganglia, cortex, and ventricles all show atrophy or other alterations.

How Can I Help?

In order to conduct HD research, investigators require samples of tissue or blood from families with HD. Access to individuals with HD and their families may be difficult however, because families with HD are often scattered across the country or around the world. A research project may need individuals of a particular age or gender or from a certain geographic area. Some scientists need only statistical data while others may require a sample of blood, urine, or skin from family members. All of these factors complicate the task of finding volunteers. The following NINDS-supported efforts bring together families with HD, voluntary health agencies, and scientists in an effort to advance science and speed a cure.

The NINDS-sponsored HD Research Roster at the Indiana University Medical Center in Indianapolis, which was discussed earlier, makes research possible by matching scientists with patient and family volunteers. The first DNA bank was established through the roster. Although the gene has already been located, DNA from individuals who have HD is still of great interest to investigators. Of continuing interest are twins, unaffected individuals who have affected offspring, and individuals with two defective HD genes, one from each parent—a very rare occurrence. Participation in the roster and in specific research projects is voluntary and confidential. For more information about the roster and DNA bank, contact:

Indiana University Medical Center
Department of Medical and Molecular Genetics
Medical Research and Library Building
975 W. Walnut Street
Indianapolis, IN 46202-5251

Brain tissue is also critical to the HD research effort, and many individuals are willing to donate their brains and other organs to research after they die. The NINDS supports two national human brain specimen banks, one at the Greater Los Angeles Health Care System, and the other at McLean Hospital near Boston. These banks supply investigators around the world with tissue not only from individuals with HD but also from those with other neurological or psychiatric diseases. Both banks need brain tissue to enable scientists to study these disorders more intensely. Prospective donors should contact:

Harvard Brain Tissue Resource Center
McLean Hospital
115 Mill Street
Belmont, MA 02178
Toll-Free: 800-BRAIN-BANK (800-272-4622)
Phone: 617-855-2400
Fax: 617-855-3199
Website: http://www.brainbank.mclean.org
E-mail: btrc@mclean.harvard.edu

Human Brain and Spinal Fluid Resource Center
Greater Los Angeles Health Care System
11301 Wilshire Boulevard
Los Angeles, CA 90073
Phone: 310-268-3536
Fax: 310-269-4768
Website: http://www.loni.ucla.edu/%7Ennrsb/NNRSB
E-mail: brainbnk@ucla.edu

What Is the Role of Voluntary Organizations?

Private organizations have been a mainstay of support and guidance for at-risk individuals, people with HD, and their families. These organizations vary in size and emphasis, but all are concerned with helping individuals and their families, educating lay and professional audiences about HD, and promoting medical research on the disorder. Some voluntary health agencies support scientific workshops and research and some have newsletters and local chapters throughout the country. These agencies enable families, health professionals, and investigators to exchange information, learn of available services and benefits, and work toward common goals.

Chapter 16

Inborn Errors of Metabolism

Chapter Contents

Section 16.1—Biotinidase Deficiency.................................... 172
Section 16.2—Galactosemia... 173
Section 16.3—Maple Syrup Urine Disease............................. 175
Section 16.4—Phenylketonuria (PKU) 177
Section 16.5—Tyrosinemia 182
Section 16.6—Urea Cycle Disorders 184

Section 16.1

Biotinidase Deficiency

From Genetics Home Reference, a service of the U.S. National Library of Medicine (http://ghr.nlm.nih.gov), January 2004.

What is biotinidase deficiency?

Biotinidase deficiency is an inherited disorder in which the body is not able to process the vitamin biotin properly. Biotin, sometimes called vitamin H, is an important water-soluble vitamin that aids in the metabolism of fats, carbohydrates, and proteins.

How common is biotinidase deficiency?

Approximately 1 in 60,000 newborns are affected by profound (less than 10 percent of normal enzyme activity) or partial (10–30 percent of normal enzyme activity) biotinidase deficiency.

What genes are related to biotinidase deficiency?

Mutations in the *BTD* gene cause biotinidase deficiency.

Biotinidase is the enzyme that is made by the *BTD* gene. Many mutations that cause the enzyme to be nonfunctional or to be made at extremely low levels have been identified. Biotin is a vitamin that is chemically bound to proteins. (Most vitamins are only loosely associated with proteins.) Without biotinidase activity, the vitamin biotin cannot be separated from foods and therefore cannot be used by the body. Another function of the biotinidase enzyme is to recycle biotin from enzymes that are important in metabolism. When biotin is lacking, specific enzymes called carboxylases cannot function to metabolize proteins, fats, or carbohydrates. Individuals lacking biotinidase activity can still have normal carboxylases if they ingest small amounts of biotin.

How do people inherit biotinidase deficiency?

This condition is inherited in an autosomal recessive pattern, which means two copies of the gene must be altered for a person to be affected by the disorder. Most often, the parents of a child with an autosomal recessive disorder are not affected but are carriers of one copy of the altered gene.

Section 16.2

Galactosemia

Galactosemia is a rare hereditary disease leading not only to cirrhosis in infants, but more seriously, to early devastating illness if not diagnosed quickly. This disease is caused by elevated levels of galactose (a sugar in milk) in the blood resulting from a deficiency of the liver enzyme required for its metabolism (breakdown).

Risk: To have the disease, a child must inherit the tendency from both parents. The incidence of the disease is approximately one in 20,000 live births. For each pregnancy, in such a family, there is a one in four chance a baby will be born with the deficiency. Because of the potential disastrous side effects of late diagnosis, many states have mandatory neonatal screening programs for galactosemia. The disease usually appears in the first days of life following the ingestion of breast milk or formula.

Symptoms: Vomiting, liver enlargement, and jaundice are often the earliest signs of the disease, but bacterial infections (often severe), irritability, failure to gain weight, and diarrhea may also occur. If unrecognized in the newborn period, the disease may produce liver, brain, eye and kidney damage.

Diagnosis: Blood tests can make the diagnosis. The disease is detected by measuring the level of enzyme in red blood cells, white blood cells, or the liver. Affected patients have no enzyme activity; carriers (parents) have intermediate enzyme activity (about ½ the normal level). A galactose tolerance test should never be done, as it may be harmful. Affected infants who ingest galactose will excrete it in large quantities in their urine where it can also be detected. If the infant is vomiting, and not taking milk, the test can be negative. If the disease is suspected, the diagnosis should be confirmed by blood testing.

Treatment: Treatment is based on elimination of galactose from the diet. This may be done in the early neonatal period by stopping breast feeding and by the administration of diets which contain no lactose or galactose (Nutramigen, Pregestimil). This diet should be compulsively followed, and continued for years, and possibly for life. The red blood cell levels of galactose or its metabolites (galactose-1-phosphate) may be used as a monitor to gauge the adherence to the diet and restriction of galactose. It is also recommended that mothers of affected infants be placed on a galactose-free diet during the subsequent pregnancy. This may somewhat modify symptoms present at birth.

With early therapy, any liver damage which occurred in the first few days of life will nearly completely heal. Galactosemia should be considered in any jaundiced infant because of beneficial effects of early dietary restriction.

Section 16.3

Maple Syrup Urine Disease

Description: Maple syrup urine disease (MSUD) is an inherited metabolic disorder, that, if untreated, causes mental retardation, physical disabilities, and death. First described as a disease in 1954, it is a rare disorder, believed to be in all ethnic groups worldwide. The national incidence is one in 225,000 births. Among Mennonites in eastern Pennsylvania the incidence is about one in 760 births.

MSUD derives its name from the sweet, burnt sugar, or maple syrup smell of the urine. The disorder affects the way the body metabolizes (processes) certain components of protein. These components are the three branched-chain amino acids leucine, isoleucine, and valine. These amino acids accumulate in the blood causing a toxic effect that interferes with brain functions.

Types and Symptoms: The term, maple syrup urine disease, includes a range of classic and variant types of the disorder. The symptoms of classic MSUD are usually evident within the first week of life. Variant forms of MSUD are milder, however, the symptoms can be severe during times of illness.

The first symptoms in an infant are poor appetite, irritability, and the characteristic odor of the urine. Within days they lose their sucking reflex and grow listless, have a high-pitched cry, and become limp with episodes of rigidity. Without diagnosis and treatment, symptoms progress rapidly to seizures, coma, and death. In some variant types, failure to thrive may be the first sign. The earlier these children are diagnosed and treated, the less risk of permanent damage.

Testing for MSUD: Some states test for MSUD in their newborn screening programs. MSUD should be included in all screening programs. Ideally each infant should be tested within 24 hours of birth and the test results available by two to three days of age. This should be the goal of all testing for MSUD. Early diagnosis is of paramount importance for the child with MSUD to develop normally. Unfortunately some variant types of MSUD may be missed with screening programs. However, any child at risk or suspected of having MSUD should be tested. If the result is positive, or suspected to be positive, treatment should be started immediately.

Testing to identify carriers is only available for the Mennonite classic type of MSUD. The Mennonite population from eastern Pennsylvania is at high risk for this classic form of the disorder.

Treatment: Treatment of children with MSUD must be started as soon as possible, preferably at birth. It involves a complex approach of maintaining metabolic control. A special, carefully controlled diet is the focus of daily treatment. This requires careful monitoring of protein intake and close medical supervision.

The diet centers around a synthetic formula or "medical food" which provides nutrients and all the amino acids except leucine, isoleucine, and valine. These three amino acids are added to the diet with carefully controlled amounts of food to provide the protein necessary for normal growth and development without exceeding the level of tolerance.

Various tests are available to monitor the levels of the amino acids and their keto acid derivatives in the blood and urine. Illnesses and stress, as well as consuming too much protein, raise these levels. Even mild illnesses can become life threatening. A metabolic imbalance requires dietary changes and at times hospitalization.

Heredity: Each parent of a child with MSUD carries a defective gene for MSUD along with a normal gene. The defective gene is a recessive gene; therefore, parents are called "carriers" and are not affected by the disease. Each child receives one gene from each parent.

When both parents are carriers, there is a one in four chance with each pregnancy that the baby will receive a defective gene from each parent and have MSUD; a two in four chance the baby will receive one defective and one normal gene becoming a carrier of MSUD; and a one in four chance the baby will receive two normal genes. Persons with two normal genes cannot pass MSUD to their offspring.

Section 16.4

Phenylketonuria (PKU)

Questions and Answers about PKU

PKU (phenylketonuria) is an inherited disorder of body chemistry that, if untreated, causes mental retardation. Fortunately, through routine newborn screening, almost all affected newborns are now diagnosed and treated early, allowing them to grow up with normal intelligence.

About one baby in 15,000 is born with PKU in the United States. The disorder occurs in all ethnic groups, although it is more common in individuals of Northern European and Native American ancestry than in those of African-American, Hispanic, and Asian ancestry.

What is PKU?

Due to a missing or deficient enzyme, children with PKU cannot process a part of the protein called phenylalanine, which is present in nearly all foods. Without treatment, phenylalanine builds up in the bloodstream and causes brain damage and mental retardation.

How does PKU affect a child?

Children born with PKU appear normal for the first few months. If untreated, by three to six months they begin to lose interest in their surroundings and, by the time they are a year old, they are obviously developmentally delayed. Children with untreated PKU who have suffered central nervous system damage often are irritable, restless,

177

and destructive. They may have a musty odor about them, and may have dry skin, rashes, or convulsions. They usually are physically well developed and tend to have blonder hair than their siblings.

Who gets PKU?

PKU is inherited when both parents have the PKU gene and both pass it on to their baby. A parent who has the PKU gene, but not the disease, is called a "carrier." A carrier has a normal gene as well as a PKU gene in each cell. A carrier's health is not affected in any known way.

When both parents are carriers, there is a one-in-four (25 percent) chance that both will pass the PKU gene on to a child, causing the child to be born with the disease. There also is a two in four (50-50) chance that the baby will inherit the PKU gene from one parent and the normal gene from the other, making it a carrier like its parents. There also is a one-in-four chance that both will pass on the normal gene, and the baby will neither have the disease nor be a carrier. These chances are the same in each pregnancy.

Are all babies tested for PKU?

All states and U.S. territories screen for PKU. Babies are tested before they leave the hospital. This was the nation's first newborn screening test. Developed with the help of the March of Dimes, the test has been routinely administered since the 1960s, sparing thousands of children from mental retardation.

How is the test done?

The baby's heel is pricked and a few drops of blood are taken. (The same blood sample can be used to screen for a number of other inborn errors of body chemistry.) The blood generally is sent to a regional medical laboratory to find out if it has more than a normal amount of phenylalanine, and findings are sent to the health care professional responsible for the baby's care. If results are abnormal, more tests are done to determine whether the baby has PKU or if there is some other cause of high phenylalanine levels.

The test is highly accurate when performed as recommended, when the baby is more than 24 hours of age but less than seven days. However, early discharge from the hospital is becoming more common, and many babies are tested within the first 24 hours of life. Since some cases of PKU can be missed when the test is performed this early, the American Academy of Pediatrics recommends that infants whose initial test was taken within the first 24 hours of life be tested again at one to two weeks of age.

Can PKU symptoms be prevented?

Yes. Mental retardation can be prevented if the baby is treated with a special diet that is low in phenylalanine begun within the first 7 to 10 days of life.

At first, the baby is fed a special formula that contains protein but no phenylalanine. Breast milk or infant formula is used sparingly to supply only as much phenylalanine as the baby can tolerate. Later, certain vegetables, fruits, some grain products (for example, certain cereals and noodles) and other low-phenylalanine foods are added to the diet, but no regular milk, cheese, eggs, meat, fish, and other high protein foods are ever allowed. Since protein is essential for normal growth and development, the child must continue to have one of the special formulas which are high in protein and essential nutrients, but contain little or no phenylalanine. Diet drinks and foods that contain the artificial sweetener aspartame (which contains phenylalanine and is sold as NutraSweet® or Equal®) must be strictly avoided.

Children and adults with PKU require follow-up care at a medical center or clinic that specializes in this disorder. The diet for each person must be individualized, depending upon how much phenylalanine can be tolerated, his or her age, weight, and other factors. All affected persons need regular blood tests to measure if the levels of phenylalanine are too high or too low. Testing for babies may be as often as once a week for the first year, then once or twice a month throughout childhood. The diet must then be adjusted accordingly.

Individuals with PKU must remain on a restricted diet throughout childhood and adolescence, and generally for life (although some relaxation of the diet may be possible in some cases as the individual ages). Until the 1980s, health care providers believed that children with PKU could safely discontinue their special diet around age 6 when brain growth was completed. However, high blood levels of phenylalanine in children and adolescents can lead to a decrease in IQ, to learning disabilities, and to behavioral disturbances in most—but perhaps not all—children with PKU.

Parents of children with PKU and affected adults should discuss their diet and treatment questions with health care professionals at one of the special clinics for PKU.

What is maternal PKU?

There are an estimated 3,000 healthy young women of childbearing age with successfully treated PKU in the United States. Most discontinued their special diet in childhood because, at that time, most doctors believed it was safe to do so.

If these young women are eating a normal diet, their blood phenylalanine levels are very high when they become pregnant. During pregnancy, high blood levels of phenylalanine in the mother are devastating to the fetus. In up to 90 percent of such cases, the babies will have mental retardation and/or a small head size (microcephaly). Many also will have heart defects, low birthweight, and characteristic facial features. Because most of these babies do not inherit PKU, but are suffering from brain damage entirely caused by their mothers' high phenylalanine levels during pregnancy, they cannot be helped by the PKU diet.

Fortunately, there is a way to help prevent mental retardation and other problems in babies of women with PKU. It is now clear that these young women need to resume their special diets at least three months prior to pregnancy and continue the diet throughout pregnancy. This controls the blood phenylalanine levels so they can have a healthy baby. They will need at least weekly blood tests throughout pregnancy to make sure blood phenylalanine levels are not too high.

The March of Dimes urges all young women who know or suspect that they were treated for PKU as children to contact their health care provider or clinic before they attempt to conceive, so that their blood phenylalanine levels can be measured and the special diet begun, if necessary.

Occasionally, a woman has undiagnosed PKU that can pose a risk to her baby. These women, who generally were not screened as newborns, usually are mildly affected, and may be diagnosed only following the birth of a baby with PKU-related birth defects. In order to help prevent these birth defects, some doctors recommend screening women who may be at risk of PKU, such as those with a family history of the disorder, so affected women can start the PKU diet prior to pregnancy.

What is new in PKU research?

Researchers are studying the long-term outcome for children who were born from treated maternal PKU pregnancies. While these children usually do not have birth defects, researchers want to see if these children reach their full cognitive potential.

Others are developing a genetically engineered version of the missing enzyme, which eventually may allow affected individuals to eat a more normal diet. March of Dimes and other researchers also are exploring the possibility of treating PKU using gene therapy.

References

ACOG Committee on Genetics. "Maternal phenylketonuria." Committee Opinion, number 230, January 2000.

Hanley, W.B., et al. Undiagnosed maternal phenylketonuria: the need for prenatal selective screening or case finding. *American Journal of Obstetrics and Gynecology*, volume 180, number 4, April 1999, pages 986-994.

National Institutes of Health Consensus Development Statement. "Phenylketonuria: Screening and Management." Washington, D.C., October 16–18, 2000.

Extending the Successful Prevention of Mental Retardation through Newborn Screening

When women with phenylketonuria (PKU)—a metabolic disorder diagnosed in newborns—do not follow a special diet, their babies are at risk for mental retardation. The results of a small interview study conducted by the Centers for Disease Control (CDC) were released in the February 15, 2002 edition of the *Morbidity and Mortality Weekly Report* (*MMWR*). The article, "Barriers to Successful Dietary Control Among Pregnant Women with Phenylketonuria," states that two thirds of the participants in the study were not properly managing their diets at the time they conceived.

The prevention of mental retardation associated with PKU has been successful with the aid of newborn screening. Unfortunately, preventing maternal PKU-associated mental retardation is more challenging. Although a special diet for those diagnosed with PKU is recommended for life, it is often discontinued during adolescence. When women with PKU become pregnant and do not follow their diets, their babies are very likely to be affected by mental retardation and other birth defects. These birth outcomes are not caused by PKU in the infant, but by the mother's condition. Most of the birth defects can be prevented in babies if mothers maintain PKU-specific diets before and during pregnancy.

Dr. José Cordero, Director, National Center on Birth Defects and Developmental Disabilities, said the CDC study indicates several barriers might complicate affected women's ability to follow the life-long diet, including cost, adverse tastes, and poor adherence to medical recommendations. "To ensure that women with PKU have healthy babies, it is critical that women stay on their special diets and that we find effective ways to help them and their babies," Cordero said. "To successfully prevent maternal PKU-associated mental retardation, these barriers must be addressed."

Section 16.5

Tyrosinemia

Hereditary tyrosinemia is a genetic inborn error of metabolism associated with severe liver disease in infancy. The disease is inherited in an autosomal recessive fashion which means that both parents must be carriers of the gene for the disease. In such families, there is a one out of four risk that pregnancies will produce an affected infant.

The clinical features of the disease tend to fall into two categories:

- In the so-called acute form of the disease, abnormalities appear in the first month of life. Babies may show poor weight gain, enlarged liver and spleen, distended abdomen, swelling of the legs and increased tendency to bleeding, particularly nose bleeds. Jaundice may or may not be prominent. Despite vigorous therapy, death from hepatic failure frequently occurs between three and nine months of age. Children with this form of disease are excellent candidates for liver transplantation.

- Some children have a more chronic form of tyrosinemia with a gradual onset and less severe clinical features. In these, enlargement of the liver and spleen are prominent, the abdomen is distended with fluid, weight gain may be poor, and vomiting and diarrhea occur frequently. Affected patients usually develop cirrhosis and its complications. In older patients, there is an increases risk of liver cancer. These children also require liver transplantation.

Diagnosis: Liver tests are often abnormal. Low serum albumin and clotting factors are frequently found. The transaminases (liver enzymes) may be mildly to moderately elevated, but the bilirubin is increased to a variable extent. Because of the biochemical defect, abnormal products may be measured in the urine which confirm diagnosis. These are parahydroxy phenyllactic acid and parahydroxy phenylpyruvic acid. In addition, succinylacetone and succinylacetoacetate are found in the urine.

There may be hypoglycemia (low blood sugar) and evidence of loss of certain substances in the urine including sugar, protein, and amino acids. The basic biochemical defect is an abnormality in a key enzyme in the metabolism of an essential amino acid, phenylalanine. The enzyme is fumarylacetoacetate hydrolase (FAH) which is markedly reduced in affected patients. As a consequence, toxic metabolic products in the pathway by which phenylalanine is utilized build up and damage a variety of tissues, although the major findings occur in the liver and kidneys.

Prenatal diagnosis is possible and can be performed by measuring succinylacetone in the amniotic fluid or fumarylacetoacetate hydrolase (FAH) in amniotic fluid cells. This allows for genetic counseling and consideration of termination of pregnancy in affected infants.

Treatment: Although treatment has not been shown to be of benefit, it is customary to place affected infants on diets low in phenylalanine, methionine, and tyrosine. This will lead to normal blood amino acid levels which may be of some value. Strict attention to excellent nutrition, adequate vitamin and mineral intake, prevents nutritional deterioration and helps keep the patient as well as possible for transplantation. The most effective form of therapy at the present time is liver transplantation.

Section 16.6

Urea Cycle Disorders

What is a urea cycle disorder?

A urea cycle disorder is a genetic disorder caused by a deficiency of one of six enzymes in the urea cycle which is responsible for removing ammonia from the blood stream. The urea cycle involves a series of biochemical steps in which nitrogen, a waste product of protein metabolism, is removed from the blood and converted to urea. Normally, the urea is transferred into the urine and removed from the body. In urea cycle disorders, the nitrogen accumulates in the form of ammonia, a highly toxic substance, and is not removed from the body. Ammonia then reaches the brain through the blood, where it causes irreversible brain damage and/or death.

Urea cycle disorders are included in the category of inborn errors of metabolism. There is no cure. Inborn errors of metabolism are generally considered to be rare but represent a substantial cause of brain damage and death among newborns and infants. Because many cases of urea cycle disorders remain undiagnosed and/or infants born with the disorders die without a definitive diagnosis, the exact incidence of these cases is unknown and underestimated. It is believed that many sudden infant death syndrome cases may be attributed to an undiagnosed inborn error of metabolism such a urea cycle disorder. In April 2000, research experts at the Urea Cycle Consensus Conference estimated the incidence of the disorders at one in 10,000 births. This represents a significant increase in case diagnosis in the last two years. One of the goals of the Foundation is to educate the medical community at large in the identification and treatment of urea cycle disorders in order that timely intervention will result in saving the lives of these children.

What are the symptoms?

The Neonatal Period: Children with severe urea cycle disorders typically show symptoms after the first 24 hours of life. The baby may be irritable at first, followed by vomiting and increasing lethargy. Soon after, seizures, hypotonia (poor muscle tone), respiratory distress, and coma may occur. If untreated, the child will die. These symptoms are caused by rising ammonia levels in the blood. Acute neonatal symptoms can present in all the enzyme defects, but are most common in boys with ornithine transcarbamylase (OTC) deficiency.

Childhood: Children with mild or moderate urea cycle enzyme deficiencies may not show symptoms until early childhood. Early symptoms may include hyperactive behavior, sometimes accompanied by screaming and self-injurious behavior, and refusal to eat meat or other high-protein foods. Later symptoms may include frequent episodes of vomiting, especially following high-protein meals; seizures, lethargy and delirium; and finally, if the condition is undiagnosed and untreated, coma and death. Children with this disorder may be referred to child psychologists because of their behavior and eating problems. Childhood episodes of hyperammonemia (high ammonia levels in the blood) may be brought on by viral illnesses including chicken pox, high-protein meals, or even exhaustion. The condition is sometimes misdiagnosed as Reye's syndrome. Childhood onset can be seen in both boys and girls.

Adulthood: Recently, the number of adult individuals being diagnosed with urea cycle disorders has increased at an alarming rate. Recent evidence has indicated that these individuals have survived undiagnosed to adulthood, probably due to less severe enzyme deficiencies. These individuals exhibit stroke-like symptoms, episodes of lethargy, and delirium. These adults are likely to be referred to neurologists or psychiatrists because of their psychiatric symptoms. However, without proper diagnosis and treatment, these individuals are at risk for permanent brain damage, coma, and death. Adult-onset symptoms have been observed following viral illnesses, childbirth, and use of many drugs, including valproic acid and corticosteroids.

What are the six urea cycle disorders?

There are six disorders of the urea cycle. Each is referred to by the initials of the missing enzyme.

- **NAGS:** N-acetylglutamate synthetase

- **CPS:** carbamyl phosphate synthetase
- **OTC:** ornithine transcarbamylase
- **AS:** argininosuccinic acid synthetase (citrullinemia)
- **AL/ASA:** argininosuccinase acid lyase (argininosuccinic aciduria)
- **AG:** arginase

Individuals with childhood or adult onset disease may have a partial enzyme deficiency. All of these disorders are transmitted genetically as autosomal recessive genes—each parent contributes a defective gene to the child—except for one of the defects, ornithine transcarbamylase (OTC) deficiency. This urea cycle disorder is acquired in one of three ways: as an X-linked trait from the mother, who may be an undiagnosed carrier; in some cases of female children, the disorder can also be inherited from the father's X-chromosome; and finally, OTC deficiency may be acquired as a "new" mutation occurring in the fetus uniquely. Recent research has shown that some female carriers of the disease may become symptomatic with the disorder later in life, suffering high ammonia levels or confusional states due to high levels of glutamine in the brain. Several undiagnosed women have died during childbirth as a result of high ammonia levels and on autopsy were determined to have been unknown carriers of the disorder.

What are the treatment options?

The treatment of urea cycle disorders consists of balancing dietary protein intake in order that the body receive the essential amino acids responsible for cell growth and development, but not so much protein that excessive ammonia is formed. This protein restriction is used in conjunction with medications, Buphenyl (sodium phenylbutyrate) or sodium benzoate, which provide alternative pathways for the removal of ammonia from the blood. These medications are usually given by way of tube feedings, either via gastrostomy tube (a tube surgically implanted in the stomach) or nasogastric tube through the nose into the stomach. The treatment may also include supplementation with special amino acid formulas developed specifically for urea cycle disorders, multiple vitamins, and calcium supplements. Frequent blood tests are required to monitor the disorders and optimize treatment, and frequently hospitalizations are necessary to control crises (hyperammonemia).

Recently there has been an explosion of research involving the connection between urea cycle disorders and other major diseases, such as cancer, AIDS, and sickle cell anemia. Researchers have found at least two major areas of interest in relation to urea cycle disorders. The first connection involves changes in urea cycle enzyme production in cancer patients with bone marrow transplants undergoing chemotherapy. Because the production of urea cycle enzymes takes place in the liver, drugs toxic to the liver, such as those used in chemotherapy, are observed to be causing changes in the urea cycle. Thus, these bone marrow transplant patients are developing the same accumulation of ammonia (hyperammonemia) seen in children with urea cycle disorders. Another study has found changes (polymorphisms) in these enzymes in large populations. This raises questions as to the significance of these variations on the overall health of the individual.

The second connection relates to the drugs that were developed through the Orphan Drug Act for treating the children with of urea cycle disorders. These drugs, pioneered by children with urea cycle disorders, are now being used in Phase II clinical trials at major cancer research institutions across the nation. The drugs appear to halt the production of cancer cells in numerous cancers, including melanoma and lymphoma.

Other large research institutions are now looking at urea cycle disorders, a previously limited disease, as a new key to developing treatments in other areas of medicine. This new interest will bring more resources to bear for urea cycle research, and our ultimate goal of a cure for the children suffering from these devastating disorders.

Liver transplantation is an option for severe neonatal-onset OTC and CPS deficiency and for children who suffer recurrent crises despite optimal medical management. This treatment alternative must be carefully evaluated with expert medical professionals to determine the potential for success as compared to the potential for new medical concerns, such has immunosuppression-related lymphoproliferative disease or neurodevelopmental delay. Recent advancements in technologies such as tandem mass spectrometry have made it possible to screen all newborns for argininosuccinate synthetase deficiency (citrullinemia), argininosuccinate lyase, and arginase deficiency. Research into screens for OTC and CPS deficiencies has been initiated. We believe that comprehensive newborn screening will help prevent brain damage and other severe consequences of delayed diagnoses and save children's lives.

Chapter 17

Leukodystrophies

Introduction

What is leukodystrophy?

Leukodystrophy refers to progressive degeneration of the white matter of the brain due to imperfect growth or development of the myelin sheath, the fatty covering that acts as an insulator around nerve fiber. Myelin, which lends its color to the white matter of the brain, is a complex substance made up of at least ten different chemicals. The leukodystrophies are a group of disorders that are caused by genetic defects in how myelin produces or metabolizes these chemicals. Each of the leukodystrophies is the result of a defect in the gene that controls one (and only one) of the chemicals. Specific leukodystrophies include metachromatic leukodystrophy, Krabbe disease, adrenoleukodystrophy, Pelizaeus-Merzbacher disease, Canavan disease,

This chapter includes excerpts from the following facts sheets produced by the National Institute of Neurological Disorders and Stroke (NINDS): "NINDS Leukodystrophy Information Page," reviewed December 2003; "NINDS Adreno-leukodystrophy Information Page," reviewed September 2003; "NINDS Alexander Disease Information Page," reviewed December 2003; "NINDS Canavan Disease Information Page," reviewed December 2003; "NINDS Krabbe Disease Information Page," reviewed December 2003; "NINDS Metachromatic Leukodystrophy Information Page," reviewed December 2003; "NINDS Pelizaeus-Merzbacher Disease Information Page," reviewed July 2003; "NINDS Refsum Disease Information Page," reviewed July 2001; and "NINDS Zellweger Syndrome Information Page," reviewed December 2001.

childhood ataxia with central hypomyelination or CACH (also known as vanishing white matter disease), Alexander disease, Refsum disease, and cerebrotendinous xanthomatosis. The most common symptom of a leukodystrophy disease is a gradual decline in an infant or child who previously appeared well. Progressive loss may appear in body tone, movements, gait, speech, ability to eat, vision, hearing, and behavior. There is often a slowdown in mental and physical development. Symptoms vary according to the specific type of leukodystrophy, and may be difficult to recognize in the early stages of the disease.

Is there any treatment?

Treatment for most of the leukodystrophies is symptomatic and supportive, and may include medications, physical, occupational, and speech therapies; and nutritional, educational, and recreational programs. Bone marrow transplantation is showing promise for a few of the leukodystrophies.

What is the prognosis?

The prognosis for the leukodystrophies varies according to the specific type of leukodystrophy.

What research is being done?

The National Institute of Neurological Disorders and Stroke (NINDS) supports research on genetic disorders, including the leukodystrophies. The goals of this research are to increase scientific understanding of these disorders, and to find ways to prevent, treat, and, ultimately, cure them.

Adrenoleukodystrophy

What is adrenoleukodystrophy?

Adrenoleukodystrophy (ALD) is one of a group of genetic disorders called the leukodystrophies that cause damage to the myelin sheath, an insulating membrane that surrounds nerve cells in the brain. People with ALD accumulate high levels of saturated, very long chain fatty acids (VLCFA) in the brain and adrenal cortex because they do not produce the enzyme that breaks down these fatty acids in the normal manner. The loss of myelin and the progressive dysfunction of the adrenal gland are the primary characteristics of ALD. ALD has two subtypes. The most common is the X-linked form (X-ALD), which involves an abnormal gene located on the X-chromosome. Women have two X-chromosomes and are the carriers of the disease, but since men only have one X-chromosome and lack the protective effect of the extra X-chromosome, they are more severely affected. Onset of X-ALD can occur in childhood or in adulthood.

The childhood form is the most severe, with onset between ages four and ten. The most common symptoms are usually behavioral changes such as abnormal withdrawal or aggression, poor memory, and poor school performance. Other symptoms include visual loss, learning disabilities, seizures, poorly articulated speech, difficulty swallowing, deafness, disturbances of gait and coordination, fatigue, intermittent vomiting, increased skin pigmentation, and progressive dementia.

In the milder adult-onset form, which typically begins between ages 21 and 35, symptoms may include progressive stiffness, weakness or paralysis of the lower limbs, and ataxia. Although adult-onset ALD progresses more slowly than the classic childhood form, it can also result in deterioration of brain function. The abnormal genes that cause neonatal ALD are not located on the X-chromosome, which means that both male and female babies can be affected. Symptoms include mental retardation, facial abnormalities, seizures, retinal degeneration, weak muscle tone, enlarged liver, and adrenal dysfunction. This form usually progresses rapidly. A mild form of ALD is occasionally seen in women who are carriers of the disorder. Symptoms include progressive stiffness, weakness or paralysis of the lower limbs, ataxia, excessive muscle tone, mild peripheral neuropathy, and urinary problems.

Is there any treatment?

Adrenal function must be tested periodically in all patients with ALD. Treatment with adrenal hormones can be lifesaving. Symptomatic and supportive treatments for ALD include physical therapy, psychological support, and special education. Recent evidence suggests that a mixture of oleic acid and euric acid, known as "Lorenzo's Oil," administered to boys with X-ALD can reduce or delay the appearance of symptoms. Bone marrow transplants can provide long-term benefit to boys who have early evidence of X-ALD, but the procedure carries risk of mortality and morbidity and is not recommended for those whose symptoms are already severe or who have the adult-onset or neonatal forms. Oral administration of docosahexanoic acid (DHA) may help infants and children with neonatal ALD.

What is the prognosis?

Prognosis for patients with ALD is generally poor due to progressive neurological deterioration. Death usually occurs within one to ten years after the onset of symptoms.

What research is being done?

The NINDS supports research on genetic disorders such as ALD. The aim of this research is to find ways to prevent, treat, and cure these disorders. Intensive basic research has proposed two new approaches, 4-phenylbutyrate and lovastatin, which could potentially lower levels of VLCFA in the brain. Therapeutic trials for both agents are planned.

Alexander Disease

What is Alexander disease?

Alexander disease is a rare, genetically determined degenerative disorder of the central nervous system. It is one of a group of disorders known as the leukodystrophies. In Alexander disease, the destruction of white matter in the brain is accompanied by the formation of fibrous protein deposits called Rosenthal fibers. It is caused by mutations in the gene for glial fibrillary acidic protein (GFAP). The majority of cases are sporadic (not inherited), but there are families in which more than one child will have the disorder. Alexander disease primarily affects males and usually begins at about six months of age. Symptoms may include mental and physical retardation, dementia, enlargement of the brain and head, spasticity (stiffness of arms and/or legs), and seizures. In addition to the infantile form, juvenile and adult onset forms of the disorder have been reported. These forms occur less frequently and have a longer course of progression.

Is there any treatment?

There is no cure for Alexander disease, nor is there a standard course of treatment. Treatment of Alexander disease is symptomatic and supportive.

What is the prognosis?

The prognosis for individuals with Alexander disease is generally poor. Most children with the infantile form do not survive past the age of six. Juvenile and adult onset forms of the disorder have a slower, more lengthy course.

Canavan Disease

What is Canavan disease?

Canavan disease, one of the most common cerebral degenerative diseases of infancy, is a gene-linked, neurological birth disorder in which the white matter of the brain degenerates into spongy tissue riddled with microscopic fluid-filled spaces. Canavan disease is one of a group of genetic disorders known as the leukodystrophies. Canavan disease is caused by mutations in the gene for an enzyme called aspartoacylase. Symptoms of Canavan disease, which appear in early infancy and progress rapidly, may include mental retardation, loss of previously acquired motor skills, feeding difficulties, abnormal muscle tone (floppiness or stiffness), and an abnormally large, poorly controlled head. Paralysis, blindness, or hearing loss may also occur. Children are characteristically quiet and apathetic. Although Canavan disease may occur in any ethnic group, it is more frequent among Ashkenazi Jews from eastern Poland, Lithuania, and western Russia, and among Saudi Arabians. Canavan disease can be identified by a simple prenatal blood test that screens for the missing enzyme or for mutations in the gene that controls aspartoacylase. Both parents must be carriers of the defective gene in order to have an affected child. When both parents are found to carry the Canavan gene mutation, there is a one in four (25%) chance with each pregnancy that the child will be affected with Canavan disease.

Is there any treatment?

Canavan disease causes progressive brain atrophy. There is no cure, nor is there a standard course of treatment. Treatment is symptomatic and supportive.

What is the prognosis?

The prognosis for Canavan disease is poor. Death usually occurs before age four, although some children may survive into their teens and twenties.

What research is being done?

The gene for Canavan disease has been located. Research supported by the NINDS includes studies to understand how the brain and nervous system normally develop and function and how they are affected by genetic mutations. These studies contribute to a greater understanding of gene-linked disorders such as Canavan disease, and have the potential to open promising new avenues of treatment.

Krabbe Disease

What is Krabbe disease?

Krabbe disease is a rare, degenerative disorder of the central and peripheral nervous systems that is characterized by the presence of globoid cells (cells that have more than one nucleus) in demyelinated portions of the brain. It is one of a group of genetic disorders called the leukodystrophies. Krabbe disease is caused by a deficiency of galactocerebrosidase—an essential enzyme for myelin metabolism. Infants with Krabbe disease are normal at birth. Symptoms begin between the ages of three and six months with irritability, inexplicable crying, fevers, limb stiffness, seizures, feeding difficulties, vomiting, and slowing of mental and motor development. There are also juvenile- and adult-onset cases of Krabbe disease, which have similar symptoms but slower progression.

Is there any treatment?

Although there is no cure for Krabbe disease, bone marrow transplantation has been shown to benefit mild cases early in the course of the disease. Generally, treatment for the disorder is symptomatic and supportive. Physical therapy may help maintain or increase muscle tone and circulation.

What is the prognosis?

The prognosis for infants with Krabbe disease is poor. The disorder is generally fatal before age two. Prognosis may be significantly better for children who receive early bone marrow transplantation.

Metachromatic Leukodystrophy

What is metachromatic leukodystrophy?

Metachromatic leukodystrophy (MLD) is one of a group of genetic disorders called the leukodystrophies. MLD is caused by a deficiency of the enzyme arylsulfatase A. There are three forms of MLD: late infantile, juvenile, and adult. In the late infantile form, which is the most common, affected children have difficulty walking after the first year of life. Symptoms include hypotonia (low muscle tone), speech abnormalities and loss of mental abilities, blindness, rigidity (uncontrolled muscle tightness), convulsions, impaired swallowing, paralysis, and dementia. Children with this form of MLD become bedridden, blind, and enter a vegetative state. They usually die in the first decade. Those with the juvenile form (between three and ten years of age) usually begin with emotional disturbances and dementia and then develop symptoms similar to the infantile form but with slower progression. In the adult form, MLD commonly begins around age 30 as a psychiatric disorder or progressive dementia. The illness runs a long course, usually averaging 15 years.

Is there any treatment?

There is no cure for MLD. Bone marrow transplantation may delay progression of the disease in some cases. Other treatment is symptomatic and supportive.

What is the prognosis?

The prognosis for MLD is poor. In the infantile form, death may occur between three and six years after onset. In the juvenile and adult forms, the progression of symptoms is slower and those affected may live a decade or more after diagnosis.

Pelizaeus-Marzbacher Disease

What is Pelizaeus-Merzbacher disease?

Pelizaeus-Merzbacher disease (PMD) is a rare, progressive, degenerative central nervous system disorder in which coordination, motor abilities, and intellectual function deteriorate. The disease is one of a group of gene-linked disorders known as the leukodystrophies, which affect growth of the myelin sheath—the fatty covering that wraps around and protects nerve fibers in the brain. The disease is caused by a mutation in the gene that controls the production of a myelin protein called proteolipid protein (PLP). PMD is inherited as an X-linked recessive trait, in that the affected individuals are male and the mothers are carriers of the PLP mutation. Severity and onset of the disease ranges widely, depending on the type of PLP mutation, and extends from the mild, adult-onset spastic paraplegia (SPG2) to the severe form with onset at infancy and death in early childhood. The characteristic set of neurological symptoms includes nystagmus (rapid, involuntary, rhythmic jerking of the eyes and the head), spastic paraparesis (paralysis of the legs with hyperactive tendon reflexes), and limb ataxia (lack of coordination in the arms and legs). Pronounced changes in the extent of myelination can be detected by MRI analyses. Other symptoms may include slow growth, tremor, failure to develop normal control of head movement, and deteriorating speech and mental function.

Is there any treatment?

There is no cure for Pelizaeus-Merzbacher disease, nor is there a standard course of treatment. Treatment, which is symptomatic and supportive, may include medication for movement disorders.

What is the prognosis?

The prognosis for those with the severe forms of Pelizaeus-Merzbacher disease is poor, with progressive deterioration until death. On the other end of the disease spectrum, individuals with the mild form (in which spastic paraplegia is the chief symptom) may have nearly normal activity and life span.

Refsum Disease

What is Refsum disease?

Refsum disease is one of a group of genetic disorders called the leukodystrophies that affect growth of the myelin sheath, the fatty covering—which acts as an insulator—on nerve fibers in the brain. Refsum disease is characterized by the abnormal accumulation of phytanic acid in blood plasma and tissues. (Phytanic acid is not made in the human body; it comes from the diet—dairy products, beef, lamb, and some seafood). Symptoms of the disorder may include vision impairments (retinitis pigmentosa), peripheral neuropathy, ataxia (impaired muscle coordination), impaired hearing, and bone and skin changes. Nystagmus (rapid, involuntary to-and-fro eye movements), anosmia (absence of the sense of smell), and ichthyosis (a skin disorder causing dry, rough, scaly skin) may also occur. Onset of Refsum disease varies from early childhood to age 50, however, symptoms usually appear by age 20. The disorder affects both males and females.

Is there any treatment?

Treatment for Refsum disease includes restricting foods that contain phytanic acid. Plasmapheresis (the removal and reinfusion of blood plasma) may also be required.

What is the prognosis?

The prognosis for individuals with Refsum disease varies. With treatment, symptoms of peripheral neuropathy and ichthyosis generally disappear. However, treatment cannot undo the damage to vision and hearing.

Zellweger Syndrome

What is Zellweger syndrome?

Zellweger syndrome is a rare, congenital (present at birth) disorder characterized by the reduction or absence of peroxisomes (cell structures that rid the body of toxic substances) in the cells of the liver, kidneys, and brain. Zellweger syndrome is one of a group of genetic disorders called peroxisomal diseases that affect brain development and the growth of the myelin sheath, the fatty covering—which acts as an insulator—on nerve fibers in the brain. The most common features of Zellweger syndrome include an enlarged liver, high levels of iron and copper in the blood, and vision disturbances. Some affected infants may show prenatal growth failure. Symptoms at birth may include lack of muscle tone and an inability to move. Other symptoms may include unusual facial characteristics, mental retardation, seizures, and an inability to suck and/or swallow. Jaundice and gastrointestinal bleeding may also occur.

Is there any treatment?

There is no cure for Zellweger syndrome, nor is there a standard course of treatment. Infections should be guarded against to prevent such complications as pneumonia and respiratory distress. Other treatment is symptomatic and supportive.

What is the prognosis?

The prognosis for individuals with Zellweger syndrome is poor. Death usually occurs within six months after onset and may be caused by respiratory distress, gastrointestinal bleeding, or liver failure.

Chapter 18

Lipid Storage Diseases

Chapter Contents

Section 18.1—Batten Disease 200
Section 18.2—Fabry Disease 206
Section 18.3—Gaucher Disease 210
Section 18.4—Mucolipidoses 214
Section 18.5—Mucopolysaccharidoses 216
Section 18.6—Niemann-Pick Disease 226
Section 18.7—Sandhoff Disease 234
Section 18.8—Tay-Sachs Disease 236

Section 18.1

Batten Disease

"Batten Disease Fact Sheet," National Institute of Neurological
Disorders and Stroke (NINDS), reviewed April 2003.

What is Batten disease?

Batten disease is a fatal, inherited disorder of the nervous system that begins in childhood. Early symptoms of this disorder usually appear between the ages of 5 and 10, when parents or physicians may notice a previously normal child has begun to develop vision problems or seizures. In some cases the early signs are subtle, taking the form of personality and behavior changes, slow learning, clumsiness, or stumbling. Over time, affected children suffer mental impairment, worsening seizures, and progressive loss of sight and motor skills. Eventually, children with Batten disease become blind, bedridden, and demented. Batten disease is often fatal by the late teens or twenties.

Batten disease is named after the British pediatrician who first described it in 1903. Also known as Spielmeyer-Vogt-Sjögren-Batten disease, it is the most common form of a group of disorders called neuronal ceroid lipofuscinoses (or NCLs). Although Batten disease is usually regarded as the juvenile form of NCL, some physicians use the term Batten disease to describe all forms of NCL.

What are the other forms of NCL?

There are three other main types of NCL, including two forms that begin earlier in childhood and a very rare form that strikes adults. The symptoms of these three types are similar to those caused by Batten disease, but they become apparent at different ages and progress at different rates.

- Infantile NCL (Santavuori-Haltia disease) begins between about 6 months and 2 years of age and progresses rapidly. Affected children fail to thrive and have abnormally small heads (microcephaly). Also typical are short, sharp muscle contractions called myoclonic jerks. Patients usually die before age 5, although some have survived in a vegetative state a few years longer.

- Late infantile NCL (Jansky-Bielschowsky disease) begins between ages 2 and 4. The typical early signs are loss of muscle coordination (ataxia) and seizures that do not respond to drugs. This form progresses rapidly and ends in death between ages 8 and 12.

- Adult NCL (Kufs disease or Parry's disease) generally begins before the age of 40, causes milder symptoms that progress slowly, and does not cause blindness. Although age of death is variable among affected individuals, this form does shorten life expectancy.

How many people have these disorders?

Batten disease and other forms of NCL are relatively rare, occurring in an estimated two to four of every 100,000 live births in the United States. These disorders appear to be more common in Finland, Sweden, other parts of northern Europe, and Newfoundland, Canada. Although NCLs are classified as rare diseases, they often strike more than one person in families that carry the defective genes.

How are NCLs inherited?

Childhood NCLs are autosomal recessive disorders; that is, they occur only when a child inherits two copies of the defective gene, one from each parent. When both parents carry one defective gene, each of their children faces a one in four chance of developing NCL. At the same time, each child also faces a one in two chance of inheriting just one copy of the defective gene. Individuals who have only one defective gene are known as carriers, meaning they do not develop the disease, but they can pass the gene on to their own children. Because the mutated genes that are involved in certain forms of Batten disease are known, carrier detection is possible in some instances.

Adult NCL may be inherited as an autosomal recessive or, less often, as an autosomal dominant disorder. In autosomal dominant inheritance, all people who inherit a single copy of the disease gene develop the disease. As a result, there are no unaffected carriers of the gene.

What causes these diseases?

Symptoms of Batten disease and other NCLs are linked to a buildup of substances called lipofuscins (lipopigments) in the body's tissues.

These lipopigments are made up of fats and proteins. Their name comes from the technical word lipo, which is short for lipid or fat, and from the term pigment, used because they take on a greenish-yellow color when viewed under an ultraviolet light microscope. The lipopigments build up in cells of the brain and the eye as well as in skin, muscle, and many other tissues. Inside the cells, these pigments form deposits with distinctive shapes that can be seen under an electron microscope. Some look like half-moons, others like fingerprints. These deposits are what doctors look for when they examine a skin sample to diagnose Batten disease.

The biochemical defects that underlie several NCLs have recently been discovered. An enzyme called palmitoyl-protein thioesterase has been shown to be insufficiently active in the infantile form of Batten disease (this condition is now referred to as CLN1). In the late infantile form (CLN2), a deficiency of an acid protease, an enzyme that hydrolyzes proteins, has been found as the cause of this condition. A mutated gene has been identified in juvenile Batten disease (CLN3), but the protein for which this gene codes has not been identified.

How are these disorders diagnosed?

Because vision loss is often an early sign, Batten disease may be first suspected during an eye exam. An eye doctor can detect a loss of cells within the eye that occurs in the three childhood forms of NCL. However, because such cell loss occurs in other eye diseases, the disorder cannot be diagnosed by this sign alone. Often an eye specialist or other physician who suspects NCL may refer the child to a neurologist, a doctor who specializes in diseases of the brain and nervous system.

In order to diagnose NCL, the neurologist needs the patient's medical history and information from various laboratory tests. Diagnostic tests used for NCLs include:

- **Blood or urine tests:** These tests can detect abnormalities that may indicate Batten disease. For example, elevated levels of a chemical called dolichol are found in the urine of many NCL patients.

- **Skin or tissue sampling:** The doctor can examine a small piece of tissue under an electron microscope. The powerful magnification of the microscope helps the doctor spot typical NCL deposits. These deposits are common in skin cells, especially those from sweat glands.

- **Electroencephalogram or EEG:** An EEG uses special patches placed on the scalp to record electrical currents inside the brain. This helps doctors see telltale patterns in the brain's electrical activity that suggest a patient has seizures.

- **Electrical studies of the eyes:** These tests, which include visual-evoked responses and electroretinograms, can detect various eye problems common in childhood NCLs.

- **Brain scans:** Imaging can help doctors look for changes in the brain's appearance. A commonly used imaging technique is computed tomography, or CT, which uses x-rays and a computer to create a sophisticated picture of the brain's tissues and structures. A CT scan may reveal brain areas that are decaying in NCL patients. Another imaging technique that is becoming increasingly common is magnetic resonance imaging, or MRI. MRI uses a combination of magnetic fields and radio waves, instead of radiation, to create a picture of the brain.

- **Measurement of enzyme activity:** Measurement of the activity of palmitoyl-protein thioesterase involved in CLN1 and the acid protease involved in CLN2 in white blood cells or cultured skin fibroblasts can be used to confirm these diagnoses.

- **DNA analysis:** If families where the mutation in the gene for CLN3 is known, DNA analysis can be used to confirm the diagnosis or for the prenatal diagnosis of this form of Batten disease. When the mutation is known, DNA analysis can also be used to detect unaffected carriers of this condition for genetic counseling.

Is there any treatment?

As yet, no specific treatment is known that can halt or reverse the symptoms of Batten disease or other NCLs. However, seizures can sometimes be reduced or controlled with anticonvulsant drugs, and other medical problems can be treated appropriately as they arise. At the same time, physical and occupational therapy may help patients retain function as long as possible.

Some reports have described a slowing of the disease in children with Batten disease who were treated with vitamins C and E and with diets low in vitamin A. However, these treatments did not prevent the fatal outcome of the disease.

Support and encouragement can help patients and families cope with the profound disability and dementia caused by NCLs. Often, support groups enable affected children, adults, and families to share common concerns and experiences.

Meanwhile, scientists pursue medical research that could someday yield an effective treatment.

What research is being done?

Within the federal government, the focal point for research on Batten disease and other neurogenetic disorders is the National Institute of Neurological Disorders and Stroke (NINDS). The NINDS, a part of the National Institutes of Health, is responsible for supporting and conducting research on the brain and central nervous system. Through the work of several scientific teams, the search for the genetic cause of NCLs is gathering speed.

Other investigators are also working to identify what substances the lipopigments contain. Although scientists know lipopigment deposits contain fats and proteins, the exact identity of the many molecules inside the deposits has been elusive for many years. Scientists have unearthed potentially important clues. For example one NINDS-supported scientist, using animal models of NCL, has found that a large portion of this built-up material is a protein called subunit c. This protein is normally found inside the cell's mitochondria, small structures that produce the energy cells need to do their jobs. Scientists are now working to understand what role this protein may play in NCL, including how this protein winds up in the wrong location and accumulates inside diseased cells. Other investigators are also examining deposits to identify the other molecules they contain.

In addition, research scientists are working with NCL animal models to improve understanding and treatment of these disorders. One research team, for example, is testing the usefulness of bone marrow transplantation in a sheep model, while other investigators are working to develop mouse models. Mouse models will make it easier for scientists to study the genetics of these diseases, since mice breed quickly and frequently.

How can I help research?

The NINDS supports two national human brain specimen banks. These banks supply investigators around the world with tissue from patients with neurological and psychiatric diseases. Both banks need brain tissue from Batten disease patients to enable scientists to study this disorder more intensely. Prospective donors or their families should contact:

Harvard Brain Tissue Resource Center
McLean Hospital
115 Mill Street
Belmont, MA 02178
Toll-Free: 800-BRAIN-BANK (800-272-4622)
Phone: 617-855-2400
Fax: 617-855-3199
Website: http://www.brainbank.mclean.org
E-mail: btrc@mclean.harvard.edu

Human Brain and Spinal Fluid Resource Center
Greater Los Angeles Health Care System
11301 Wilshire Boulevard
Los Angeles, CA 90073
Phone: 310-268-3536
Fax: 310-269-4768
Website: http://www.loni.ucla.edu/%7Ennrsb/NNRSB
E-mail: brainbnk@ucla.edu

Two organizations not funded by the NINDS also provide research scientists with nervous system tissue from patients with neurological disorders. Interested donors should write or call:

Brain and Tissue Bank for Developmental Disorders
University of Miami School of Medicine
Department of Neurology (D4-5)
1501 NW 9th Avenue
Miami, FL 33101
Toll-Free: 800-59-BRAIN (800-592-7246)
Phone: 305-243-6219
Website: http://pathology.med.Miami.edu/btb
E-mail: BTBcoord@med.Miami.edu

National Disease Research Interchange (NDRI)
8 Penn Center
1628 JFK Boulevard, 8th Floor
Philadelphia, PA 19103
Toll-Free: 800-222-NDRI (800-222-6374)
Phone: 215-557-7361
Fax: 215-557-7154
Website: http://www.ndriresource.org
E-mail: info@ndriresource.org

Section 18.2

Fabry Disease

"Questions and Answers about Fabry Disease," is from "Fabry Disease," *Genetics Home Reference: Your Guide to Understanding Genetic Conditions*, a service of the U.S. National Library of Medicine (http://grh.nlm .nih.gov), updated February 2004. "FDA Approves First Treatment for Fabry Disease" is from a U.S. Food and Drug Administration (FDA) press release dated April 24, 2003.

Questions and Answers about Fabry Disease

What is Fabry disease?

Fabry disease is an inherited disorder caused by a buildup of a particular type of fat (lipid) in the body's cells. This buildup results in pain and potentially life-threatening complications such as progressive kidney damage, heart attack, and stroke. Milder forms of the disorder may appear later in life and only affect the heart.

How common is Fabry disease?

This condition affects an estimated one in 40,000 to 117,000 live births. Milder forms of the disorder may be more common.

What genes are related to Fabry disease?

Mutations in the *GLA* gene cause Fabry disease.

The *GLA* gene makes an enzyme called alpha-galactosidase A. This enzyme is active in lysosomes, which are structures inside cells that digest and recycle particles that the cell doesn't need. The enzyme normally breaks down a particular molecule called globotriaosylceramide. Mutations in the *GLA* gene prevent alpha-galactosidase A from breaking down globotriaosylceramide, allowing it to build up in the body's cells. Over time, this buildup damages cells throughout the body, particularly blood vessels in the skin, kidneys, heart, and nervous system.

How do people inherit Fabry disease?

This condition is inherited in an X-linked pattern. A condition is considered X-linked if the gene that causes the disorder is located on the X chromosome (one of the two sex chromosomes). A striking characteristic of X-linked inheritance is that fathers cannot pass X-linked traits to their sons.

Specifically, this condition is most often described as having an X-linked recessive pattern of inheritance. In males, who have only one X chromosome, one altered copy of the gene is necessary to cause the condition. In females, who have two X chromosomes, a mutation usually must be present in both copies of the gene to cause the disorder. Males are more frequently affected than females by X-linked recessive disorders.

In some cases, females with one altered copy of the *GLA* gene may have mild signs and symptoms related to the condition. Other women with one altered copy of the gene experience severe features of the disorder and require treatment.

FDA Approves First Treatment for Fabry Disease

In April 2003, the U.S. Food and Drug Administration (FDA) approved the first treatment for patients with Fabry disease, a serious metabolic genetic disorder affecting approximately one in 40,000 males. While it is believed that fewer females suffer the most serious consequences of the disease, they can be similarly and seriously affected as well. Because of a deficiency in an enzyme, alpha-galactosidase A, Fabry disease causes certain fats to accumulate in the blood vessels over many years, leading to the involvement of various tissues and organs of the body, including the kidneys and the heart, which can then cause organ failure. As a result, patients with Fabry disease often must cope with significant pain and disability and typically have a shortened life span.

The new product, called Fabrazyme (agalsidase beta), is a version of the human form of the natural enzyme produced by recombinant DNA technology. It is given intravenously. This replacement of the missing enzyme reduces a particular type of lipid (fat) accumulation in many types of cells, including blood vessels in the kidney and other organs. It is believed likely that this reduction of fat deposition will prevent the development of life-threatening organ damage and have a positive health effect on patients.

"This priority approval of an orphan drug illustrates FDA's commitment to approving innovative new therapies for patients with serious and life-threatening diseases quickly, based on response to treatment of biological markers likely to predict long-term clinical benefit." said FDA Commissioner Mark B. McClellan, M.D., Ph.D. "The orphan drugs program provides crucial incentives for innovators to develop new treatments for rare diseases. By approving this new biotechnology therapy under the 'accelerated approval' process, we are making this product available more quickly to patients who need it."

Fabrazyme was approved under an accelerated or early approval mechanism. This policy allows for expediting the approval of therapies that treat serious or life-threatening illnesses when studies of the products indicate early favorable outcomes that are likely to predict clinical benefit. The approval is based on surrogate endpoints—laboratory measurements or physical signs—for evidence of effectiveness. The surrogate endpoints are believed to be likely to predict benefit for the patient.

In this case, the manufacturer of Fabrazyme (Genzyme Corporation, Cambridge, Massachusetts) has performed biopsies looking at the cells lining the blood vessels within the kidney and other organs in patients with Fabry disease. Many (but not all) of the cells examined have shown significant clearance of lipid deposits in patients treated with Fabrazyme.

"A key part of our accelerated approval process involves further study of the new treatment after approval, to confirm clinical benefit," said Dr. Jesse Goodman, Director of FDA's Center for Biologics Evaluation and Research (CBER). "In this case, FDA has worked closely with the product developer to make sure that, despite the relatively small number of patients with this disease, all reasonable steps will be pursued to make sure that we learn more about the product's clinical benefits and long-term safety once it is on the market."

One of the requirements of an accelerated approval is that the sponsor completes a post-market study verifying that patients will benefit from the product. Genzyme has committed to continue conducting their ongoing randomized placebo-controlled trial to verify Fabrazyme's benefit to patients and by assessing the drug's effects on the progression of kidney and heart disease and the incidence of strokes.

In addition, Genzyme is taking further steps to assure the availability of information to determine long-term effects of treatment with Fabrazyme. Genzyme has set up a patient registry to follow the long-term progress of patients who have been treated to better understand

Fabry disease and to evaluate the long-term effects of treatment. Enrollment in this registry is voluntary.

FDA and Genzyme are also discussing a variety of novel statistical approaches to analyze data and better assess the effectiveness of the treatment, to augment the data collected through the clinical trial. The potential approaches being evaluated include measures such as within-patient analyses of trends in creatinine levels (a measure of kidney function) on placebo and on Fabrazyme, and modeling utilizing historical information from matched patients.

"Effective studies after approval are essential for collecting valuable evidence on the clinical benefits and longer-term effects of products approved on an accelerated basis," said FDA Commissioner McClellan. "FDA intends to evaluate whether the continuation of the Fabrazyme clinical trial, potentially coupled with additional analyses of data from patients who many not complete the trial and of data from patients receiving long-term treatment, represents the most effective approach to acquiring important confirmatory evidence after approval."

In clinical studies of Fabrazyme, the main safety concern in patients receiving Fabrazyme was infusion reactions, some of which were severe. These include fever, chest tightness, blood pressure changes, abdominal pain and headache. Most patients also develop antibodies to the product and some patients who experience allergic reactions may need to be further evaluated. Because of the potential for these severe reactions, appropriate medical observation and support should be available when Fabrazyme is administered.

Orphan products are developed to treat rare diseases, or conditions that affect fewer than 200,000 people in the U.S. such as Fabry disease. Under the Orphan Drug Act, FDA provides modest grants to organizations to develop products to treat orphan diseases. The act provides a seven-year period of exclusive marketing to the first sponsor who obtains marketing approval for a designated orphan drug.

Section 18.3

Gaucher Disease

Gaucher disease is the most common lipid-storage disorder, and is the most common genetic disease affecting Jewish people of Eastern European ancestry.

Gaucher disease results from a specific enzyme deficiency in the body, caused by a genetic mutation received from both parents. The disease course is quite variable, ranging from no outward symptoms to severe disability and death.

Fortunately, testing is available to identify potential parents who are carriers of the gene and to accurately diagnose those people who have the disease. And even more fortunately, an effective enzyme replacement therapy is available for one of the variants of the disease.

Prevalence and Transmission of Gaucher Disease

Gaucher disease is an inborn error of metabolism. Inborn metabolic disorders are those conditions resulting from a specific malfunction in one or more of the body's many individual chemical processes. Although there are at least 34 mutations known to cause Gaucher disease, there are four genetic mutations which account for 95% of the Gaucher disease in the Ashkenazi Jewish population, and 50% of the Gaucher disease in the general population. These can be identified through a blood test.

The carrier rate for the mutations which cause Gaucher disease may be as high as one in 14 Jewish people of Eastern European ancestry, and one in 100 of the general population. Gaucher disease is transmitted as an autosomal recessive; that is, it occurs equally among males and females, and both parents must carry the mutation for the child to have the disease. If both parents are carriers, then there is a one in four chance that the child will have Gaucher disease, a one in two chance that the child will not have the disease but will be a carrier, and a one in four chance that the child will neither have the disease nor be a carrier.

Symptoms of Gaucher Disease

In 1882, a French physician named Philippe Charles Ernest Gaucher (pronounced: go-SHAY) first described a clinical syndrome in a 32-year-old woman whose liver and spleen were enlarged. The most common symptoms of Gaucher disease are enlargement of the liver and spleen, anemia, reduced platelets (resulting in easy bruising and long clotting times), bone pain (bone crises), bone infarctions often leading to damage to the shoulder or hip joints, and a generalized demineralization of the bones (osteoporosis). The weakening of the bones can then lead to spontaneous fractures. The course of the disease is quite variable, ranging from no overt symptoms to skeletal problems, liver or spleen damage, bleeding, or other problems. There are indications of an increased risk of multiple myeloma, a type of slow growing cancer in the bones, in older individuals with Gaucher disease. Because enzyme therapy has only been available since 1991, there are no data regarding this finding in individuals who are receiving the enzyme replacement therapy.

The characteristics just listed refer primarily to the type 1 form of the disease. This is often called the adult form, although the cause is present from the time of conception. Type 1 Gaucher disease occurs worldwide in all populations, but is most prevalent in the Ashkenazi Jewish population (the Jews of Eastern European ancestry). Within this population, type 1 Gaucher disease occurs at a rate of one in 450 live births, and is the most common genetically based disease affecting Jewish people.

There are other forms of Gaucher disease which, in addition to the liver, spleen, and bone complications characteristic of type 1 Gaucher disease, also result in acute neurological symptoms. Type 2 Gaucher disease, called the acute neuropathic form, is characterized by brainstem abnormalities and is usually fatal during the first three years of life. Type 2 Gaucher disease shows no ethnic predilection, and occurs rarely, with an incidence of one in 100,000 live births. Type 3 Gaucher disease, the chronic neuropathic form, also shows no ethnic predilection, and is estimated to occur in one in 50,000 live births. The neurologic symptoms of type 3 Gaucher disease are slowly progressive and appear later in childhood than the symptoms of type 2 Gaucher disease. Neurologic symptoms of type 3 Gaucher disease include incoordination, mental deterioration, and myoclonic seizures.

211

There is a subclassification of type 3, called Norbottnian Gaucher disease, named for the region in Sweden where it has been identified. The slowly progressive neurologic symptoms of Norbottnian Gaucher disease may not occur until early adulthood.

Testing for Gaucher Disease

Gaucher disease can be detected through a simple blood test. There are Gaucher specialists throughout the country who can diagnose, evaluate and recommend proper treatment. The testing process can be done at a hospital, Gaucher specialist's office, or through your family physician. Your physician can draw blood that would then be sent to a specific laboratory for testing. For more information on the testing process and for testing kit information, visit the University of Pittsburgh's Generin Diagnostics website (http://www.generindiagnostics.com).

An enzyme assay test measures glucocerebrosidase (GC) activity in leukocytes, fibroblasts, or urine. Individuals who are affected with Gaucher disease will have very low levels of enzyme activity. There are four common mutations of the GC gene: N370S, L444P, 84gg and IVS2[+1]. DNA analysis for these four mutations detects 90% to 95% of the mutations associated with Gaucher disease in the Ashkenazi Jewish population, and 50% to 75% of the associated mutations in the general population. Neither disease type nor severity of disease is defined by enzyme assay. DNA analysis is used in combination with the enzyme assay test to diagnose Gaucher disease and is helpful in defining the subtype.

Carrier Testing

Approximately one in 60,000 people have Gaucher disease. However, among Jews of Eastern European (Ashkenazi) descent, one in 450 people will have the disorder, and the carrier rate is approximately one in 14. Carrier status can be detected through a simple blood test. The testing process can be done at a hospital, Gaucher specialist's office, or through your family physician. Laboratory assay tests use chromosomes, DNA, RNA, and genes to determine the genetic status of a person who is at high risk for a particular condition. For detailed information on genetic testing, visit the University of Pittsburgh's Generin Diagnostics website (http://www.generindiagnostics.com).

Prevention and Treatment of Gaucher Disease

Carrier testing is reliable and readily available.

An enzyme replacement therapy is available, which provides the missing enzyme. Much outcome assessment has yet to be completed, but indications are that the symptoms can be entirely reversed in children with type 1 Gaucher disease. It would be important to begin treatment before there is significant organ or bone damage. Current data strongly suggest that enzyme replacement therapy is an effective treatment for type 1 Gaucher disease in all age groups, with a treatment effect occurring most readily in children, and over a longer period of time in adults. It is not clear whether the neurological symptoms of Gaucher disease respond to the enzyme replacement therapy, but initial reports have been disappointing.

Standard of Care

The current treatment for Gaucher disease is Cerezyme, however, due to many variables, method of care for each individual may vary. For information about specific Standards of Care for Gaucher Disease, please contact:

National Gaucher Foundation
5410 Edson Lane, Suite 260
Rockville, MD 20852-3130
Toll-Free: 800-428-2437
Phone: 301-816-1515
Fax: 301-816-1516
Website: http://www.gaucherdisease.org
E-mail: ngf@gaucherdisease.org

Human trials have begun with a gene therapy, using technology developed for other diseases, which will give the Gaucher patient the ability to produce the enzyme not produced by the defective gene.

Research is ongoing into various treatments and supplemental therapies for Gaucher disease.

Clinical Course of Gaucher Disease

The symptoms associated with Gaucher disease result from the accumulation of a fatty substance, a lipid called glucocerebroside. This lipid is a byproduct of the normal recycling of red blood cells. When the gene with the instructions for producing an enzyme to break down this byproduct is defective, the lipid accumulates. Gaucher disease is, therefore, a lipid storage disease, and is the most common disease of this type. The lipid is found in many places in the body, but most commonly in the macrophages (big-eater cells) in the bone marrow. There it interferes with normal bone marrow functions, such as production of platelets (leading to bleeding and bruising) and red blood cells (leading to anemia).

The presence of glucocerebroside seems to also trigger the loss of minerals in the bones, causing the bones to weaken, and can interfere with the bone's blood supply, causing areas of bone-death, or infarctions. The most immediate human cost of type I Gaucher disease is related to the loss of function when a hip or shoulder becomes infarcted or a long bone fractures, the great pain experienced during reduced blood flow to the bones (bone crises), abdominal problems related to massive enlargement of the liver and spleen, poor blood clotting, and anemia. Type 2 and type 3 Gaucher disease result in severe neurological impairment or early demise.

Section 18.4

Mucolipidoses

"NINDS Mucolipidoses Information Page," National Institute of Neurological Disorders and Stroke (NINDS), reviewed July 2003.

What are the mucolipidoses?

The mucolipidoses are a group of inherited diseases characterized by genetic defects that cause problems with the metabolism of enzymes. These deficiencies result in bone and joint damage, and may cause severe complications in the organ systems of the body. The group includes four diseases:

- Mucolipidosis I (sialidosis)
- Mucolipidosis II (I-cell disease)
- Mucolipidosis III (pseudo-Hurler polydystrophy)
- Mucolipidosis IV

Symptoms of the mucolipidoses include: mental retardation, impairment in the development of psychomotor skills, stiff or deformed joints, short stature, spinal curvature, claw-like hands, hip joint deterioration, fatigue, abnormalities of the skull and face, frequent respiratory infections, and clouding of the cornea. Mucolipidoses can be detected before birth, using prenatal screening tests. Some forms are more common among Ashkenazi Jews and French Canadians.

Is there any treatment?

Treatment for the mucolipidoses disorders is symptomatic and depends upon the severity of the disease. In some cases, surgery is necessary to correct bone or joint damage. Complications accompanying mucolipidoses are often treated with antibiotics.

What is the prognosis?

The prognosis for anyone with a mucolipidoses disorder is based on the severity of the symptoms, which can range from relatively moderate to life threatening. Some forms of mucolipidoses can be fatal.

What research is being done?

The NINDS supports research on genetic disorders such as the mucolipidoses. This research includes studies to understand how genetic defects can cause neurological diseases. NINDS-funded studies contribute to a greater understanding of the brain in sickness and health and can open promising new avenues for the development of successful treatments.

Section 18.5

Mucopolysaccharidoses

"Questions and Answers about Mucopolysaccharidoses" is from "The Mucopolysaccharidoses Fact Sheet," National Institute of Neurological Disorders and Stroke (NINDS), NIH Pub. No. 03-5115, January 2003. "FDA Approves First Treatment for Genetic Metabolic Disorder Including Hurler Dystrophy," is from a U.S. Food and Drug Administration (FDA) press release dated April 30, 2003.

Questions and Answers about Mucopolysaccharidoses

What are the mucopolysaccharidoses?

The mucopolysaccharidoses are a group of inherited metabolic diseases caused by the absence or malfunctioning of certain enzymes needed to break down molecules called glycosaminoglycans—long chains of sugar carbohydrates in each of our cells that help build bone, cartilage, tendons, corneas, skin, and connective tissue. Glycosaminoglycans (formerly called mucopolysaccharides) are also found in the fluid that lubricates our joints.

People with a mucopolysaccharidosis either do not produce enough of one of the 11 enzymes required to break down these sugar chains into proteins and simpler molecules or they produce enzymes that do not work properly. Over time, these glycosaminoglycans collect in the cells, blood, and connective tissues. The result is permanent, progressive cellular damage that affects the individual's appearance, physical abilities, organ and system functioning, and, in most cases, mental development.

Who is at risk?

It is estimated that one in every 25,000 babies born in the United States will have some form of the mucopolysaccharidoses. It is an autosomal recessive disorder, meaning that only individuals inheriting the defective gene from both parents are affected. (The exception is MPS II, or Hunter syndrome, in which the mother alone passes along the defective gene to a son.) When both people in a couple have the defective gene, each pregnancy carries with it, a one in four chance that the child will be affected. The parents and siblings of an affected child may have no sign of the disorder. Unaffected siblings and select relatives of a child with one of the mucopolysaccharidoses may carry the recessive gene and could pass it to their own children.

In general, the following factors may increase the chance of getting or passing on a genetic disease:

• A family history of a genetic disease.

• Parents who are closely related or part of a distinct ethnic or geographic circle.

• Parents who do not show disease symptoms but carry a disease gene.

The mucopolysaccharidoses are classified as lysosomal storage diseases. These are conditions in which large numbers of molecules that are normally broken down or degraded into smaller pieces by intracellular units called lysosomes accumulate in harmful amounts in the body's cells and tissues, particularly in the lysosomes.

What are the signs and symptoms?

The mucopolysaccharidoses share many clinical features but have varying degrees of severity. These features may not be apparent at birth but progress as storage of glycosaminoglycans affects bone, skeletal structure, connective tissues, and organs. Neurological complications may include damage to neurons (which send and receive signals throughout the body) as well as pain and impaired motor function. This results from compression of nerves or nerve roots in the spinal cord or in the peripheral nervous system, the part of the nervous system that connects the brain and spinal cord to sensory organs such as the eyes and to other organs, muscles, and tissues throughout the body.

Depending on the mucopolysaccharidoses subtype, affected individuals may have normal intellect or may be profoundly retarded, may experience developmental delay, or may have severe behavioral problems. Many individuals have hearing loss, either conductive (in which pressure behind the ear drum causes fluid from the lining of the middle ear to build up and eventually congeal), neurosensitive (in which tiny hair cells in the inner ear are damaged), or both. Communicating hydrocephalus—in which the normal circulation of cerebrospinal fluid becomes blocked over time and causes increased pressure inside the head—is common in some of the mucopolysaccharidoses. Surgically inserting a shunt into the brain can drain fluid. The eye's cornea often becomes cloudy from intracellular storage, and degeneration of the retina and glaucoma also may affect the patient's vision.

Physical symptoms generally include coarse or rough facial features (including a flat nasal bridge, thick lips, and enlarged mouth and tongue), short stature with disproportionately short trunk (dwarfism), dysplasia (abnormal bone size and/or shape) and other skeletal irregularities, thickened skin, enlarged organs such as liver or spleen, hernias, and excessive body hair growth. Short and often claw-like hands, progressive joint stiffness, and carpal tunnel syndrome can restrict hand mobility and function. Recurring respiratory infections are common, as are obstructive airway disease and obstructive sleep apnea. Many affected individuals also have heart disease, often involving enlarged or diseased heart valves.

Another lysosomal storage disease often confused with the mucopolysaccharidoses is mucolipidosis. In this disorder, excessive amounts of fatty materials known as lipids (another principal component of living cells) are stored, in addition to sugars. Persons with mucolipidosis may share some of the clinical features associated with the mucopolysaccharidoses (certain facial features, bony structure abnormalities, and damage to the brain), and increased amounts of the enzymes needed to break down the lipids are found in the blood.

What are the different types of the mucopolysaccharidoses?

Seven distinct clinical types and numerous subtypes of the mucopolysaccharidoses have been identified. Although each mucopolysaccharidosis (MPS) differs clinically, most patients generally experience a period of normal development followed by a decline in physical and/or mental function.

MPS I is divided into three subtypes based on severity of symptoms. All three types result from an absence of, or insufficient levels of, the enzyme alpha-L-iduronidase. Children born to an MPS I parent carry the defective gene.

MPS I

- *MPS I H, Hurler syndrome,* is the most severe of the MPS I subtypes. Developmental delay is evident by the end of the first year, and patients usually stop developing between ages 2 and 4. This is followed by progressive mental decline and loss of physical skills. Language may be limited due to hearing loss and an enlarged tongue. In time, the clear layers of the cornea become clouded and retinas may begin to degenerate. Carpal tunnel syndrome (or similar compression of nerves elsewhere in the body) and restricted joint movement are common.

Affected children may be quite large at birth and appear normal but may have inguinal (in the groin) or umbilical (where the umbilical cord passes through the abdomen) hernias. Growth in height may be faster than normal but begins to slow before the end of the first year and often ends around age 3. Many children develop a short body trunk and a maximum stature of less than 4 feet. Distinct facial features (including flat face, depressed nasal bridge, and bulging forehead) become more evident in the second year. By age 2, the ribs have widened and are oar-shaped. The liver, spleen, and heart are often enlarged. Children may experience noisy breathing and recurring upper respiratory tract and ear infections. Feeding may be difficult for some children, and many experience periodic bowel problems. Children with Hurler syndrome often die before age 10 from obstructive airway disease, respiratory infections, or cardiac complications.

- *MPS I S, Scheie syndrome,* is the mildest form of MPS I. Symptoms generally begin to appear after age 5, with diagnosis most commonly made after age 10. Children with Scheie syndrome have normal intelligence or may have mild learning disabilities; some may have psychiatric problems. Glaucoma, retinal degeneration, and clouded corneas may significantly impair vision. Other problems include carpal tunnel syndrome or other nerve compression, stiff joints, claw hands and deformed feet, a short neck, and aortic valve disease. Some affected individuals also have obstructive airway disease and sleep apnea. Persons with Scheie syndrome can live into adulthood.

- *MPS I H-S, Hurler-Scheie syndrome,* is less severe than Hurler syndrome alone. Symptoms generally begin between ages 3 and 8. Children may have moderate mental retardation and learning difficulties. Skeletal and systemic irregularities include short stature, marked smallness in the jaws, progressive joint stiffness, compressed spinal cord, clouded corneas, hearing loss, heart disease, coarse facial features, and umbilical hernia. Respiratory problems, sleep apnea, and heart disease may develop in adolescence. Some persons with MPS I H-S need continuous positive airway pressure during sleep to ease breathing. Life expectancy is generally into the late teens or early twenties.

Although no studies have been done to determine the frequency of MPS I in the United States, studies in British Columbia estimate that one in 100,000 babies born has Hurler syndrome. The estimate for Scheie syndrome is one in 500,000 births and for Hurler-Scheie syndrome, it is one in 115,000 births.

MPS II

- *MPS II, Hunter syndrome,* is caused by lack of the enzyme iduronate sulfatase. Hunter syndrome has two clinical subtypes and is the only one of the mucopolysaccharidoses in which the mother alone can pass the defective gene to a son. The incidence of Hunter syndrome is estimated to be one in every 100,000 to 150,000 male births.

- Children with *MPS II A*, the more severe form of Hunter syndrome, share many of the same clinical features associated with Hurler syndrome (MPS I H) but with milder symptoms. Onset of the disease is usually between ages 2 and 4. Developmental decline is usually noticed between the ages of 18 and 36 months, followed by progressive loss of skills. Other clinical features include coarse facial features, skeletal irregularities, obstructive airway and respiratory complications, short stature, joint stiffness, retinal degeneration (but no corneal clouding), communicating hydrocephalus, chronic diarrhea, enlarged liver and spleen, and progressive hearing loss. Whitish skin lesions may be found on the upper arms, back, and upper legs. Death from upper airway disease or cardiovascular failure usually occurs by age 15.

- Physical characteristics of *MPS II B* are less obvious and progress at a much slower rate. Diagnosis is often made in the second decade of life. Intellect and social development are not affected. Skeletal problems may be less severe, but carpal tunnel syndrome and joint stiffness can restrict movement and height is somewhat less than normal. Other clinical symptoms include hearing loss, poor peripheral vision, diarrhea, and sleep apnea, although respiratory and cardiac complications can contribute to premature death. Persons with MPS II B may live into their 50s or beyond.

MPS III

MPS III, Sanfilippo syndrome, is marked by severe neurological symptoms. These include progressive dementia, aggressive behavior, hyperactivity, seizures, some deafness and loss of vision, and an inability to sleep for more than a few hours at a time. This disorder tends to have three main stages. During the first stage, early mental and motor skill development may be somewhat delayed. Affected children show a marked decline in learning between ages 2 and 6, followed by eventual loss of language skills and loss of some or all hearing. Some children may never learn to speak. In the syndrome's second stage, aggressive behavior, hyperactivity, profound dementia, and irregular sleep may make children difficult to manage, particularly those who retain normal physical strength. In the syndrome's last stage, children become increasingly unsteady on their feet and most are unable to walk by age 10.

Thickened skin and mild changes in facial features, bone, and skeletal structures become noticeable with age. Growth in height usually stops by age 10. Other problems may include narrowing of the airway passage in the throat and enlargement of the tonsils and adenoids, making it difficult to eat or swallow. Recurring respiratory infections are common.

There are four distinct types of Sanfilippo syndrome, each caused by alteration of a different enzyme needed to completely break down the heparan sulfate sugar chain. Little clinical difference exists between these four types but symptoms appear most severe and seem to progress more quickly in children with type A. The average duration of Sanfilippo syndrome is 8 to 10 years following onset of symptoms. Most persons with MPS III live into their teenage years, and some live longer.

- Sanfilippo A is the most severe of the MPS III disorders and is caused by the missing or altered enzyme heparan N-sulfatase. Children with Sanfilippo A have the shortest survival rate among those with the MPS III disorders.

- Sanfilippo B is caused by the missing or deficient enzyme alpha-N-acetylglucosaminidase.

- Sanfilippo C results from the missing or altered enzyme acetyl-CoA alpha-glucosaminide acetyltransferase.

- Sanfilippo D is caused by the missing or deficient enzyme N-acetylglucosamine 6-sulfatase.

The incidence of Sanfilippo syndrome (for all four types combined) is about one in 70,000 births.

MPS IV

MPS IV, Morquio syndrome, is estimated to occur in one of every 200,000 births. Its two subtypes result from the missing or deficient enzymes N-acetylgalactosamine 6-sulfatase (type A) or beta-galactosidase (type B) needed to break down the keratan sulfate sugar chain. Clinical features are similar in both types but appear milder in Morquio type B. Onset is between ages 1 and 3. Neurological complications include spinal nerve and nerve root compression resulting from extreme, progressive skeletal changes, particularly in the ribs and chest; conductive and/or neurosensitive loss of hearing; and clouded corneas. Intelligence is normal unless hydrocephalus develops and is not treated.

Physical growth slows and often stops around age 8. Skeletal abnormalities include a bell-shaped chest, a flattening or curvature of the spine, shortened long bones, and dysplasia of the hips, knees, ankles, and wrists. The bones that stabilize the connection between the head and neck can be malformed (odontoid hypoplasia); in these cases, a surgical procedure called spinal cervical bone fusion can be lifesaving. Restricted breathing, joint stiffness, and heart disease are also common. Children with the more severe form of Morquio syndrome may not live beyond their twenties or thirties.

MPS VI

Children with *MPS VI, Maroteaux-Lamy syndrome,* usually have normal intellectual development but share many of the physical symptoms found in Hurler syndrome. Caused by the deficient enzyme N-acetylgalactosamine 4-sulfatase, Maroteaux-Lamy syndrome has a variable spectrum of severe symptoms. Neurological complications include clouded corneas, deafness, thickening of the dura (the membrane that surrounds and protects the brain and spinal cord), and pain caused by compressed or traumatized nerves and nerve roots.

Growth is normal at first but stops suddenly around age 8. By age 10 children have developed a shortened trunk, crouched stance, and restricted joint movement. In more severe cases, children also develop a protruding abdomen and forward-curving spine. Skeletal changes (particularly in the pelvic region) are progressive and limit movement. Many children also have umbilical or inguinal hernias. Nearly all children have some form of heart disease, usually involving valve dysfunction.

MPS VII

MPS VII, Sly syndrome, one of the least common forms of the mucopolysaccharidoses, is estimated to occur in fewer than one in 250,000 births. The disorder is caused by deficiency of the enzyme beta-glucuronidase. In its rarest form, Sly syndrome causes children to be born with hydrops fetalis, in which extreme amounts of fluid are retained in the body. Survival is usually a few months or less. Most children with Sly syndrome are less severely affected. Neurological symptoms may include mild to moderate mental retardation by age 3, communicating hydrocephalus, nerve entrapment, corneal clouding, and some loss of peripheral and night vision. Other symptoms include short stature, some skeletal irregularities, joint stiffness and restricted movement, and umbilical and/or inguinal hernias. Some patients may have repeated bouts of pneumonia during their first years of life. Most children with Sly syndrome live into the teenage or young adult years.

MPX IX

As of 2001, only one case of *MPS IX* had been reported. The disorder results from hyaluronidase deficiency. Symptoms included nodular soft-tissue masses located around joints, with episodes of painful swelling of the masses and pain that ended spontaneously within 3 days. Pelvic radiography showed multiple soft-tissue masses and some bone erosion. Other traits included mild facial changes, acquired short stature as seen in other MPS disorders, and normal joint movement and intelligence.

How are the mucopolysaccharidoses diagnosed?

Diagnosis often can be made through clinical examination and urine tests (excess mucopolysaccharides are excreted in the urine). Enzyme assays (testing a variety of cells or body fluids in culture for enzyme deficiency) are also used to provide definitive diagnosis of one of the mucopolysaccharidoses. Prenatal diagnosis using amniocentesis and chorionic villus sampling can verify if a fetus either carries a copy of the defective gene or is affected with the disorder. Genetic counseling can help parents who have a family history of the mucopolysaccharidoses determine if they are carrying the mutated gene that causes the disorders.

How are the mucopolysaccharidoses treated?

Currently there is no cure for these disorders. Medical care is directed at treating systemic conditions and improving the person's quality of life. Physical therapy and daily exercise may delay joint problems and improve the ability to move.

Changes to the diet will not prevent disease progression, but limiting milk, sugar, and dairy products has helped some individuals experiencing excessive mucus.

Surgery to remove tonsils and adenoids may improve breathing among affected individuals with obstructive airway disorders and sleep apnea. Sleep studies can assess airway status and the possible need for nighttime oxygen. Some patients may require surgical insertion of an endotracheal tube to aid breathing. Surgery can also correct hernias, help drain excessive cerebrospinal fluid from the brain, and free nerves and nerve roots compressed by skeletal and other abnormalities. Corneal transplants may improve vision among patients with significant corneal clouding.

Enzyme replacement therapies are currently in use or are being tested. Enzyme replacement therapy has proven useful in reducing non-neurological symptoms and pain.

Bone marrow transplantation (BMT) and umbilical cord blood transplantation (UCBT) have had limited success in treating the mucopolysaccharidoses. Abnormal physical characteristics, except for those affecting the skeleton and eyes, may be improved, but neurologic outcomes have varied. BMT and UCBT are high-risk procedures and are usually performed only after family members receive extensive evaluation and counseling.

What research is being done?

Research funded by the National Institute of Neurological Disorders and Stroke (NINDS) has shown that viral-delivered gene therapy in animal models of the mucopolysaccharidoses can stop the buildup of storage materials in brain cells and improve learning and memory. Researchers are planning additional studies to understand how gene therapy prompts recovery of mental function in these animal models. It may be years before such treatment is available to humans.

Scientists are working to identify the genes associated with the mucopolysaccharidoses and plan to test new therapies in animal models and in humans. Animal models are also being used to investigate therapies that replace the missing or insufficient enzymes needed to break down the sugar chains.

Gene therapy trials in humans are studying the effects of enzyme replacement on enlarged organs (such as the liver or spleen) and on cardiac and pulmonary dysfunction. Additional trials will determine the extent and immediate cause(s) of hearing loss and inner ear dysfunction common to many storage diseases, and will identify possible methods to correct structural and functional problems contributing to hearing and balance disturbance.

FDA Approves First Treatment for Genetic Metabolic Disorder Including Hurler Disorder

In April 2003, the Food and Drug Administration (FDA) approved the first treatment for patients with certain forms of a rare genetic disease called MPS I, which includes Hurler syndrome. This disease results from the absence or malfunctioning of an enzyme that breaks down molecules called glycosaminoglycans (GAG) in the cells. The build up of GAG in the cells of patients with MPS I results in progressive cellular damage that affects appearance, physical abilities, organ functions and, in some cases, mental development.

The new biotechnology product, Aldurazyme (laronidase), is a version of the human form of the deficient enzyme. This new biotechnology product helps prevent the build-up of GAG in the cells and has been shown to improve lung function and exercise ability. It was designated as a priority new drug under FDA's prescription drug user fee program; the initial review was completed within six months of application receipt, and it was approved within 9 months of application receipt. Aldurazyme's approval is for patients with Hurler and Hurler-Scheie forms of MPS I as well as patients with the Scheie form with moderate to severe symptoms.

Aldurazyme was studied in a randomized, placebo-controlled study of 45 MPS I patients, most of whom had Hurler-Scheie. After 26 weeks, patients receiving the product had improved lung function and walking capacity based on a six-minute walk test. There is no evidence that the new product has any positive effects on central nervous system (CNS) symptoms such as developmental delay and hydrocephalus.

The most serious adverse reaction reported with Aldurazyme was an anaphylactic (allergic) reaction occurring approximately three hours after the product was infused that required an emergency tracheostomy (an opening in the neck to help breathing) in a patient with severe lung problems.

The most common adverse reactions were upper respiratory tract infection, rash, and injection site reactions. The main safety concerns related to infusion reactions included flushing, fever, headache and rash.

In addition to its designation as a priority new drug, Aldurazyme is an orphan drug. The orphan drugs program provides incentives for companies to develop new treatments for rare diseases that affect fewer than 200,000 people in the U.S. The Orphan Drug Act provides a seven-year period of exclusive marketing to the first sponsor who obtains marketing approval for a designated orphan drug.

Aldurazyme is manufactured by BioMarin Pharmaceuticals of Novato, California.

Section 18.6

Niemann-Pick Disease

This chapter includes the following articles reprinted with permission from the National Niemann-Pick Disease Foundation: "What Is Niemann-Pick Disease?" © 2002; "What are the Signs and Symptoms of NPD?" © 2002; "How Is NPD Transmitted?" © 2000; "How Is NPD Diagnosed?" © 2003; and "What Treatment Is Available for NPD?" © 2003. All rights reserved. For additional information, visit http://www.nnpdf.org.

What Is Niemann-Pick Disease?

Niemann-Pick disease (Niemann-Pick) is actually a term for a group of diseases which affect metabolism and which are caused by specific genetic mutations. The three most commonly recognized forms of the disease are types A, B and C.

Types A and B Niemann-Pick are both caused by the deficiency of a specific enzyme activity, acid sphingomyelinase (ASM). This enzyme is ordinarily found in special compartments within cells called lysosomes and is required to metabolize a special lipid, called sphingomyelin. If ASM is absent or not functioning properly, this lipid cannot be metabolized properly and is accumulated within the cell, eventually causing cell death and the malfunction of major organ systems.

Types A and B are both caused by the same enzymatic deficiency and there is a growing consensus that the two forms represent opposite ends of a continuous scale. People with type A generally have little or no ASM production (less than 1% of normal) while those with type B have approximately 10% of the normal level of ASM.

While both type A and B have ASM activity that is significantly lower than normal, the clinical prognosis for these two groups of patients is very different. Type A Niemann-Pick is a severe neurologic disease which generally leads to death by 2 to 3 years of age. It is believed that the majority of Niemann-Pick cases are type A.

In contrast, patients with type B generally have little or no neurologic involvement and may survive into late childhood or adulthood. Type B individuals usually have enlarged livers and spleens, and respiratory problems are common. The enlargement of organs and the respiratory problems both can cause cardiovascular stress and can lead to heart disease later in life.

Patients with intermediate ASM activity tend to have more neurological problems than type B but fewer problems than type A. Because there is not a precise correlation between ASM activity and neurological involvement, it is not possible to accurately predict the severity of the disease by enzyme testing.

Type C Niemann-Pick, although similar in name to types A and B, is very different at the biochemical and genetic level. Patients are not able to metabolize cholesterol and other lipids properly within the cell. Consequently, excessive amounts of cholesterol accumulate within the liver and spleen and excessive amounts of other lipids accumulate in the brain.

Because the defect in metabolism in type C occasionally leads to a secondary reduction in ASM activity in some cells, all three types were originally called Niemann-Pick disease.

Type C Niemann-Pick has 300 to 400 cases diagnosed world wide. It is believed that the number of people affected is higher but it is often difficult for the correct diagnosis to be made. Niemann-Pick type C (NPC) has been initially diagnosed as a learning disability, mild retardation, clumsiness, and delayed development of fine motor skills. Vertical gaze palsy (the inability to move the eyes up and down), enlarged liver, or enlarged spleen are strong indications that NPC should be considered.

There is considerable variation in when symptoms first appear and in the progression of the disease. Symptoms may appear as early as a few months old or as late as adulthood. In most cases, neurological symptoms begin appearing between the ages of 4 and 10. Generally, the later neurological symptoms begin, the slower the progression of the disease.

Type C is always fatal. The vast majority of children die before age 20 (and many die before the age of 10). Late onset of symptoms can lead to longer life spans but it is extremely rare for any person to reach 40.

In the past, other types of Niemann-Pick were identified. The older forms include:

- Type D Niemann-Pick was described in the French Canadian population of Yarmouth County, Nova Scotia. Genealogical evidence indicates that Joseph Muise (c. 1679–1729) and Marie Amirault (1684–c. 1735) are common ancestors to all of the Nova Scotia cases. This is now recognized as a variation of type C.

- Type E Niemann-Pick was described for cases of adults onset. This is now considered a variation of type C where the metabolic processes are only partially dysfunctional, slowing the onset and progression of symptoms.

Niemann-Pick affects all segments of the population with cases reported from North America, South America, Europe, Africa, Asia, and Australia. However a higher incidence of has been found in certain populations:

- Ashkenazi Jewish population (types A and B)
- French Canadian population of Nova Scotia (type D)
- Maghreb region (Tunisia, Morocco, and Algeria) of North Africa (type B)
- Spanish American population of southern New Mexico and Colorado (type C)

Pick's disease is sometimes confused with Niemann-Pick but it is a different disease.

What Are the Signs and Symptoms of Niemann-Pick Disease (NPD)?

Symptoms of all forms of Niemann-Pick are variable—no single symptom should be used to include or exclude Niemann-Pick as a diagnosis. A person in the early stages of the disease may exhibit only a few of the symptoms. Even in the later stages of the disease, not all symptoms may be present.

Type A Niemann-Pick begins in the first few months of life. Symptoms may include:

- feeding difficulties
- a large abdomen within 3 to 6 months
- progressive loss of early motor skills
- cherry red spot in the eye

228

- (generally) a very rapid decline leading to death by two to three years of age.

Type B is biochemically similar to type A but the symptoms are more variable. Abdominal enlargement may be detected in early childhood but there is almost no neurological involvement, such as loss of motor skills. Some patients may develop repeated respiratory infections.

Type C Niemann-Pick usually affects children of school age, but the disease may strike at any time from early infancy to adulthood. Symptoms may include:

- jaundice at (or shortly after) birth

- an enlarged spleen and/or liver

- difficulty with upward and downward eye movements (vertical supranuclear gaze palsy)

- unsteadiness of gait, clumsiness, problems in walking (ataxia)

- difficulty in posturing of limbs (dystonia)

- slurred, irregular speech (dysarthria)

- learning difficulties and progressive intellectual decline (dementia)

- sudden loss of muscle tone which may lead to falls (cataplexy)

- tremors accompanying movement and, in some cases, seizures.

Type C is the most variable form of the disease. Symptoms may appear and then disappear. Some symptoms may never appear. The rate the disease progresses is different from person to person. The rate of progress for an individual will change over time.

Type C is often incorrectly diagnosed. Some of the common errors are:

- Attention deficit disorder (ADD)

- Learning disability

- Retardation

- Delayed development

Vertical supranuclear gaze palsy (VSGP or VGP) is highly suggestive of type C. VSGP is the inability to move the eyes up and down. Parents often notice this when their child walks up and down stairs, watches TV while sitting on the floor, or in similar situations—the child tilts their head to see instead of moving their eyes. Liver or spleen problems in the first few months after birth are also highly suggestive of type C.

How Is NPD Transmitted?

All types of Niemann-Pick are autosomal recessive. This means that both parents carry one copy of the abnormal gene, without having any signs of the disease themselves. (They are carriers or heterozygotes.) Children with Niemann-Pick disease have two copies of the abnormal gene.

When both parents are carriers, there is a one in four chance that a child will be affected with the disease and one in two chance that a child will be a carrier.

Carrier detection testing for all families is not yet reliable. The mutations for types A and B have been extensively studied, particularly among the Ashkenazi Jewish population, and DNA tests for these forms of Niemann-Pick are available. Antenatal diagnosis (diagnosis in the fetus) of NPD is available in a limited number of centers. Carrier detection is possible for other families only after their specific mutation is identified.

The Ara Parseghian Medical Research Center has funded a Genetic Testing and Counseling Center for type C at the Mayo Clinic. The National Niemann-Pick Disease Foundation (NNPDF) funded continuing research in 1999 to identify and describe all known mutations in the type C gene. To date, over 100 mutations have been identified and a description of the *NPC1* gene has been developed.

Dr. Wenda Greer of Dalhousie University has discovered that the type D appears to be a specific mutation of the *NPC1* gene. This discovery will allow for genetic testing of families with this form of Niemann-Pick.

How Is NPD Diagnosed?

Type A and B Niemann-Pick are diagnosed by measuring the ASM (acid sphingomyelinase) activity in white blood cells. The test can be performed after taking a small blood sample from suspected individuals. While this test will identify persons with type A and B (two mutated genes), it is not very reliable for detecting persons who are carriers (only one mutated gene).

It is possible to diagnose types A and B carriers by DNA testing because the gene containing the blueprint for ASM has been cloned and many of its mutations identified. The Mount Sinai Department of Human Genetics has identified certain populations where specific mutations account for a high percentage of cases (Table 18.1.). In other populations, the mutations must first be identified for the individual before DNA carrier testing can be performed.

Table 18.1. High Percent of Mutations Identified in Certain Populations

Population	Mutations	Percentage	NP Type
Ashkenazi Jewish	R496L, L302P	53%	A
Saudi Arabian	H421Y, K576N	85%	B
Turkish	L137P, fsP189, L549P	75%	B
Portuguese/Brazilian	S379P, R441X, R474W, F480L	55%	B
English/Scottish	A196P	42%	B
Other	Delta R608	12%	B

Type B statistics are from "The Demographics and Distribution of Type B Niemann-Pick Disease: Novel Mutations Lead to New Genotype/Phenotype Correlations" by Simonaro CM, Desnick RJ, McGovern MM, Wasserstein MP, Schuchman EH in the *American Journal of Human Genetics,* Oct 4, 2002.

Type A statistics are from "Identification and expression of a common missense mutation (L302P) in the acid sphingomyelinase gene of Ashkenazi Jewish type A Niemann-Pick disease patients" by Levran O, Desnick RJ, Schuchman EH in *Blood,* Oct 15, 1992.

The Mount Sinai School of Medicine (website: http://www.mssm .edu/nieman-pick), University of Pittsburgh (website: http://www .pitt.edu/~edugene/neimann,html), and UCSF-Stanford Lysosomal Disease Center (website: http://www.som.ucsf.edu/departments/lyso-somal) can assist with DNA testing and diagnosis for types A and B.

Type C Niemann-Pick is initially diagnosed by taking a small piece of skin (skin biopsy), growing the cells (fibroblasts) in the laboratory, and then studying their ability to transport and store cholesterol. The transport of cholesterol in the cells is studied by measuring conversion of the cholesterol from one form to another (esterification). The storage of cholesterol is assessed by staining the cells with a compound

231

(filipin), which glows under ultraviolet light. It is important that both of these tests be performed, since reliance on one or the other may lead to the diagnosis being missed in some cases.

Since 1997, research funded by the NNPDF has cataloged over 100 of the genetic mutations related to type C, representing 95% of the known cases of type C. This research led to the establishment of a Genetic Counseling and Carrier Testing Center in December 1999. Located at the Mayo Clinic, and funded in part by the Ara Parseghian Medical Research Foundation, the Center provides DNA testing and counseling for patients and families with NP type C.

Research published in December 2000 identified the cause of the remaining 5% of NPC cases as the gene *HE1*. Mutations of the gene have not been cataloged yet but knowledge of the gene will allow for future testing.

Because Niemann-Pick type C is rare and its symptoms are quite variable, it is not widely known even in the medical community. While education efforts by National Niemann-Pick Disease Foundation (NNPDF) have increased awareness of the disease, there are still instances of misdiagnosis and/or delayed diagnosis. If your child is exhibiting symptoms of Niemann-Pick, you may need to ask your doctor to consider the possibility of NP.

What Treatment Is Available for NPD?

The news concerning treatments for all forms of Niemann-Pick is improving but there is still much to do before definitive therapies are available. Just a few years ago, the cause of Niemann-Pick was unknown. Now the genetic sources of Niemann-Pick have been identified and research is focusing on how the biochemical mechanisms work and how they can be corrected.

Potential treatments are described for informational purposes only. You should consult with your physician for medical advice about individual cases.

Types A and B

Research into definitive therapies has progressed rapidly since the early 1990's. Mount Sinai School of Medicine is conducting research on bone marrow transplantation, enzyme replacement therapy, and gene therapy. These therapies have proven effective against type B NPD in the laboratory but they have not been effective against the progressive neurological decline found in type A NPD.

Bone marrow transplantation has proven effective in mouse models for many aspects of type B when the transplant occurs early in life. Because bone marrow transplant is a complex medical procedure, it has only been done a few times on humans with type B. The results of these transplants has been mixed.

Enzyme replacement has been tested on mice and shown to be effective for type B. It has also been used successfully in other storage diseases, such as Gaucher type I.

Gene therapy would allow the defective gene to be replaced by normal genes. Positive results have been obtained with individual cells but testing on Niemann-Pick mice is just beginning.

Supportive treatment can help manage the symptoms of type B NPD and improve the quality of life for type A NPD. Support may be needed from:

- Pulmonologist for respiratory problems
- Cardiologist for heart problems
- Liver and spleen specialist
- Nutritionist
- Physical therapist
- Learning specialist (if neurological difficulties are identified)
- Gastroenterologist

Type C

There is no definitive therapy for type C Niemann-Pick. Research is continuing to identify potential treatments that would either slow or stop the progression of the disease.

A clinical trial of Zavesca (or OGT-918) for type C Niemann-Pick is underway in the U.S. and Europe. Zavesca slowed, but did not stop, the neurological decline when tested on NPC mice. Current information on this trial can be found on our OGT-918 web page at http://www.nnpdf.org/ogt918.htm.

A drug assay is being conducted by Dr. Laura Liscum. Nearly 50,000 compounds were tested by Bristol Meyers Squibb for potential effectiveness with type C. Fifty compounds were identified as candidates for further testing but none has proven suitable for human use. Work is continuing on related compounds.

Laboratory studies of neurosteroids have had encouraging results when tested on mice but more work needs to be done before a clinical trial can be considered.

Many of the symptoms of Niemann-Pick type C can be controlled or tempered by drugs and supportive treatment. Each patient must be considered individually, depending on symptoms. Supportive treatments should be re-evaluated on a regular basis as the disease progresses.

For more information about treatment for NPD, contact:

National Niemann-Pick Disease Foundation
P.O. Box 49
415 Madison Ave.
Ft. Atkinson, WI 53538
Toll-Free: 877-CURE-NPC (877-287-3672)
Phone: 920-563-0930
Fax: 920-563-0931
Website: http://www.nnpdf.org
E-mail: nnpdf@idcnet.com

Section 18.7

Sandhoff Disease

"NINDS Sandhoff Disease Information Page," National Institute of Neurological Disorders and Stroke (NINDS), reviewed December 2001.

What is Sandhoff disease?

Sandhoff disease is a rare, genetic, lipid storage disorder resulting in the progressive deterioration of the central nervous system. It is caused by a deficiency of the enzyme hexosaminidase which results in the accumulation of certain fats (lipids) in the brain and other organs of the body. Although Sandhoff disease is a severe form of Tay-Sachs disease—which is prevalent primarily in people of European Jewish descent—it is not limited to any ethnic group. Onset of the disorder usually occurs at 6 months of age. Symptoms may include motor weakness, startle reaction to sound, early blindness, progressive mental and motor deterioration, frequent respiratory infections, macrocephaly (an abnormally enlarged head), doll-like facial appearance, cherry-red spots in the back of the eyes, seizures, and myoclonus (shock-like contractions of a muscle).

Is there any treatment?

There is no specific treatment for Sandhoff disease. Treatment is symptomatic and supportive.

What is the prognosis?

The prognosis for individuals with Sandhoff disease is poor. Death usually occurs by age 3 and is generally caused by respiratory infections.

What research is being done?

The NINDS supports research on genetic disorders such as Sandhoff disease. The goals of this research are to increase scientific understanding of these disorders, and to find ways to prevent, treat, and, ultimately, cure them. Scientists have had some limited success in studies using the mouse model of this disorder by inhibiting the formation of the accumulating lipid. The animals fare better but the treatment is still far from life saving.

Section 18.8

Tay-Sachs Disease

"Tay-Sachs Disease (Classical Infantile Form)" is excerpted from *What Every Family Should Know, 6th Edition*, with permission from the National Tay-Sachs and Allied Diseases Association, Inc. Copyright © 2003. All rights reserved. For additional information, visit http://www.ntsad.org. "What Is Late Onset Tay-Sachs" is reprinted with permission from the Late Onset Tay-Sachs Foundation, http://www.lotsf.org. © 2002. All rights reserved.

Tay-Sachs Disease (Classical Infantile Form)

What is Tay-Sachs disease?

The classical form of Tay-Sachs disease (TSD) is a fatal genetic disorder in children that causes progressive destruction of the central nervous system. The disease is named for Dr. Warren Tay (1843–1927), a British ophthalmologist who in 1881 described a patient with a cherry-red spot on the retina of the eye. It is also named for Bernard Sachs (1858–1944), a New York neurologist whose work several years later provided the first description of the cellular changes in Tay-Sachs disease. Sachs also recognized the familial nature of the disorder and, by observing numerous cases, he noted that most babies with Tay-Sachs disease were of eastern European Jewish origin.

Tay-Sachs disease is caused by the absence of a vital enzyme called hexosaminidase A (Hex-A). Without Hex-A, a fatty substance or lipid called GM2 ganglioside accumulates abnormally in cells, especially in the nerve cells of the brain. This ongoing accumulation causes progressive damage to the cells. The destructive process begins in the fetus early in pregnancy, although the disease is not clinically apparent until the child is several months old. By the time a child with TSD is three or four years old, the nervous system is so badly affected that life itself cannot be supported. Even with the best of care, all children with classical TSD die early in childhood, usually by the age of five.

A baby with Tay-Sachs disease appears normal at birth and seems to develop normally until about six months of age. The first signs of

TSD can vary and are evident at different ages in affected children. Initially, development slows; there is a loss of peripheral vision, and the child exhibits an abnormal startle response. By about two years of age, most children experience recurrent seizures and diminishing mental function. The infant gradually regresses, losing skills one by one, and is eventually unable to crawl, turn over, sit, or reach out. Other symptoms include increasing loss of coordination, progressive inability to swallow, and breathing difficulties. Eventually, the child becomes blind, mentally retarded, paralyzed, and nonresponsive to his or her environment.

To date, there is no cure or effective treatment for TSD. However, there is active research being done in many investigative laboratories in the U.S. and around the world. The use of enzyme replacement therapy to provide the Hex-A which is missing in babies with TSD has been explored. Although this approach is theoretically promising, scientists face serious obstacles. Because the disease affects brain cells that are protected by the blood-brain barrier, enzymes like Hex-A are blocked from entering the brain from the blood. Bone marrow transplantation has also been attempted but, to date, has been only partially successful in reversing or slowing damage to the central nervous system in babies with TSD. Other approaches that may prove more promising in the future include gene therapy targeted to cells in the central nervous system and/or the introduction of functional neural stem cells into the brains of affected children.

Although a cure for Tay-Sachs disease does not exist at the present time, support for families of affected children is available through organizations such as the National Tay-Sachs and Allied Diseases Association (NTSAD).

How is Tay-Sachs disease transmitted?

All of us carry genes, in pairs, located along 23 pairs of chromosomes. TSD is controlled by a pair of genes on chromosome 15; these are the genes that code for the enzyme Hex-A. If either or both Hex-A genes are active, the body produces enough of the enzyme to prevent the abnormal build-up of the GM2 ganglioside lipid. Carriers of TSD—people who have one copy of the inactive gene along with one copy of the active gene—are healthy. They do not have Tay-Sachs disease. The only significance of being a carrier is the possibility of passing the inactive gene to one's children. A carrier has a 50% chance of passing the inactive gene on to his or her children; any child who inherits one inactive gene is a Tay-Sachs carrier like the parent. If both parents are carriers and their child inherits the inactive TSD gene from each of them, the child will have Tay-Sachs disease since he or she has inherited two inactive genes and, therefore, cannot make any functional Hex-A.

When both parents are carriers of the inactive Tay-Sachs gene, they have a one in four chance (25%) with each pregnancy that their child will have Tay-Sachs disease, and a three in four chance (75%) that their child will be healthy. Of their unaffected children, there is a two in three chance that each child will be a carrier, like the parents. This pattern of inheritance is called autosomal recessive.

Are certain populations at higher risk?

Recessive diseases such as Tay-Sachs often occur more frequently, though not exclusively, in a defined population. A person's chances of being a TSD carrier are significantly higher if he or she is of eastern European (Ashkenazi) Jewish descent. Approximately one in every 27 Jews in the United States is a carrier of the TSD gene. There is also a noticeable incidence of TSD in non-Jewish French Canadians living near the St. Lawrence River, in the Cajun community in Louisiana and in the Irish community in the United States. By contrast, the carrier rate in the general population as well as in Jews of Sephardic origin is about one in 250.

While there are certain populations known to be at higher risk for carrying an altered Hex-A gene, anyone in any population can be a carrier of TSD. If two such individuals have children, they will have the same one in four chance, with each pregnancy, of having a child with TSD. In fact, over the past 25 years, carrier screening and genetic counseling within high-risk populations have greatly reduced the number of children born with TSD in these groups. At the same time, the number of children born with TSD to couples not known a priori to be at high risk of being carriers of TSD has remained more or less constant. Therefore a great percentage of the babies born with Tay-Sachs disease today are born to couples who were not previously thought to be at significant risk.

Is there a test to identify carriers?

Tay-Sachs most often appears in families with no prior history of the disease. The TSD gene can be carried without being expressed through many generations. Before 1970, the only way to learn if one was a Tay-Sachs carrier was to be the parent of a baby with TSD. Now, safe and reliable carrier testing is available to identify Tay-Sachs carriers. Most important, testing can identify carrier couples who are at risk for bearing a child with TSD—before a tragedy occurs. With this vital information, couples can explore the various options that will enable them to protect their families from this devastating disease.

A simple blood test can distinguish Tay-Sachs carriers from non-carriers. Blood samples can be analyzed by either enzyme assay or DNA studies. The enzyme assay is a biochemical test that measures the level of Hex-A in a person's blood. Carriers have less Hex-A in their body fluid and cells than non-carriers. (Babies with Tay-Sachs disease have a total absence of Hex-A in their cells.) The biochemical test is able to detect all Tay-Sachs carriers of all ethnic backgrounds.

Accurate biochemical testing requires laboratories to be proficient in specialized laboratory procedures and experienced in the interpretation of test results. To ensure accuracy, persons seeking such carrier testing for TSD should verify that the analysis is being performed at a laboratory that participates in the International Tay-Sachs Laboratory Quality Control Program supported by NTSAD. A complete list of laboratories affiliated with the Quality Control Program is available through NTSAD (Website: http://www.ntsad.org; complete contact information is provided in the end section of this book).

DNA-based carrier testing looks for specific mutations, or changes, in the gene that codes for Hex-A. Since 1985, when the Hex-A gene was isolated, over 75 different mutations in this gene have been identified. Some are more prevalent than others; a few are associated with a later-onset form of the disease, rather than with the infantile form described here.

The limitation of DNA-based carrier testing is that not all known mutations in the Hex-A gene are detected by the test, and others have yet to be identified. The tests currently available detect about 95% of carriers of Ashkenazi Jewish background and about 60% of non-Jewish individuals. Therefore, some people who are carriers will not be identified by DNA analysis alone.

DNA testing can provide very important information when used in conjunction with biochemical testing, especially in cases where both members of a couple are determined to be carriers. Knowing information about the mutations carried by each parent, and whether they are classical or late-onset Tay-Sachs mutations, is important if a couple chooses to undergo prenatal diagnosis.

Tay-Sachs carrier testing is vital for individuals in high-risk populations who are planning to have children. Even if your childbearing years are over, your carrier status can be an extremely important piece of information. If you are a carrier, your close relatives (children, brothers, sisters, cousins, aunts, uncles) should be alerted to be tested as well. Tay-Sachs carrier testing is also vital for the close relatives of families with an affected child, regardless of ethnic background, since all parents of children with Tay-Sachs are, by definition, carriers.

Note: Some special considerations are involved in Tay-Sachs carrier testing of pregnant women when using a biochemical assay. The best advice for women is to be tested before pregnancy. The blood serum test used to test males and non-pregnant women cannot be used in pregnant women because of changes in serum enzyme levels during pregnancy. Pregnant women must instead be tested using leukocytes (white blood cells). The leukocyte test is as reliable as the blood serum test, but is considerably more complex and costly. In addition, testing before pregnancy allows a couple time to consider the information they are given. If a couple is found to be at risk, they can review their options and make the necessary decisions about planning and protecting their families.

If there is no cure, is there a way to prevent the tragedy of Tay-Sachs disease?

Tay-Sachs today is largely a preventable tragedy for those in high-risk populations such as the Ashkenazi Jews, the French Canadians, the Cajuns, and the Irish. The implementation of population based carrier screening programs to identify carrier-carrier couples, coupled with other medical advances, offer high risk couples the means of having full, healthy families. In other populations where the carrier frequency is much lower and screening programs for TSD are not in place, parents do not have the chance to learn their carrier status prior to the birth of an affected child so, each year, a small number of children are born with TSD. Once identified as carriers, these couples, too, can go on to have full, healthy families.

Today, at-risk couples can choose from two available prenatal diagnostic procedures: amniocentesis and chorionic villus sampling (CVS). Amniocentesis involves removing and testing a small quantity of the fluid that bathes the fetus in the uterus. This procedure is done at approximately the sixteenth week of pregnancy. If Hex-A is found to be present, the fetus is not affected by TSD. On the other hand, if Hex-A is missing in fetal cells, the infant will have TSD. If the fetus is affected, the family may elect to have a therapeutic abortion. In this way, even at-risk couples can be helped to have children, as many as they wish, who are free of Tay-Sachs disease.

Chorionic villus sampling (CVS) is a newer technique. It is performed earlier in pregnancy, in the tenth or eleventh week, and usually provides a test answer much sooner than amniocentesis. The cell sample is obtained by withdrawing a small bit of the developing placenta (afterbirth). Because the procedure is performed earlier than amniocentesis—often before the pregnancy shows—CVS gives couples more privacy in their decision making as well as a safer pregnancy termination, should a therapeutic abortion be necessary.

Recently, assisted reproductive technologies have become available to at-risk couples who wish to have children but for whom abortion is not an option. One option available to them is artificial insemination by a non-carrier sperm donor. Another option, available only for couples with identified DNA mutations in the Hex-A gene, involves in-vitro fertilization using the couple's own eggs and sperm. Here, in-vitro fertilization is followed by an analysis of the DNA of the newly formed embryos to determine which carry two copies of the TSD gene and which do not; only those embryos determined not to be affected with TSD are implanted in the woman. This latter method, called preimplantation genetic diagnosis or PGD for short, is complex and quite expensive but is sometimes, although not often, covered by insurance.

Genetic counseling is an important service available to all carrier couples to assist them in assessing their reproductive options. In addition to reviewing the various options for family planning which are currently available to high-risk couples (prenatal diagnosis by amniocentesis or CVS and selective termination of affected fetuses; adopting children; assisted reproductive technologies such as in-vitro fertilization followed by reimplantation diagnosis or artificial insemination by a non-carrier donor; or taking a 25% risk of bearing a child with TSD) the genetic counselor can help carriers fulfill their responsibility of informing family members that they, too, may be carriers and should be tested.

What Is Late Onset Tay-Sachs?

Late onset Tay-Sachs disease is a degenerative genetic disorder which causes debilitating physical and/or mental symptoms.

Physical manifestations may include hand tremors, clumsiness, speech impediments, swallowing difficulties, problems with gait and balance, and muscle weakness. Not all physical symptoms are present in every affected person. Psychiatric disorders may also be present in some cases.

Many of these symptoms first become apparent in childhood, getting progressively more severe as the affected person gets older. Most of the affected people identified so far have been previously misdiagnosed as having one of the better-known neuromuscular disorders such as muscular dystrophy, multiple sclerosis, or amyotrophic lateral sclerosis (Lou Gehrig's disease).

How is it caused?

Late onset Tay-Sachs disease is caused by a deficiency of an enzyme called Hexosaminidase A (Hex A) which breaks down a particular lipid or fatty substance in the nerve cells of the brain. The fat is created naturally in the body and is not connected with fats in the diet. The lipids build up, leading to a gradual degeneration of the central nervous system, particularly in the cerebellum, accounting for the atrophy of the cerebellum seen by magnetic resonance imaging (MRI).

How is it related to infantile Tay-Sachs?

Late onset Tay-Sachs is genetically similar to the more common infantile Tay-Sachs disease. The latter causes rapid degeneration of the central nervous system, leading to death in very early childhood. Late onset Tay-Sachs is compatible with a normal life span reflecting a slower degeneration.

Who is vulnerable?

Carriers and people with late onset Tay-Sachs disease can be from any ethnic group, most identified carriers of the gene are of either Eastern European Jewish or French Canadian background. However, the gene has been identified in people of several diverse ethnic backgrounds.

How is it diagnosed?

Although at present there is no cure for any form of Tay-Sachs disease, a simple blood test identifies carriers and people affected with the condition. People affected with Tay-Sachs disease inherit Tay-Sachs genes from both parents. People who inherit the gene from only one parent are carriers, but are unaffected by either form of Tay-Sachs.

Chapter 19

Nerofibromatoses

What are the neurofibromatoses?

The neurofibromatoses are genetic disorders of the nervous system that primarily affect the development and growth of neural (nerve) cell tissues. These disorders cause tumors to grow on nerves and produce other abnormalities such as skin changes and bone deformities. The neurofibromatoses occur in both sexes and in all races and ethnic groups. Scientists have classified the disorders as neurofibromatosis type 1 (NF1) and neurofibromatosis type 2 (NF2). Other or variant types of the neurofibromatoses may exist, but are not yet identified.

What is NF1?

NF1 is the more common type of the neurofibromatoses, occurring in about one in 4,000 individuals in the United States. Although many affected persons inherit the disorder, between 30 and 50 percent of new cases arise spontaneously through mutation (change) in an individual's genes. Once this change has taken place, the mutant gene can be passed on to succeeding generations.

Previously, NF1 was known as peripheral neurofibromatosis (or von Recklinghausen's neurofibromatosis) because some of the symptoms—skin spots and tumors—seemed to be limited to the outer

"Neurofibromatosis Fact Sheet," National Institute of Neurological Disorders and Stroke (NINDS), reviewed May 2003.

nerves, or peripheral nervous system, of the affected person. This name is no longer technically accurate because central nervous system tumors are now known to occur in NF1.

What are the signs and symptoms of NF1?

In diagnosing NF1, a physician looks for two or more of the following:

- five or more light brown skin spots (cafe-au-lait macules) measuring more than five millimeters in diameter in patients under the age of puberty or more than 15 millimeters across in adults and children over the age of puberty;

- two or more neurofibromas (tumors that grow on a nerve or nerve tissue, under the skin) or one plexiform neurofibroma (involving many nerves);

- freckling in the armpit or groin areas;

- benign growths on the iris of the eye (known as Lisch nodules or iris hamartomas);

- a tumor on the optic nerve (optic glioma);

- severe scoliosis (curvature of the spine);

- enlargement or deformation of certain bones other than the spine; and

- a parent, sibling, or child with NF1.

When do symptoms appear?

Symptoms, particularly those on the skin, are often evident at birth or during infancy, and almost always by the time a child is about 10 years old. Neurofibromas become evident at around 10 to 15 years of age. In most cases, symptoms are mild and patients live normal and productive lives. In some cases, however, NF1 can be severely debilitating.

Symptoms and severity of the disorder may vary among members of affected families.

How is NF1 treated?

Treatments are presently aimed at controlling symptoms. Surgery can help some bone malformations. For scoliosis, bone surgery may be combined with back braces. Surgery can also remove painful or disfiguring tumors; however, there is a chance that the tumors may grow back and in greater numbers. In the rare instances when tumors become malignant (three to five percent of all cases), treatment may include surgery, radiation, or chemotherapy.

What is NF2?

This less common variant of the neurofibromatoses affects about one in 40,000 persons. NF2 is characterized by bilateral (occurring on both sides of the body) tumors on the eighth cranial nerve. It was formerly called bilateral acoustic neurofibromatosis or central neurofibromatosis because the tumors, which cause progressive hearing loss, were thought to grow primarily on the auditory nerve, a branch of the eighth cranial nerve responsible for hearing. Scientists now know that the tumors typically occur on the vestibular nerve, another branch of the eighth cranial nerve near the auditory nerve. The tumors, called vestibular schwannomas for their location and for the type of cells in them, cause pressure damage to neighboring nerves. In some cases, the damage to nearby vital structures, such as other cranial nerves and the brainstem, can be life-threatening.

What are the signs and symptoms of NF2?

To determine if an individual has NF2, a physician looks for the following:

1. bilateral eighth nerve tumors,
2. a parent, sibling, or child with NF2 and a unilateral eighth nerve tumor, or
3. a parent, sibling, or child with NF2 and any two of the following:

   - glioma,
   - meningioma,
   - neurofibroma,
   - schwannoma, or
   - cataract at an early age.

When do symptoms appear?

Affected individuals may notice hearing loss as early as the teen years. In addition to changes in hearing that may occur in one or both ears, other early symptoms may include tinnitus (ringing noise in the ear) and poor balance. Headache, facial pain, or facial numbness, caused by pressure from the tumors, may also occur.

How is NF2 treated?

Treatments for NF2 are aimed at controlling the symptoms. Improved diagnostic technologies, such as MRI (magnetic resonance imaging), can reveal tumors as small as a few millimeters in diameter, thus allowing early treatment. Surgery to remove tumors completely is one option, but may result in hearing loss. Other options include partial removal of tumors, radiation, and, if the tumors are not progressing rapidly, the conservative approach of watchful waiting.

Are there prenatal tests for the neurofibromatoses?

Genetic testing is available for families with documented cases of NF1 and NF2. Genetic analysis can be used to confirm clinical diagnosis if the disease is a result of familial inheritance. New (spontaneous) mutations cannot be confirmed genetically. Prenatal diagnosis of familial NF1 or NF2 is also possible utilizing amniocentesis or chorionic villus sampling procedures. Genetic counselors can provide information about these procedures and offer guidance in coping with the neurofibromatoses.

What do scientists know about the neurofibromatosis?

Formerly the neurofibromatoses were grouped as one disorder with at least two variations. Scientists now know that NF1 and NF2 are two distinct entities because the genes believed to be responsible for them are located on different chromosomes. The NF1 gene is on chromosome 17, while the gene for NF2 is on chromosome 22.

Humans have 23 pairs of chromosomes, receiving one set of 23 chromosomes from each parent. Chromosomes carry genes that determine an individual's characteristics, such as sex, stature, hair and eye color, and distinctive family traits. Genes produce proteins that control an individual's development and health. If an inherited gene is defective, or a gene becomes defective spontaneously before birth, a genetic disorder may result. The neurofibromatoses are inherited as dominant disorders, which means that if either parent has the defective gene, each child born to that parent has a 50 percent chance of inheriting the defective gene.

What research is being done on the neurofibromatosis?

National Institute of Neurological Disorders and Stroke (NINDS), a unit of the federal government's National Institutes of Health (NIH), has primary responsibility for conducting and supporting research on neurological disorders. The Institute sponsors basic studies aimed at understanding normal and abnormal development of the brain and nervous system and clinical studies to improve diagnosis and treatment of neurological disorders. In conjunction with the NIH's National Cancer Institute, the NINDS encourages research specifically targeted on the neurofibromatoses.

Several years ago, research teams supported by the NINDS located the exact position of the NF1 gene on chromosome 17. The NF1 gene has been cloned and its structure analyzed. The product of the NF1 gene is a large and complex protein called neurofibromin. One portion of this protein is similar to a family of proteins called GAP (guanosine triphosphatase-activating protein). Scientists have demonstrated that GAP proteins play a significant role in tumor suppression in certain cancers. The proteins act as switches that regulate the complex chemical interactions and sequences of cell growth. The similarity of the NF1 protein to GAP proteins suggests that the NF1 protein may have a similar switching role in the development of neurofibromas. Scientists theorize that defects in the gene may lessen or inhibit the normal output of its protein and allow the irregular cell growth that may lead to tumor development.

In addition to the work on NF1, intensive efforts have led to the identification of the NF2 gene on chromosome 22. As in NF1, the NF2 gene product is a tumor suppressor protein (termed merlin or schwannomin). Basic studies in molecular genetics may lead one day to nonsurgical or pharmacologic treatments aimed at retarding or suppressing tumors associated with the neurofibromatoses.

The NINDS also encourages research aimed at developing improved methods of diagnosing the neurofibromatoses and at identifying factors that contribute to the wide variations of symptoms and severity of the disorders. Early diagnosis of the neurofibromatoses is essential so that affected individuals can obtain treatment, counseling, and referral to specialized facilities.

The Interinstitute Medical Genetics Research Program at the NIH Clinical Center conducts NF2 family history research, including a study involving individuals and families with NF2. With information from this study, investigators have confirmed the location of the NF2 gene on chromosome 22. Also, using specimens from some of the families, scientists have isolated and sequenced the NF2 gene, and have described two different patterns of clinical features in NF2 patients. Investigators are continuing to study these patterns to see if they correspond to specific types of gene mutations.

How can I help research?

NINDS contributes to the support of two national human specimen banks, one at the Veterans Administration Medical Center in Los Angeles and the other at McLean Hospital near Boston. These banks supply investigators around the world with tissue from patients with neurological and other disorders. Both banks need tissue from individuals with NF1 or NF2 to enable scientists to study these disorders more intensely. Prospective donors may write to:

Harvard Brain Tissue Resource Center
McLean Hospital
115 Mill Street
Belmont, MA 02178
Toll-Free: 800-BRAIN-BANK (800-272-4622)
Phone: 617-855-2400
Fax: 617-855-3199
Website: http://www.brainbank.mclean.org
E-mail: btrc@mclean.harvard.edu

Human Brain and Spinal Fluid Resource Center
Greater Los Angeles Health Care System
11301 Wilshire Boulevard
Los Angeles, CA 90073
Phone: 310-268-3536
Fax: 310-269-4768
Website: http://www.loni.ucla.edu/%7Ennrsb/NNRSB
E-mail: brainbnk@ucla.edu

Chapter 20

Neuromuscular Disorders

Chapter Contents

Section 20.1—Barth Syndrome 250
Section 20.2—Charcot-Marie-Tooth Disease 251
Section 20.3—Mitochondrial Myopathies 257
Section 20.4—Muscular Dystrophies 258
Section 20.5—Spinal Muscular Atrophy 273

Section 20.1

Barth Syndrome

"NINDS Barth Syndrome Information Page," National Institute of
Neurological Disorders and Stroke (NINDS), reviewed March 2003.

What is Barth syndrome?

Barth syndrome is a rare congenital metabolic and neuromuscular disorder that affects boys. It is passed from mother to son through
the sex-linked, or X, chromosome. Symptoms affect multiple systems
of the body and may include changes to metabolism, motor delays,
hypotonia (reduced muscle tone), delayed growth, cardiomyopathy
(leading to a poorly functioning heart), weakened immune system,
chronic fatigue, lack of stamina, hypoglycemia (low blood sugar),
mouth ulcers, diarrhea, and varying degrees of physical and learning disability. Boys with the disorder also have fewer white blood cells
(a condition called neutropenia), which may lead to an increased risk
for serious bacterial infections.

Barth syndrome affects at least 50 families worldwide, but there
is evidence that it is underdiagnosed. On average 50 percent of children born to a carrier mother will inherit the defective gene, but only
boys will have symptoms. All daughters born to an affected male will
be carriers.

Is there any treatment?

There is no specific treatment for Barth syndrome. Bacterial infections caused by neutropenia can be effectively treated with antibiotics. The drug granulocyte colony stimulating factor, or GCSF, can
stimulate white cell production by the bone marrow and help combat
infection. Medicines may be prescribed to control heart problems. The
dietary supplement carnitine has aided some Barth children but in
others it has caused increasing muscle weakness and even precipitated heart failure. Only careful dietary monitoring directed by a
physician or nutritionist familiar with the disorder can ensure proper
caloric and nutritional intake.

What is the prognosis?

Early and accurate diagnosis is key to prolonged survival for boys born with Barth syndrome. Severe infections and cardiac failure are common causes of death in affected children.

What research is being done?

The National Institute of Neurological Disorders and Stroke (NINDS) supports research on genetic disorders such as Barth syndrome, including basic research on mitochondrial dysfunction and investigations of other inborn errors of metabolism. The 1996 discovery of the Barth gene, called *G4.5* or *TAZ1*, is helping scientists and physicians better understand the metabolic and biochemical abnormalities seen in the disease and learn how genes cause heart disease, muscle weakness, and other problems in the body. The ultimate goal of this research is to find ways to prevent, treat, and cure these disorders.

Section 20.2

Charcot-Marie-Tooth Disease

"Charcot-Marie-Tooth Disease Fact Sheet," National Institute of Neurological Disorders and Stroke (NINDS), reviewed April 2003.

What is Charcot-Marie-Tooth disease?

Charcot-Marie-Tooth disease (CMT) is one of the most common inherited neurological disorders, affecting approximately one in 2,500 people in the United States. The disease is named for the three physicians who first identified it in 1886—Jean-Martin Charcot and Pierre Marie in Paris, France, and Howard Henry Tooth in Cambridge, England. CMT, also known as hereditary motor and sensory neuropathy (HMSN) or peroneal muscular atrophy, comprises a group of disorders that affect peripheral nerves. The peripheral nerves lie outside the brain and spinal cord and supply the muscles and sensory organs in the limbs. Disorders that affect the peripheral nerves are called peripheral neuropathies.

What are the symptoms of Charcot-Marie-Tooth disease?

The neuropathy of CMT affects both motor and sensory nerves. A typical feature includes weakness of the foot and lower leg muscles, which may result in foot drop and a high-stepped gait with frequent tripping or falls. Foot deformities, such as high arches and hammer-toes (a condition in which the middle joint of a toe bends upwards) are also characteristic due to weakness of the small muscles in the feet. In addition, the lower legs may take on an "inverted champagne bottle" appearance due to the loss of muscle bulk. Later in the disease, weakness and muscle atrophy may occur in the hands, resulting in difficulty with fine motor skills. Although sensory nerves are also involved, patients rarely notice significant numbness or pain.

Onset of symptoms is most often in adolescence or early adulthood, however presentation may be delayed until mid-adulthood. The severity of symptoms is quite variable in different patients and some people may never realize they have the disorder. Progression of symptoms is very gradual. CMT is not fatal and people with most forms of CMT have a normal life expectancy.

What are the types of Charcot-Marie-Tooth disease?

There are many forms of CMT disease. The principal types include CMT1, CMT2, CMT3, CMT4, and CMTX. CMT1 is the most frequent and results from abnormalities in the myelin sheath. There are three main types of CMT1. CMT1A is an autosomal dominant disease resulting from a duplication of the gene on chromosome 17 that carries the instructions for producing the peripheral myelin protein-22 (PMP-22). The PMP-22 protein is a critical component of the myelin sheath. An overabundance of this gene causes the structure and function of the myelin sheath to be abnormal. Patients experience weakness and atrophy of the muscles of the lower legs beginning in adolescence; later they experience hand weakness and sensory loss. Interestingly, a different neuropathy distinct from CMT1A called hereditary neuropathy with predisposition to pressure palsy (HNPP) is caused by a deletion of one of the PMP-22 genes. In this case abnormally low levels of the PMP-22 gene result in episodic, recurrent demyelinating neuropathy. CMT1B is an autosomal dominant disease caused by mutations in the gene that carries the instructions for manufacturing the myelin protein zero (P0) which is another critical component of the myelin sheath. Most of these mutations are point mutations, meaning a mistake occurs in only one letter of the DNA genetic code. To date, scientists have identified more than 30 different point mutations in the P0 gene. As a result of abnormalities in P0, CMT1B produces symptoms similar to those found in CMT1A. The gene defect that causes CMT1C, which also has symptoms similar to those found in CMT1A, has not yet been identified.

CMT2 is less common than CMT1 and results from abnormalities in the axon of the peripheral nerve cell rather than the myelin sheath. Recently a mutation was identified in the gene that codes for the kinesin family member 1B-beta protein in families with CMT2A. Kinesins are proteins that act as motors to help power the transport of materials along the train tracks (microtubules) of the cell. Another recent finding is a mutation in the neurofilament-light gene, identified in a Russian family with CMT2E. Neurofilaments are structural proteins that help maintain the normal shape of a cell. Genes that cause other forms of CMT2 have not yet been identified.

CMT3 or Dejerine-Sottas disease is a severe demyelinating neuropathy that begins in infancy. Infants have severe muscle atrophy, weakness, and sensory problems. This rare disorder can be caused by a specific point mutation in the P0 gene or a point mutation in the PMP-22 gene.

CMT4 comprises several different subtypes of autosomal recessive demyelinating motor and sensory neuropathies. Each neuropathy subtype is caused by a different genetic mutation, may affect a particular ethnic population, and produces distinct physiologic or clinical characteristics. Patients with CMT4 generally develop symptoms of leg weakness in childhood and by adolescence they may not be able to walk. The gene abnormalities responsible for CMT4 have yet to be identified.

CMTX is an X-linked dominant disease and is caused by a point mutation in the connexin-32 gene on the X chromosome. The connexin-32 protein is expressed in Schwann cells—cells that wrap around nerve axons, making up a single segment of the myelin sheath. This protein may be involved in Schwann cell communication with the axon. Males who inherit one mutated gene from their mothers show moderate to severe symptoms of the disease beginning in late childhood or adolescence (the Y chromosome that males inherit from their fathers does not have the connexin-32 gene). Females who inherit one mutated gene from one parent and one normal gene from the other parent may develop mild symptoms in adolescence or later or may not develop symptoms of the disease at all.

What causes Charcot-Marie-Tooth disease?

A nerve cell communicates information to distant targets by sending electrical signals down a long, thin part of the cell called the axon. In order to increase the speed at which these electrical signals travel, the axon is insulated by myelin, which is produced by another type of cell called the Schwann cell. Myelin twists around the axon like a jelly-roll cake and prevents dissipation of the electrical signals. Without an intact axon and myelin sheath, peripheral nerve cells are unable to activate target muscles or relay sensory information from the limbs back to the brain.

CMT is caused by mutations in genes that produce proteins involved in the structure and function of either the peripheral nerve axon or the myelin sheath. Although different proteins are abnormal in different forms of CMT disease, all of the mutations affect the normal function of the peripheral nerves. Consequently, these nerves slowly degenerate and lose the ability to communicate with their distant targets. The degeneration of motor nerves results in muscle weakness and atrophy in the extremities (arms, legs, hands, or feet), and the degeneration of sensory nerves results in a reduced ability to feel heat, cold, and pain.

The gene mutations in CMT disease are usually inherited. Each of us normally possesses two copies of every gene, one inherited from each parent. Some forms of CMT are inherited in an autosomal dominant fashion, which means that only one copy of the abnormal gene is needed to cause the disease. Other forms of CMT are inherited in an autosomal recessive fashion, which means that both copies of the abnormal gene must be present to cause the disease. Still other forms of CMT are inherited in an X-linked fashion, which means that the abnormal gene is located on the X chromosome. The X and Y chromosomes determine an individual's sex. Individuals with two X chromosomes are female and individuals with one X and one Y chromosome are male. In rare cases the gene mutation causing CMT disease is a new mutation which occurs spontaneously in the patient's genetic material and has not been passed down through the family.

How is Charcot-Marie-Tooth disease diagnosed?

Diagnosis of CMT begins with a standard patient history, family history, and neurological examination. Patients will be asked about the nature and duration of their symptoms and whether other family members have the disease. During the neurological examination a physician will look for evidence of muscle weakness in the arms, legs, hands, and feet, decreased muscle bulk, reduced tendon reflexes, and sensory loss. Doctors look for evidence of foot deformities, such as high arches, hammertoes, inverted heel, or flat feet. Other orthopedic problems, such as mild scoliosis or hip dysplasia, may also be present. A specific sign that may be found in patients with CMT1 is nerve enlargement that may be felt or even seen through the skin. These enlarged nerves, called hypertrophic nerves, are caused by abnormally thickened myelin sheaths.

If CMT is suspected, the physician may order electrodiagnostic tests for the patient. This testing consists of two parts: nerve conduction studies and electromyography (EMG). During nerve conduction studies, electrodes are placed on the skin over a peripheral motor or sensory nerve. These electrodes produce a small electric shock that may cause mild discomfort. This electrical impulse stimulates sensory and motor nerves and provides quantifiable information that the doctor can use to arrive at a diagnosis. EMG involves inserting a needle electrode through the skin to measure the bioelectrical activity of muscles. Specific abnormalities in the readings signify axon degeneration. EMG may be useful in further characterizing the distribution and severity of peripheral nerve involvement.

If all other tests seem to suggest that a patient has CMT, a neurologist may perform a nerve biopsy to confirm the diagnosis. A nerve biopsy involves removing a small piece of peripheral nerve through an incision in the skin. This is most often done by removing a piece of the nerve that runs down the calf of the leg. The nerve is then examined under a microscope. Patients with CMT1 typically show signs of abnormal myelination. Specifically, "onion bulb" formations may be seen which represent axons surrounded by layers of demyelinating and remyelinating Schwann cells. Patients with CMT2 usually show signs of axon degeneration.

Genetic testing is available for some types of CMT and may soon be available for other types; such testing can be used to confirm a diagnosis. In addition, genetic counseling is available to parents who fear that they may pass mutant genes to their children.

How is Charcot-Marie-Tooth disease treated?

There is no cure for CMT, but physical therapy, occupational therapy, braces and other orthopedic devices, and even orthopedic surgery can help patients cope with the disabling symptoms of the disease.

Physical and occupational therapy, the preferred treatment for CMT, involves muscle strength training, muscle and ligament stretching, stamina training, and moderate aerobic exercise. Most therapists recommend a specialized treatment program designed with the approval of the patient's physician to fit individual abilities and needs. Therapists also suggest entering into a treatment program early; muscle strengthening may delay or reduce muscle atrophy, so strength training is most useful if it begins before nerve degeneration and muscle weakness progress to the point of disability.

Stretching may prevent or reduce joint deformities that result from uneven muscle pull on bones. Exercises to help build stamina or increase endurance will help prevent the fatigue that results from performing everyday activities that require strength and mobility. Moderate aerobic activity can help to maintain cardiovascular fitness and overall health. Most therapists recommend low-impact or no-impact exercises, such as biking or swimming, rather than activities such as walking or jogging, which may put stress on fragile muscles and joints.

Many CMT patients require ankle braces and other orthopedic devices to maintain everyday mobility and prevent injury. Ankle braces can help prevent ankle sprains by providing support and stability during activities such as walking or climbing stairs. High-top shoes or boots can also give the patient support for weak ankles. Thumb splints can help with hand weakness and loss of fine motor skills. Assistive devices should be used before disability sets in because the devices may prevent muscle strain and reduce muscle weakening. Some CMT patients may decide to have orthopedic surgery to reverse foot and joint deformities.

What research is being done?

The NINDS supports research on CMT and other peripheral neuropathies in an effort to learn how to better treat, prevent, and even cure these disorders. Ongoing research includes efforts to identify more of the mutant genes and proteins that cause the various disease subtypes, efforts to discover the mechanisms of nerve degeneration and muscle atrophy with the hope of developing interventions to stop or slow down these debilitating processes, and efforts to find therapies to reverse nerve degeneration and muscle atrophy.

One promising area of research involves gene therapy experiments. Research with cell cultures and animal models has shown that it is possible to deliver genes to Schwann cells and muscle. Another area of research involves the use of trophic factors or nerve growth factors, such as the hormone androgen, to prevent nerve degeneration.

Section 20.3

Mitochondrial Myopathies

"NINDS Mitochondrial Myopathies Information Page," National Institute of Neurological Disorders and Stroke (NINDS), reviewed November 2003.

What are mitochondrial myopathies?

Mitochondrial myopathies are a group of neuromuscular diseases caused by damage to the mitochondria—small, energy-producing structures found in every cell in the body that serve as the cells' "power plants." Nerve cells in the brain and muscles require a great deal of energy, and thus appear to be particularly damaged when mitochondrial dysfunction occurs. Some of the more common mitochondrial myopathies include Kearns-Sayre syndrome, myoclonus epilepsy with ragged-red fibers, and mitochondrial encephalomyopathy with lactic acidosis and stroke-like episodes. The symptoms of mitochondrial myopathies include muscle weakness or exercise intolerance, heart failure or rhythm disturbances, dementia, movement disorders, stroke-like episodes, deafness, blindness, droopy eyelids, limited mobility of the eyes, vomiting, and seizures. The prognosis for these disorders ranges in severity from progressive weakness to death. Most mitochondrial myopathies occur before the age of 20, and often begin with exercise intolerance or muscle weakness. During physical activity, muscles may become easily fatigued or weak. Muscle cramping is rare, but may occur. Nausea, headache, and breathlessness are also associated with these disorders.

Is there any treatment?

Although there is no specific treatment for any of the mitochondrial myopathies, physical therapy may extend the range of movement of muscles and improve dexterity. Vitamin therapies such as riboflavin, coenzyme Q, and carnitine (a specialized amino acid) may provide subjective improvement in fatigue and energy levels in some patients.

What is the prognosis?

The prognosis for patients with mitochondrial myopathies varies greatly, depending largely on the type of disease and the degree of involvement of various organs. These disorders cause progressive weakness and can lead to death.

What research is being done?

The NINDS conducts and supports research on mitochondrial myopathies. The goals of this research are to increase scientific understanding of these disorders and to find ways to effectively treat, prevent, or potentially cure them.

Section 20.4

Muscular Dystrophies

This section includes excerpts reprinted with permission from "Facts about Rare Muscular Dystrophies: Congenital, Distal, Emery-Dreifuss and Oculopharyngeal Muscular Dystrophies," © 2002 Muscular Dystrophy Association (MDA); "Facts about Duchenne and Becker Muscular Dystrophies (DMD and BMD)," © 2000 MDA; "Facts about Limb-Girdle Muscular Dystrophy (LGMD)," © 2000 MDA; "Facts About Facioscapulohumeral Muscular Dystrophy," © 2004 MDA; and "Facts about Myotonic Muscular Dystrophy," © 2000 MDA. For additional information, call the Muscular Dystrophy Association National Headquarters toll-free at (800) 572-1717. To find an MDA office in your area, look in your local telephone book, or click on "Clinics and Services" on the MDA website, http://www.mdausa.org.

What is muscular dystrophy?

The muscular dystrophies are a group of genetic diseases that cause weakness and muscle wasting, primarily in the skeletal or voluntary muscles (those we control such as the muscles of the arms and legs).

Most people with muscular dystrophy experience some degree of muscle weakness during their lifetimes, but each of the disorders affects different muscle groups and may have different accompanying symptoms. Because muscle weakness usually progresses over time in the muscular dystrophies, lifestyle changes, assistive devices and occupational therapy may be needed to help a person adapt to new situations.

What causes muscular dystrophy?

All the forms of muscular dystrophy are inherited—that is, they're caused by mutations (changes) in a person's genes. Our genes are made of DNA and they reside in our chromosomes. Each gene contains the "recipe" for a different protein and its variations, and these proteins are necessary for our bodies to function correctly.

When a gene has a mutation, it may make a defective protein or none at all. Most commonly, missing or defective proteins in the muscles prevent muscle cells from working properly, leading to symptoms of muscular dystrophy, including muscle weakness and wasting over time.

What happens to someone with muscular dystrophy?

Most forms of muscular dystrophy are progressive and they tend to worsen with time. However, age of onset and rate of progression can vary widely from one disorder to the next. Some, but not all, of these disorders can affect life expectancy. In many cases, advancing knowledge allows for treatment of the symptoms that are most likely to decrease life expectancy.

In most cases of muscular dystrophy, muscle mass in the affected regions may become visibly wasted (decrease in size), and the arms, legs, or trunk may become so weak they eventually can't move. Some forms of muscular dystrophy are accompanied by contractures, or stiff joints, and some are accompanied by scoliosis, or spinal curvature.

The diaphragm and other muscles that operate the lungs may weaken, making them less effective in moving air in and out. Problems that may indicate poor respiratory function include headaches, mental dullness, difficulty concentrating or staying awake, and nightmares. Anyone with a weakened respiratory system is also subject to more infections and difficulty in coughing. A simple cold can quickly progress to pneumonia. During infections, it's important to get prompt treatment before a respiratory emergency occurs. If breathing ability declines, the family can get a coughing machine or learn procedures to assist with coughing and keep the bronchial system free from secretions. A respiratory therapist or pulmonologist can be consulted for the needed information.

Forms of muscular dystrophy that affect the muscles used for swallowing may require that precautions be taken when eating or drinking so that food isn't aspirated into the lungs. Although most muscular dystrophies don't affect the brain, some are accompanied by brain changes that cause learning disabilities that range from slight to severe.

Finally, some forms of muscular dystrophy also affect the heart, and special precautions must be taken to monitor heart function. Each disorder has its own special areas of concern.

What can be done to treat muscular dystrophy?

There are currently no cures for any form of muscular dystrophy, but there are many therapies designed to help deal with common symptoms of the disease group. For instance, contractures may be helped by physical therapy and sometimes tendon-release surgery, while scoliosis may respond to bracing or surgery, and heart problems may respond to medication or an implanted pacemaker. (Physical and occupational therapies can be arranged through your child's school or through your Muscular Dystrophy Association [MDA] clinic.)

Many people with these forms of muscular dystrophy live very full lives. Your MDA clinic director will help you plan the best strategy for coping with your or your child's specific needs.

Does it run in the family?

On being told they have a genetic disorder such as muscular dystrophy, bewildered patients often ask, "But it doesn't run in the family, so how could it be genetic?"

Muscular dystrophy can run in a family, even if only one person in the biological family has it. This is because of the ways in which genetic diseases are inherited.

Each form of muscular dystrophy follows one of three patterns of inheritance: recessive, dominant or X-linked. In brief, if a disease is recessive, two copies of the defective gene (one from each parent) are required to produce the disease. Each parent would be a carrier of the gene flaw, but wouldn't usually have the disease.

If a disease is dominant, then only one copy of the genetic defect is needed to cause the disease. Anyone with the gene flaw will have disease symptoms and can pass the disorder to children. If a disease is X-linked, it's passed from mother to son, while daughters can be carriers but don't generally get the disease.

Many times MD appears to have occurred "out of the blue," but in reality, one or both parents may be carriers, silently harboring the genetic mutation (a flaw in the gene). Many parents have no idea they're carriers of a disease until they have a child who has the disease.

In rare cases, muscular dystrophy actually can occur "out of the blue" when a new mutation appears with a baby's conception, though neither parent carries the gene flaw. These are called spontaneous mutations, and, after they occur, they can be passed on to the next generation, thereby introducing the gene for a specific MD into the family.

What are Duchenne and Becker muscular dystrophies?

Duchenne muscular dystrophy (DMD) was first described by the French neurologist Guillaume Benjamin Amand Duchenne in the 1860s. Becker muscular dystrophy (BMD) is named after the German doctor Peter Emil Becker, who first described this variant of DMD in the 1950s.

In DMD, boys begin to show signs of muscle weakness as early as age three. The disease gradually weakens the skeletal, or voluntary, muscles, those in the arms, legs and trunk. By the early teens or even earlier, the boy's heart and respiratory muscles may also be affected. Many boys with DMD have mild learning impairments. Death in DMD usually comes by the mid to late 20s and is usually due to either cardiac or respiratory failure.

BMD is a much milder version of DMD. Its onset is usually in the teens or early adulthood, and the course is slower and far less predictable than that of DMD. Effects on the heart can be severe, even if other muscles are not greatly affected. Life expectancy is not necessarily shortened, but it can be if the heart is involved.

Though DMD and BMD affect boys almost exclusively, in rare cases they can affect girls.

What happens to the voluntary muscles of someone with DMD or BMD?

Duchenne: The course of DMD is fairly predictable. Children with the disorder are often late in learning to walk. In toddlers, parents may notice enlarged calf muscles, or pseudohypertrophy. A preschooler with DMD may seem clumsy and fall often. Soon, he has trouble climbing stairs, getting up from the floor, or running.

By school age, the child may walk on his toes or the balls of his feet, with a slightly rolling gait. He has a waddling and unsteady gait and can easily fall over. To try to keep his balance, he sticks his belly out and puts his shoulders back. He also has difficulty raising his arms.

Nearly all children with DMD lose the ability to walk sometime between ages seven and 12. In the teen years, activities involving the arms, legs, or trunk require assistance or mechanical support.

Becker: Often, the diagnosis of Becker muscular dystrophy isn't made until adolescence or even adulthood, possibly when a young man finds he can't keep up in physical education classes or military training. To compensate for his weakening muscles, the young man begins walking with a waddling gait, walking on his toes or sticking out his abdomen.

As with Duchenne, the pattern of muscle loss in BMD usually begins with the hips and pelvic area, the thighs and the shoulders. But in BMD, the rate of muscle degeneration varies a great deal from one person to another. Some men require wheelchairs by their 30s or later, while some manage for many years with minor aids, such as canes.

What is limb-girdle muscular dystrophy?

Limb-girdle muscular dystrophy (LGMD) isn't really one disease. It's a group of disorders affecting voluntary muscles, mainly those around the hips and shoulders—the pelvic and shoulder girdles, also known as the limb girdles. You may also hear the term proximal used to describe the muscles that are most affected in LGMD. The proximal muscles are those closest to the center of the body; distal muscles are farther away from the center (for example, in the hands and feet). The distal muscles are affected late in LGMD, if at all. Over time (usually many years), the person with LGMD loses muscle bulk and strength. Eventually, he may need a power wheelchair or scooter, especially for long distances.

LGMD can begin in childhood, adolescence, young adulthood or even later. Both genders are affected equally. When limb-girdle muscular dystrophy begins in childhood, some physicians say, the progression is usually faster and the disease more disabling. When the disorder begins in adolescence or adulthood, they say, it's generally not as severe and progresses more slowly.

In what ways is a person affected by LGMD?

LGMD, like other muscular dystrophies, is primarily a disorder of skeletal muscle. Other names for skeletal muscle are voluntary and striated muscle (because of its microscopic appearance). These are the muscles you use to move the limbs, neck, trunk, and other parts of the body that are under voluntary control. Heart muscle, which is slightly different from skeletal muscle, and respiratory muscles, which are actually skeletal muscles, are sometimes also involved in LGMD.

The involuntary or smooth muscles, such as those that control the body's digestive and elimination processes, usually aren't affected in LGMD. Recent research in animals suggests that some forms of LGMD may affect the involuntary muscles responsible for normal blood vessel contraction and relaxation, and that this involvement could be a factor in some of the heart problems occasionally seen in LGMD.

Pain isn't a major part of LGMD, but limited mobility sometimes leads to muscle soreness and joint pain. Exercises to keep joints limber, moving around as much as possible, warm baths and, if needed, medication can keep this kind of discomfort to a minimum.

The brain, the intellect and the senses are unaffected in LGMD. People with LGMD can think, see, hear and feel sensations as well as those without muscular dystrophy. They maintain control over their bowel and bladder functions, and sexual function is normal.

What is facioscapulohumeral muscular dystrophy?

Facioscapulohumeral muscular dystrophy (FSHD) is a genetic muscle disorder in which the muscles of the face, shoulder blades, and upper arms are among the most severely affected.

The long name comes from facies, the Latin word and medical term for face; scapula, the Latin word and anatomical term for shoulder blade; and humerus, the Latin word for upper arm and the anatomical term for the bone that goes from the shoulder to the elbow.

The term muscular dystrophy means slowly progressive muscle degeneration, with increasing weakness and wasting (loss of bulk) of muscles. In FSHD, weakness first and most seriously affects the face, shoulders, and upper arms, but the disease usually also causes weakness in other muscles.

Because FSHD is a disease that usually progresses very slowly and rarely affects the heart or respiratory system, it isn't considered life-threatening. Most people with the disease have a normal life span.

What happens to someone with FSHD?

The age of onset, progression and severity of FSHD vary a great deal.

Usually, symptoms develop during the teen years, with most people noticing some problems by age 20, although weakness in some muscles can begin as early as infancy and as late as the 50s. In some people, the disease can be so mild that no symptoms are noticed. In these cases, the disease may only be diagnosed after another, more affected member of the family comes to medical attention.

Usually, people don't go to the doctor until their shoulder or leg muscles become involved and they experience difficulty reaching over their heads or going up and down stairs. When questioned closely, many people can remember having symptoms in childhood, such as shoulder blades that stuck out or trouble throwing a ball. Very often, people say they've never been able to whistle or blow up a balloon, or that they've had trouble drinking through a straw, but they may not have associated these problems with muscular dystrophy.

In most people with FSHD, the disease progresses very slowly. It can take as long as 30 years for the disease to become seriously disabling, and that doesn't happen to everyone. Estimates are that about 20 percent of people with FSHD eventually use a wheelchair at least some of the time.

Facial Weakness: Facial weakness is often the first sign of FSHD, but it may not be noticed right away by the person with the disorder. It's usually brought to his or her attention by someone else or by a doctor.

The muscles most affected are those that surround the eyes and mouth. It's hard to pucker up or to get much strength in the mouth, which is why people with the disease have trouble with balloons, straws and whistling.

Of somewhat more concern is the weakness in the eye muscles, which can keep the eyes from closing completely during the night. As the disease progresses, the eyes can sometimes dry out overnight, which can injure them. Waking up in the morning with gritty, burning, or dry eyes may be a sign that eye closure isn't complete. Wearing an eye shield or patching the eyes during sleep may be necessary.

Shoulder Weakness: Most people with FSHD notice weakness in the area of the shoulder blades—the scapulae—as the first sign that something is amiss.

The shoulder blades are normally fairly fixed in their position. They act as fulcrums that allow the arm muscles to get leverage for lifting things, including their own weight.

In FSHD, the muscles that hold the shoulder blades in place weaken, allowing these bones to move excessively. The shoulder blades stick out and rise up toward the neck as they move, which is called scapular winging, because the protruding bone resembles a wing. Leverage is at least partially lost. The weakness often isn't the same on both sides of the body.

Early on, the person with FSHD notices things like being unable to throw a ball effectively. Later, it may be hard to lift the arms over the head to do one's hair or reach a high shelf or hang something. These problems are due to weakening of the muscles around the shoulder and in the upper arm.

Lower Leg Weakness: As FSHD progresses, the muscles on the front and sides of the lower legs often weaken. These are the muscles that allow us to raise the front of the foot when walking so we don't trip over our toes.

When these muscles weaken, the foot stays down after pushing off during walking, sometimes tripping the walker. This condition is called foot drop.

The doctor may say, "Walk on your heels, like a penguin" to test the strength of these foot-lifting muscles.

When questioned, people will say, "I seem to catch my foot when I walk" or "I seem to fall over my own feet." Trouble with stairs and with uneven surfaces is common.

Not everyone with FSHD develops this lower leg problem.

Abdominal Muscle Weakness: In many people with FSHD, weakness develops in the muscles of the abdomen. These can weaken early in the disorder. As abdominal weakness progresses, the person develops a lordosis, an exaggerated curve in the lumbar (lower) region of the spine.

Hip Weakness: In some people, weakness of the hip muscles that surround the pelvis (doctors call this the pelvic girdle) also occurs. This doesn't happen to everyone. Weakness of the hips seems to start most often in middle adulthood, if it happens at all. Hip weakness causes trouble with rising from a chair or negotiating stairs and can lead to the need for a wheelchair, especially for long distances. Upper leg muscles are sometimes also affected. Pelvic girdle weakness may result in a waddling gait and contribute to the lordosis so often seen in FSHD.

In children with FSHD, hip weakness may be the first thing parents notice, since it causes trouble with walking and running.

Unequal (Nonsymmetrical) Weakness: In most people with FSHD, weakness differs at least a little bit between the left and right sides of the body. In some people with FSHD, this difference between sides can be quite striking. The reason for this lack of symmetry, which is not seen in most types of muscular dystrophy, is not clear.

What is myotonic muscular dystrophy?

Myotonic muscular dystrophy (MMD) is a form of muscular dystrophy that affects muscles and many other organs in the body. Unlike some forms of muscular dystrophy, MMD often doesn't become a problem until adulthood and usually allows people to walk and be pretty independent throughout their lives.

The infant form of MMD is more severe. Unfortunately, it can occur in babies born to parents who have the adult form, even if they have very mild cases.

The word myotonic is the adjective for the word myotonia, an inability to relax muscles at will. In MMD, the myotonia is usually mild. In fact, many people attribute it to "stiffness" or think they have arthritis. If anything is noticeable, it's usually difficulty with one's grip, for example when using a tool or writing instrument.

Myotonia isn't a feature of any other form of muscular dystrophy (although it occurs in other kinds of muscle diseases, where it can be severe). When a person suspected of having muscular dystrophy has myotonia, the diagnosis is likely to be MMD.

The term muscular dystrophy means slowly progressive muscle degeneration, with increasing weakness and wasting (loss of bulk) of muscles. The weakness and wasting of muscles generally present much more of a problem to people with MMD than does the myotonia. However, they usually aren't as severe as in some other types of muscular dystrophy.

MMD symptoms sometimes begin at birth. Infants with this disorder, congenital MMD, have severe muscle weakness, including weakening of muscles that control breathing and swallowing. These problems can be life-threatening and need intensive care. Myotonia isn't part of the picture in infants with MMD.

MMD symptoms can also begin in children past infancy but not yet adolescents, although this is unusual. Generally, the earlier MMD begins, the more severe the disease is. Myotonic muscular dystrophy is often known simply as myotonic dystrophy and is occasionally called Steinert's disease, after a doctor who originally described the disorder in 1909. It's also called dystrophia myotonica, a Latin name, and therefore often abbreviated "DM."

MMD varies greatly in severity, even within the same family. Not everyone has all the symptoms and not everyone has them to the same degree.

There is, however, a distinct difference between the type that affects newborn infants—congenital MMD—and the type that begins in adolescence or adulthood—adult-onset MMD.

What happens in adult-onset MMD?

It's reassuring to know that when MMD begins in the teen years or during adulthood, it's often only a moderately disabling condition with very slow progression. As one doctor put it, "Some people with MMD go through much of their lives without troubling or being troubled by the medical profession."

There can be troubling symptoms, however, for many people. Although many different parts of the body can be affected by MMD, most people with the disease have only some of the following symptoms. Most of the problems can be lessened with medical treatment.

- **Limb Muscles:** Weakness of the voluntary muscles, such as those that control the arm and legs, is usually the most noticeable symptom for people with adult-onset MMD.

- **Head, Neck and Face Muscles:** A long, thin face with hollow temples, drooping eyelids and, in men, balding in the front, is typical in myotonic dystrophy. The muscles of the neck, jaw and parts of the head and face may weaken in MMD.

- **Breathing and Swallowing Muscles:** Respiratory muscles can become weak in MMD, affecting lung function and depriving the body of needed oxygen. Swallowing muscles, if weakened, can lead to choking, or "swallowing the wrong way," with food or liquid going down the trachea (windpipe) instead of the esophagus (tube from the throat to the stomach).

- **Myotonia:** The myotonia of voluntary muscles can make it hard for someone with MMD to relax the grip, especially in cold temperatures. Myotonia can affect other muscles, but usually it isn't noticeable.

- **Heart Problems:** The heart can be affected in adult MMD. Oddly, since MMD is mostly a muscle disease, it isn't the muscle part of the heart (which pumps blood) that's most affected, but rather the part that sets the rate and rhythm of the heartbeat—the heart's conduction system. It's common in MMD, especially after many years, to develop a conduction block, a block in the electricity-like signal that keeps the heart beating at a safe rate.

- **Internal Organs:** In MMD, many of the involuntary muscles that surround the hollow organs can weaken and can also have myotonia. These include the muscles of the digestive tract, the uterus and the blood vessels.

- **The Brain:** First, as with other aspects of MMD, there's a wide range in severity of the mental and emotional symptoms of the disorder. Some people function very well, others poorly, many somewhere in between. Children born with the severe, congenital form of MMD have a lot of learning problems and may even be mentally retarded. They often need special education because of these disabilities. In adults, severe mental impairment is less common, but an overall inability to "settle down to something," apply oneself to work or family life, concentrate or become engrossed in a task is often reported.

- **The Eyes:** Cataracts—cloudy areas of the lens of the eye that can eventually interfere with vision—are extremely common in MMD. The muscles that move the eyes, as well as those that open and close them, can also be affected in MMD, and other eye problems can sometimes occur.

- **Diabetes:** Most people with MMD don't have severe diabetes, but they may develop a mild type sometimes referred to as insulin resistance with high blood sugar.

- **Anesthesia:** An unusually high rate of complications and even deaths associated with general anesthesia (given during any surgery) have been reported in people with MMD. This can occur even if the MMD is mild. In fact, these cases can be particularly dangerous, because the surgeon, anesthesiologist and patient may be less likely to pay much attention to the MMD when planning the surgery. Surgery can usually be safely undertaken these days with careful monitoring of cardiac and respiratory functions before, during and after the surgery.

What happens in congenital MMD?

The most serious form of MMD is the congenital (at birth) form of the disease. When a child with congenital MMD is born, it's almost always found that the mother has adult-onset MMD—even though her symptoms may be so mild that she doesn't even know she has the disorder.

Mothers with MMD can also pass on the adult-onset form. When fathers with MMD have children, the child can also inherit the disease, but it's almost always the adult-onset form. These unusual features of MMD aren't seen in other genetic disorders.

- **Weak Muscles:** Babies born with congenital MMD have very weak muscles and a lack of muscle tone (hypotonia). They appear floppy, have trouble breathing, and suck and swallow poorly.

- **Mental Retardation:** Infants born with congenital MMD are likely to be mentally retarded, although this isn't always the case. This seems to be related to maldevelopment of parts of the brain, presumably caused by genetic abnormalities.

- **Speech and Hearing Difficulties:** The muscles involved in talking are often affected in congenital MMD. Hearing can also be impaired.

- **Vision Problems:** The eye muscles in congenital MMD are affected and can cause the eyes not to work together; this condition is called strabismus. Cataracts, common in adult-onset MMD, aren't a feature of congenital MMD during early childhood. However, children with MMD are likely to develop them later.

What is congenital muscular dystrophy?

The term congenital muscular dystrophy (CMD) is actually the name for a group of muscular dystrophies that are united by the fact that muscle weakness begins in infancy or very early childhood (typically before age two). Congenital diseases are those in which the symptoms are present at or soon after birth.

A diagnosis of CMD can be confusing because for many years the term was used as a "catchall" name to describe conditions that looked like other muscular dystrophies, but started much earlier or followed different patterns of inheritance. In recent years doctors have agreed that there are several different categories of "true" CMD, caused by specific gene mutations, and they're distinct from other muscular dystrophies. It's possible that some people who received diagnoses of CMD many years ago may actually have some other known form of muscular dystrophy with an unusually early onset.

Although children with CMD can have different associated symptoms, degrees of severity and rates of progression, most exhibit some progressive muscle weakness. This weakness, usually first identified as hypotonia, or lack of muscle tone, can make an infant seem "floppy." Later, infants and toddlers may be slow to meet motor milestones such as rolling over, sitting up or walking, or may not meet some milestones at all.

Some of the rarer forms of CMD are also accompanied by significant learning disabilities, or mental retardation.

What is distal muscular dystrophy?

First described in 1902, distal muscular dystrophy (DD), or distal myopathy, is the name of a group of disorders that primarily affect distal muscles, those farthest away from the hips and shoulders such as muscles in the hands, feet, lower arms or lower legs. Although muscle weakness is usually first detected in the distal muscles, with time, other muscle groups may become affected as well. Intellect isn't affected in these diseases.

What is Emery-Dreifuss muscular dystrophy?

Emery-Dreifuss muscular dystrophy (EDMD) is characterized by wasting and weakness of the muscles that make up the shoulders and upper arms and those of the calf muscles of the legs. Another prominent aspect of this disease is the appearance of contractures (stiff joints) in the elbows, neck, and heels very early in the course of the disease. Finally, and very importantly, a type of heart problem called a conduction block is a common feature of EDMD and requires monitoring.

What is oculopharyngeal muscular dystrophy?

Oculopharyngeal muscular dystrophy (OPMD) is characterized by weakness of the muscles that control the eyelids (leading to droopy eyelids, a condition also known as ptosis), and by weakness of the facial muscles and pharyngeal muscles (those in the throat used for swallowing). It also affects limb muscles. Symptoms of the disease usually don't begin until the mid 40s or 50s, but can occur earlier.

OPMD is usually inherited as a dominant disease, but rare cases may show a recessive pattern of inheritance. When muscle tissue from a person with OPMD is examined under the microscope, clumps of proteins called inclusions are seen in the muscle cell nuclei (the cellular compartments that contain the chromosomes).

The disease is most common in French-Canadian families or families of French-Canadian descent. Research into the genealogy of these families has suggested that a single couple, Zacharie Cloutier and Saincte Dupont, who immigrated to Canada from France in 1634, may have harbored the genetic defect responsible for the majority of today's French-Canadian cases. There's also a high incidence of OPMD among Hispanic residents of northern New Mexico.

OPMD can also affect people who aren't of French-Canadian or Hispanic background.

What tests are used to diagnose muscular dystrophy?

In diagnosing any form of muscular dystrophy, a doctor usually begins by taking a patient and family history and performing a physical examination. Much can be learned from these, including the pattern of weakness. The history and physical go a long way toward making the diagnosis, even before any complicated diagnostic tests are done.

The doctor also wants to determine whether the patient's weakness results from a problem in the muscles themselves or in the nerves that control them. Problems with muscle-controlling nerves, or motor nerves, originating in the spinal cord and reaching out to all the muscles, can cause weakness that looks like a muscle problem but really isn't.

Usually, the origin of the weakness can be pinpointed by a physical exam. Occasionally, special testing called electromyography (EMG) is done. In this kind of test, electricity and very fine pins are used to stimulate the muscles or nerves individually to see where the problem lies. Electromyography is uncomfortable, but not usually very painful.

Early in the diagnostic process doctors often order a special blood test called a CK level. CK stands for creatine kinase, an enzyme that leaks out of damaged muscle. When elevated CK levels are found in a blood sample, it usually means muscle is being destroyed by some abnormal process, such as a muscular dystrophy or an inflammation. Therefore, a high CK level suggests that the muscles themselves are the likely cause of the weakness, but it doesn't tell exactly what the muscle disorder might be.

To determine which disorder is causing CK elevation, a doctor may order a muscle biopsy, the surgical removal of a small sample of muscle from the patient. By examining this sample, doctors can tell a great deal about what's actually happening inside the muscles. Modern techniques can use the biopsy to distinguish muscular dystrophies from infections, inflammatory disorders, and other problems.

Other tests on the biopsy sample can provide information about which muscle proteins are present in the muscle cells, and whether they're present in the normal amounts and in the right locations. This can tell the doctor and patient what's wrong with the cells' proteins and provide likely candidates as to which genes are responsible for the problem. The correlation between missing proteins on the muscle biopsy and genetic flaws isn't perfect, however. An MDA clinic physician can help you understand these results.

An MR (magnetic resonance) scan may also be ordered. These scans, which are painless, allow doctors to visualize what's going on inside weakening muscles.

Genetic tests, using a blood sample, can analyze the person's genes for particular defects that cause the rare muscular dystrophies, but these tests often aren't necessary for diagnosis or for determining treatment.

Section 20.5

Spinal Muscular Atrophy

This text is to serve as a source of information and support to those involved with children and adults with spinal muscular atrophy (SMA). Whether you have a family member or close friend, your interest in this is probably based on the fact that you or someone you care about is awaiting diagnosis of SMA or has been diagnosed with SMA.

We understand the concern that you might have upon hearing the terms, Werdnig-Hoffmann, Kugelberg-Welander, or spinal muscular atrophy. We've all heard of leukemia, AIDS, and cystic fibrosis, but spinal muscular atrophy is an unknown. It is relatively unknown despite the fact that one in 40 people are carriers, and one in every 6,000 live births is affected—which is why so much research is being conducted to discover its cause(s) and cure.

What Is Spinal Muscular Atrophy?

Spinal muscular atrophy (SMA) is a disease of the anterior horn cells. Anterior horn cells are located in the spinal cord. SMA affects the voluntary muscles for activities such as crawling, walking, head and neck control, and swallowing.

It mainly affects the proximal muscles, or in other words the muscles closest to the point of origin, in this case those closest to the trunk of one's body. Weakness in the legs is generally greater than weakness in the arms. Some abnormal movements of the tongue, called tongue fasciculations, may be present in patients with type I and in some patients with type II. The senses and feelings are normal as is intellectual activity. In fact it is often observed that patients with SMA are unusually bright and sociable.

273

Type I Acute (Severe)

Type I SMA is also called Werdnig-Hoffmann Disease. The diagnosis of children with this type is usually made before six months of age and in the majority of cases before three months. There may be lack of fetal movement in the final months of pregnancy.

Usually a child with type I, (Werdnig-Hoffmann) is never able to lift his/her head or accomplish normal physical milestones. Swallowing and feeding may be difficult, and the child may show some difficulties with their own secretions. There is a general weakness in the intercostals and accessory respiratory muscles (the muscles situated between the ribs). The chest may appear concave (sunken in) due to the diaphragmatic (tummy) breathing.

Note: Although diagnosis may be made before six months of age it does not necessarily follow the same course of severity for each patient.

Type II (Chronic)

Diagnosis of type II is almost always made before two years of age with the majority of cases diagnosed by 15 months. Children with this type may sit unsupported although they are usually unable to come to a sitting position without assistance. At some point they may be able to stand. This is most often accomplished with the aid of bracing and/or a parapodium/standing frame.

Feeding and swallowing problems are not usually characteristic of type II, although in some patients this can occur and a feeding tube may become necessary.

Tongue fasciculations are less often found in children with type II, but a fine tremor in the outstretched fingers is common. Children with type II are also diaphragmatic breathers.

Type III (Mild)

Diagnosis of type III, often referred to as Kugelberg-Welander or juvenile spinal muscular atrophy, is made sometime after 18 months of age and as late as adolescence. The patient with type III can stand alone and walk, but may show difficulty with walking and/or getting up from a sitting or bent over position. With type III, a fine tremor can be seen in the outstretched fingers but tongue fasciculations are seldom seen.

Note: Patients with spinal muscular atrophy types I, II and III will lose function over time. The explanation for this loss is unclear based on recent research.

Type IV (Adult Onset)

Typically in the adult form symptoms begin after age 35. It is very rare for spinal muscular atrophy to begin between the ages of 18 and 30. Adult SMA is characterized by insidious onset and very slow progression. The bulbar muscles, those muscles used for swallowing and respiratory function, are rarely affected in type IV.

Adult Onset X-Linked SMA

This form, also known as Kennedy's syndrome or bulbo-spinal muscular atrophy, occurs only in males, although females can be carriers. This form of SMA is associated with a mutation in the gene that codes for part of the androgen receptor; and, therefore, these male patients often have breast enlargement known as gynecomastia. Also noticeably affected are the facial and tongue muscles. Like all forms of SMA the course of the disease is variable but, in general, tends to be slowly progressive or nonprogressive.

Diagnosing Spinal Muscular Atrophy

Genetic Testing

Probes that detect deletions in types I, II, and III SMA have been reported. One of these probes is for a gene called survival motor neuron (SMN), and it detects the absence of gene sequences in approximately 90–94% of SMA patients. This information makes this SMN gene test very useful for the diagnosis of SMA. However, the defect in this gene cannot be used to indicate the severity of the disease. Also, the results may show that there is no deletion of the SMN gene. If this is the case, then a muscle biopsy and/or electromyography (EMG) would be necessary to confirm the diagnosis.

Serum Enzymes

This is a regular blood test. The enzyme most commonly studied is CPK (creatine-phosphokinase). In type I (Werdnig-Hoffmann) this enzyme tends to be normal, but moderate elevation may occur in the milder forms.

EMG (Electromyography)

This test measures the electrical activity of muscle. In this procedure small needles are inserted into the patient's muscles, usually the arms and thighs, while an electrical pattern is observed and recorded. The readout is similar to that of an EKG (ECK; electrocardiograph). In addition, a nerve conduction velocity (NVC) may also be performed. In this test the response of a nerve to an electrical stimulus is measured.

When this test is performed on a child, if at all possible, seek a doctor experienced in dealing with children. Also be sure to bring lots of things with which to keep your child occupied. Hold your child on your lap during the procedure, as it is a tremendous help in making an unpleasant procedure somewhat bearable. Ask your doctor whether your child, the patient, should be given a mild pain killer or sedative prior to the test.

Muscle Biopsy

This is a surgical procedure where an incision (approximately three inches long) is made and a small section of muscle is removed, usually from the thigh. The biopsy is used to check for degeneration. This procedure can be done with a local anesthetic. It is an especially important point when dealing with children who may be suffering from a neuromuscular disorder and may have weak respiratory function.

Note: There is an alternative to the biopsy; it is a procedure known as a needle biopsy. Instead of a two-to-three inch incision, only a small nick in the skin is necessary. Be sure to inquire about this procedure.

Parents' Concerns

Parents often do not remember to ask for an explanation of all the tests, or because of other concerns, they may not be clearheaded enough to hear or understand the explanations. Remember:

- No matter what, you—as a parent or as a patient—have rights and that you are not alone.

- Most hospitals have social service departments that can give you a shoulder to lean on.

- Don't be afraid to say NO if something doesn't seem right.

- Don't be intimidated or afraid to ask questions.

- If you forget to ask something call your doctor or contact Families of SMA for suggestions.

Prognosis: What Does it Mean? What Are We to Expect?

Each type of SMA has variability among individual patients. Please keep this in mind when reading this section.

Type I Acute

In the acute type of this disease the bulbar muscles are often affected, and this may make feeding and swallowing extremely difficult. Breathing is often labored due to reduced strength of the chest muscles, and most breathing can be seen in the abdominal areas, with the chest appearing sunken in.

Because of increasing overall weakness or repeated respiratory infections, the prognosis is poor. Death in the majority of children with type I SMA usually occurs by two years of age.

Note: Again, it is important to note the overlap of types I and II.

Type II Intermediate

Because of the range of progression seen in patients with type II it is hard to tell how fast, if at all, the weakness will progress. Some children may learn to walk with the aid of bracing and may survive into adulthood. However, others, due to weakened chest and respiratory muscles may become increasingly weak with probable respiratory infections, such as pneumonia. There are many cases in which the initial progressive weakness may remain the same, or there may be periods of worsening followed by long periods of stability. With such variables, age of death can vary greatly. It can take place as early as three years or not until adulthood.

Although not all children diagnosed with type II develop respiratory weakness, respiratory failure is usually the cause of death following a bout of pneumonia or other respiratory infection.

Type III Mild

Patients with type III will again vary greatly. However, the prognosis is very good. Often walking will be possible, or the patient will be fully functional for years before assistance is necessary. As with type I and type II respiratory infections should be prevented and necessary precautions taken.

Type IV Adult Onset

There is nothing unusual or distinctive about the current management of the adult forms of spinal muscular atrophy. Proper diagnosis, genetic counseling, and appropriate physical therapy remain mainstays.

Taking the Diagnosis Home: What Can We Do?

Type I (and Some Type II)

While most children diagnosed with type I are still infants there are a myriad of things that can be done to assist in the cognitive and emotional health of your child. Using balloons and feathers as toys makes for wonderful stimulation and allows them that feeling of independence and accomplishment. Reaching games are a form of physical therapy that can be very helpful. Instructions in range of motion and other physical therapy ideas by a licensed physical therapist are important no matter how young the child. Your physical therapist can also suggest ideal seating systems that will be most helpful in the comfort and maximum mobility of your child.

Also getting in touch with a respiratory therapist is very important especially so you can be instructed in CPT (chest physiotherapy). CPT is a means of clearing the lungs of accumulated mucus by using a series of procedures to assist in coughing.

Saliva can settle in the nasopharynx causing a faint gurgling sound. Often the secretions or mucus can not be cleared with these noninvasive measures and the use of a suction machine may be necessary. Activities such as blowing raspberries, or bubbles, or anything that encourages respiratory strength can be beneficial.

Water therapy can be very helpful as the buoyancy of the water allows movement of the arms and legs that may otherwise not be there. Be sure that the water temperature is at least 90°F and that the child's head does not go under the water or into the water. You must watch so that the child has no possibility of aspirating (getting fluid into their lungs).

Aspirating can also become a problem with children when eating. Sometimes the child may even aspirate his/her own secretions. As this becomes a problem, loss of weight may also be noted and assistive feeding may be necessary. Two possible options are:

- **Naso Gastric Tube:** A tube inserted through the nose which goes directly into the stomach.

- **Gastric Tube:** A more permanent option. It involves a surgical procedure to insert a tube or button directly into the stomach. It may be possible to do this procedure with a local anesthetic and an intravenous (IV) sedation drip.

It will be necessary to monitor respiratory distress by measuring the level of oxygen and to determine if oxygen from an outside source is necessary. The tool used to measure this is called a Biox-oximeter. This is a small clip which is usually placed on the patient's index finger to determine the oxygen saturation.

To help the child with breathing a ventilator can be used. There are several possibilities when considering ventilation.

- **Negative Pressure Ventilation** can be achieved by placing the patient in a Port-A-Lung. This is a much smaller version of the old fashioned iron lung. It works by using external ventilation to create negative pressure to set the rate of breathing.

- **Bi-Pap (Biphasic Positive Airway Pressure):** This ventilation unit uses a nasal mask with a cap, which fits over the head to hold it in place over the nose. A small hose is attached that feeds oxygen. This unit allows maximum inspiration and expiration. A small alarm is also attached to detect for leaks.

For long term ventilation a tracheotomy is usually performed. There may be other options available. Consult your physicians and respiratory therapists or contact Families of SMA for literature.

It is important to understand your rights when it comes to making life-sustaining decisions for your child. Be sure that both parents discuss their feelings about this very delicate topic. It is a decision that cannot be made lightly, and all options should be covered. Talking to a counselor in the department of social services at your hospital may be helpful. Once your decision has been reached be sure that you put it in writing and that all necessary medical personal and family members are aware of your wishes. This is your decision, one you have reached with great care and anguish, and under no circumstances should you allow others to judge you or place their values upon you.

Type II (and Some Type III)

Raising a child with SMA should be no different than raising a child who is not affected. Do as many things as possible that are age appropriate. Many times this means making adaptations. It is very important that children with SMA are assisted in reaching their utmost potential. This includes getting the child upright at the earliest possible age.

Standing is important in the development of all children. It allows for better respiratory function, greater bowel function, and encourages greater mobility. Talk to your child's physician about a prescription for standing aids.

There are several options to consider when choosing the appropriate standing aid. Among them are a standing frame and a parapodium. For added mobility and independence a standing wheelchair is ideal. A child as young as 13 months can use this. Bracing is also an option. Reciprocating gait orthosis (RGOs) have been found to work for children with type II, and these children have been able to take some steps.

The use of a light weight manual wheelchair can be an exciting addition for the SMA child. It can provide mobility, independence, and a taste of adventure, while still allowing them to use some of their own strength. However, it should be understood that for true independence and mobility, a power wheelchair is necessary.

Scoliosis (curvature of the spine) occurs at some point in all children with SMA type I and II and some type III. The degree of the scoliosis will be a factor in deciding how to treat it. Because scoliosis can restrict breathing and pulmonary function, necessary precautions should be taken early. Among these options are custom seating systems, seating aids, and a body jacket. Later spinal fusion may need to be considered.

If your child is having continuous upper respiratory infections you may want to inquire about an IPPB (intermittent positive pressure breathing) machine. The IPPB may assist with respiratory function and help prevent the lungs from becoming stiff. IPPB is also helpful in eliminating secretions. Using an incentive spirometer daily allows you to measure lung capacity. When volumes are low it usually indicates an increase in mucus and/or a cold developing.

Diet, as with any growing child, is very important. Your child's diet deserves careful consideration. Excessive weight can make mobility more difficult. Good eating habits help contribute to strong minds and strong bodies. Constant contact with your physician and a nutritionist is very important in this aspect of maintenance.

Type III

Because children with type III walk at some point unassisted, it is important that they be monitored so that any difficulty may be detected at an early stage. The use of a walker and bracing may become necessary. The use of a lightweight manual wheelchair may be considered for distance as well as an electric scooter or other motorized chair. Physical and occupational therapists should be consulted. Diet should also be watched.

Type IV: Adult Onset

As an adult you are aware of your weaknesses and limitations. You should work together with your physician, and physical and occupational therapists to work out the best possible program for you. As with types I, II, and III, diet and nutrition are an important factor in your well being. It is important to keep your body and mind healthy.

What Causes Spinal Muscular Atrophy?

Spinal muscular atrophy is an autosomal recessive disease, which means that both parents must be carriers—both parents must have the gene responsible and these genes must be passed onto the child. When a child has received this gene from each of its parents it will than be affected by SMA. Although both parents are carriers, the likelihood of affected child is 25%, or one in four, for each pregnancy.

Familial forms (affecting other family members) of spinal muscular atrophy in the older age group can occur as a result of autosomal recessive, mutation, or autosomal dominant transmission. The genetic defects underlying these diseases make it necessary to be precise regarding the inheritance pattern in a particular family.

I Am a Carrier of the SMA Gene: What Can I Do?

If you find you are a carrier of the SMA gene it is necessary that you seek the advice of a genetic counselor. This counselor will assist biological parents to better understand the risks and chances of having another affected child. The genetic counselor will take a complete family history which will include any diseases, deaths, causes of death, still births, and miscarriages of each family member. This information helps them to identify persons likely to carry a defective gene. Sometimes laboratory studies will follow.

The information presently available allows for prenatal testing with 98% reliability. The decision to have prenatal testing performed and the options available once the results of the testing are back can be difficult. These are individual decisions and very personal. It is important that both parents have discussed their feelings together and with their genetic counselor. A family may also wish to consult with their clergyman.

Once a decision has been made it is important to be supportive of one another and to allow any necessary time to grieve. This is a difficult decision, one that has taken great anguish and thought. Under no circumstances should you allow others' values or judgment to affect you

Ongoing Research

The Indiana University Roster, which is funded by Families of SMA, was instrumental in locating the chromosome that carries the SMA gene. The gene has been identified and the protein discovered. Now through the collaborative efforts of the North American Spinal Muscular Atrophy Research Group, funded totally by Families of SMA, research moves forward to the next stages.

- continued development of SMA mouse models

- development of therapeutic strategies by either gene replacement or gene activation

- clinical trials

Major researchers throughout the world are being funded by Families of SMA in efforts to not only alleviate but to cure the spinal muscular atrophy diseases. It is an exciting thought that as research progresses we will reach our goal for a treatment and cure in the not too distant future.

How Families of SMA Can Help

Families of SMA was founded by a group of parents of children with SMA type II. They all continue to be actively involved working to raise money to distribute educational materials, provide patient services and support research, which will lead to a treatment and cure.

As caring parents and professionals who have experienced the day to day trials and tribulations of raising a child with spinal muscular atrophy or have had to deal with the loss of a child or family member with spinal muscular atrophy, we can offer support and understanding when it is most needed. By phone and networking Families of SMA volunteer staff and members are there when you need them or just a friendly ear to listen and share.

The publishing of a quarterly newsletter keeps families and professionals up to date on the latest in research, technology, and day to day coping in regards to spinal muscular atrophy.

The sponsoring of annual conferences allows families and professionals hands on techniques and family to family support, while also giving the children a great opportunity to make new friends and have a great time.

Because Families of SMA understands the financial hardship living with spinal muscular atrophy can cause, they have a very large equipment pool which is available free of charge to members of Families of SMA.

Most of all Families of SMA can offer friendship and hope. Please contact us so that we can help you with any questions you may have or support you may need. We are all here for each other. For more information contact:

Families of SMA (Spinal Muscular Atrophy)
National Headquarters
P.O. Box 196
Libertyville, IL 60048-0196
Toll-Free: 800-886-1762
Website: http://www.fsma.org
E-mail: info@fsma.org

Chapter 21

Rett Syndrome

In October 1999, scientists sponsored by the National Institute of Child Health and Human Development (NICHD) made a remarkable announcement—they discovered that a change in the sequence of a single gene can cause Rett syndrome. Rett syndrome is one of many conditions classified as an autism spectrum disorder, which means it is not autism but has features that are similar to autism. This disorder causes autism-like symptoms, such as poor language skills, repeated hand motions, and decreased social contact in girls. These symptoms begin sometime between ages six months and 18 months after apparently normal development.

With this discovery, NICHD researchers have their first glimpse into this baffling disease. These researchers join parents, families, and communities affected by the disorder in hoping that the discovery will lead to better diagnosis, treatment, and maybe even prevention of Rett syndrome.

What is Rett syndrome?

Imagine you are the parent of a baby girl. When she is born, the doctor tells you she is normal and healthy. You watch her start to become a little person. She smiles at you and your family when she's six weeks old. She picks things up with her thumb and first finger when she is seven months old. At ten months, she is rolling and

National Institute of Child Health and Human Development (NICHD), NIH Pub. No. 01-4960, June 2001.

crawling her way into everything. You take pictures of her first birthday, where she is sitting up without your help and smiling at the camera. She can even say her own version of "cheese."

Now imagine that same daughter at age two. She can no longer sit up and doesn't grasp with her fingers. She starts having seizures. By the time she's three, she is always grinding her teeth and stops talking. When she turns six, her spine starts to curve, which limits how well she can move. She screams and laughs during the night for no reason, but doesn't respond to or interact with others. By her eighth birthday, she can't move on her own and can't talk.

The nightmare you just read is real for parents of girls with Rett syndrome. This tragic disorder causes some girls, whose growth, language skills, and personalities seemed normal before, to stop developing.

Sometime between their sixth and 18th month of life, these girls' development actually goes backward. They stop talking. They can't control their feet when they walk. They stop using their hands to do things, or start wringing their hands all the time. These girls stop responding to their parents and pull away from social contact with others.

Rett syndrome is a challenging disease for most of the families who are touched by it. Although many girls with the disorder live into their 40s, their lives are often not easy. Many of them can't walk or talk, but have to communicate with their eyes. They need special education, diets, and treatments for their various problems. Most girls with Rett syndrome can't care for themselves and need someone to care for them all of their lives.

What happens to girls with Rett syndrome as they get older?

In some girls with Rett syndrome, the body and mind keep growing and developing, but at a much slower rate. They have coordination problems, so they may not be able to walk backward or walk up the stairs. They also have learning disabilities, including problems remembering facts, understanding ideas, and solving problems. The lives of these girls are similar to the lives of people with other developmental disabilities, such as autism or Down syndrome.

Other girls with Rett syndrome lose more of their motor skills. They stop being able to sit up or use their hands. Some of them have seizures; others have trouble breathing while they are awake. Still others laugh or scream during the night for no apparent reason. A number of these girls develop scoliosis, which is a curving of the spine. By the time they reach their 20s, many of these girls are left completely helpless. They can't move and can't speak. These girls are at greater risk for dying suddenly and from unexplained causes.

What causes Rett syndrome?

As mentioned earlier, Rett syndrome is caused by a change in a single gene. Because this condition is relatively rare, affecting one female out of 10,000 to 15,000, researchers have long felt it probably involved genes.

Genes are very small pieces of hereditary material, which means that parents pass them on to their children. Every person gets half their genes from their mother and half from their father.

The pattern, or sequence, of your genes is like a blueprint that tells your body how to build its different parts. Your gene sequence controls how tall you are, what color your hair and eyes are, and other features of your body and mind. Changes in that blueprint can cause changes in how your body or mind develops.

Genes are found on chromosomes. Almost every cell in your body contains 23 pairs of chromosomes, 46 in all. Genes and chromosomes give the body all the information it needs to "build" a person. Of your 46 chromosomes, 44 help make your body and two control whether you're a female or a male. Females have two X chromosomes, and males have one X chromosome and one Y chromosome. Because Rett syndrome occurs only in girls, and girls have only X chromosomes, doctors decided to focus their research on the X chromosome.

Scientists found that girls with Rett syndrome have a change in the pattern of one of their genes, specifically the gene that makes a protein called methyl cytosine binding protein 2 or MECP2. Normally, girls use the genes on only one of their X chromosomes; the genes on the other X chromosome are "switched off" by a complex set of chemical reactions in the body. MECP2 is the starting point of the process that "switches off" certain genes at certain times. Without it, these other genes aren't switched off.

In Rett syndrome, the body keeps making these materials, in large amounts, even when they are no longer needed. After several months, large amounts of these materials actually start to hurt the nervous system, instead of helping it to grow. This is why girls with Rett syndrome seem to grow normally until they are between six and 18 months old, but then stop developing and eventually lose developmental ground.

Because they have only one X chromosome, boys with Rett syndrome have only the changed gene for MECP2. Since they lack the "backup" or unchanged copy of the gene that girls have on their second X chromosome, boys with Rett syndrome die before birth.

Is there any cure or treatment for Rett syndrome?

There is currently no cure for Rett syndrome. However, girls with the condition can be treated for some of the problems associated with Rett syndrome. For example, physical and occupational therapists can help these girls overcome problems of coordination and movement, while speech therapists can help these girls learn to talk or communicate. There are also a number of medicines that can help prevent seizures and breathing problems that many girls with Rett syndrome experience.

How does the information about MECP2 affect girls with Rett syndrome?

Because doctors know that MECP2 is missing in girls with Rett syndrome, and what MECP2 does in the body, they can explore ways to correct the problem. For instance, doctors might find a way to switch off genes that doesn't rely on MECP2. If doctors can slow or stop the progress of Rett syndrome, they may also be able to reverse its effects. This new information could also lead to ways to screen for Rett syndrome—to detect it before the girls start to feel the effects. In this way, doctors could start treating the girls much earlier, which could improve the lives of these girls.

The NICHD continues its efforts to understand Rett syndrome, in hopes of learning to slow, stop, and reverse its effects. The researchers involved, from both the Howard Hughes Medical Institute at Baylor College of Medicine and Stanford University, feel that the new information about MECP2 is a big step forward.

This new information also gives some insight into autism spectrum disorders, the group of conditions with similar symptoms that includes Rett syndrome. With an understanding of how these disorders affect the body, doctors will be better able to treat them. This knowledge is important not just for those affected by Rett syndrome, but also for any person touched by a developmental disorder.

Chapter 22

Tuberous Sclerosis

What is tuberous sclerosis?

Tuberous sclerosis—also called tuberous sclerosis complex (TSC; tuberous sclerosis is often referred to as tuberous sclerosis complex [TSC] in medical literature to help distinguish it from Tourette's syndrome, an unrelated neurological disorder)—is a rare, multi-system genetic disease that causes benign tumors to grow in the brain and on other vital organs such as the kidneys, heart, eyes, lungs, and skin. It commonly affects the central nervous system and results in a combination of symptoms including seizures, developmental delay, behavioral problems, skin abnormalities, and kidney disease.

The disorder affects as many as 25,000 to 40,000 individuals in the United States and about one to two million individuals worldwide, with an estimated prevalence of one in 6,000 newborns. TSC occurs in all races and ethnic groups, and in both genders.

The name tuberous sclerosis comes from the characteristic tuber or root-like growths in the brain, which calcify with age and become hard or sclerotic. The disorder—once known as epiloia or Bourneville's disease—was first identified by a French physician more than 100 years ago.

TSC may be present at birth, but signs of the disorder can be subtle and full symptoms may take some time to develop. As a result, TSC is frequently unrecognized and misdiagnosed for years.

"Tuberous Sclerosis Fact Sheet," National Institute of Neurological Disorders and Stroke (NINDS), December 2001.

What causes tuberous sclerosis?

TSC is caused by defects, or mutations, on two genes—*TSC1* and *TSC2*. Only one of the genes needs to be affected for TSC to be present. The *TSC1* gene, discovered in 1997, is on chromosome 9 and produces a protein called hamartin. The *TSC2* gene, discovered in 1993, is on chromosome 16 and produces the protein tuberin. Scientists believe these proteins act as tumor growth suppressors, agents that regulate cell proliferation and differentiation—the processes in which nerve cells divide to form new generations of cells and acquire individual characteristics.

Is TSC inherited?

Although some individuals may inherit the disorder from a parent with TSC, most cases occur as spontaneous mutations. In these situations, neither parent has the disorder or the faulty gene(s). Instead, a faulty gene first occurs in the affected individual.

In other cases, TSC is an autosomal dominant disorder, which means that the disease is carried by a dominant gene. In those cases where it is passed from parent to child, only one parent needs to have the gene in order to produce the disease in a child. If a parent has the TSC gene, each offspring has a 50 percent chance of developing the disorder. Children who inherit TSC may not have the same symptoms as their parent and they may have either a milder or a more severe form of the disorder.

Some individuals acquire TSC through a process called gonadal mosaicism. These patients have parents with no apparent defects in the two genes that cause the disorder. Yet these parents can have a child with TSC because a portion of one of the parent's reproductive cells (sperm or eggs) can contain the genetic mutation without the other cells of the body being involved. In cases of gonadal mosaicism, genetic testing of a blood sample might not reveal the potential for passing the disease to offspring.

What are the signs and symptoms of TSC?

TSC can affect any or all systems of the body, causing a variety of signs and symptoms. Signs of the disorder vary depending on which system and which organs are involved. The natural course of TSC varies from individual to individual, with symptoms ranging from very mild to quite severe. In addition to the benign tumors that frequently occur in TSC, other common symptoms include seizures, mental retardation, behavior problems, and skin abnormalities. Tumors can grow on any organ, but they most commonly occur on the brain, kidneys, heart, lungs, and skin. Malignant tumors are rare in TSC. Those that do occur primarily affect the kidneys.

Kidney problems such as cysts and angiomyolipomas occur in an estimated 40 to 80 percent of individuals with TSC, usually occurring between ages 20 and 30. Cysts are usually small, appear in limited numbers, and cause no serious problems. Approximately two percent of individuals with TSC develop large numbers of cysts in a pattern similar to polycystic kidney disease (polycystic kidney disease is a genetic disorder characterized by the growth of numerous fluid-filled cysts in the kidneys) during childhood. In these cases, kidney function is compromised and kidney failure occurs. In rare instances, the cysts may bleed, leading to blood loss and anemia.

Angiomyolipomas—benign growths consisting of fatty tissue and muscle cells—are the most common kidney lesions in TSC. These growths, which are not rare or unique to TSC, are found in about one in 300 people without TSC. Angiomyolipomas caused by TSC are usually found in both kidneys and in most cases they produce no symptoms. However, they can sometimes grow so large that they cause pain or kidney failure. Bleeding from angiomyolipomas may also occur, causing both pain and weakness. If severe bleeding does not stop naturally, there may severe blood loss, resulting in profound anemia and a life-threatening drop in blood pressure, warranting urgent medical attention.

Other rare kidney problems include renal cell carcinoma, developing from an angiomyolipoma, and oncocytomas, benign tumors unique to individuals with TSC.

Three types of brain tumors are associated with TSC: cortical tubers, for which the disease is named, generally form on the surface of the brain, but may also appear in the deep areas of the brain; subependymal nodules, which form in the walls of the ventricles—the fluid-filled cavities of the brain; and giant-cell astrocytomas, a type of tumor that can grow and block the flow of fluids within the brain, causing a buildup of fluid and pressure and leading to headaches and blurred vision.

Tumors called cardiac rhabdomyomas sometimes are found in the hearts of infants and young children with TSC. If the tumors are large or there are multiple tumors, they can block circulation and cause death. However, if they do not cause problems at birth—when in most cases they are at their largest size—they usually do not grow and probably will not affect the individual in later life.

Benign tumors called phakomas are sometimes found in the eyes of individuals with TSC, appearing as white patches on the retina. Generally they do not cause vision loss or other vision problems, but they can be used to help diagnose the disease.

Additional tumors and cysts may be found in other areas of the body, including the liver, lung, and pancreas. Bone cysts, rectal polyps, gum fibromas, and dental pits may also occur.

A wide variety of skin abnormalities may occur in individuals with TSC. Most cause no problems but are helpful in diagnosis. Some cases may cause disfigurement, necessitating treatment. The most common skin abnormalities include:

- Hypomelanotic macules ("ash leaf spots"), which are white or lighter patches of skin that may appear anywhere on the body and are caused by a lack of skin pigment or melanin—the substance that gives skin its color.

- Reddish spots or bumps called facial angiofibromas (also called adenoma sebaceum), which appear on the face (sometimes resembling acne) and consist of blood vessels and fibrous tissue.

- Raised, discolored areas on the forehead called forehead plaques, which are common and unique to TSC and may help doctors diagnose the disorder.

- Areas of thick leathery, pebbly skin called shagreen patches, usually found on the lower back or nape of the neck.

- Small fleshy tumors called ungual or subungual fibromas that grow around and under the toenails or fingernails and may need to be surgically removed if they enlarge or cause bleeding.

- Other skin features that are not unique to individuals with TSC, including molluscum fibrosum or skin tags, which typically occur across the back of the neck and shoulders, café au lait spots or flat brown marks, and poliosis, a tuft or patch of white hair that may appear on the scalp or eyelids.

TSC can cause seizures and varying degrees of mental disability. Seizures of all types may occur, including infantile spasms; tonic-clonic seizures (also known as grand mal seizures); or tonic, akinetic, atypical absence, myoclonic, complex partial, or generalized seizures.

Approximately one-half to two-thirds of individuals with TSC have mental disabilities ranging from mild learning disabilities to severe mental retardation. Behavior problems, including aggression, sudden rage, attention deficit hyperactivity disorder, acting out, obsessive-compulsive disorder, and repetitive, destructive, or self-harming behavior, may occur in children with TSC. Some individuals with TSC may also have a developmental disorder called autism.

How is TSC diagnosed?

In most cases the first clue to recognizing TSC is the presence of seizures or delayed development. In other cases, the first sign may be white patches on the skin (hypomelanotic macules). Diagnosis of the disorder is based on a careful clinical exam in combination with computed tomography (CT) or magnetic resonance imaging (MRI) of the brain, which may show tubers in the brain, and an ultrasound of the heart, liver, and kidneys, which may show tumors in those organs. Doctors should carefully examine the skin for the wide variety of skin features, the fingernails and toenails for ungual fibromas, the teeth and gums for dental pits and/or gum fibromas, and the eyes for dilated pupils. A Wood's lamp or ultraviolet light may be used to locate the hypomelanotic macules which are sometimes hard to see on infants and individuals with pale or fair skin.

In infants TSC may be suspected if the child has cardiac rhabdomyomas or seizures (infantile spasms) at birth. With a careful examination of the skin and brain, it may be possible to diagnose TSC in a very young infant. However, most children are not diagnosed until later in life when their seizures begin and other symptoms such as facial angiofibromas appear.

How is TSC treated?

There is no cure for TSC, although treatment is available for a number of the symptoms. Antiepileptic drugs may be used to control seizures, and medications may be prescribed for behavior problems. Intervention programs including special schooling and occupational therapy may benefit individuals with special needs and developmental issues. Surgery including dermabrasion and laser treatment may be useful for treatment of skin lesions. Because TSC is a lifelong condition, individuals need to be regularly monitored by a doctor to make sure they are receiving the best possible treatments. Due to the many varied symptoms of TSC, care by a clinician experienced with the disorder is recommended.

What is the prognosis?

The prognosis for individuals with TSC depends on the severity of symptoms, which range from mild skin abnormalities to varying degrees of learning disabilities and epilepsy to severe mental retardation, uncontrollable seizures, and kidney failure. Those individuals with mild symptoms generally do well and live long productive lives, while individuals with the more severe form may have serious disabilities.

In rare cases, seizures, infections, or tumors in vital organs may cause complications in some organs such as the kidneys and brain that can lead to severe difficulties and even death. However, with appropriate medical care, most individuals with the disorder can look forward to normal life expectancy.

What research is being done?

Within the federal government, the leading supporter of research on TSC is the National Institute of Neurological Disorders and Stroke (NINDS). The NINDS, part of the National Institutes of Health (NIH), is responsible for supporting and conducting research on the brain and the central nervous system. NINDS conducts research in its laboratories at NIH and also supports studies through grants to major medical institutions across the country. The National Heart, Lung, and Blood Institute and the National Cancer Institute, also components of the NIH, support and conduct research on TSC.

Scientists who study TSC seek to increase our understanding of the disorder by learning more about the *TSC1* and *TSC2* genes that can cause the disorder and the function of the proteins—tuberin and hamartin—produced by these genes. Scientists hope knowledge gained from their current research will improve the genetic test for TSC and lead to new avenues of treatment, methods of prevention, and, ultimately, a cure for this disorder.

In one study researchers defined the mutations in the *TSC1* and *TSC2* genes in a large (more than 300) group of individuals with TSC in an effort to find correlations between types of mutations and clinical features of the disorder. Mechanisms of mutation occurrence and the effects of other genes on clinical severity are also being studied. These same scientists are also developing mouse models of TSC, which will provide a unique opportunity to examine how the disease develops, discover the critical cell types that are affected in TSC, and provide the opportunity for therapeutic intervention.

Another study focuses on two major brain disorders—autism and epilepsy—that occur in children with TSC. Information from this study could lead to a better understanding of all three disorders, as well as to the development of new drug treatments.

Other scientists are trying to determine what causes skin tumors to develop in individuals with TSC and to find the molecular basis of these tumors. Findings from this study could shed new light on the genetics of TSC.

Chapter 23

Wilson Disease

Wilson disease causes the body to retain copper. The liver of a person who has Wilson disease does not release copper into bile as it should. Bile is a liquid produced by the liver that helps with digestion. As the intestines absorb copper from food, the copper builds up in the liver and injures liver tissue. Eventually, the damage causes the liver to release the copper directly into the bloodstream, which carries the copper throughout the body. The copper buildup leads to damage in the kidneys, brain, and eyes. If not treated, Wilson disease can cause severe brain damage, liver failure, and death.

Wilson disease is hereditary. Symptoms usually appear between the ages of 6 and 20 years, but can begin as late as age 40. The most characteristic sign is the Kayser-Fleischer ring—a rusty brown ring around the cornea of the eye that can be seen only through an eye exam. Other signs depend on whether the damage occurs in the liver, blood, central nervous system, urinary system, or musculoskeletal system. Many signs can be detected only by a doctor, like swelling of the liver and spleen; fluid buildup in the lining of the abdomen; anemia; low platelet and white blood cell count in the blood; high levels of amino acids, protein, uric acid, and carbohydrates in urine; and softening of the bones. Some symptoms are more obvious, like jaundice, which appears as yellowing of the eyes and skin; vomiting blood; speech and language problems; tremors in the arms and hands; and rigid muscles.

"Wilson's Disease," National Digestive Diseases Information Clearinghouse (NDDIC), a service of the National Institute of Diabetes and Digestive and Kidney Diseases (NIDDK), NIH Pub. No. 03-4684, March 2003.

Wilson disease is diagnosed through tests that measure the amount of copper in the blood, urine, and liver. An eye exam would detect the Kayser-Fleischer ring.

The disease is treated with lifelong use of D-penicillamine or trientine hydrochloride, drugs that help remove copper from tissue, or zinc acetate, which stops the intestines from absorbing copper and promotes copper excretion. Patients will also need to take vitamin B_6 and follow a low-copper diet, which means avoiding mushrooms, nuts, chocolate, dried fruit, liver, and shellfish.

Wilson disease requires lifelong treatment. If the disorder is detected early and treated correctly, a person with Wilson disease can enjoy completely normal health.

For More Information

Wilson's Disease Association
1802 Brookside Drive
Wooster, OH 44691
Phone: 800-399-0266 or 330-264-1450
Website: http://www.wilsonsdisease.org

American Liver Foundation
75 Maiden Lane, Suite 603
New York, NY 10038-4810
Toll-Free Helpline (24 hours, 7 days a week):
800-465-4837 or 888-443-7222
Phone: 800-676-9340 or 212-668-1000
Fax: 212-483-8179
Website: http://www.liverfoundation.org
E-mail: info@liverfoundation.org

Additional Information on Wilson Disease

The National Digestive Diseases Information Clearinghouse collects resource information on digestive diseases for the Combined Health Information Database (CHID). CHID is a database produced by health-related agencies of the Federal Government. This database provides titles, abstracts, and availability information for health information and health education resources. For additional information from CHID visit http://chid.nih.gov.

Part Three

Chromosome Disorders

Chapter 24

Chromosome Abnormalities

What are chromosomes?

Chromosomes are the structures that hold our genes. Genes are the individual instructions that tell our bodies how to develop and function; they govern our physical and medical characteristics, such as hair color, blood type, and susceptibility to disease.

Each chromosome has a **p** and **q** arm; **p** is the shorter arm and **q** is the longer arm. The arms are separated by a pinched region known as the centromere.

Where are chromosomes found in the body?

The body is made up of individual units called cells. Your body has many different kinds of cells, such as skin cells, liver cells, and blood cells. In the center of most cells is a structure called the nucleus. This is where chromosomes can be found.

How many chromosomes do humans have?

The typical number of chromosomes in a human cell is 46—two pairs of 23—holding an estimated 30,000 to 35,000 genes. One set of 23 chromosomes is inherited from the biological mother (from the egg), and the other set is inherited from the biological father (from the sperm).

"Chromosome Abnormalities Fact Sheet," National Human Genome Research Institute (NHGRI), reviewed March 2004.

How do scientists study chromosomes?

In order for chromosomes to be seen with a microscope, they need to be stained. Once stained, the chromosomes look like strings with light and dark "bands" and their picture can be taken. A picture, or chromosome map, of all 46 chromosomes is called a karyotype. The karyotype can help identify chromosome abnormalities that are evident in either the structure or the number of chromosomes.

To help identify chromosomes, the pairs have been numbered from one to 22, with the 23rd pair labeled "X" and "Y." In addition, each chromosome arm is defined further by numbering the bands that appear after staining; the higher the number, the further that area is from the centromere.

The first 22 pairs of chromosomes are called "autosomes" and the final pair is called the "sex chromosomes." The sex chromosomes an individual has determines that person's gender; females have two X chromosomes (XX), and males have an X and a Y chromosome (XY).

What are chromosome abnormalities?

A chromosome abnormality reflects an abnormality of chromosome number or structure. There are many types of chromosome abnormalities. However, they can be organized into two basic groups:

Numerical Abnormalities: When an individual is missing either a chromosome from a pair (monosomy) or has more than two chromosomes of a pair (trisomy). An example of a condition caused by numerical abnormalities is Down syndrome, also known as Trisomy 21 (an individual with Down syndrome has three copies of chromosome 21, rather than two). Turner syndrome is an example of monosomy 13—the individual is born with only one sex chromosome, an X.

Structural Abnormalities: When the chromosome's structure is altered. This can take several forms:

- *Deletions:* A portion of the chromosome is missing or deleted.

- *Duplications:* A portion of the chromosome is duplicated, resulting in extra genetic material.

- *Translocations:* When a portion of one chromosome is transferred to another chromosome. There are two main types of translocations. In a reciprocal translocation, segments from two different chromosomes have been exchanged. In a Robertsonian translocation, an entire chromosome has attached to another at the centromere.

- *Inversions:* A portion of the chromosome has broken off, turned upside down and reattached; therefore the genetic material is inverted.

- *Rings:* A portion of a chromosome has broken off and formed a circle or ring. This can happen with or without loss of genetic material.

Most chromosome abnormalities occur as an accident in the egg or sperm. Therefore, the abnormality is present in every cell of the body. Some abnormalities, however, can happen after conception, resulting in mosaicism (where some cells have the abnormality and some do not).

Chromosome abnormalities can be inherited from a parent (such as a translocation) or be "de novo" (new to the individual). This is why chromosome studies are often performed on parents when a child is found to have an abnormality.

How do chromosome abnormalities happen?

Chromosome abnormalities usually occur when there is an error in cell division. There are two kinds of cell division.

- *Mitosis* results in two cells that are duplicates of the original cell. In other words, one cell with 46 chromosomes becomes two cells with 46 chromosomes each. This kind of cell division occurs throughout the body, except in the reproductive organs. This is how most of the cells that make up our body are made and replaced.

- *Meiosis* results in cells with half the number of chromosomes, 23 instead of the normal 46. These are the eggs and sperm.

In both processes, the correct number of chromosomes is supposed to end up in the resulting cells. However, errors in cell division can result in cells with too few or too many copies of a chromosome. Errors can also occur when the chromosomes are being duplicated.

Other factors that can increase the risk of chromosome abnormalities are:

Maternal Age: Women are born with all the eggs they will ever have. Therefore, when a woman is 30 years old, so are her eggs. Some researchers believe that errors can crop up in the eggs' genetic material as they age over time. Therefore, older women are more at risk of giving birth to babies with chromosome abnormalities than younger women. Since men produce new sperm throughout their life, paternal age does not increase risk of chromosome abnormalities.

Environment: Although there is no conclusive evidence that specific environmental factors cause chromosome abnormalities, it is still a possibility that the environment may play a role in the occurrence of genetic errors.

Chapter 25

Angelman Syndrome

Introduction

In 1965, Dr. Harry Angelman, an English physician, first described three children with characteristics now known as the Angelman syndrome (AS). He noted that all had a stiff, jerky gait, absent speech, excessive laughter, and seizures.

AS has been reported throughout the world among divergent racial groups. In North America, the great majority of known cases seem to be of Caucasian origin. Although the exact incidence of AS is unknown, an estimate of between one in 15,000 to one in 30,000 seems reasonable.

Developmental and Physical Features

Angelman syndrome is usually not recognized at birth or in infancy since the developmental problems are nonspecific during this time. Parents may first suspect the diagnosis after reading about AS or meeting a child with the condition. The most common age of diagnosis is between three and seven years when the characteristic behaviors and features become most evident.

Excerpted with permission from, *Facts about Angelman Syndrome: Information for Families*, by the Angelman Syndrome Foundation. © 2002. All rights reserved. To view the complete text of this document, including references, visit the Angelman Syndrome Foundation website at http://www.angelman.org.

Genetic Basis of AS

For several decades the chromosome study of AS individuals revealed no abnormalities, but with the development of improved methods a very small deleted area was found in chromosome 15. Molecular methods such as FISH (fluorescence in situ hybridization) now demonstrate a deletion in about 70% of individuals with AS. The deleted area, although extremely small, is actually quite large when viewed at the molecular level. It is believed to be about 4 million base pairs in length, enough to contain many genes.

The deleted region on chromosome 15 is known to contain genes that are activated or inactivated depending upon the chromosome's parent of origin (for example, a gene may be turned on, on the chromosome 15 inherited from the mother but off on the chromosome 15 inherited from the father). This parent-specific gene activation is referred to as genetic imprinting. Because the deletions seen in AS only occur on the chromosome 15 inherited from the mother, the gene(s) responsible for AS were predicted to be active only on the maternal chromosome 15. Disruption of genes that are active on the paternally derived chromosome 15 is now known to cause another developmental disorder termed the Prader-Willi syndrome (PWS). The PWS gene(s) are actually located close to the AS gene, but they are different.

In 1997, a gene within the AS deletion region called *UBE3A* was found to be mutated in approximately 5% of AS individuals. These mutations can be as small as one base pair. This gene encodes a protein called a ubiquitin protein ligase, and *UBE3A* is believed to be the causative gene in AS. All mechanisms known to cause AS appear to cause inactivation or absence of this gene. *UBE3A* is an enzymatic component of a complex protein degradation system termed the ubiquitin-proteasome pathway. This pathway is located in the cytoplasm of all cells. The pathway involves a small protein molecule, ubiquitin that can be attached to proteins thereby causing them to be degraded. In the normal brain, the copy of *UBE3A* inherited from the father is almost completely inactive, so the maternal copy performs most of the *UBE3A* function in the brain. Inheritance of a *UBE3A* mutation from the mother causes AS; inheritance of a *UBE3A* mutation from the father has no detectable effect on the child. In some families, AS caused by a *UBE3A* mutation can recur in more than one family member.

Another cause of AS (2–3% of cases) is paternal uniparental disomy (UPD), where the child inherits both copies of chromosome 15 from the father, with no copy inherited from the mother. In this case, there is no deletion or mutation, but the child is still missing the active

UBE3A gene because the paternal-derived chromosomes only have brain-inactivated *UBE3A* genes.

A fourth class of AS individuals (3–5% of cases) have inherited chromosome 15 copies from both mother and father, but the copy inherited from the mother functions in the same way that a paternal chromosome 15 should function. This is referred to as an imprinting defect. Some AS individuals with imprinting defects have very small deletions of a region called the imprinting center (IC). The IC regulates the activity of *UBE3A* from a distant location, but how this regulation occurs is not known. In some cases, AS caused by imprinting defects can recur in more than one member of a family.

These discoveries have led to the realization that there are several genetic classes or mechanisms that can cause AS. All of these mechanisms lead to the typical clinical features of AS, although minor differences may occur between and within groups. These mechanisms are summarized in Table 25.1.

Table 25.1. Genetic Classes of Angelman Syndrome

Genetic Class	% of AS Cases	Comments
Large typical deletion	70%	Hypopigmentation is common
UBE3A mutation	5–7%	Possibility of normal carrier mother
Paternal uniparental disomy	2–3%	Inheritance of both 15s from father
Imprinting defect	3–5%	Some have IC deletion, some do not
Other chromosome abnormalities	2%	Unusual chromosome rearrangements
Unknown	15%	All diagnostic tests negative (FISH, methylation, *UBE3A* mutation analysis)

Medical and Developmental Problems

Seizures: More than 90% are reported to have seizures but this may be an over-estimation because medical reports tend to dwell on the more severe cases. Less than 25% develop seizures before 12 months of age. Most have onset before 3 years, but occurrence in older children or in teenagers is not exceptional. The seizures can be of any seizure type (such as major motor involving jerking of all extremities

305

or absence type involving brief periods with lack of awareness), and may require multiple anticonvulsant medications. Seizures may be difficult to recognize or distinguish from the child's usual tremulousness, hyperkinetic limb movements or attention deficits. The typical EEG is often more abnormal than expected, and it may suggest seizures when in fact there are none.

Gait and movement disorders: Hyperkinetic movements of the trunk and limbs have been noted in early infancy and jitteriness or tremulousness may be present in the first 6 months of life. Voluntary movements are often irregular, varying from slight jerkiness to uncoordinated coarse movements that prevent walking, feeding, and reaching for objects. Gross motor milestones are delayed; sitting usually occurring after age 12 months and walking often delayed until age 3 or 4 years.

Hyperactivity: Hyperactivity is probably the most typical behavior in AS. It is best described as hypermotoric with a short attention span. Essentially all young AS children have some component of hyperactivity and males and females appear equally affected. Infants and toddlers may have seemingly ceaseless activity, constantly keeping their hands or toys in their mouth, moving from object to object. In extreme cases, the constant movement can cause accidental bruises and abrasions. Grabbing, pinching, and biting in older children have also been noted and may be heightened by the hypermotoric activity. Persistent and consistent behavior modification helps decrease or eliminate these unwanted behaviors.

Attention span can be so short that social interaction is prevented because the AS child cannot attend to facial and other social cues. In milder cases, attention may be sufficient enough to learn sign language and other communication techniques. For these children, educational and developmental training programs are much easier to structure and are generally more effective. Observations in young adults suggest that the hypermotoric state decreases with age. Most AS children do not receive drug therapy for hyperactivity although some may benefit from use of medications such as methylphenidate (Ritalin). Use of sedating agents such as phenothiazines is not recommended due to their potency and side effects.

Laughter and happiness: It is not known why laughter is so frequent in AS. Even laughter in normal individuals is not well understood. Studies of the brain in AS, using MRI or CT scans, have not shown any defect suggesting a site for a laughter-inducing abnormality.

The first evidence of this distinctive behavior may be the onset of early or persistent social smiling at the age of 1–3 months. Giggling, chortling, and constant smiling soon develop and appear to represent normal reflexive laughter but cooing and babbling are delayed or reduced. Later, several types of facial or behavioral expressions characterize the infant's personality. A few have pronounced laughing that is truly paroxysmal or contagious and bursts of laughter occurred in 70% in one study. More often, happy grimacing and a happy disposition are the predominant behaviors. In rare cases, the apparent happy disposition is fleeting as irritability and hyperactivity are the prevailing personality traits; crying, shrieking, screaming, or short guttural sounds may then be the predominant behaviors.

Speech and language: Some AS children seem to have enough comprehension to be able to speak, but in even the highest functioning, conversational speech does not develop.

The speech disorder in AS has a somewhat typical evolution. Babies and young infants cry less often and have decreased cooing and babbling. A single apparent word, such as "mama," may develop around 10–18 months but it is used infrequently and indiscriminately without symbolic meaning. By 2–3 years of age, it is clear that speech is delayed but it may not be evident how little the AS child is verbally communicating; crying and other vocal outbursts may also be reduced. By 3 years of age, higher functioning AS children are initiating some type of non-verbal language. Some point to body parts and indicate some of their needs by use of simple gestures, but they are much better at following and understanding commands. Others, especially those with severe seizures or extreme hyperactivity cannot be attentive enough to achieve the first stages of communication, such as establishing sustained eye contact. The nonverbal language skills of AS children vary greatly; with the most advanced ones able to learn some sign language and to use such aids as picture-based communication boards.

Mental retardation and developmental testing: It is known that the cognitive abilities in AS are higher than indicated from developmental testing. The most striking area where this is evident is in the disparity between understanding language and speaking language. Because of their ability to understand language, AS children soon distinguish themselves from other severe mental retardation conditions. Young adults with AS are usually socially adept and respond to most personal cues and interactions. Because of their interest in people they establish rewarding friendships and communicate a broad repertoire of feelings and sentiments, enriching their relationship to families and friends. They participate in group activities, household chores, and in the activities and responsibilities of daily living. Like others, they enjoy most recreational activities such as TV, sports, going to the beach, etc.

There is a wide range however in the developmental outcome so that not all individuals with AS attain the above noted skills. A few will be more impaired in terms of their mental retardation and lack of attention, and this seems especially the case in those with difficult-to-control seizures or those with extremely pronounced ataxia and movement problems. Fortunately, most children with AS do not have these severe problems, but even for the less impaired child, inattentiveness and hyperactivity during early childhood often give the impression that profound functional impairment is the only outcome possible. However, with a secure home and consistent behavioral intervention and stimulation, the AS child begins to overcome these problems and developmental progress occurs.

Hypopigmentation: When AS is caused by the large deletion, skin and eye hypopigmentation usually result. This occurs because there is a pigment gene (the *P* gene) located close to the AS gene that is also missing.

Strabismus and ocular albinism: Surveys of AS patients demonstrate 30–60% incidence of strabismus. This problem appears to be more common in children with eye hypopigmentation, since pigment in the retina is crucial to normal development of the optic nerve pathways.

CNS structure: The brain in AS is structurally normal although occasional abnormalities have been reported. The most common MRI or CT change, when any is detected, is mild cortical atrophy (for example, a small decrease in the thickness of the cortex of the cerebrum) and/or mildly decreased myelination (for example, the more central parts of the brain appear to have a slight degree of diminished white matter).

Sleep disorders: Parents report that decreased need for sleep and abnormal sleep/wake cycles are characteristic of AS. Sleep disturbances have been reported in AS infants and abnormal sleep/wake cycles have been studied in one AS child who benefited from a behavioral treatment program.

Feeding problems and oral-motor behaviors: Feeding problems are frequent but not generally severe and usually manifest early as difficulty in sucking or swallowing. Tongue movements may be uncoordinated with thrusting and generalized oral-motor incoordination. There may be trouble initiating sucking and sustaining breast feeding, and bottle feeding may prove easier. Frequent spitting up may be interpreted as formula intolerance or gastroesophageal reflux. The feeding difficulties are often first present to the physician as a problem of poor weight gain or as a failure to thrive concern. Infrequently, severe gastroesophageal reflux may require surgery.

Physical growth: Newborns appear to be physically well formed, but by 12 months of age some show a deceleration of cranial growth which may represent relative or absolute microcephaly (absolute microcephaly means having a head circumference in the lower 2.5 percentile).

Education: The severe developmental delay in AS mandates that a full range of early training and enrichment programs be made available. Unstable or nonambulatory children may also benefit from physical therapy. Occupational therapy may help improve fine motor and oral-motor control. Special adaptive chairs or positioners may be required at various times, especially for hypotonic or extremely ataxic children. Speech and communication therapy is essential and should focus on nonverbal methods of communication. Augmentative communication aids, such as picture cards or communication boards, should be used at the earliest appropriate time.

Young adulthood: During adolescence, puberty may be delayed by 1–3 years but sexual maturation occurs with development of normal secondary sexual characteristics. Some weight gain can be evident in this period but frank obesity is rare. Young AS adults continue to learn and are not known to have significant deterioration in their mental abilities. Physical health in AS appears to be remarkably good. For some, seizure medications can be discontinued in the early adolescent or adult years. AS individuals with severe ataxia may lose their ability to walk if ambulation is not encouraged. Scoliosis can develop in adolescence and is especially a problem in those that are non-ambulatory. Scoliosis is treated with early bracing to prevent progression, and surgical correction or stabilization may be necessary for severe cases. Life span does not appear to be dramatically shortened and we are aware of a 58-year-old woman with AS and know of many in their third or fourth decades of life.

Chapter 26

Cri du Chat Syndrome

A Message to Parents

Children with cri du chat syndrome can lead happy, fulfilling lives as valued members of their families and communities. Many aspects of the condition described in this chapter will worry new parents a great deal but they must remember that not every child has every one of these, many are minor problems which can be dealt. You will overcome your initial shock and fear of the future as you find ways to help your child develop and learn.

What Is Cri du Chat Syndrome?

Cri du chat syndrome is a genetic disorder, it is not an illness or a disease. A child born with this disorder has specific physiological problems which result in their development being delayed both physically and intellectually. They may also have health problems because parts of their physiology have not developed correctly.

There are a number of genetic mishaps that can result in a child being born with cri du chat syndrome and all involve a missing or deleted part of the short arm of one of the pair of number five chromosomes. A chromosome has a narrow point called a centromere separating the two segments or arms which are called the short and the long arms. The short arm is named p for the French word petite which means small, and the long arm is named q because it follows p in the alphabet. Cri du chat syndrome is also called 5p- or 5p minus syndrome because part of the p arm is missing.

It is called a deletion syndrome because part of the short arm is missing or deleted. That missing piece must contain a certain region of the short arm for cri du chat syndrome to result. This critical region is known to be in the area called band 15.2. The bands are distinct areas which show up as stripes when the chromosome is stained and viewed under a microscope.

A variety of genetic arrangements can result in a child having cri du chat syndrome. These include:

Unbalanced Translocation: A translocation occurs when a piece of one chromosome breaks off and attaches to another, different chromosome. When no material is lost or gained the translocation is said to be balanced and the individual is not affected. An unbalanced translocation results in the loss or gain of genetic material which may result in a genetic disorder.

When a parent has a balanced translocation the child can be born with an unbalanced translocation. This happens in about 10% of cases of cri du chat syndrome. In a few cases the unbalanced translocation is spontaneous or de novo (new) in the child.

Ring Chromosome: In this rare situation the chromosome loses a piece from each end and the ends join to form a ring. In the child with cri du chat syndrome, this can result in additional problems depending on the amount of material lost from the long arm of the chromosome.

Interstitial Deletion: A section from within the short arm is deleted and the broken ends rejoin. The deleted section may be lost or attach itself to another chromosome.

Inversion: This occurs sometimes when a chromosome breaks at two points within the arm. The broken section flips or inverts before reattaching. It can result in a disorder because the code is reversed in that section.

Duplication or Partial Trisomy: A part of the short arm of the number five chromosome containing the critical region duplicates itself. This can be attached within the chromosome or at the tip. It also results in the code being misread.

Mosaicism: In a very few cases, the deleted chromosome is present in only some cells in the body, for example 20%, 50%, or 75% etc.

Children with this type of condition can be severely to very mildly affected depending on the percentage of cells with the deletion and which type of body cells are most involved. It is usually very difficult to diagnose since the cells containing the deletion can be hard to find and often missed in the process of taking blood or tissue samples. Children who are mosaic for cri du chat syndrome can be diagnosed with other conditions and syndromes by mistake. It is important that a correct diagnosis is made since it is possible for them to produce a child with cri du chat syndrome when they are adults if the deletion occurs in the cells of the reproductive organs.

Characteristics of the Syndrome

The most distinctive characteristic, and the one for which the syndrome was originally named in 1963 by geneticist Jerome Lejeune, is the distinctive high-pitched, monotone, cat-like cry. *Cri du chat* is French for cat's cry. The cry is thought to be the result of structural abnormality and low muscle tone. Although the voice will naturally lower as the child grows, the characteristic high pitch often persists into adulthood.

In addition to the cry, there are a number of distinguishing characteristics present in infancy which aid in recognition of the syndrome. Not every child will have every feature. Those only mildly affected may have very few or they may be less obvious.

The size and location of the deletion appears to have some correlation with the degree of disability caused by the syndrome. At present however, there is no way to determine with any accuracy how severely a particular child will be affected. All we can say at present is that those with very large deletions tend to be more severely affected and those with very small ones in and above band 15.2 tend to be more mildly affected. In general, babies with an unbalanced translocation are likely to be more severely affected.

Babies are often of low birth weight and many require help with feeding in infancy. Feeding difficulties often persist for the first few years with many experiencing reflux and swallowing problems.

Following are some major identifying characteristics:

- Monotone, weak, cat-like cry

- Small head (microcephaly)

- High palate

- Round face

- Small receding chin (micrognathia)

- Widely spaced eyes (hypertelorism)

- Low set ears

- Low broad nasal ridge

- Folds of skin over the upper eyelid (epicanthic folds)

- Distinctive palmar creases (creases on the palms of the hands)

Some of the features change as the child ages. The cry may become less distinctive and the voice lower whilst still retaining its characteristic tone and pitch. Males usually undergo the same voice changes as other males in adolescence but most females with the syndrome retain the higher pitched, monotone voice throughout life. In adolescence the face becomes more elongated, the nasal bridge high, and the epicanthic folds less distinct. The head remains smaller than normal throughout life becoming more evident in the first years, however, it is not particularly noticeable to the layperson.

Problems Reported in Those with Cri du Chat Syndrome

Following are the medical problems found in a minority of children:

- Heart defects (commonly ventral septal defects and atrial septal defects and rarely tetralogy of Fallot and endocardial cushion defects)

- Cleft palate occurs but is rare

- Kidney abnormalities are also rare

- Minor skeletal problems including hip dislocation and deformities of the feet

- Scoliosis develops in some children

- Hernias (inguinal and abdominal) are sometimes present at birth

- Bowel abnormalities

- Epilepsy is not common

- Swallowing and sucking problems are often present in the newborn and swallowing problems may persist

- Problems with intubation for anesthesia have been reported in a small number of cases due to malformations of the larynx and epiglottis

The following additional problems may be noticed as the child gets older:

- Minor hearing impairments. Hearing impairment is occasionally severe and requires hearing aids.

- Strabismus or turned eye is fairly common and should be attended to as most do not grow out of it and it does affect vision. Treatment may help.

- Other visual problems.

- Low muscle tone (hypotonia) is common in infancy and may change to high muscle tone (hypertonia) later in life. Physiotherapy is an important aspect of intervention.

- Difficulty with sucking and swallowing (dysphagia). Sucking may be very weak and the child may gag and cough when swallowing. Swallowing problems should be investigated since aspiration pneumonia may occur and treatment is possible.

- Gastrointestinal abnormalities are present in some babies.

- Gastric reflux is common in infancy and usually requires treatment.

- Chronic constipation is common. It often starts in the first year or two and usually persists throughout life. It can be well managed in most cases.

- Frequent ear infections—many children with cri du chat syndrome have ear infections often requiring treatment in childhood.

- Saliva control problems (drooling). In severe cases that have not resolved when the child is older, surgery is available to help correct this.

- Sexual development is usually normal and female fertility is possible since some instances of pregnancy have been reported.

- Dental problems are common.

- Feeding problems—children are often not interested in eating.

- Failure to thrive can be due to illness, refusal to eat or drink, or severe reflux.

The following problems have been reported by parents but have not been reported as a feature of the syndrome:

- Sudden, transient, high temperatures without obvious infection or illness. These should be reported to your doctor for further investigation.

- Apnea (breathing stops occasionally, usually during sleep). This may not be related to the syndrome but is occasionally reported by parents. If this condition exists it must be monitored as it can lead to other problems with health and behavior.

- Frequent upper respiratory infections. The increased rate of infection has not yet been identified as the result of a specific immune abnormality in this syndrome. Babies and children may develop pneumonia either from infection or from aspiration of food or liquids. Tests are available to determine if swallowing is likely to be causing infection or pneumonia.

- Sleep disorders. Early intervention and management is important to prevent long term difficulties. Behavior problems can be exaggerated in children who are getting insufficient sleep.

- Sensory defensiveness including one or more of the following:

  - Sensitivity to sound (often only particular frequencies)

  - Tactile defensiveness (sensitivity to touch on parts of the body usually the hands, feet, head and face)

  - Oral defensiveness (also called oral aversion or oral tactile sensitivity)

Life expectancy cannot be predicted and although a few children with serious health problems may have a reduced life-span, it is thought that most live well into adulthood. The oldest person reported to us to date was in her sixties.

In the past, doctors believed this syndrome resulted in severe to profound disability in all cases, however, early researchers like Professor Erik Niebuhr of Denmark, discovered that this is an extremely variable syndrome. The level of disability can range from very mild developmental delay to profound physical and intellectual disability. Most cases at present appear to fall into the moderate to severe range but even this is uncertain since more mild cases are being diagnosed.

The development of more sophisticated genetic testing technology has uncovered an increasing number of children who are only mildly affected but would not previously have been diagnosed. They have fewer of the features or problems usually associated with cri du chat syndrome and those features are usually less obvious. They also have greater developmental potential than was previously thought possible for children with this syndrome.

Development

The effects of this syndrome on the child are extremely variable but almost all children with this syndrome have a degree of intellectual disability, delayed speech and language acquisition, and slow development of motor skills. Although problematic behaviors are not uncommon, they are usually bright, loving, and sociable children with a great sense of humor who occupy a valued position within their families and communities.

Major Developmental Issues in Cri du Chat Syndrome

- Intellectual disability ranging from mild to profound with the majority being moderate to severe.

- Speech and language impairment varying from mild to profound. Research has shown children with cri du chat syndrome have better receptive than expressive language which means they can understand more complex language than you would expect based on their ability to speak. A small number do not speak at all but all can communicate with one or a combination of methods. Early consultation with a speech pathologist is important as is the early introduction of alternate means of communication.

- Low muscle tone and delayed motor development. The majority walk, most between 2 and 6 years of age. Physiotherapy is an important part of early intervention.

- Short attention span (almost 100%).

- Hyperactivity (approximately 25%).

- Challenging behaviors including obsessive, repetitive, and sometimes self-harming behaviors such as head-banging and hitting, biting, or scratching self.

No one can determine at birth how much a child will be affected by this syndrome and the best course of action is to do as much as possible to maximize the child's developmental potential and provide him or her with as many opportunities to live as normal a life as possible.

Treatment

Gene therapy is in its infancy and no techniques have yet been developed to treat these types of large chromosomal abnormalities. Although it is possible that some of the effects of this genetic deletion may eventually be treated by this method, it is unlikely in the near future.

Most of the medical problems can be treated successfully with current medical treatments. Early intervention programs, using a variety of therapies and educational strategies, focus on enhancing physical, intellectual, sensory, and social development and have been shown to greatly improve the future outlook for the child.

Early intervention programs should include:

- Physiotherapy

- Speech therapy

- Occupational therapy

- Behavioral management (if necessary)

Since most children with the syndrome experience severe speech development problems, speech and language therapy are vital. The early introduction of alternative means of communication, including a sign language such as Makaton along with a pictorial symbol system, will enhance the child's speech development, language acquisition, and behavior. Children with cri du chat syndrome are usually keen to communicate and many will develop their own signs and gestures to get what they want often preferring these to the more difficult formal signs. Children who cannot communicate effectively experience a great deal of frustration and behavior problems can develop as a result.

Improving a child's ability to communicate by any means not only helps them to make their needs known, but also helps them to develop intellectually and socially, improving the quality of their lives immeasurably.

Older children and adults who have not acquired adequate speech may benefit from using a communication device.

The level of independence a particular child achieves depends on their own inborn potential combined with the skill of those training them. Those most severely affected require full-time care throughout their lives. Most people with cri du chat syndrome are capable of achieving a degree of independent self-care but require supervision and care for life. Some of those least affected by the syndrome are be able to live independently (or with minimal assistance) in the community.

Chapter 27

DiGeorge Syndrome

22q11 Deletion Disorders: DiGeorge and Velocardiofacial Syndromes

What are DiGeorge syndrome and velocardiofacial syndrome?

DiGeorge syndrome is a disorder described in the 1960s by Dr. Angelo DiGeorge. He observed the combination of a lack of the thymus gland (which is important for certain aspects of immunity) and a lack of parathyroid glands (which results in low calcium levels in the blood). Subsequently, it was found that a high percentage of children with DiGeorge syndrome have certain forms of congenital heart disease.

Velocardiofacial syndrome (VCFS) is related disorder, first described by Dr. Robert Sprintzen in 1978. "Velo" refers to the palate in the mouth. Among children with VCFS, some will have a cleft palate. Like children with DiGeorge syndrome, children with VCFS often have congenital heart defects. There is a typical facial appearance among children with VCFS, which also resembles that observed among children with DiGeorge syndrome. Unlike DiGeorge syndrome, the immune system is not severely affected in VCFS although it can be slightly abnormal and the thymus may not be in its normal position in the chest. Low calcium levels sometimes occur in VCFS, just as in

DiGeorge syndrome. Learning problems, particularly with speech and language, are also common. VCFS was also described independently in Japan by Dr. Atsuyoshi Takao, who called it the conotruncal anomaly face syndrome. The word "conotruncal" refers to the portion of heart that includes the aorta and pulmonary artery, which is most frequently abnormal in the types of heart defects observed in VCFS.

Over time, it has become apparent that DiGeorge syndrome and VCFS overlap in many ways. This includes many of the large number of other problems that children with these diagnoses may encounter. In addition, we now know that the disorders overlap in being caused by chromosome 22q11 deletions and that both syndromes can be observed within one family (for example, a mother with VCFS may have a child with DiGeorge syndrome).

What is a 22q11 deletion?

In humans, DNA, which encodes the master plan for our bodies, is organized as 23 pairs of chromosomes. One pair, the sex chromosomes, consists of either two X chromosomes (XX), resulting in a girl, or one X and one Y chromosome (XY), resulting in a boy. The other 22 pairs of chromosomes, referred to as the autosomes, are numbered 1 through 22. While some of the DNA code can vary between individuals, the overall appearance of each chromosome is unique when viewed under a microscope with staining. Each chromosome is organized into two or three parts: a short arm (not present for some chromosomes), a central portion called the centromere, and a long arm. The arms contain the DNA sequences that encode the genes. The long arm is called by the number of the autosome and "q." Therefore, the long arm of chromosome 22 is called 22q. Chromosomal arms also have sections that appear as light or dark bands after special staining, which are numbered. Thus, 22q11 refers to the 11 band (pronounced one-one) on the long arm of chromosome 22.

Several years ago, investigators observed rare patients with DiGeorge syndrome who had changes affecting 22q11. These included some for whom that band was missing from one of their two copies of chromosome 22. Missing portions of chromosomes, which can be small or large, are referred to as deletions. With further work, a molecular test called fluorescence in situ hybridization (abbreviated as FISH) was developed that tested for deletions of 22q11 that were too small to be seen under the microscope. Using the FISH test for 22q11, it was discovered that about 90% of patients with DiGeorge syndrome and VCFS have a deletion. This special FISH test for 22q11 deletions is available in many clinical laboratories that look at chromosomes (referred to as cytogenetics laboratories). This test is performed only when physicians instruct the laboratory that they suspect a 22q11 deletion in a person or fetus. That is, this FISH test is not done routinely for every amniocentesis (procedure where fluid and cells surrounding a developing fetus are sampled) or from every blood sample from patients.

If the FISH test for 22q11 deletion is negative, can my child still have DiGeorge syndrome or VCFS?

Yes! As noted in the previous section, approximately 90% of patients with DiGeorge syndrome or VCFS will have a positive FISH test. For those with a normal test, a small percentage may have a deletion affecting the short arm of chromosome 10 (which can be tested with a different FISH test), but most have no chromosomal abnormality that can be found currently. If the doctors caring for your child make the diagnosis of DiGeorge syndrome or VCFS on the basis of certain typical features (facial appearance, heart disease, etc.), then that remains true even if the FISH tests are normal.

Does the diagnosis of DiGeorge syndrome or VCFS change the care of my child's heart problem?

Babies born with DiGeorge syndrome or VCFS frequently have heart defects. Those defects range in severity from mild to life-threatening. Those with the more serious forms of heart involvement will require surgery in the newborn and infancy period. In general, decisions about the timing and the type of surgery that these young patients require is not affected by the diagnosis of a 22q11 deletion syndrome.

Once the physicians caring for an infant with a 22q11 deletion make that diagnosis, they will perform tests to check on the immune system and on blood calcium levels. Varying degrees of immune system dysfunction may be present. If the immune system is abnormal, there is a somewhat higher risk of certain types of infection after the heart surgery. In addition, if babies who require heart surgery need a blood transfusion, the blood is typically treated with radiation (irradiated) before it is given to the baby. This treatment kills any living white blood cells in the unit of blood. These white blood cells, if alive, could harm the body of a child with 22q11 deletion syndrome if the immune system is weak. This is called graft-versus-host disease and is prevented with the radiation of the blood prior to transfusion. In addition, physicians caring for young infants after heart surgery routinely monitor for low calcium levels in the blood and would be even more vigilant in a child with a 22q11 deletion syndrome. If this occurs, it is easy to treat by infusing some calcium-containing solution through an intravenous line.

If my child has a 22q11 deletion syndrome, what is the risk for my other children or others in our family?

Most children with a 22q11 deletion are the first person in their family to have that problem. Through some elegant scientific studies, we now understand that this area of chromosome 22 is prone to loss. Thus, there will always be a small risk of new 22q11 deletion for any pregnancy.

When someone with a 22q11 deletion has children of their own, there is a 50-50 chance of passing along a copy of chromosome 22 with that deletion with each pregnancy. This also means, of course, that there is an equal chance that their next child will not inherit the deletion. Like flipping coins for heads or tails, the results of previous pregnancies do not affect the next one. So, a person with a 22q11 deletion and a first child who did not inherit the deletion has the same 50-50 risk with their second child.

In a small percentage of cases, a parent of a child with a 22q11 deletion is also found to have that problem. Once an infant or child is identified as having the deletion, the geneticists will often take a history concerning the parents and examine them in order to decide whether or not one of the parents has it too. Since the severity of the disorder observed in individuals with 22q11 deletions can vary, a parent may have gone without a diagnosis if the disorder is mild in them. When in doubt, the geneticist can test for the deletion in a blood sample using the same FISH test. If a parent is found to have the deletion, the geneticists will then turn their attention to others in the family who might have it too. These could include other children as well as the siblings and parents of the affected parent.

If the doctors decide that neither parent has a 22q11 deletion syndrome, then the risk for others in the family including their other children (siblings of the child with the 22q11 deletion) is no greater than anyone else in the world, which is estimated at one in 2,000 births.

If a sibling of a child with 22q11 deletion does not have the deletion, then they cannot pass it along to their children. The 22q11 deletion syndromes do not skip generations.

If a parent has a 22q11 deletion syndrome, what will their child who inherits the deletion be like?

The deletions of chromosome 22q11 that cause DiGeorge syndrome and VCFS are identical. Scientists are actively trying to figure out why the disease varies if the loss of the piece of chromosome 22 is the same, but we do not know at this point. It is clear, however, that a parent with VCFS can have a child inheriting the deletion who turns out to have DiGeorge syndrome. Similarly, a parent with VCFS and no heart problem can have a child with VCFS and a significant heart defect. Other aspects of the disorder also vary among family members with 22q11 deletions. The only reliable thing is that any child inheriting the deletion will have some disease features.

If my fetus has a 22q11 deletion, what will he or she be like?

As described in the previous answer, there is a lot of variability in the disease among patients with 22q11 deletions. This creates uncertainty about the status of a developing fetus if the amniocentesis reveals that there is a 22q11 deletion. Using ultrasound testing, specially trained obstetricians can look at the developing fetus and define certain aspects of the 22q11 disorders such as the number of kidneys. Similarly, specially trained pediatric cardiologists can look carefully at the heart of a developing fetus in order to detect serious heart defects. Some of the milder heart defects that babies with 22q11 deletions might be born with are not readily seen with this test. Fortunately, the most serious heart defects can be seen in nearly all fetuses. Definition of the heart defects enables physicians and parents to plan properly for the remaining pregnancy and the care of the baby after birth.

Developmental delay/learning issues are an important concern for children with 22q11 deletions although many children with them have minimal or mild learning problems. At present, there are no tools for predicting this aspect of the 22q11 deletion disorders in fetuses or newborns.

Chapter 28

Down Syndrome

Chapter Contents

Section 28.1—Basic Facts about Down Syndrome 326
Section 28.2—Understanding the Different Types of
      Down Syndrome 329
Section 28.3—How Is Down Syndrome Diagnosed in
      a Newborn? 331
Section 28.4—Health Issues in Down Syndrome 332
Section 28.5—Early Intervention and Down Syndrome 333

Section 28.1

Basic Facts about Down Syndrome

"Down Syndrome," National Dissemination Center for Children with Disabilities (NICHCY), Fact Sheet 4, January 2004. Additional information is available online at www.nichcy.org.

Definition

Down syndrome is the most common and readily identifiable chromosomal condition associated with mental retardation. It is caused by a chromosomal abnormality: for some unexplained reason, an accident in cell development results in 47 instead of the usual 46 chromosomes. This extra chromosome changes the orderly development of the body and brain. In most cases, the diagnosis of Down syndrome is made according to results from a chromosome test administered shortly after birth.

Incidence

Approximately 4,000 children with Down syndrome are born in the U.S. each year, or about one in every 800 to 1,000 live births. Although parents of any age may have child with Down syndrome, the incidence is higher for women over 35. Most common forms of the syndrome do not usually occur more than once in a family.

Characteristics

There are over 50 clinical signs of Down syndrome, but it is rare to find all or even most of them in one person. Some common characteristics include:

- Poor muscle tone;
- Slanting eyes with folds of skin at the inner corners (called epicanthal folds);
- Hyperflexibility (excessive ability to extend the joints);
- Short, broad hands with a single crease across the palm on one or both hands;

- Broad feet with short toes;

- Flat bridge of the nose;

- Short, low-set ears;

- Short neck;

- Small head;

- Small oral cavity; and/or

- Short, high-pitched cries in infancy.

Individuals with Down syndrome are usually smaller than their non-disabled peers, and their physical as well as intellectual development is slower.

Besides having a distinct physical appearance, children with Down syndrome frequently have specific health-related problems. A lowered resistance to infection makes these children more prone to respiratory problems. Visual problems such as crossed eyes and far- or nearsightedness are higher in those with Down syndrome, as are mild to moderate hearing loss and speech difficulty.

Approximately one third of babies born with Down syndrome have heart defects, most of which are now successfully correctable. Some individuals are born with gastrointestinal tract problems that can be surgically corrected.

Some people with Down syndrome also may have a condition known as atlantoaxial instability, a misalignment of the top two vertebrae of the neck. This condition makes these individuals more prone to injury if they participate in activities which overextend or flex the neck. Parents are urged to have their child examined by a physician to determine whether or not their child should be restricted from sports and activities which place stress on the neck. Although this misalignment is a potentially serious condition, proper diagnosis can help prevent serious injury.

Children with Down syndrome may have a tendency to become obese as they grow older. Besides having negative social implications, this weight gain threatens these individuals' health and longevity. A supervised diet and exercise program may help reduce this problem.

Educational and Employment Implications

Shortly after a diagnoses of Down syndrome is confirmed, parents should be encouraged to enroll their child in an infant development/

early intervention program. These programs offer parents special instruction in teaching their child language, cognitive, self-help, and social skills, and specific exercises for gross and fine motor development. Research has shown that stimulation during early developmental stages improves the child's chances of developing to his or her fullest potential. Continuing education, positive public attitudes, and a stimulating home environment have also been found to promote the child's overall development.

Just as in the normal population, there is a wide variation in mental abilities, behavior, and developmental progress in individuals with Down syndrome. Their level of retardation may range from mild to severe, with the majority functioning in the mild to moderate range. Due to these individual differences, it is impossible to predict future achievements of children with Down syndrome.

Because of the range of ability in children with Down syndrome it is important for families and all members of the school's education team to place few limitations on potential capabilities. It may be effective to emphasize concrete concepts rather than abstract ideas. Teaching tasks in a step-by-step manner with frequent reinforcement and consistent feedback has been proven successful. Improved public acceptance of persons with disabilities along with increased opportunities for adults with disabilities to live and work independently in the community, have expanded goals for individuals with Down syndrome. Independent living centers, group shared and supervised apartments, and support services in the community have proven to be important resources for persons with disabilities.

Section 28.2

Understanding the Different Types of Down Syndrome

Down syndrome is usually caused by an error in cell division called non-disjunction. However, two other types of chromosomal abnormalities, mosaicism and translocation, are also implicated in Down syndrome—although to a much lesser extent. Regardless of the type of Down syndrome which a person may have, all people with Down syndrome have an extra, critical portion of the number 21 chromosome present in all, or some, of their cells. This additional genetic material alters the course of development and causes the characteristics associated with the syndrome.

Nondisjunction

Nondisjunction is a faulty cell division which results in an embryo with three number 21 chromosomes instead of two. Prior to, or at, conception, a pair of number 21 chromosomes, in either the sperm or the egg, fail to separate. As the embryo develops, the extra chromosome is replicated in every cell of the body. This faulty cell division is responsible for 95 percent of all cases of Down syndrome.

Why nondisjunction occurs is currently unknown, although it does seem to be related to advancing maternal age. Many people are surprised to find out that 80 percent of children born with Down syndrome are born to women under 35 years of age. This is because younger women have higher fertility rates. It does not contradict the fact that the incidence of births of children with Down syndrome increases with the age of the mother.

Although nondisjunction can be of paternal origin, this occurs less frequently. Because this error in cell division is often present in the egg prior to conception, and women are born with their complete store of eggs, it has been postulated that some environmental factors may be implicated in nondisjunction. However, despite years of research, the cause (or causes) of nondisjunction, is still unknown. There seems to be no connection between any type of Down syndrome and parents' activities before or during pregnancy.

Mosaicism

Mosaicism occurs when nondisjunction of the 21st chromosome takes place in one of the initial cell divisions after fertilization. When this occurs, there is a mixture of two types of cells, some containing 46 chromosomes and some containing 47. Those cells with 47 chromosomes contain an extra 21st chromosome. Because of the "mosaic" pattern of the cells, the term mosaicism is used. Mosaicism is rare, being responsible for only one to two percent of all cases of Down syndrome.

Some research has shown that individuals with mosaic Down syndrome are less affected than those with trisomy 21; however, broad generalizations are not possible due to the wide range of abilities that people with Down syndrome possess.

Translocation

Translocation is a different type of chromosomal problem and occurs in only three to four percent of people with Down syndrome. Translocation occurs when part of the number 21 chromosome breaks off during cell division and attaches to another chromosome. While the total number of chromosomes in the cells remains 46, the presence of an extra part of the number 21 chromosome causes the features of Down syndrome. As with nondisjunction trisomy 21, translocation occurs either prior to or at conception.

Unlike nondisjunction, maternal age is not linked to the risk of translocation. Most cases are sporadic, chance events. However, in about one-third of cases, one parent is a carrier of a translocated chromosome. For this reason, the risk of recurrence for translocation is higher than that of nondisjunction. Genetic counseling can be sought to determine the origin of the translocation.

Section 28.3

How Is Down Syndrome Diagnosed in a Newborn?

The diagnosis of Down syndrome is usually suspected after birth as a result of the baby's appearance. It is a particularly difficult time, coupled with the natural stresses of childbirth. Although there is no easy way to be informed, most families agree that having the baby present, being together, and being told as soon as possible is the best way to proceed.

There are many physical characteristics which form the basis for suspecting an infant has Down syndrome. Many of these characteristics are found, to some extent, in the general population of individuals who do not have Down syndrome. Hence, if Down syndrome is suspected, a karyotype will be performed to ascertain the diagnosis. Some infants with Down syndrome have only a few of these traits, while others have many. Among the most common traits are:

- Muscle hypotonia, low muscle tone

- Flat facial profile, a somewhat depressed nasal bridge and a small nose

- Oblique palpebral fissures, an upward slant to the eyes

- Dysplastic ear, an abnormal shape of the ear

- A single deep crease across the center of the palm

- Hyperflexibility, an excessive ability to extend the joints

- Dysplastic middle phalanx of the fifth finger, fifth finger has one flexion furrow instead of two

- Epicanthal folds, small skin folds on the inner corner of the eyes

- Excessive space between large and second toe

- Enlargement of tongue in relationship to size of mouth

Section 28.4

Health Issues in Down Syndrome

Health Issues

Many children with Down syndrome have health complications beyond the usual childhood illnesses. Approximately 40% of the children have congenital heart defects. It is very important that an echocardiogram be performed on all newborns with Down syndrome in order to identify any serious cardiac problems that might be present. Some of the heart conditions require surgery while others only require careful monitoring. Children with Down syndrome have a higher incidence of infection, respiratory, vision, and hearing problems as well as thyroid and other medical conditions. However, with appropriate medical care most children and adults with Down syndrome can lead healthy lives. The average life expectancy of individuals with Down syndrome is 55 years, with many living into their sixties and seventies.

Pre-Natal Diagnosis

Two types of procedures are available to pregnant women: screening tests and diagnostic tests. The screening tests estimate the risk of the baby having Down syndrome. Diagnostic tests tell whether or not the baby actually has Down syndrome.

Screening Tests

- At this time the most commonly used screening test is "The Triple Screen." This is a combination of three tests that measure quantities of various substances in the blood. These tests are usually done between 15 and 20 weeks of gestation.

- Sonograms (ultrasounds) are usually performed in conjunction with other screenings. These can show some physical traits that are helpful in calculating the risk of Down syndrome.

- Screening tests do not accurately confirm the diagnosis of Down syndrome. In fact, false positives and false negatives frequently occur.

Diagnostic Tests

Three diagnostic tests are currently available:

- Amniocentesis is performed between 12 and 20 weeks gestation.
- Chorionic villus sampling (CVS) is conducted between 8 and 12 weeks.
- Percutaneous umbilical blood sampling (PUBS) is performed after 20 weeks.

Section 28.5

Early Intervention and Down Syndrome

"Clinical Info: Early Intervention and Down Syndrome," by Valentine Dmitriev, Ph.D. Reprinted with permission from the National Down Syndrome Society, http://www.ndss.org. © 2004 National Down Syndrome Society. All rights reserved.

Among the many developmental stages through which growing children will pass, the most rapid and developmentally significant changes occur during the first three years of life. It is during this transitional period between infancy and early childhood that children achieve their basic physical, cognitive, language, social, and self-help skills. Furthermore, it is expected that these skills will be attained according to predictable developmental patterns, thus laying the foundation for future progress. As a rule, these developmental goals are reached in an orderly manner, seemingly spontaneously, with more successes than failure. Children with Down syndrome, however, may face some potential difficulties in certain areas of development. Children with Down syndrome do progress through the same developmental stages, but they do so on their own timetables.

What is early intervention?

Based upon patterns of development, early intervention is a systematic program of physical therapy, exercise, and activity designed to remedy developmental delays that may be experienced by children with Down syndrome. In many instances, the program is individualized to meet the specific needs of each child, and to help all infants and children reach growth milestones in every area of development. Early intervention helps in each of the four main areas of development: gross motor and fine motor skills, language, social development, and self-help skills.

When should early intervention start?

Early intervention should begin any time shortly after birth and continue until the child reaches age three. The sooner early intervention begins, the better; however, it's never too late to start. Once it is determined that your baby has Down syndrome, you may contact your local early intervention specialist and arrange for an evaluation and assessment.

What do the terms "milestones" and "key ages" mean?

Milestones refer to a series of skills in the four areas of development which a child is expected to achieve at a designated time, also referred to as a key age which may be calculated in terms of weeks, months or years. It must be remembered that development is a continuous process that begins at conception and which proceeds stage by stage in an orderly sequence. Each milestone represents a skill which is prerequisite to the next stage in development. In monitoring the development of a child with Down syndrome, it is more useful to look at the sequence of milestones achieved, rather than the age at which the milestone is reached.

How can early intervention benefit a child with Down syndrome?

Early intervention can help in many ways. During the first three to four months of life, for example, an infant is expected to gain head control and the ability to pull to a sitting positions (with help) with no head lags and enough strength in the upper torso to maintain an erect posture. Appropriate physical therapy may assist a baby with Down syndrome, who may have low muscle tone, in achieving this milestone.

One of the fine motor skills that an infant is expected to achieve is the ability to hold and reach for objects. Here again, the baby with Down syndrome may need help before mastering these tasks. Physical therapy and practice in achieving these and subsequent milestones can assist a baby with Down syndrome. Early intervention can also prevent a child with Down syndrome from reaching a plateau at some point in development. Thus, the goal of early intervention programs is to enhance and accelerate development by building on a child's strengths and by strengthening those areas that are weaker, in all areas of development.

Why is gross motor development so important?

All areas of development are equally important, although the emphasis changes as the child grows. Nevertheless, before birth and in the first months of life, physical development remains the underlying foundation for all future progress. Babies learn through interaction with their environment. In order to do so, an infant must have the ability to move freely and purposefully. The ability to explore one's surroundings, the ability to reach and grasp toys, to turn one's head in order to follow a moving object with one's eyes, the ability to roll over, and to crawl in pursuit of a desired objective. All of these behaviors are dependent upon gross as well as fine motor development. These physical, interactive activities foster understanding and mastery of the environment, stimulating cognitive, language, and social development.

Why does health affect development?

Health plays a major role in everyone's well-being and progress, and this holds true for children with Down syndrome. For this reason, early intervention should begin with a thorough assessment of an infant's health. All health concerns should receive prompt attention to prevent them from interfering with a child's development. Generally, doctors have become much more sensitive to the health needs of children with Down syndrome than they were in the past. Early diagnosis and proper treatment promise better health, and as a result, better developmental progress.

What can I expect in terms of my child's potential and future development?

Early intervention, research, and case histories have shown that children with Down syndrome have a far greater potential for learning and for functioning as contributing members of society than it was believed to be possible even 10 to 15 years ago. At the same time, we must remember that each child, whether he has Down syndrome or not, is a unique individual with his own strengths and weaknesses, his own abilities, as well as his own rate of development. Even when milestones are reached on schedule, expectations must be balanced. Low expectations will set limits on what a child can achieve. At the same time, unrealistically high expectations place undue burdens on a child, which may lead to failure. Acceptance of your child is the best approach. Optimistic, yet realistic, expectations plus the ability to recognize and reinforce the smallest increments of progress are the attitudes that are most likely to have a positive effect on development. In this way, early interventions succeed in maximizing achievement.

How can parents benefit from early intervention programs?

Programs of early intervention have a great deal to offer to parents in terms of support, encouragement, and information. The programs teach parents how to interact with their infant and toddler, how to meet their child's specific needs, and how to enhance development. Furthermore, early intervention centers give parents the opportunity to share their concerns with other parents.

How can I find an early intervention program?

Today, every state in the U.S. has a center that coordinates early intervention services in the state. Information can be obtained through the National Down Syndrome Society (NDSS) and other organizations about the center nearest you. Public schools and community colleges are other resources. If there are no developmental centers in your area, many helpful books are available.

Who pays for early intervention?

The evaluation to determine whether your child is eligible for early intervention is free of charge if performed by a state authorized entity. No child deemed eligible can be denied services based on ability to pay, but insurance companies may be billed and/or a sliding scale payment may be required, depending on what state you reside in. Check with your state's early intervention center for information about authorized service providers and financial obligations. Frequently, there is little or no cost to parents for these services.

Summary

- Children develop according to their individual timetables.

- Early intervention may help encourage and accelerate development.

- The four main areas of development are gross and fine motor skills, language, self help, and social development.

- Milestones are essential as prerequisite stepping stones to each new level of maturity.

- Early intervention benefits children with Down syndrome by helping to prevent developmental delays that may occur.

- Gross and fine motor development is important because it facilitates progress in language, cognition, and self-help by enabling children to interact with their environment.

- Health factors play a major role in a child's achievement. Early assessment of an infant's health is essential. Health problems must be treated as soon as they are recognized.

- Parental expectations influence a child's development. Unrealistically high, or low, expectations can be damaging to a child's self esteem and progress. An accepting, optimistic, yet realistic attitude creates a nurturing environment for optimum progress.

- Early intervention programs help parents by providing support, encouragement, training, and companionship.

- Nearly every area in the U.S. has developmental centers that serve children with special needs. Information can be obtained from NDSS, similar organizations, schools, colleges, and books.

—by Valentine Dmitriev, Ph.D.

Chapter 29

Edwards Syndrome

Definition

Trisomy 18 (alternative name: Edwards syndrome) is a syndrome associated with the presence of a third (extra) number 18 chromosome.

Causes, Incidence, and Risk Factors

Trisomy 18 is a relatively common syndrome affecting approximately one out of 3,000 live births and affecting girls more than three times as often as boys. Multiple abnormalities are associated with the presence of an extra number 18 chromosome. Many of these abnormalities are not compatible with more than a few months of life. Few infants survive beyond the first year.

Common findings include low birth weight, mental retardation, low-set ears, malformed ears, small jaw (micrognathia), hand abnormalities, congenital heart disease, hernias, and undescended testicle (cryptorchidism). There may be many other abnormalities noted.

Symptoms

- Unusually large uterus during pregnancy
- Low birth weight infant
- Mental deficiency

"Trisomy 18," © 2003 A.D.A.M., Inc.; reprinted with permission.

- Low-set ears

- Small jaw (micrognathia)

- Clenched hands

- Hypoplastic (underdeveloped) fingernails

- Umbilical hernia or inguinal hernia

- Diastasis recti

- Cryptorchidism

- Crossed legs (preferred position)

- Congenital heart disease

  - VSD (ventricular septal defect)

  - ASD (atrial septal defect)

  - PDA (patent ductus arteriosus)

- Congenital kidney abnormalities

  - Horseshoe kidney

  - Hydronephrosis

  - Polycystic kidney

- Coloboma of iris

- Microcephaly

- Motormental retardation

- Pectus carinatum

Signs and Tests

Examination of the pregnant woman may show polyhydramnios (extra amniotic fluid). At the birth of the child, an unusually small placenta may be noted.

Physical examination may show an excess of arched type finger print patterns. X-rays may reveal a short breast bone (sternum). Chromosome studies show trisomy 18, partial trisomy, or translocation.

Treatment

Treatment is supportive, but life-sustaining measures are not recommended.

Support Groups

Support Organization for Trisomy 18, 13 and Related Disorders (SOFT)

2982 S. Union St.
Rochester, NY 14624
Toll-Free: 800-716-7638
Phone: 716-594-4621
Website: http://www.trisomy.org

Expectations (Prognosis)

The abnormalities of trisomy 18 are generally not compatible with more than a few months of life. Fifty percent of the affected infants do not survive beyond the first week of life. More than ten children have survived to teenage years, but usually with marked handicaps.

Complications

Complications depend on the specific abnormalities that affect the infant.

Calling Your Health Care Provider

Call your health care provider and genetic counselor if you have had a child with Trisomy 18 and you plan to have another child.

Prevention

Prenatal diagnosis of trisomy 18 is possible with an amniocentesis and chromosome studies on amniotic cells. Parents who have a child with translocational trisomy 18 should have chromosome studies because they are at increased risk for another child with trisomy 18.

Chapter 30

Fragile X Syndrome

What is fragile X syndrome?

Fragile X syndrome (also called fragile X) is the most common inherited form of mental retardation after Down syndrome. It results from a change, or mutation, in a single gene, which can be passed from one generation to the next. Fragile X appears in families of every ethnic group and income level.

Symptoms of fragile X syndrome occur because the mutated gene cannot produce enough of a protein that is needed by the body's cells—especially cells in the brain—to develop and function normally. The amount and usability of this protein, in part, determine how severe the effects of fragile X are.

The most noticeable and consistent effect of fragile X is on intelligence. More than 80 percent of males with fragile X have an IQ (intelligence quotient) of 75 or less. The effect of fragile X on intelligence is more variable in females. Some females have mental impairment, some have learning disabilities, and some have a normal IQ.

People with fragile X syndrome also share certain medical problems as well as many common physical characteristics, such as large ears and a long face. In addition, having fragile X is often associated with problems with sensation, emotion, and behavior.

Excerpted from "Families and Fragile X Syndrome," National Institute on Child Health and Human Development (NICHD), NIH Pub. No. 96-3402, revised 2003.

What causes fragile X syndrome?

The underlying cause of fragile X is a change in a single gene, the fragile X mental retardation 1 (*FMR1*) gene, which is found on the X chromosome.

Genes contain the information used by other parts of a cell to make proteins. Proteins are the body's building blocks. Each protein performs a specific job. They make up the structure of your organs and tissues and are needed for all of your body's chemical functions.

Each gene contains information for making at least one protein. If this information is changed, then the cell may not be able to make that protein, or it may not be able to make a form of the protein that the body can use. Fragile X occurs because the *FMR1* gene is unable to make normal amounts of usable fragile X mental retardation protein, or FMRP.

The amount of FMRP in the body is one factor that determines how severe the effects of having fragile X are. A person with nearly normal levels of FMRP usually has mild or no symptoms, while a person with very little or no normal FMRP has more severe symptoms.

Scientists are still studying the role of FMRP in the body. One current research study revealed that certain cell processes brain cells use to communicate with one another occur in excess in mice that have little or no FMRP; that is, the brain cells may communicate too much or may communicate inappropriately. Researchers believe that FMRP may regulate the amount of communication between cells and keep it under control. Scientists are hopeful that they can identify a similar function for FMRP in humans.

What keeps the FMR1 gene from producing FMRP in fragile X syndrome?

The information for making a protein has two parts: the introduction, and the instructions for the protein itself. Scientists call the introduction "the promoter region" of the gene because of its role in starting the protein-building process. The promoter region of the *FMR1* gene contains repeats of a specific sequence (cytosine-guanine-guanine or CGG) that, when normal, controls the activity level of the gene in building FMRP.

The number of repeated sequences in the promoter region varies from person to person. Most people who do not have fragile X have between six and 40 CGG repeats, with the average being about 30 repeats in the promoter region. However, in a mutated *FMR1* gene, the promoter may have hundreds of repeated sequences. A gene with

55 to 200 repeats is generally considered a "premutation." A gene with more than about 200 repeats is called a "full mutation." (The number of repeats and their effects are still being studied. You may encounter differences in the number of repeats for a premutation depending on your source.) The larger number of repeats (more than 200) inactivates the gene. This inactivation process is called methylation. When the gene is inactivated, the cell may make little or none of the needed FMRP.

What goes wrong in a mutated gene?

A number of things can go wrong in a gene that can result in a mutation. The mutation affects the gene's ability to make the needed amount of protein or to make enough usable protein. In the case of fragile X, usually the *FMR1* gene is present, and its chemical sequence is correct, however, a mutated *FMR1* gene includes repeats of a specific sequence in its promoter region.

One interesting aspect of fragile X is that, even with a full mutation gene, the body may be able to make some FMRP. Three things affect how much FMRP is produced:

- **The number of CGG repeats:** People with a full mutation (200 or more repeats) usually have many of the more severe symptoms associated with fragile X. In contrast, people with a premutation gene may have few, if any, symptoms and may not even know they carry a mutated gene. Researchers are still trying to sort out any, patterns or trends in the symptoms of people with a premutation gene.

- **Being mosaic.** Not every cell in the body is exactly the same. In fragile X, this means that some cells may have 200 or more repeats in the FMR1 promoter, while other cells, premutation cells, may have fewer than 200 repeats. This is called being "mosaic," meaning either that the mutation is in some of the cells, but not all of them, or that it is not in all of the cells to the same degree. The premutation cells may be able to make FMRP. Similarly, methylation may not happen at all, or to the same degree, in every cell. If enough cells produce FMRP, the symptoms of fragile X will be milder than if none of the cells produce FMRP.

- **Being female:** Because females have two X chromosomes, females with fragile X have one normal *FMR1* gene and one mutated *FMR1* gene in most of their cells. But, only one X chromosome is active in each cell, and only the genes on the active chromosome are used to build proteins. The cell seems to randomly choose which chromosome is used. In some cells, then, the X chromosome that contains the normal *FMR1* gene is active, and the cell uses it to make FMRP. As a result, even females with a full mutation are often able to make some of the needed protein. For this reason, the symptoms of fragile X usually affect females less often and less seriously than males.

How many people are affected by fragile X syndrome?

Currently, researchers don't know exactly how many people have either the full mutation or the premutation form of the *FMR1* gene. Even though researchers can estimate the number of people affected by fragile X, these estimates can be very different and the number of people affected by a full mutation or a premutation of the *FMR1* gene is still being studied.

A summary of existing research conducted by the Centers for Disease Control and Prevention in 2001 estimated that approximately one in 3,500 to 8,900 males is affected by the full mutation of the *FMR1* gene, and that one in 1,000 males has the premutation form of the *FMR1* gene. This study also estimated that one in 250 to 500 females in the general population has the premutation. Another study estimated that one in 4,000 females is affected by the full mutation.

How is fragile X syndrome inherited?

The gene for fragile X is carried on the X chromosome. Because both males (XY) and females (XX) have at least one X chromosome, both can pass on the mutated gene to their children.

A father with the altered gene for fragile X on his X chromosome will only pass that gene on to his daughters. He passes a Y chromosome on to his sons, which doesn't transmit the condition. Therefore, if the father has the altered gene on his X chromosome, but the mother's X chromosomes are normal, all of the couple's daughters would have the altered gene for fragile X, while none of their sons would have the mutated gene.

Current research indicates that a father can pass on the premutation form of the *FMR1* gene only to his daughters. In other words, if a daughter inherits the mutated *FMR1* gene from her father, she will get only the premutation from him, not the full mutation. Even if the father himself has a full mutation, it appears that sperm can carry only the premutation. Scientists don't understand how or why fathers can only pass on the milder form of fragile X to their daughters. This remains an area of focused research.

Because mothers pass on only X chromosomes to their children, if the mother has the altered gene for fragile X, she can pass that gene to either her sons or her daughters. If the mother has the mutated gene on one X chromosome and has one normal X chromosome, and the father has no genetic mutations, all the children have a 50–50 chance of inheriting the mutated gene.

The odds noted here apply to each child the parents have. Having one child who receives an X chromosome with the *FMR1* mutation does not increase or decrease the chances of having another child with the mutated *FMR1* gene. Nor do these odds influence the severity of the symptoms. Having one child with mild symptoms does not mean that the other children will have severe symptoms, and having a child with severe symptoms does not mean that other children will have mild symptoms.

A premutation gene is less stable than a full mutation. In some cases, the mutated gene may expand from the premutation to the full mutation as it is passed on from mother to child. The chances of expansion depend on the number of repeats in the promoter of the premutation gene; the higher the number of repeats, the more likely it is that the gene will expand. These chances also increase with each generation. Children of a mother who has the premutation, then, may have no genetic mutation, the premutation, or the full mutation.

Further, because an altered *FMR1* gene can be passed on without symptoms, many people are unaware that they have it. As a result, a premutation form of the *FMR1* gene can be silently passed through a family for generations, with no one ever showing any symptoms. However, with each generation, it becomes more likely that the premutation gene will expand its number of repeats to become a full mutation gene, which would also increase the number of and seriousness of symptoms.

What are the signs and symptoms of fragile X syndrome?

Not everyone with fragile X has the same signs and symptoms, or to the same degree. Even affected children in the same family can have different signs and symptoms. These differences often make fragile X hard to diagnose. However, because everyone with fragile X has too little FMRP, they do share a pattern of certain physical, social, mental, and sensory characteristics. Although most of the fragile X research to date has focused on children, adults with fragile X also have most of these signs and symptoms.

Intelligence and learning: Many people with fragile X have impaired intellectual functioning, which affects their ability to think, reason, and learn. In most cases, researchers use an intelligence test to measure intellectual functioning, resulting in an IQ (intelligence quotient) score. Researchers consider people who score between 85 and 115 on an IQ test to have "average" intelligence. On the whole, less than 20 percent of males with fragile X have an IQ in this range. At the same time, few people with fragile X are severely or profoundly impaired, with IQs below 40 or 25, respectively. In general, those with a full mutation tend to have an IQ somewhere in between 40 and 85, which is considered mild to moderate mental impairment.

Among females who have full-mutation *FMR1* genes, only about one-third have an IQ in the mental retardation range. Females with fragile X are more likely to have relatively normal cognitive development, or they may show a learning disability where their academic achievement in some areas is lower than their overall ability to learn. For example, a female with a learning disability in math might score several grades below her grade level in math, even though her IQ is within the normal range.

Physical: Many infants and young children with fragile X have no distinctive physical features. Some children have very soft, velvety skin, a broad forehead, or a slightly larger head than other children their age. However, when these children enter puberty, usually around age 11, they may begin to develop certain features that are typical of teens and adults with fragile X, such as a longer face or jaw and larger, more noticeable ears. Most do not grow as tall as their peers, or as tall as one might expect them to grow, based on the height of their family members.

Other physical changes also come with puberty for those who have fragile X. Many males develop enlarged testicles, a condition called macro-orchidism. With this condition, the testicles may grow to twice their normal size. This condition is not due to hormonal imbalance and does not affect sexual development.

One job of FMRP may be to help the body maintain its connective tissues. Connective tissues support the body, inside and out. Many people with fragile X have loose, flexible joints. They may have flat feet and be able to extend joints like the thumb, knee, and elbow further than normal. Weak connective tissue can predispose a person to certain medical conditions, such as hernia and frequent middle ear infections. Weak connective tissue can also affect the valves and vessels of the heart, so that blood in the heart may not flow smoothly, which creates a heart murmur (called mitral valve prolapse). Although it involves the heart, this condition is usually not life threatening, but it is a good idea for a person with a heart murmur to be monitored by a health care professional on a regular basis.

Late in life, some males who have a premutation may develop hand tremors and problems with walking.

Fragile X affects females in some different ways. About 16–19 percent of females who have a premutation gene experience premature ovarian failure (POF), meaning their ovarian function stops before normal menopause, sometimes well before the age of 40. Some may experience POF as early as their mid-twenties. POF affects a woman's ability to get pregnant. It is important, then, for women to know whether or not they have a premutation gene, and to have this knowledge early enough, so that they can consider their options for having a family. In contrast, POF occurs in only 1 percent of women who have two normal *FMR1* genes, and the average age of menopause for women who are not affected by fragile X is 51. Women who have a full mutation gene do not lose ovarian function as early as women with a premutation gene, but they still tend to begin menopause earlier than women who are not affected by fragile X. Scientists do not know why the effect is milder in women who have a full mutation form of the gene than in women with a premutation form of the gene.

Social and emotional: Most children with fragile X—especially boys—feel a great deal of social anxiety; that is, they aren't completely comfortable in new situations, meeting new people, or doing new things. Their level of anxiety can be so high that they may avoid social situations. When these children do seek contact with others, they are often extremely nervous or uncomfortable. Their anxiety may show up as a lack of eye contact and/or fast, choppy speech. Although all children feel some degree of social anxiety, this discomfort usually doesn't keep them from being social, as it may for children with fragile X.

In addition to being anxious, males with fragile X tend to be easily upset. They are easily overwhelmed with sights and sounds, and can become very distressed in a busy store or restaurant. Unexpected changes in routine, like entering a new class or classroom, can also upset them. Some children respond by becoming extremely rigid or tense, while others whine or cry. At times, their reactions can spill over into tantrums or repetitive actions, such as rocking back and forth and biting themselves. In adolescence, changes, such as rising hormone levels, may make these outbursts more extreme. In one study of teenage males with fragile X, about one-third showed angry, aggressive behavior. Such behavior can get them into trouble at school. Providing medication and a calm environment can help keep such behaviors from getting worse.

In addition, males with fragile X tend to experience much longer periods of anxiety than their peers. Like other males, their heart rate and other signs of nervousness increase when they do challenging tasks, but many males with fragile X stay highly anxious for much longer time frame. So, in addition to having a level of anxiety that is often higher than their peers, males with fragile X also take longer to calm down than other males do.

Females with fragile X may have social problems, too, but theirs tend to be milder. A female with fragile X may feel uneasy around strangers or have trouble making friends, but these females don't tend to be aggressive as adolescents.

Speech and language: Language difficulties in children who have fragile X range from mild stuttering to more severe problems with basic language skills. Basic language skills include the ability to pronounce words clearly, to speak and write using words and grammar correctly, and to communicate in meaningful ways.

Females with fragile X rarely have severe problems with speech or language. In fact, many have vocabulary and grammar skills that are appropriate for their age, which can help them learn to read and write. However, their social anxiety and shyness may get in the way of communication. Some females with fragile X speak in a rambling, disorganized way or often get off the subject. Most males with fragile X have more serious problems expressing themselves. These difficulties typically include problems speaking clearly and other problems with language that can be moderate to severe. In terms of speech, males with fragile X often have problems coordinating the structures, vocal processes (such as pitch, loudness, and tone), and movements needed for clear speech. They often have difficulty receiving and processing spoken information, such as following spoken directions, storing words and concepts for future use, and creating their own meaningful responses to questions or comments.

Males with fragile X may stutter or leave sounds out of their words. Many repeat themselves, restart the same sentence many times, or ask the same question again and again. Some may talk too fast, mumble, or speak in a loud, high voice. Some of these difficulties may be due to sensory overload or social anxiety, rather than a problem with the parts of the brain that control speech and language.

Perhaps most importantly, males with fragile X usually have difficulty using speech and language in social contexts. They often seem unaware of conversational "clues," such as facial expressions, tone of voice, and body language. As a result, they may speak out of turn, fail to answer a question, or turn away because they aren't sure what to do. Unlike males with other developmental disorders, like autism, males with fragile X seem to be very interested in communicating, but may experience sensory overload or social overload when they try to hold a conversation.

For some children, language problems are more severe. Many children with fragile X begin talking later than expected. Most begin using words around age four, but some may not talk until age of six or eight. Most talk eventually, but some may remain nonverbal throughout life. For these nonverbal children, a wide variety of picture-based and computer-based devices may help them to communicate, which could also reduce behavior difficulties that result from not being able to talk. Pictures, sign language, and generic gestures can also be helpful for all children with fragile X, before they start talking.

Sensory: Many children with fragile X are sensitive to certain sensations. They may become frantic at the sound of a loud noise or may be easily distracted by slight sounds in the room. They may be bothered by the texture of their clothes against their skin, or they may be unable to focus on the parts of their environment that are important, such as the sound of the teacher's voice. Infants with fragile X may have problems drinking from a bottle, perhaps because the feel of the nipple upsets them. Some children try to avoid being touched, and even a brief tickle or hug may be overwhelming. Even though many of these symptoms are often life-long, most people affected by fragile X, with the proper intervention, can find ways to handle or avoid the discomfort.

Children with fragile X may also have problems with balance. A sense of balance helps keep the body upright and stable. Problems with balance, coordination, and connective tissue can cause difficulties for children with fragile X as they learn to sit, stand, and walk, or later, to ride a bike. Even so, most children with fragile X learn to do these tasks.

Is there a cure for fragile X syndrome?

Although research continues and knowledge about fragile X and its characteristics grows, there is no cure for fragile X at this time.

351

Are there treatments for fragile X syndrome?

Currently there is no definitive, single treatment for fragile X. However, there are a variety of ways to help minimize the symptoms of the condition. Children with fragile X who receive appropriate education, behavioral or physical therapy, and medication have the best chance of using their individual capabilities and skills. Even those with significant mental retardation can learn to master many self-help skills.

One important factor in developing a child's long-term potential is early intervention. The sooner a child begins to get help, the more opportunity for learning. Because a young child's brain is still forming, early intervention gives children the best start possible and the best chance of developing their full potential. Even so, no matter when a person is diagnosed with fragile X, it's never too late to benefit from treatment.

Educational options: Most children with fragile X, including those with severe mental retardation, are guaranteed free, appropriate public education under federal law. Public Law 105-17: The Individuals with Disabilities Education Act—IDEA (1997) makes it possible for children with disabilities to get free educational services and educational devices to help them learn as much as they can. Each child is entitled to these services from age three through high school, or until age 21, whichever comes first. Also, every state operates an early intervention program for children from birth to age three; children with fragile X should qualify for these services. The law also states that children must be taught in the least restrictive environment, appropriate for that individual child. This statement does not mean that each child will be placed in a regular classroom, but instead, that the best combination of one-to-one tutoring, small group work, and regular classroom work will be arranged.

Because not all children or adolescents with fragile X have mental impairment or special needs, a medical diagnosis of fragile X does not guarantee access to special education services. The child must have certain cognitive or learning deficits. Parents can contact a local school principal or special education coordinator to learn how to have their child examined to see if he or she qualifies for services under the IDEA.

If a child qualifies for special services, a team of people, including the child's parents or caregivers, teachers, school psychologist, and other child development specialists, will work together to design an Individualized Education Plan (IEP) for the child. The IEP includes specific learning goals for that child, based on his or her needs and capabilities. The team also decides how best to carry out the IEP, such as making choices about classroom placement for the child, determining any devices or special assistance the child needs, and identifying the developmental specialists who will work with the child.

A child with fragile X should be evaluated and re-evaluated on a regular basis by his or her special services team. In this way, the team can determine how the child is doing and whether any changes are needed in his or her treatment (for instance, changes to the IEP, changes in classroom placement, or changes in other services) to ensure the child is getting the best possible care.

In general, there are three classroom placement options for a child with fragile X, based on his or her specific abilities and needs:

- **Full inclusion in a regular classroom.** The child spends the full day in the regular classroom rather than just among children with special needs. This situation is sometimes called "mainstreaming." Specialists work with the child in the classroom, with other students present. There may be an aide assigned to help the child with certain kinds of tasks.

- **Inclusion with "pull-out" services.** In this type of placement, the child spends most of the day in the regular classroom. However, for part of the day, he or she attends small-group classes with one or more developmental specialists, such as a speech-language therapist or a physical therapist. This arrangement gives the child exposure to children who do not have special needs, as well as more individual attention to his or her areas of special needs.

- **Full-time, special education classroom.** Some children with fragile X may do better in a smaller special education class than in a regular classroom. Special education classrooms usually have fewer children and offer more individualized attention from the teacher. Such programs may be offered at the school or in central locations that serve a larger area. Regional special education centers often have facilities and equipment designed for children with special needs. For some children, a special school for children with similar disabilities may be the best option.

Placement decisions should be based on each child's needs and abilities. In most cases, these decisions require a balance of various priorities to maximize the chances for the best possible outcome for the child.

Therapeutic options: A variety of professionals can help individuals with fragile X and their families deal with symptoms of the disorder. Such assistance is usually most effective when provided by health care professionals experienced with fragile X.

- Speech-language therapists can help people with fragile X to improve their pronunciation of words and sentences, slow down speech, and use language more effectively.

- Occupational therapists help find ways to adjust tasks and conditions to match a person's needs and abilities.

- Physical therapists design activities and exercises to build motor control and to improve posture and balance.

- Behavioral therapists try to identify why a child acts in negative ways and then seek ways to prevent these distressing situations, and to teach the child to cope with the distress.

The services of these specialists may be available to pre-school and school-aged children, as well as to teens, through the local public school system. In a school setting, several specialists often work together to assess each child's particular strengths and weaknesses, and to plan a program that is specially tailored to meet the child's needs. These services are often free. More intense and individualized help is available through private clinics, but the family usually has to pay for private services, although some health insurance plans may help cover the cost.

Medication options: Currently, there is no medication that can cure fragile X. Further, the Food and Drug Administration (FDA) has not approved any drugs specifically for the treatment of fragile X or its causes. But, in many cases, medications have been used to treat many of the symptoms associated with fragile X, as shown in Table 30.1. Please note that the National Institute of Child Health and Human Development (NICHD) does not endorse or support the use of any of these medications in treating symptoms of fragile X syndrome, or for other conditions for which the medications are not FDA approved.

Medication is most effective when paired with therapy designed to teach new coping skills or behavior. Not every medication helps every child with behavioral symptoms related to fragile X. Doctors usually prescribe these kinds of medications on a trial basis, to see if they help. If so, the doctor may need to adjust the dose to meet the needs of each child.

Table 30.1. Medications Used to Treat Symptoms Associated with Fragile X

<ins>Symptoms</ins>	<ins>Generic Medications</ins> (Brand names in parentheses)
Seizures or *Mood instability*	• Carbamazepine (Tegretol) • Valproic acid or divalproex (Depakote) • Lithium carbonate • Gabapentin (Neurontin) • Lamotrigine (Lamictal) • Topiramate (Topamax), tiagabine (Gabitril), and vigabatrin (Sabril) Phenobarbital and primidone (Mysoline)
Attention deficit (With or without hyperactivity)	• Methylphenidate (Ritalin, Concerta) and dexamethamphetamine (Adderall, Dexedrine) • L-acetylcarnitine • Venlafaxine (Effexor) and nefazodone (Serzone) • Amantadine (Symmetrel) • Folic acid
Hyperarousal or Sensory *over-stimulation* (Often occurs with ADD/ADHD)	• Clonidine (Catapres TTS patches) • Guanfacine (Tenex)
Aggression; *Intermittent explosive* *disorder; Obsessive-* *compulsive disorder* (Often occurs with anxiety and/or depression)	• Fluoxetine (Prozac) • Sertraline (Zoloft) and citalopram (Celexa) • Paroxetine (Paxil) • Fluvoxamine (Luvox) • Risperidone (Risperdal) • Quetiapine (Seroquel) • Olanzapine (Zyprexa)
Sleep disturbances	• Trazodone • Melatonin

Note: This table is meant for reference ONLY and should not take the place of your health care provider's advice. You should discuss any questions you may have about medication with your health care provider directly. Some of these medications have serious risks involved with their use; others may make symptoms worse at first or may take several weeks to become effective. Doctors may have to try different dosages or different combinations of medications to find the most effective plan. Families, caregivers, and doctors need to work together to ensure that a medication is working, and that a medication plan is safe.

What are the options for adults who have fragile X syndrome?

IDEA requires transition plans for moving from one phase of life to another, and the move from teenager to young adult to adult is no exception. The special services team, which can include family, teachers, a school psychologist, and other developmental specialists, makes the transition plan based on the individual's needs, interests, and skills. These plans may include vocational assessment and training, additional education, supported employment, and community participation. IDEA requires that the plan be in place by the time the individual is 16 years old. The plan will also consider the individual's level of independence to determine what type of living arrangements he or she might benefit from in the future.

As the teenager with fragile X gets closer to finishing high school, or to his or her 21st birthday, the structure of his or her day may change to include work/study programs, job-related behavior training, and independent living classes. With the proper treatment and training, a young person with fragile X may be able to live on his or her own, hold a job, and be an active member of his or her community.

What should I do if I find out someone in my family has fragile X syndrome?

If someone in your family, a child or an adult, is diagnosed with fragile X, you may also want to be tested to see if you have a mutated *FMR1* gene. It is now possible to test for fragile X in people of any age, as well as before birth. These tests are simple and accurate.

At present, testing for fragile X is not done routinely. The tests are often done to help diagnose a child who is developmentally delayed or shows signs of autism or mental retardation. Couples who have one or more relatives with mental retardation of unknown cause may also want to be evaluated before deciding to have a child.

Health care professionals may also recommend an evaluation for fragile X in a person with one of the following traits:

- Any person who has mental retardation of unknown cause, developmental delay, or learning disability

- Any person with autism or showing autistim-like behaviors

- Any person with a relative who has fragile X or mental retardation of unknown cause

- Anyone who was previously assessed for fragile X using the chromosome test (Because this test is older, costly, and often inaccurate, it is recommended that another type of test be used to diagnose fragile X.)

- Women with premature ovarian failure (POF) or with a family history of POF

Can we prevent or cure fragile X?

Two decades ago, researchers might have said "No." Now scientists are exploring several promising possibilities, including:

- **Gene repair, gene reactivation, and gene therapy.** Scientists may be able to induce certain brain chemicals to repair defective *FMR1* genes. Researchers are also seeking ways to prevent or reverse methylation, the process that interferes with the instructions for making FMRP and inactivates the *FMR1* gene. Still other scientists are trying to determine if it is possible to replace defective genes with stable, working copies of the *FMR1* gene. This type of gene research involves a number of challenges. First, it is important that researchers learn how many cells are needed to produce the right amount of protein. Too much of the protein may be as harmful as too little, so finding the right balance is crucial. Another difficulty lies in targeting only the defective *FMR1* genes for repair or reactivation, without affecting other healthy genes. Further, replacing genes, especially those involved in brain function, carries additional problems and risks. However, researchers continue to pursue these avenues. NICHD-supported and other sponsored research is already underway to study the possibility of reversing methylation on the *FMR1* promoter sequence, prenatally. Success in this area may allow scientists to "reactivate" FMRP production before a child is born. Other gene research is also underway.

- **Protein replacement.** Scientists already make FMRP in the lab. At present, however, they are unable to get FMRP to the brain, partly because the FMRP molecule is too large to pass through the structures that protect the brain. Someday people with fragile X may be able to take a pill or injection of FMRP to relieve many of the symptoms of fragile X.

- **Protein substitute through medication.** Scientists may be able to use other substances to take the place of FMRP in certain brain processes. Using these substitutes, brain processes and other functions of FMRP may be able to occur normally. For example, new drugs may be able to regulate processes in the brain, like communication between neurons, that seem to be affected by low levels of FMRP.

While these research avenues are promising, none of them has progressed enough to provide immediate help to someone with fragile X. Parents, families, and caregivers should work together with health care professionals, educators, and therapists to ensure that those affected by fragile X receive the care that they need.

This is an exciting time in fragile X research. Dr. James Watson, who received the Nobel Prize in Physiology or Medicine for the co-discovery of the double-helix structure of DNA, believes that science will be able to defeat the negative effects of fragile X. He predicts, "Our wealth of research strategies and technologies may soon lead to new forms of therapy and medication. Someday we may be able to prevent the mental retardation and other symptoms of fragile X."

Chapter 31

Klinefelter Syndrome

What is Klinefelter syndrome?

In 1942, Harry Klinefelter, Fuller Albright, and their coworkers at the Massachusetts General Hospital published a report about 9 men who had enlarged breasts, sparse facial and body hair, small testes, and the inability to produce sperm. This combination of features has come to be recognized as Klinefelter syndrome.

What causes Klinefelter syndrome?

Klinefelter syndrome is caused by the presence of an extra sex chromosome. Males with the syndrome have a sex chromosome composition of XXY instead of the usual XY male sex chromosome complement.

What causes XXY?

XXY is caused by a biological accident during a process called meiosis. Meiosis is a process experienced by all cells, which are destined to develop into sperm or eggs. In this process, the 46 chromosomes in the cell divide to make two new cells with 23 chromosomes each. Before meiosis is completed, however, chromosomes pair with their corresponding chromosomes and exchange bits of genetic material. In women, the X chromosomes from each parent pair, and in men, the X and Y chromosomes pair. After the exchange, the chromosomes separate, and meiosis continues. In some cases, the two X chromosomes or the X and Y chromosomes fail to pair and fail to exchange genetic material. Occasionally, this results in their moving independently to the same cell, producing either an egg with two Xs, or a sperm having both an X and a Y chromosome. When a sperm having both an X and a Y chromosome fertilizes an egg having a single X chromosome, or a normal sperm bearing a Y chromosome fertilizes an egg having two X chromosomes, an XXY male is conceived.

About 50 percent of the time, the extra chromosome comes from the father and the other 50 percent of the time, it comes from the mother. Older mothers have a slightly increased risk of having a boy with XXY.

How common is Klinefelter syndrome?

In the early 1970s, it was found that the XXY was one of the most common chromosomal abnormalities, occurring as frequently as one in 500 male births.

Who are XXY males?

Although XXY is common, the syndrome itself—the set of signs and symptoms that may result from having the extra chromosome—is quite uncommon. Many men with XXY live out their lives without ever suspecting that they have an additional chromosome. For this reason, some experts prefer to describe boys and men with the extra chromosome as "XXY males" rather than Klinefelter syndrome males.

What problems do XXY males have?

In addition to occasional breast enlargement, lack of facial and body hair, and a rounded body type, XXY males are more likely than other males to be overweight, and tend to be taller than their fathers and brothers.

A far more serious problem is one that is not always readily apparent. Although XXY males are not usually mentally retarded, most have some degree of language impairment. As children, they often learn to speak much later than do other children and may have difficulty learning to read and write. And while they eventually do learn to speak and converse normally, the majority tends to have some degree of difficulty with language throughout their lives.

If untreated, this language impairment can lead to school failure and its attendant loss of self-esteem. Fortunately, however, this language disability usually can be compensated for. Chances for success are greatest if treatment for the language difficulty is begun in early childhood.

How is the diagnosis of XXY made?

A study of the person's chromosomes is done to make the diagnosis of XXY. The test is commonly called a karyotype (a standard layout of the chromosomes).

To perform a karyotype of the blood cells, a small blood sample is drawn. White blood cells are separated from the sample, mixed with a tissue culture medium, incubated, and checked for chromosomal abnormalities, such as an extra X chromosome.

When is the diagnosis of XXY typically made?

Because they often don't appear any different from anyone else, many XXY males never learn of their extra chromosome. However, if they are diagnosed, this most likely occurs before birth, early childhood, adolescence, or in adulthood (as a result of testing for infertility).

Before birth: In recent years, many XXY males have been diagnosed before birth through amniocentesis or chorionic villus sampling (CVS). In amniocentesis, a sample of the fluid surrounding the fetus is withdrawn. Fetal cells in the fluid are then examined for chromosomal abnormalities. CVS is similar to amniocentesis, except that the procedure is done in the first trimester of the pregnancy and the fetal cells needed for examination are taken from the placenta. Neither procedure is used routinely except when there is a family history of genetic defects, the pregnant woman is older than 35, or when other medical indications are present.

Early childhood: The next most likely opportunity for diagnosis is when the child begins school. A physician may suspect a boy is an XXY male if he is delayed in learning to talk and has difficulty with reading and writing. XXY boys may also be tall and thin and somewhat passive and shy. Again, however, there are no guarantees. Some of the boys who fit this description will have the XXY chromosome count, but many others will not.

Adolescence: A few XXY males are diagnosed at adolescence, when excessive breast development compels them to seek medical attention. Like some chromosomally normal males, many XXY males undergo slight breast enlargement at puberty. Of these, only a fraction of XXY males develop breasts large enough to embarrass them.

Adulthood: A diagnosis of XXY in adulthood is usually the result of testing for infertility. At this time, an examining physician may note the undersized testes which are characteristic of an XXY male. In addition to infertility tests, the physician may order tests to detect increased levels of hormones known as gonadotropins, which are common in XXY males.

What are XXY boys like in childhood?

XXY babies differ little from other children their age. They tend to start life as what many parents call "good" babies—quiet, undemanding, and perhaps even a little passive. As toddlers, they may be somewhat shy and reserved. They usually learn to walk later than most other children do.

XXY boys may have delays in learning to speak. The language delays for some boys may be severe, with the child not fully learning to talk until about age 5. Others may learn to speak at a normal rate, and not meet with any problems until they begin school, where they may experience reading difficulties. A few may not have any problems at all in learning to speak or read.

XXY males usually have difficulty with expressive language—the ability to put thoughts, ideas, and emotions into words. In contrast, their faculty for receptive language—understanding what is said—is close to normal.

XXY boys, like other language-disabled children, may need help with social skills. Language is essential not only for learning the school curriculum, but also for building social relationships. By talking and listening, children make friends in the process, sharing information, attitudes, and beliefs. Through language, they also learn how to behave not just in the schoolroom, but also on the playground. If their sons' language disability seems to prevent them from fitting in socially, the parents of XXY boys may want to ask school officials about a social skills training program.

XXY boys tend to retain the same temperament and disposition they first displayed as infants and toddlers. As a group, they tend to be shy, somewhat passive, and unlikely to take a leadership role. Although they do make friends with other children, they tend to have only a few friends at a time. They also tend as a group to be cooperative and eager to please.

What are XXY boys like in adolescence?

In general, XXY boys enter puberty normally, without any delay of physical maturity. But as puberty progresses, they fail to keep pace with other males. In chromosomally normal teenaged boys, the testes gradually increase in size, from an initial volume of about 2 ml, to about 15 ml. In XXY males, while the penis is usually of normal size, the testes remain at 2 ml, and cannot produce sufficient quantities of the male hormone, testosterone. As a result, many XXY adolescents, although taller than average, may not be as strong as other teenaged boys, and may lack facial or body hair.

As they enter puberty, many boys will undergo slight breast enlargement. For most teenaged males, this condition, known as gynecomastia, tends to disappear in a short time. About one-third of XXY boys develop enlarged breasts in early adolescence, slightly more than do chromosomally normal boys. In XXY boys, this condition may be permanent. However, only about 10 percent of XXY males have breast enlargement great enough to require surgery.

Most XXY adolescents benefit from receiving an injection of testosterone every 2 weeks, beginning at puberty. The hormone increases strength and brings on a more muscular, masculine appearance. (See information about testosterone treatment below.)

Adolescence and the high school years can be difficult for XXY boys and their families, particularly in neighborhoods and schools where the emphasis is on athletic ability and physical prowess. Lack of strength and agility, combined with a history of learning disabilities, may damage self-esteem. Unsympathetic peers, too, may sometimes make matters worse through teasing or ridicule. While XXY males share many characteristics, they cannot be pigeonholed into rigid categories. Several have played football, and one, in particular, is an excellent tennis player.

The damage to self-esteem may be more severe in XXY teenagers who are diagnosed in early or late adolescence. Teachers and even parents may have dismissed their learning difficulties as laziness. Lack of athletic prowess and their inability to use language properly in social settings may have resulted in isolating these teens from their peers. Some may react by sliding quietly into depression and withdrawing from contact with other people. Others may try to find acceptance in a dangerous crowd.

For these reasons, XXY males who are diagnosed as teenagers may need psychological counseling as well as help in overcoming their learning disabilities. Assistance with learning disabilities is available through public school systems for XXY males high-school age and under. Referrals to qualified mental health specialists can be obtained from family physicians.

Is testosterone treatment advisable for XXY males?

Ideally, XXY males should begin testosterone treatment as they enter puberty. XXY males diagnosed in adulthood are also likely to benefit from the hormone. A regular schedule of testosterone injections increases strength and muscle size, and promotes the growth of facial and body hair.

Testosterone injections often induce beneficial psychological changes as well. As they begin to develop a more masculine appearance, the self-confidence of XXY males tends to increase. Many become more energetic and stop having sudden, angry mood changes. What is not clear is whether these psychological changes are a direct result of the testosterone treatment or are a side benefit of the increased self-confidence that the treatment may bring. As a group, XXY boys tend to suffer from depression, principally because of their scholastic difficulties and problems fitting in with other males their age. Sudden, angry mood changes are typical of depressed people.

Other benefits of testosterone treatment may include a decreased need for sleep, an enhanced ability to concentrate, and improved relations with others. However, in order to benefit from the treatment, an XXY male must decide on his own that he is ready to commit to a regular schedule of injections.

Sometimes, younger adolescents, who may be somewhat immature, seem not quite ready to take the shots. It is an inconvenience, and many don't like needles. Most physicians do not push the young men to take the injections. Instead, they usually recommend informing XXY adolescents and their parents about the benefits of testosterone injections and letting them take as much time as they need to make their decision.

Individuals can respond to testosterone treatment in different ways. Although the majority of XXY males ultimately benefit from testosterone, a few do not. To ensure that the injections will provide the maximum benefit, XXY males who are ready to begin testosterone injections should consult a qualified endocrinologist (a medical doctor who is a specialist on hormones) who has experience treating XXY males.

What are the possible side effects of testosterone treatment?

Side effects of testosterone injections are few. Some individuals may develop a minor allergic reaction at the injection site, resulting in an itchy welt resembling a mosquito bite. Applying a non-prescription hydrocortisone cream to the area will reduce swelling and itching.

Testosterone injections may also result in a condition known as benign prostatic hyperplasia (BPH). This condition is also common in chromosomally normal males, affecting more than 50 percent of men in their sixties, and as many as 90 percent in their seventies and eighties. In XXY males receiving testosterone injections, this condition may begin sometime after age 40. In BPH, the prostate increases in size, sometimes squeezing the bladder and urethra and causing difficulty urinating, "dribbling" after urination, and the need to urinate frequently. XXY males receiving testosterone injections should consult their physicians about a regular schedule of prostate examinations.

Are there variations of the XXY chromosome complement?

Variations of the XXY chromosome count can occur. The most common is XY/XXY mosaicism in which some cells have the additional X chromosome and others do not. The percentage of cells containing the extra chromosome varies from case to case. In some instances, XY/XXY mosaics may have enough normally functioning cells in the testes to allow them to father children.

Males with 2, 3, or 4 extra X chromosomes have also been reported in the medical literature—XXY, XXXY, or XXXXY. In these individuals, the features of Klinefelter syndrome may be exaggerated, with a low IQ or moderate to severe mental retardation. In rare instances, an individual may possess both an additional X and an additional Y chromosome.

What is the sexual behavior of XXY boys?

There is no evidence that XXY males are any more inclined toward homosexuality than are other men. The only significant sexual difference between XXY men and teenagers and other males their age is that the XXY males may have less interest in sex. However, regular injections of the male sex hormone testosterone can bring sex drive up to normal levels.

In some cases, testosterone injections lead to a false sense of security. After receiving the hormone for a time, XXY males may conclude they have derived as much benefit from it as possible and discontinue the injections. But when they do, their interest in sex almost invariably diminishes until they resume the injections.

What is the fertility of XXY males?

The vast majority of XXY males do not produce enough sperm to allow them to become biological fathers. If these men and their wives wish to become parents, they should seek counseling from their family physician regarding infertility and adoption.

No XXY male should automatically assume he is infertile without further testing. In a very small number of cases, XXY males have been able to father children. In addition, a few individuals who believe themselves to be XXY males may actually be XY/XXY mosaics. Along with having cells with the XXY chromosome count, these males may also have cells with the normal XY chromosome count. If the number of XY cells in the testes is great enough, the individual should be able to father children. Karyotyping, the method traditionally used to identify an individual's chromosome count, may sometimes fail to identify XY/XXY mosaics. For this reason, a karyotype should never be used to predict whether an individual would be infertile or not.

Are there special health concerns for XXY males?

Compared with other males, XXY males have a slightly increased risk of autoimmune disorders. In this group of diseases, the immune system, for unknown reasons, attacks the body's organs or tissues. The most well known of these diseases are type I (insulin dependent) diabetes, autoimmune thyroiditis, and systemic lupus erythematosus. Most of these conditions can be treated with medication. XXY males with enlarged breasts have the same risk of breast cancer as do women—roughly 50 times the risk XY males have. For this reason, these XXY adolescents and men need to practice regular breast self-examination. XXY males may also wish to consult their physicians about the need for more thorough breast examinations by medical professionals.

XXY males who do not receive testosterone injections may have an increased risk of developing osteoporosis in later life. In this condition, which usually afflicts women after the age of menopause, the bones lose calcium, becoming brittle and more likely to break.

What are XXY males like in adulthood?

Relatively little is known about XXY adults. Studies in the U.S. have focused largely on XXY males identified in infancy from large random samples. Only a few of these individuals have reached adulthood; most are still in adolescence.

Comparatively few studies of XXY males diagnosed in adulthood have been conducted. By and large, the men who took part in these studies were not selected at random but identified by a particular characteristic, such as height. For this reason, it is not known whether these individuals are truly representative of XXY men as a whole or simply represent a particular segment.

One study found a group of XXY males diagnosed between the ages of 27 and 37 to have suffered a number of setbacks in comparison to a similar group of XY males. The XXY men were more likely to have had histories of scholastic failure, depression, and other psychological problems, and to lack energy and enthusiasm. But by the time the XXY men had reached their forties, most had surmounted their problems. The majority said that their energy and activity levels had increased, they were more productive on the job, and their relationships with other people had improved. In fact, the only difference between the XY males and the XXY males was that the latter were less likely to have been married.

That these men eventually overcame their troubled pasts is encouraging for all XXY males and particularly encouraging for those diagnosed in childhood. Had they received counseling, support, and testosterone treatments beginning in childhood, these men might have avoided the difficulties of their twenties and thirties.

Although a supportive environment through childhood and adolescence appears to offer the greatest chance for a well-adjusted adulthood, it is not too late for XXY men diagnosed as adults to seek help. Research has shown that testosterone injections, begun in adulthood, can be beneficial. Psychological counseling also offers the best hope of overcoming depression and other psychological problems. For referrals to endocrinologists qualified to administer testosterone or to mental health specialists, XXY men should consult their physicians.

Chapter 32

Patau Syndrome

Definition

Trisomy 13 (alternative name: Patau syndrome) is a syndrome associated with the presence of a third (extra) number 13 chromosome.

Causes, Incidence, and Risk Factors

Trisomy 13 occurs in about one out of every 5,000 live births. It is a syndrome with multiple abnormalities, many of which are not compatible with more than a few months of life. Almost half of the affected infants do not survive beyond the first month, and about three quarters die within six months.

Trisomy 13 is associated with multiple abnormalities, including severe mental defects and defects of the brain that lead to seizures (hypsarrhythmia), apnea, deafness, and ocular (relating to the eye) abnormalities.

The eyes are small with defects in the iris (coloboma). Most infants have a cleft lip and cleft palate, and low-set ears. Congenital heart disease is present in approximately 80% of affected infants. Hernias and genital abnormalities are common.

Symptoms

* Mental retardation, severe

"Trisomy 13," © 2003 A.D.A.M., Inc.; reprinted with permission.

- Seizures
- Small head (microcephaly)
- Scalp defects (absent skin)
- Small eyes (microphthalmia)
- Cleft lip and/or palate
- Eyes close set (hypotelorism)—eyes may actually fuse together into one
- Iris defects (coloboma)
- Pinna abnormalities and low set ears
- Simian crease
- Extra digits (polydactyly)
- Hernias: umbilical hernia, inguinal hernia
- Undescended testicle (cryptorchidism)
- Hypotonia
- Micrognathia
- Motormental retardation
- Skeletal (limb) abnormalities

Signs and Tests

The infant may have a single umbilical artery at birth. There are often signs of congenital heart disease:

- Ventricular septal defect (VSD)
- Atrial septal defect (ASD)
- Patent ductus arteriosus (PDA)
- Abnormal placement of the heart (dextroversion—the heart is placed toward the right side of the chest instead of the left)

Gastrointestinal X-rays or ultrasound may reveal abnormal rotation of the internal organs.

MRI or CT scans of the head may reveal a structural abnormality of the brain, called holoprosencephaly, where the two cerebral hemispheres are fused.

Chromosome studies show trisomy 13, partial trisomy, trisomy 13 mosaic, or translocation.

Treatment

Because of the severity of congenital defects, life-sustaining procedures are generally not attempted.

Support Groups

Support Organization for Trisomy 18, 13 and Related Disorders (SOFT)
2982 S. Union St.
Rochester, NY 14624
Toll-Free: 800-716-SOFT (7638)
Phone: 716-594-4621
Website: http://www.trisomy.org

Expectations (Prognosis)

Extremely short survival time is expected—80% of babies die in the first month of life. Survivors have severe mental defects. Rarely, affected persons survive to adulthood.

Complications

Complications begin almost immediately. They include breathing difficulty or lack of breathing (apnea), deafness, vision problems, feeding problems, seizures, heart failure, and others.

Calling Your Health Care Provider

Call for an appointment with your health care provider if you have had a child with trisomy 13 and you plan to have another child.

Prevention

Trisomy 13 can be diagnosed prenatally by amniocentesis with chromosome studies of the amniotic cells. Trisomy 13 mosaicism and partial trisomy 13 also occur. Parents of infants with translocation type trisomy 13 should also have translocation studies.

Chapter 33

Prader-Willi Syndrome

What is Prader-Willi syndrome (PWS)?

PWS is a complex genetic disorder that typically causes low muscle tone, short stature, incomplete sexual development, cognitive disabilities, problem behaviors, and a chronic feeling of hunger that can lead to excessive eating and life-threatening obesity.

Is PWS inherited?

Most cases of PWS are attributed to a spontaneous genetic error that occurs at or near the time of conception for unknown reasons. In a very small percentage of cases (2 percent or less), a genetic mutation that does not affect the parent is passed on to the child, and in these families more than one child may be affected. A PWS-like disorder can also be acquired after birth if the hypothalamus portion of the brain is damaged through injury or surgery.

How common is PWS?

It is estimated that one in 12,000 to 15,000 people has PWS. Although considered a "rare" disorder, Prader-Willi syndrome is one of the most common conditions seen in genetics clinics and is the most common genetic cause of obesity that has been identified. PWS is found in people of both sexes and all races.

How is PWS diagnosed?

Suspicion of the diagnosis is first assessed clinically, then confirmed by specialized genetic testing on a blood sample. Formal diagnostic criteria for the clinical recognition of PWS have been published as have laboratory testing guidelines for PWS.

What is known about the genetic abnormality?

Basically, the occurrence of PWS is due to lack of several genes on one of an individual's two chromosome 15s—the one normally contributed by the father. In the majority of cases, there is a deletion—the critical genes are somehow lost from the chromosome. In most of the remaining cases, the entire chromosome from the father is missing and there are instead two chromosome 15s from the mother (uniparental disomy). The critical paternal genes lacking in people with PWS have a role in the regulation of appetite. This is an area of active research in a number of laboratories around the world, since understanding this defect may be very helpful not only to those with PWS but to understanding obesity in otherwise normal people.

What causes the appetite and obesity problems in PWS?

People with PWS have a flaw in the hypothalamus part of their brain, which normally registers feelings of hunger and satiety. While the problem is not yet fully understood, it is apparent that people with this flaw never feel full; they have a continuous urge to eat that they cannot learn to control. To compound this problem, people with PWS need less food than their peers without the syndrome because their bodies have less muscle and tend to burn fewer calories.

Does the overeating associated with PWS begin at birth?

No. In fact, newborns with PWS often cannot get enough nourishment because low muscle tone impairs their sucking ability. Many require special feeding techniques or tube feeding for several months after birth, until muscle control improves. Sometime in the following years, usually before school age, children with PWS develop an intense interest in food and can quickly gain excess weight if calories are not restricted.

Do diet medications work for the appetite problem in PWS?

Unfortunately, no appetite suppressant has worked consistently for people with PWS. Most require an extremely low-calorie diet all their lives and must have their environment designed so that they have very limited access to food. For example, many families have to lock the kitchen or the cabinets and refrigerator. As adults, most affected individuals can control their weight best in a group home designed specifically for people with PWS, where food access can be restricted without interfering with the rights of those who don't need such restriction.

What kinds of behavior problems do people with PWS have?

In addition to their involuntary focus on food, people with PWS tend to have obsessive/compulsive behaviors that are not related to food, such as repetitive thoughts and verbalizations, collecting and hoarding of possessions, picking at skin irritations, and a strong need for routine and predictability. Frustration or changes in plans can easily set off a loss of emotional control in someone with PWS, ranging from tears to temper tantrums to physical aggression. While psychotropic medications can help some individuals, the essential strategies for minimizing difficult behaviors in PWS are careful structuring of the person's environment and consistent use of positive behavior management and supports.

Does early diagnosis help?

While there is no medical prevention or cure, early diagnosis of Prader-Willi syndrome gives parents time to learn about and prepare for the challenges that lie ahead and to establish family routines that will support their child's diet and behavior needs from the start. Knowing the cause of their child's developmental delays can facilitate a family's access to important early intervention services and may help program staff identify areas of specific need or risk. Additionally, a diagnosis of PWS opens the doors to a network of information and support from professionals and other families who are dealing with the syndrome.

What does the future hold for people with PWS?

With help, people with PWS can expect to accomplish many of the things their "normal" peers do—complete school, achieve in their outside areas of interest, be successfully employed, even move away from their family home. They do, however, need a significant amount of support from their families and from school, work, and residential service providers to both achieve these goals and avoid obesity and the serious health consequences that accompany it. Even those with IQs in the normal range need lifelong diet supervision and protection from food availability.

Although in the past many people with PWS died in adolescence or young adulthood, prevention of obesity can enable those with the syndrome to live a normal lifespan. New medications, including psychotropic drugs and synthetic growth hormone, are already improving the quality of life for some people with PWS. Ongoing research offers the hope of new discoveries that will enable people affected by this unusual condition to live more independent lives.

How can I get more information about PWS?

A strong national organization of families and professionals, PWSA (USA) offers a toll-free helpline, a bimonthly member newsletter and numerous publications about PWS, a World Wide Web page (http://www.pwsausa.org), an annual family conference and scientific meeting, and chapters throughout the country to provide local family support and advocacy.

Prader-Willi Syndrome Association (USA)
5700 Midnight Pass Road
Sarasota, FL 34242
Toll-Free: 800-926-4797
Phone: 941-312-0400
Fax: 941-312-0142
Website: http://www.pwsausa.org

Chapter 34

Triple X Syndrome

What is XXX or triple X syndrome?

XXX syndrome (also called triple X syndrome or trisomy X) affects females who have three X chromosomes, instead of the usual two. It is the most common X-chromosome disorder in females. Triple X is a random mutation, usually inherited from the mother. Parents who have a daughter with triple X usually do not have to worry about their later children having the syndrome. The mutation occurs in 1 in every 1,000 to 3,000 newborn girls, but it is often not diagnosed until later in life.

What are the features of triple X syndrome?

Many girls and women with triple X have no signs or symptoms. Signs and symptoms vary a lot between individuals, but can include:

- Increased space between the eyes
- Vertical skin folds that may cover the inner corners of the eyes (epicanthal folds)
- Tall stature (height)
- Small head

"XXX Syndrome (Trisomy X)," reprinted with permission from, *Your Child: Development and Behavior Resources*, http://www.med.umich.edu/1libr/yourchild/, a website of the University of Michigan Health System. Copyright © 2004 Regents of the University of Michigan.

- Speech and language delays and learning disabilities
- Delayed development of certain motor skills
- Behavioral problems
- Seizures
- Delayed puberty
- Infertility
- Rarely, mental retardation

How is triple X diagnosed and treated?

XXX syndrome is diagnosed by a blood test that looks at a person's chromosomes (karyotype.) There is no cure for XXX syndrome, and treatment is mainly supportive. Girls with XXX syndrome may need to be seen by specialists if they have certain problems, such as:

- An endocrinologist if there is a delay in puberty
- A pediatric psychologist or neurologist if there is developmental delay
- A speech and language pathologist if there is speech delay

Genetic counseling may also be helpful, although no XXX daughter of an XXX mother has yet been reported. Women with XXX syndrome have a normal life span.

Chapter 35

Turner Syndrome

Clinical Features of Turner Syndrome

Turner syndrome affects approximately one out of every 2,500 female live births worldwide. It embraces a broad spectrum of features, from major heart defects to minor cosmetic issues. Some individuals with Turner syndrome may have only a few features, while others may have many. Almost all people with Turner syndrome have short stature and loss of ovarian function, but the severity of these problems varies considerably amongst individuals.

Appearance

Individuals with Turner syndrome may have a short neck with a webbed appearance, a low hairline at the back of the neck, and low-set ears. Hands and feet of affected individuals may be swollen or puffy at birth, and often have soft nails that turn upward at the ends when they are older. All these features appear to be due to obstruction of the lymphatic system during fetal development. Another characteristic cosmetic feature is the presence of multiple pigmented nevi, which are colored spots on the skin.

Text in this chapter is from "Clinical Features of Turner Syndrome," and "Genetic Features of Turner Syndrome," National Institute of Child Health and Human Development, (NICHD), 2001; available online at http://turners .nichd.nih.gov.

Short Stature

Almost all individuals with Turner syndrome have short stature. This is partially due to the loss of action of the *SHOX* gene on the X-chromosome. This particular gene is important for long bone growth. The loss of *SHOX* may also explain some of the skeletal features found in Turner syndrome, such as short fingers and toes, and irregular rotations of the wrist and elbow joints. Linear growth is attenuated in utero, and statural growth lags during childhood and adolescence, resulting in adult heights of 143–145 cm (approximately 4 feet 8 inches). Final adult height in Turner syndrome can be increased by a few inches if growth hormone (GH) treatment is given relatively early in childhood. However, not all individuals with Turner syndrome get a good growth response to GH.

Puberty/Reproduction

Unknown genes on the X-chromosome regulate the development and functions of the ovary. Most individuals with Turner syndrome experience loss of ovarian function early in childhood, and thus do not enter puberty at the normal age.

Some teenagers may undergo some breast development and begin menstruating, but cease further development and menses during the later teen years. A few women with Turner syndrome have apparently normal ovarian function with regular menses until the mid-20s before ovarian failure occurs.

It is standard medical practice to treat girls with Turner syndrome with estrogen to induce breast development and other features of puberty if menses has not occurred by age 15 years at the latest. Girls and women with Turner syndrome should be maintained on estrogen-progesterone treatment to maintain their secondary sexual development and to protect their bones from osteoporosis until at least the usual age of menopause (50 years).

Most women with Turner syndrome do not have ovaries with healthy oocytes capable of fertilization and embryo formation. Current assisted reproductive technology, however, may allow women to become pregnant with donated oocytes.

Cardiovascular

From 5–10% of children with Turner syndrome are found to have a severe constriction of the major blood vessel coming out from the heart, a condition known as coarctation of the aorta. This defect is thought to be the result of an obstructed lymphatic system compressing the developing aorta during fetal life. This can be surgically corrected as soon as it is diagnosed.

Other major defects in the heart and its major vessels are reported to a much lesser degree. As many as 15% of adults with Turner syndrome are reported to have bicuspid aortic valves, meaning that the major blood vessel from the heart has only two rather than three components to the valve regulating blood flow. This condition has been discovered mainly by medical imaging studies on women without symptoms, and may not be clinically obvious. It requires careful medical monitoring, since bicuspid aortic valves can deteriorate or become infected. In general, it is advised that all persons with Turner syndrome undergo annual cardiac evaluations.

Many women with Turner syndrome have high blood pressure, which may be apparent even in childhood. In some cases this high blood pressure may be due to aortic constriction, or to kidney abnormalities. In a majority of women, however, no specific cause for the high blood pressure has been found.

Kidney

Kidney problems are present in approximately one third of individuals with Turner syndrome and may contribute to high blood pressure. Three types of kidney problems have been reported: a single horseshoe-shaped kidney, as opposed to two distinct, bean-shaped structures; an abnormal urine collecting system; or an abnormal artery supply to the kidneys. While these problems may be corrected surgically and the kidneys usually function normally, they may be associated with a tendency towards high blood pressure and infections.

Osteoporosis

There is a high incidence of osteoporosis—meaning thin or weak bones—in women with Turner syndrome. Osteoporosis leads to loss of height, curvature of the spine and increased bone fractures.

The primary cause of osteoporosis in individuals with Turners appears to be inadequate circulating estrogen in the body. Turner women who have low levels of estrogen due to ovarian failure can take estrogen treatments, which will help prevent osteoporosis. It is possible that other factors contribute to the severity of osteoporosis in Turner syndrome. For example, there may be defects in bone structure or strength related to

381

the loss of unknown X-chromosome genes. This is an area of major medical significance, which demands further study to help prevent osteoporosis and fractures in women with Turner syndrome.

Diabetes

Type 2 diabetes, also known as insulin resistant diabetes (glucose intolerance), has a high occurrence rate in individuals with Turner syndrome.

Individuals with Turner syndrome have twice the risk of the general population for developing this disease. It appears that the muscles of many persons with Turner syndrome fail to utilize glucose efficiently, and this may contribute to the development of high blood sugar (diabetes). The reason for the high risk of diabetes amongst individuals with Turner syndrome is unknown.

Diabetes type 2 can be controlled through careful monitoring of blood-sugar levels, diet, exercise, regular doctor visits and sometimes medication.

Thyroid

Approximately one third of individuals with Turner syndrome have a thyroid disorder, usually hypothyroidism. Symptoms of this condition include decreased energy, dry skin, cold-intolerance, and poor growth.

In most cases, it is caused by an immune system attack on the thyroid gland (also known as Hashimoto's thyroiditis). Although it is not known why thyroid disorders occur with a high frequency in Turner syndrome, the condition is easily treated with thyroid hormone supplements.

Cognitive Function/Educational Issues

In general, individuals with Turner syndrome have normal intelligence. This is in contrast to other chromosomal syndromes such as Down's syndrome (Trisomy 21). However, girls and women with Turner syndrome may have difficulty with specific visual-spatial coordination tasks (for example, mentally rotating objects in space) and learning math (geometry, arithmetic). This very specific learning problem has been termed the Turner neurocognitive phenotype and appears due to loss of X-chromosome genes important for selected aspects of nervous system development.

Some girls and women with Turner syndrome experience difficulties with memory and motor coordination. These problems may be related to estrogen deficiency and individuals often improve when given estrogen treatment. The verbal skills of individuals with Turner syndrome are usually normal.

Genetic Features of Turner Syndrome

Turner syndrome is a disorder caused by the loss of genetic material from one of the sex chromosomes.

Humans normally have a total of 46 chromosomes (which are tiny, DNA-containing elements) that are present in every cell of the body. DNA encodes genes, which specify all the proteins that make up the body and control its functions.

In humans, there are 23 matched pairs of chromosomes in every cell. Each cell contains 22 pairs of chromosomes called autosomes that are the same in males and females. The remaining pair of chromosomes, the X and Y chromosomes, are not shaped similarly, and thus are not matched in the same way as the autosomes.

The X and Y chromosomes are called sex chromosomes. They are responsible for the difference in development between males and females. A Y chromosome contains genes responsible for testis development; and the presence of a X chromosome paired with a Y chromosome will determine male development. On the other hand, two X chromosomes are required for normal ovarian development in females.

X Chromosome Monosomy

During the process in which oocytes (eggs) or sperm are formed, one of the sex chromosomes is sometimes lost. An embryo receiving only a Y chromosome can not survive, but an embryo receiving only a X chromosome may survive and develop as a female with Turner syndrome.

In order to examine the matching pairs of chromosomes for a person, doctors can perform a blood test and look at the chromosomes found in the lymphocytes, a particular type of blood cell. This will determine the karyotype of that individual.

The karyotype of X monosomy is termed, 45X meaning that an individual has 44 autosomes and a single X chromosome. The usual female karyotype is 46, XX.

X Chromosome Mosaicism

A sex chromosome may also be lost during early stages of embryonic development, such that some cells of the growing body receive a single X chromosome. This condition is called mosaicism, and the clinical features of Turner syndrome correlate with the relative percentage of 45X cells within the body.

If only a small percentage of cells have been affected, the phenotypes of Turner syndrome may be relatively mild. In other words, mosaicism may lessen the severity of certain clinical features. An example of the lessened effects due to mosaicism is if a woman with Turner syndrome experiences regular menstrual cycles until her late 20's rather than not having any menstrual cycle at all.

The genetic diagnosis in such cases may require the examination of many, many blood cells, and/or the examination of other cell types such as skin cells. The genotype is usually specified as 45X(10)/46XX (90) to indicate for example, that 10% of cells examined were found to have X monosomy.

X Chromosome Defects

A third cause of Turner syndrome involves X chromosome defects rather than complete loss. For example, one X chromosome may be fragmented, have portions deleted or other structural problems such as ring formation preventing the normal expression of X chromosome genes.

The clinical consequences of having one normal and one structurally defective X chromosome vary widely. A small deletion may result in a single feature such as ovarian failure or short stature and no other effects. Larger deletions or deletions affecting critical areas regulating the whole chromosome may result in a full spectrum of Turner syndrome problems.

Moreover, the presence of small ring X chromosome causes severe consequences, because in addition to absence of some important genes, there may be deleterious expression of X chromosome genes that are normally silenced, or inactivated in the second X chromosome. The diagnosis of abnormal X chromosomes may require specialized, molecular cytogenetic studies to identify small deletions or inversions of X chromosome material.

Is Turner Syndrome Hereditary?

While Turner syndrome is genetic in that it involves the loss or abnormal expression of X chromosome genes, it is not usually hereditary in the conventional sense. That is, it does not typically run in families. The one exception to this observation are families with a X chromosome deletion which is stable enough to be passed down through the generations and which also allows fertility.

Turner syndrome affects all races, nationalities and regions of the world equally, and parents who have produced many unaffected children may still have a child with Turner syndrome. There are no known toxins or environmental hazards that increase the chances of Turner syndrome.

A woman with Turner syndrome has a low probability of being fertile, since the ovaries are negatively impacted in this disorder. However, if she does become pregnant and passes on her normal X chromosome to her offspring, no continuation of the syndrome is expected.

Chapter 36

Williams Syndrome

What Is Williams Syndrome?

Williams syndrome is a rare genetic condition (estimated to occur in one in 20,000 births) which causes medical and developmental problems.

Williams syndrome was first recognized as a distinct entity in 1961. It is present at birth, and affects males and females equally. It can occur in all ethnic groups and has been identified in countries throughout the world.

Common Features of Williams Syndrome

Characteristic facial appearance: Most young children with Williams syndrome are described as having similar facial features. These features, which tend to be recognized by only a trained geneticist or birth defects specialist, include a small upturned nose, long philtrum (upper lip length), wide mouth, full lips, small chin, and puffiness around the eyes. Blue and green-eyed children with Williams syndrome can have a prominent starburst or white lacy pattern on their iris. Facial features become more apparent with age.

Heart and blood vessel problems: The majority of individuals with Williams syndrome have some type of heart or blood vessel problem. Typically, there is narrowing in the aorta (producing supravalvular aortic stenos is SVAS), or narrowing in the pulmonary arteries. There is a broad range in the degree of narrowing, ranging from trivial to severe (requiring surgical correction of the defect). Since there is an increased risk for development of blood vessel narrowing or high blood pressure over time, periodic monitoring of cardiac status is necessary.

Hypercalcemia (elevated blood calcium levels): Some young children with Williams syndrome have elevations in their blood calcium level. The true frequency and cause of this problem is unknown. When hypercalcemia is present, it can cause extreme irritability or colic-like symptoms. Occasionally, dietary or medical treatment is needed. In most cases, the problem resolves on its own during childhood, but lifelong abnormality in calcium or vitamin D metabolism may exist and should be monitored.

Low birth-weight/low weight gain: Most children with Williams syndrome have a slightly lower birth-weight than their brothers or sisters. Slow weight gain, especially during the first several years of life, is also a common problem and many children are diagnosed as failure to thrive. Adult stature is slightly smaller than average.

Feeding problems: Many infants and young children have feeding problems. These problems have been linked to low muscle tone, severe gag reflex, poor suck/swallow, tactile defensiveness, etc. Feeding difficulties tend to resolve as the children get older.

Irritability (colic during infancy): Many infants with Williams syndrome have an extended period of colic or irritability. This typically lasts from 4 to 10 months of age, then resolves. It is sometimes attributed to hypercalcemia. Abnormal sleep patterns with delayed acquisition of sleeping through the night may be associated with the colic.

Dental abnormalities: Slightly small, widely spaced teeth are common in children with Williams syndrome. They also may have a variety of abnormalities of occlusion (bite), tooth shape or appearance. Most of these dental changes are readily amenable to orthodontic correction.

Kidney abnormalities: There is a slightly increased frequency of problems with kidney structure and/or function.

Hernias: Inguinal (groin) and umbilical hernias are more common in Williams syndrome than in the general population.

Hyperacusis (sensitive hearing): Children with Williams syndrome often have more sensitive hearing than other children. Certain frequencies or noise levels can be painful an/or startling to the individual. This condition often improves with age.

Musculoskeletal problems: Young children with Williams syndrome often have low muscle tone and joint laxity. As the children get older, joint stiffness (contractures) may develop. Physical therapy is very helpful in improving muscle tone, strength and joint range of motion.

Overly friendly (excessively social) personality: Individuals with Williams syndrome have a very endearing personality. They have a unique strength in their expressive language skills, and are extremely polite. They are typically unafraid of strangers and show a greater interest in contact with adults than with their peers.

Developmental delay, learning disabilities and attention deficit: Most people with Williams syndrome have some degree of intellectual handicap. Young children with Williams syndrome often experience developmental delays; milestones such as walking, talking, and toilet training are often achieved somewhat later than is considered normal. Distractibility is a common problem in mid-childhood, which appears to get better as the children get older.

Older children and adults with Williams syndrome often demonstrate intellectual strengths and weaknesses. There are some intellectual areas (such as speech, long term memory, and social skills) in which performance is quite strong, while other intellectual areas (such as fine motor and spatial relations) are significantly deficient.

Diagnosing Williams Syndrome

The diagnosis of Williams syndrome generally has two parts:

- Clinical diagnosis based on a variety of characteristics.

- Medical/genetic test confirmation through a blood test: the FISH test.

The FISH Test

You can obtain a blood test to confirm the clinical diagnosis of Williams syndrome. A laboratory can use the technique known as fluorescent in situ hybridization (FISH).

FISH is a type of specialized chromosome analysis utilizing specially prepared elastin probes. If a patient has two copies of the elastin gene (one on each of their number 7 chromosomes), they probably do not have WS. If the individual only has one copy, the diagnosis of WS will be confirmed.

Virtually all (98–99%) persons with typical features of WS will have a deletion of the elastin gene. In more technical terms, Williams syndrome is the result of a deletion of the 7q11.23 region of chromosome 7 containing the elastin gene and is believed to be a contiguous gene syndrome. Diagnosis of Williams syndrome is confirmed by dual color FISH using a specific probe and a control probe.

The laboratory will need 5 ml of blood drawn in a sodium heparin tube. The sample should arrive in the lab the same day it was drawn or on the following day. Results are usually available in two to four weeks.

The FISH test is readily available at major hospitals and cytogenetics laboratories around the country, but it is not a routine test. Therefore not all labs will do FISH-based diagnosis. Families or their physicians should call the lab in advance to make sure they can perform the test.

If you have any doubts that a child may have Williams syndrome, the FISH test will give you a clear cut answer in most cases.

It may be possible, however, that an individual has most of the characteristics of Williams syndrome yet does not show that an elastin gene is missing. In such cases, only an experienced medical geneticist will be able to assess whether or not the questioned individual may have Williams syndrome.

Note: It is extremely unlikely that any other family member also has Williams syndrome. On the other hand, if the individual with Williams syndrome plans to become a parent, there is a 50/50 chance that his or her child will have Williams syndrome. If such a situation should arise, consult an obstetrician about using the FISH test for prenatal testing of the embryonic cells.

Part Four

Complex Disorders with a Genetic Component

Chapter 37

The Interplay of Genes and the Environment

Information from the Human Genome Project has caused scientists to re-examine the role of genetics and other risk factors involved in the development of disease. Understanding this complex interplay of genes and environment will lead us to new methods of disease detection and prevention.

Gene Environment Interaction

Virtually all-human diseases result from the interaction of genetic susceptibility factors and modifiable environmental factors, broadly defined to include infectious, chemical, physical, nutritional, and behavioral factors.

This is perhaps the most important fact in understanding the role of genetics and environment in the development of disease. Many people tend to classify the cause of disease as either genetic or environmental. Indeed, some rare diseases, such as Huntington or Tay-Sachs disease, may be the result of a deficiency of a single gene product, but these diseases represent a very small proportion of all human disease. Common diseases, such as diabetes or cancer, are a result of the complex interplay of genetic and environmental factors.

"Gene-Environment Interaction Fact Sheet," Office of Genetics and Disease Prevention, Centers for Disease Control and Prevention (CDC), updated January 2004. Available online at http://www.cdc.gov/genomics/info/factshts/geneenviro.htm.

Genetic Variations

Variations in genetic makeup are associated with almost all disease. Even so-called single-gene disorders actually develop from the interaction of both genetic and environmental factors. For example, phenylketonuria (PKU) results from a genetic variant that leads to deficient metabolism of the amino acid phenylalanine; in the presence of normal protein intake, phenylalanine accumulates and is neurotoxic. PKU occurs only when both the genetic variant (phenylalanine hydroxylase deficiency) and the environmental exposure (dietary phenylalanine) are present.

Environmental Factors

Genetic variations do not cause disease but rather influence a person's susceptibility to environmental factors. We do not inherit a disease state per se. Instead, we inherit a set of a susceptibility factors to certain effects of environmental factors and therefore inherit a higher risk for certain diseases. This concept also explains why individuals are differently affected by the same environmental factors. For example, some health conscious individuals with acceptable cholesterol levels suffer myocardial infarction at age 40. Others individuals seem immune to heart disease in spite of smoking, poor diet, and obesity. Genetic variations account, at least in part, for this difference in response to the same environmental factors.

Intervention Strategies

Genetic information can be used to target interventions. We all carry genetic variants that increase our susceptibility to some diseases. By identifying and characterizing gene-environment interactions, we have more opportunities to effectively target intervention strategies. Many of the genetic risk factors for diseases have not been identified, and the complex interaction of genes with other genes and genes with environmental factors is not yet understood. Clinical and epidemiological studies are necessary to further describe these factors and their interactions. However, as our understanding of genetic variations increases, so should our knowledge of environmental factors, so that ultimately, genetic information can be used to plan appropriate intervention strategies for high-risk individuals.

Chapter 38

Cancer Genetics

Chapter Contents

Section 38.1—Cancer Genetics Overview 396
Section 38.2—Heredity and Breast Cancer 407
Section 38.3—Heredity and Colon Cancer 409
Section 38.4—Heredity and Skin Cancer 411
Section 38.5—Heredity and Prostate Cancer 414

Section 38.1

Cancer Genetics Overview

PDQ® Cancer Information Summary. National Cancer Institute; Bethesda, MD. Cancer Genetics Overview (PDQ®): Genetics - Health Professional. Updated 12/2003. Available at: http://cancergov. Accessed April 1, 2004.

Knowledge about cancer genetics is rapidly expanding, with implications for all aspects of cancer management, including prevention, screening, and treatment.

Significance of the Terms Mutation and Carrier

A mutation is a change in the usual DNA sequence of a particular gene. Mutations can have harmful, beneficial, or neutral effects on health, and may be inherited as autosomal dominant, autosomal recessive, or X-linked traits. Mutations that cause serious disability early in life are usually rare in the population, because of their adverse effect on life expectancy and reproduction. However, if the mutation is autosomal recessive, that is, if the health effect of the mutation is caused only when two copies of the mutation are inherited, carriers (healthy people carrying one copy of the mutation) may be relatively common. Common in this context generally refers to a prevalence of 1% or more.

Mutations that cause health effects in middle and old age, including several mutations known to cause a predisposition to cancer, may also be relatively common. Many cancer-predisposing mutations are autosomal dominant, that is, the cancer susceptibility occurs when only one copy of the mutation is inherited. For autosomal dominant conditions, the term carrier is often used in a different way, to denote people who have inherited the genetic predisposition conferred by the mutation.

Assumptions Concerning the Identification of People with an Increased Susceptibility to Cancer

Genetic information, including information from family history and from DNA-based testing, provides a means to identify people who have an increased risk of cancer. Family history often identifies people with a moderately increased risk of cancer, and in some cases may be an indicator of the presence of polymorphisms that influence cancer susceptibility, through such mechanisms as changes in the rate of metabolism of agents that predispose to cancer or catabolism of carcinogens, or effects on DNA repair or regulation of cell division. Less often, family history indicates the presence of an inherited cancer predisposition conferring a high lifetime risk of cancer. In some cases, DNA-based testing can be used to confirm a specific mutation as the cause of the inherited risk, and to determine whether family members have inherited the mutation.

Identifying a person with an increased risk of cancer can reduce the occurrence of cancer through clinical management strategies (for example, tamoxifen for breast cancer, colonoscopy for colon cancer) or improve that person's health outcome or quality of life through intrinsic benefits of the information itself (for example, no genetic predisposition). Intrinsic benefits may include better ability to plan for the future (having children, career, retirement or other decisions) with improved knowledge about cancer risk. Methods of genetic risk assessment include assessment of personal and family history of disease and genetic testing; the latter is generally undertaken only when family history of disease or other clinical characteristics, such as early onset of cancer, indicate a substantial likelihood of an inherited predisposition to cancer.

Genetic testing may also be sought by people affected with cancer, both newly diagnosed individuals and survivors of earlier cancers. Testing may be desired to define personal cancer etiology, to clarify risk to offspring, to define the appropriateness of particular surveillance approaches, or to aid in decision-making about risk-reducing prophylactic surgery.[1] While there are effective interventions specific for some cancer genetic syndromes (for example, multiple endocrine neoplasia type 2A [MEN 2A], familial adenomatous polyposis [FAP], retinoblastoma [RB]), genetic testing is still being integrated into the management of patients with hereditary forms of common cancers (for example, breast cancer).[2] Some patients and physicians may wish to include genetic risk status as a factor in consideration of treatment options.

A genetic assessment is likely to aid clinical decision-making only when management is based on genetic information (for example, when the clinical interventions being considered would be offered to genetically susceptible people but not to those of average risk, or when interventions that are effective in people of average risk are ineffective in those with genetic susceptibility). Intrinsic benefits of genetic information, for example, improvement in quality of life as a result of knowledge about genetic susceptibility, may be accompanied by potential personal and social risks as well (for example, reduced self-worth; guilt; family disruption; stigmatization; or loss of health, disability, or life insurance). Genetic information may sometimes provide a direct health benefit by demonstrating the lack of an inherited cancer susceptibility. For example, if a family is known to carry a cancer-predisposing mutation, a family member may experience reduced worry and lower health care costs if his/her genetic test indicates that he/she does not carry the mutation. The family member may be able to forego certain medical tests, such as early use of colonoscopy for persons at high risk of an HNPCC (hereditary nonpolyposis colon cancer) mutation.

Evaluation of Evidence

Creating evidence-based summaries in cancer genetics is challenging because the rapid evolution of new information often results in evidence that is incomplete or of limited quality. In addition, established methods for evaluating the quality of the evidence are available for some but not all aspects of cancer genetics. Varying levels of evidence are available for different topics. As in other aspects of medicine, testing and treatment decisions must be based on information that sometimes falls short of the optimal level of evidence, for example, data from randomized trials.

Evidence Related to the Clinical Value of Genetic Tests and Family History Information

In assessing a genetic test (or other method of genetic assessment, including family history), the analytic validity, clinical validity, and clinical utility of the test need to be considered.[3]

Analytic Validity: Analytic validity refers to how well the genetic assessment performs in measuring the property or characteristic it is intended to measure. In the case of family history, analytic validity refers to the accuracy of the family history information. In the case of a test for a specific mutation, analytic validity refers to the accuracy of a genetic test in identifying the presence or absence of the mutation. Analytic validity of a genetic test is affected by the technical accuracy and reliability of the testing procedure, and also by the quality of the laboratory processes (including specimen handling).

The evaluation of analytic validity is complex for some genetic tests. A panel test, for example, tests for the presence of a particular set of mutations (for example, the known deleterious mutations in the *BRCA1* gene), and the analytic validity of the different components of the test may vary. Some genetic tests involve the evaluation of the DNA sequence of portions of a gene, to determine whether any mutations are present (including mutations not previously identified). The sensitivity and specificity of these sequencing tests may vary with the laboratory techniques employed, the proportion of the gene tested, and the structural nature of the mutations present in the gene.

Clinical Validity: Clinical validity refers to the predictive value of a test for a given clinical outcome (for example, the likelihood that cancer will develop in someone with a positive test), and is in large measure determined by the sensitivity and specificity with which a test identifies people with a defined clinical condition. Sensitivity of a test refers to the proportion of persons who test positive from among those with a clinical condition; specificity refers to the proportion of persons who test negative from among those without the clinical condition. In the case of genetic susceptibility to cancer, clinical validity can be thought of at two levels: (1) Does a positive test identify a person as having an increased risk of cancer? (2) If so, how high is the cancer risk associated with a positive test? Thus, the clinical validity of a genetic test is the likelihood that cancer will develop in someone with a positive test result. This likelihood is affected not only by the presence of the gene itself, but also by any modifying factors that affect the penetrance of the mutation, for example, the carrier's environment or behaviors (or perhaps by the presence or absence of mutations in other genes). For this reason, the clinical validity of a genetic test for a specific mutation may vary in different populations. If the cancer risk associated with a given mutation is unknown or variable, a test for the mutation will have uncertain clinical validity. A summary of definitions of concepts relevant to understanding clinical validity and other aspects of cancer genetics testing has been published.[4]

The test should be evaluated in the population in which the test will be used. Evidence that a particular genetic mutation results in a cancer predisposition often derives initially from linkage studies that use samples of families meeting stringent criteria for autosomal dominant inheritance of cancer risk. The demonstration of strong linkage of cancer to a pattern of autosomal dominant inheritance supports a causal molecular mechanism for the inherited cancer predisposition. Once linkage is established, a strong case for association between the genetic trait and disease can be made, even though the families used in the study are not representative of the general population. The genetic trait measured in linkage studies is not always the causal function itself, but may instead be a genetic trait closely linked to it. Additional molecular studies are required to identify the specific gene associated with inherited risk, after linkage studies have determined its chromosomal location.

Linkage studies, however, provide only limited evidence concerning either the range of cancer types associated with a mutation or the magnitude of risk and lifetime probability of cancer conferred by a mutation in less selected populations. In addressing these questions, the best information for clinical decisions comes from naturally occurring populations in which people with all degrees of risk are represented, similar to those in which clinical or public health decisions must be made. Thus, observations about cancer risk in families having multiple members with early breast cancer are applicable only to other families meeting those same clinical criteria. Ideally, the families tested should also have similar exposures to factors that can modify the expression of the gene(s) being studied. The mutation-associated risk in other populations, such as families with less dramatic cancer aggregation, or the general population, can best be assessed by direct study of those populations.

Clinical Utility: The clinical utility of the test refers to the likelihood that the test will, by prompting an intervention, result in an improved health outcome. The clinical utility of a genetic test is based on the health benefits of the interventions offered to persons with positive test results. Three strategies are available to improve the health outcome of people with a genetic susceptibility to cancer: screening to detect early cancer or precancerous lesions, interventions to reduce the risk of developing cancer, and interventions to improve quality of life. Evaluation of interventions should consider their efficacy (capacity to produce an improved health outcome) and effectiveness (likelihood that the improved outcome will occur, taking into account actual use of the intervention and recommended follow-up). Sometimes genetic information may lead to consideration of changes in the approach to clinical management, based on expert opinion, in the absence of proof of clinical utility.

Genetic Counseling

Genetic counseling has been defined by the American Society of Human Genetics as "a communication process which deals with the human problems associated with the occurrence or risk of occurrence of a genetic disorder in a family. The process involves an attempt by one or more appropriately trained persons to help the individual or family to:

- comprehend the medical facts, including the diagnosis, probable course of the disorder, and the available management;

- appreciate the way that heredity contributes to the disorder and to the risk of recurrence in specific relatives;

- understand the alternatives for dealing with the risk of recurrence;

- choose a course of action which seems to them appropriate in view of their risk, their family goals, and their ethical and religious standards and act in accordance with that decision; and

- make the best possible adjustment to the disorder in an affected family member and/or to the risk of recurrence of that disorder."[5]

Central to genetic counseling philosophy and practice are the principles of: voluntary utilization of services, informed decision-making, nondirective and noncoercive counseling when the medical benefits of one course of action are not demonstrably superior to another, attention to psychosocial and affective dimensions of coping with genetic risk, and protection of client confidentiality and privacy. Genetic counseling generally involves some combination of rapport building and information gathering; establishing or verifying diagnoses; risk assessment and calculation of quantitative occurrence/recurrence risks; education and informed consent processes; psychosocial assessment, support, and counseling appropriate to a family's culture and ethnicity. Readers interested in the nature and history of genetic counseling are referred to a number of comprehensive reviews.[6–9]

In the past decade, genetic counseling has expanded to include discussion of genetic testing for cancer risk as more genes associated with inherited cancer risk have been discovered. Cancer genetic counseling often involves a multidisciplinary team of health professionals who have expertise in this area. The team may include a genetic counselor, genetic advanced practice nurse or medical geneticist, mental health professional, and medical expert such as oncologist, surgeon, or internist. The process of counseling may require a number of visits in order to address the medical, genetic testing, and psychosocial issues. Even when cancer risk counseling is initiated by an individual, inherited cancer risk has implications for the entire family. Because genetic risk affects biological relatives, contact with these relatives is often essential to collect an accurate family and medical history. Cancer genetic counseling may involve several family members, some of whom may have had cancer, and others who have not.

Quality of Evidence

The quality of evidence depends on the appropriateness of the type of study to the question being evaluated and on how well the study is designed and implemented. In evaluating interventions, the strongest evidence is obtained from a well-designed and well-conducted randomized clinical trial. Other questions, particularly those related to the prevalence and clinical validity of genetic information, and emotional and familial outcomes, require well-designed descriptive studies. For some studies, particular elements of study design, such as the nature of the population studied or the duration of observation, may be crucial in assessing the quality of the study.

During early phases of research in a new area, information relevant to the needs of patients and clinicians may come from work at all levels of evidence. These include well-designed quasi-experimental (nonrandomized, controlled single-group, pre/post, cohort, time, or matched case-control series) or nonexperimental studies (case reports, clinical examples, qualitative or narrative studies, or theoretical work). Such research may yield information important to patients and clinicians who must make decisions before full data are available on the risks and benefits of cancer genetic testing. In addition, such work helps to focus future research using rigorous designs with adequate statistical power.

Study Populations

Studies assessing the clinical validity of genetic information from population-based data are not biased by common selection factors. The level of evidence required for informed decision-making about genetic testing, however, depends on the circumstances of testing. Evidence from a sample of high-risk families may be sufficient to provide useful information for testing decisions among people with similar family histories, but it may be insufficient to inform early recommendations for or decisions about testing in the general public. Even among people with similar family histories, however, other contributing genes or different exposures could modify the effect of the mutation for which testing is done. In evaluating evidence, the most important consideration is the relevance of the available data to the patient for whom a genetic assessment is being considered. In summaries addressing the cancer risk associated with polymorphisms and mutations, the study populations used for each risk assessment will be noted, according to the following categories.

1. Population-based.

2. Proxy for population-based. (The study population selected is assumed to be generally representative of the population from which it is drawn. Example: Persons participating in a community-based Tay-Sachs screening program, as a proxy for persons of Jewish descent.)

3. Public recruitment of volunteers, for example, using a newspaper ad.

4. Sequential case series.

5. Convenience sample.

6. An affected family or several families.

Evidence Related to Screening

The PDQ (Physician Data Query) Cancer Genetics Editorial Board has adopted the following definitions related to screening:

- Screening is a means of accomplishing early detection of disease in people without symptoms of the disease being sought.

- Detection examinations, tests, or procedures used in screening are usually not diagnostic, but sort out persons suspicious for the presence of cancer from those who are not.

- Diagnosis of disease is made following a work-up, biopsy, or other tests in pursuing symptoms or positive detection procedures.

Five requirements should be met before it is considered appropriate to screen for a medical condition:[10,11]

1. The medical condition being sought causes a substantial burden of suffering, measured both as mortality and the frequency and severity of morbidity and loss of function;

2. A screening test or procedure exists that will detect cancers earlier in their natural history than diagnosis prompted by symptoms, and is acceptable to patients and society in terms of convenience, comfort, risk, and cost;

3. Strong evidence exists that early detection and treatment improve disease outcomes;

4. The harms of screening are known and acceptable; and

5. Screening is judged to do more good than harm, considering all benefits and harms it induces as well as the cost, and cost-effectiveness of the screening program.

In order of strength of evidence, the levels are as follows:

1. Evidence obtained from at least one well-designed and conducted randomized controlled trial;

2. Evidence obtained from well-designed and conducted nonrandomized controlled trials;

3. Evidence obtained from well-designed and conducted cohort or case-control analytic studies, preferably from more than one center or research group;

4. Evidence obtained from multiple-time series with or without intervention;

5. Opinions of respected authorities based on clinical experience, descriptive studies, or reports of expert committees.

Evidence Related to Cancer Prevention

Evidence related to cancer prevention is evaluated using the same criteria developed for other PDQ summaries. Refer to the PDQ screening and prevention summaries for more information.

Prevention is defined as a reduction in the incidence of cancer and, therefore, cancer-related morbidity and mortality. Examples of prevention strategies are a diet high in fiber, fruits and vegetables; regular exercise; smoking cessation; and drugs such as aspirin and folic acid. The strongest evidence is obtained from a well-designed and well-conducted randomized clinical trial with cancer-specific mortality as the end point. It is, however, not always practical to conduct such a trial to address every question in the field of cancer prevention. For each summary of evidence statement, the associated levels of evidence are listed. In order of strength of evidence, the levels are as follows:

1. Evidence obtained from at least one well-designed and conducted randomized controlled trial that has:

    a. cancer mortality endpoint;

    b. cancer incidence endpoint;

    c. generally accepted intermediate endpoint (for example, large adenomatous polyps for studies of colorectal cancer prevention; high-grade squamous intraepithelial lesions of the cervix for studies of cervical cancer prevention).

2.   Evidence obtained from well-designed and conducted nonrandomized controlled trials that have:

    a. cancer mortality endpoint;

    b. cancer incidence endpoint;

    c. generally accepted intermediate endpoint (for example, large adenomatous polyps for studies of colorectal cancer prevention; high-grade squamous intraepithelial lesions of the cervix for studies of cervical cancer prevention).

3.   Evidence obtained from well-designed and conducted cohort or case-control studies, preferably from more than one center or research group, that have:

    a. cancer mortality endpoint;

    b. cancer incidence endpoint;

    c. generally accepted intermediate endpoint (for example, large adenomatous polyps for studies of colorectal cancer prevention; high-grade squamous intraepithelial lesions of the cervix for studies of cervical cancer prevention).

4.   Ecologic (descriptive) studies (for example, international patterns studies, migration studies) that have:

    a. cancer mortality endpoint;

    b. cancer incidence endpoint;

    c. generally accepted intermediate endpoint (for example, large adenomatous polyps for studies of colorectal cancer prevention; high-grade squamous intraepithelial lesions of the cervix for studies of cervical cancer prevention).

5.   Opinions of respected authorities based on clinical experience or reports of expert committees (for example, any of the above study designs using nonvalidated surrogate endpoints).

References

1. MacDonald, D.J., Choi, J., Ferrell, B., et al.: Concerns of women presenting to a comprehensive cancer centre for genetic cancer risk assessment. *J Med Genet* 39 (7): 526–30, 2002.

2. Statement of the American Society of Clinical Oncology: genetic testing for cancer susceptibility, Adopted on February 20, 1996. *J Clin Oncol* 14 (5): 1730–6; discussion 1737–40, 1996.

3. Holtzman, N.A., Watson, M.S., eds.: Promoting Safe and Effective Genetic Testing in the United States: Final Report of the Task Force on Genetic Testing. Baltimore, MD: Johns Hopkins Press, 1998.

4. Grann, V.R., Jacobson, J.S.,: Population screening for cancer-related germline gene mutations. *Lancet Oncol* 3 (6): 341–8, 2002.

5. Genetic counseling. *Am J Hum Genet* 27 (2): 240–2, 1975.

6. Baker, D.L., Schuette, J.L., Uhlmann, W.R., eds.: *A Guide to Genetic Counseling.* New York, NY: Wiley-Liss, 1998.

7. Bartels, D.M., LeRoy, B.S., Caplan, A.L., eds.: *Prescribing Our Future: Ethical Challenges in Genetic Counseling.* New York, NY: Aldine de Gruyter, 1993.

8. Kenen, R.H.: Genetic counseling: the development of a new inter-disciplinary occupational field. *Soc Sci Med* 18 (7): 541–9, 1984.

9. Kenen, R.H., Smith, A.C.: Genetic counseling for the next 25 years: models for the future. *J Genet Couns* 4(2): 115–124, 1995.

10. Woolf, S.H.: Screening for prostate cancer with prostate-specific antigen. An examination of the evidence. *N Engl J Med* 333 (21): 1401–5, 1995.

11. Winawer, S.J., Fletcher, R.H., Miller, L., et al.: Colorectal cancer screening: clinical guidelines and rationale. *Gastroenterology* 112 (2): 594–642, 1997.

Section 38.2

Heredity and Breast Cancer

"Learning About Breast Cancer," National Human Genome Research
Institute, 2004; available online at http://www.genome.gov.

What do we know about heredity and breast cancer?

Breast cancer is a common disease. Each year, approximately
200,000 women in the United States are diagnosed with breast cancer, and one in nine American women will develop breast cancer in
her lifetime. But hereditary breast cancer—caused by a mutant gene
passed from parents to their children—is rare. Estimates of the incidence of hereditary breast cancer range from between 5 to 10 percent
to as many as 27 percent of all breast cancers.

In 1994, the first gene associated with breast cancer—*BRCA1* (for
Breast Cancer 1) was identified on chromosome 17. A year later, a second gene associated with breast cancer—*BRCA2*—was discovered on
chromosome 13. When individuals carry a mutated form of either
BRCA1 or *BRCA2*, they have an increased risk of developing breast
or ovarian cancer at some point in their lives. Children of parents with
a *BRCA1* or *BRCA2* mutation have a 50 percent chance of inheriting
the gene mutation.

What do we know about hereditary breast cancer in Ashkenazi Jews?

In 1995 and 1996, studies of DNA samples revealed that Ashkenazi
(Eastern European) Jews are 10 times more likely to have mutations
in *BRCA1* and *BRCA 2* genes than the general population. Approximately 2.65 percent of the Ashkenazi Jewish population has a mutation in these genes, while only 0.2 percent of the general population
carries these mutations.

Further research showed that three specific mutations in these
genes accounted for 90 percent of the *BRCA1* and *BRCA2* variants
within this ethnic group. This contrasts with hundreds of unique
mutations of these two genes within the general population. However,

despite the relatively high prevalence of these genetic mutations in Ashkenazi Jews, only seven percent of breast cancers in Ashkenazi women are caused by alterations in *BRCA1* and *BRCA2*.

What other genes may cause hereditary breast cancer?

Not all hereditary breast cancers are caused by *BRCA1* and *BRCA2*. In fact, researchers now believe that at least half of hereditary breast cancers are not linked to these genes. Scientists also now think that these remaining cases of hereditary breast cancer are not caused by another single, unidentified gene, but rather by many genes, each accounting for a small fraction of breast cancers.

Is there a test for hereditary breast cancer?

Hereditary breast cancer is suspected when there is a strong family history of breast cancer: occurrences of the disease in at least three first or second-degree relatives (sisters, mothers, aunts). Currently the only tests available are DNA tests to determine whether an individual in such a high-risk family has a genetic mutation in the *BRCA1* or *BRCA2* genes.

When someone with a family history of breast cancer has been tested and found to have an altered *BRCA1* or *BRCA2* gene, the family is said to have a known mutation. Positive test results only provide information about the risk of developing breast cancer. The test cannot tell a person whether or when cancer might develop. Many, but not all, women and some men who inherit an altered gene will develop breast cancer. Both men and women who inherit an altered gene, whether or not they develop cancer themselves, can pass the alteration on to their sons and daughters.

But even if the test is negative, the individual may still have a predisposition to hereditary breast cancer. Currently available technique can't identify all cancer-predisposing mutations in the *BRCA1* and *BRCA2* genes. Or, an individual may have inherited a mutation caused by other genes. And, because most cases of breast cancer are not hereditary, individuals may develop breast cancer whether or not a genetic mutation is present.

How do I decide whether to be tested?

Given the limitations of testing for hereditary breast cancer, should an individual at high risk get tested? Genetic counselors can help individuals and families make decisions regarding testing.

For those who do test positive for the *BRCA1* or *BRCA2* gene, surveillance (mammography and clinical breast exams) can help detect the disease at an early stage. A woman who tests positive can also consider taking the drug tamoxifen, which has been found to reduce the risk of developing breast cancer by almost 50 percent in women at high risk. Clinical trials are now under way to determine whether another drug, raloxifene, is also effective in preventing breast cancer.

What are research results on hereditary breast cancer?

Gene test differentiates cancer types: National Human Genome Research Institute (NHGRI) scientists have developed a new genetic test that, for the first time, can easily distinguish between hereditary and sporadic forms of breast cancer. Sporadic forms of breast cancer are those caused by genetic changes that occur during a woman's life, rather than an inherited genetic mutation.

Section 38.3

Heredity and Colon Cancer

"Learning About Colon Cancer," National Human Genome Research Institute, 2004; available online at http://www.genome.gov.

What do we know about heredity and colon cancer?

Colon cancer, a malignant tumor of the large intestine, affects both men and women. In the year 2000, there were an estimated 130,200 cases diagnosed.

The vast majority of colon cancer cases are not hereditary. However, approximately 5 percent of individuals with colon cancer have a hereditary form. In those families, the chances of developing colon cancer is significantly higher than in the average person.

Scientists have discovered several genes contributing to a susceptibility to two types of colon cancer:

FAP (familial adenomatous polyposis): So far, only one FAP gene has been discovered—the *APC* gene on chromosome 5. But over 300 different mutations of that gene have been identified. Individuals with this syndrome develop many polyps in their colon. People who inherit mutations in this gene have a nearly 100 percent chance of developing colon cancer by age 40.

HNPCC (hereditary nonpolyposis colorectal cancer): Individuals with an HNPCC gene mutation have an estimated 80 percent lifetime risk of developing colon or rectal cancer. However, these cancers account for only three to five percent of all colorectal cancers. So far, four HNPCC genes have been discovered:

- *hMSH2* on chromosome 2, which accounts for 60 percent of HNPCC colon cancer cases.

- *hMLH1* on chromosome 3, which accounts for 30 percent of HNPCC colon cancer cases.

- *hPMSI* on chromosome 2, which accounts for 5 percent of HNPCC colon cancer cases.

- *hPMS2* on chromosome 7, which accounts for 5 percent of HNPCC colon cancer cases.

Together, FAP and HNPCC gene mutations account for approximately 5 percent of all colorectal cancers. These hereditary cancers typically occur at an earlier age than sporadic (non-inherited) cases of colon cancer. The risk of inheriting these mutated genes from an affected parent is 50 percent for both males and females.

The genes that cause these two syndromes were relatively easy to discover because they exert strong effects. Other genes that cause susceptibility to colon cancer are harder to discover because the cancers are caused by an interplay among a number of genes, which individually exert a weak effect.

Is there a test for hereditary colon cancer?

Gene testing can identify some individuals who carry genes for FAP and some HPNCC cases of colon cancer. However, the tests are not perfect at this point in time. So, some families may have alterations in the FAP or HNPCC gene that can not be detected.

The test for FAP syndrome involves examining DNA in blood cells called lymphocytes (white blood cells), looking for mutations in the *APC* gene. No treatment to reduce cancer risk is currently available for people with FAP. But for those who test positive, frequent surveillance can detect the cancer at an early, more treatable stage. Because of the early age at which this syndrome appears, the test may be offered to people under 18 who have a parent known to carry the mutated gene.

Researchers hope that an easier test, now experimental, will become available in three to five years. This new test examines a stool sample and looks for cancer cells sloughed off by the *APC* gene.

Genetic tests for HNPCC are of limited value since the current test can identify only a few mutations on two genes that cause HNPCC (*hMSH2* and *hMLH1*). There are no clinical tests for the other two HNPCC genes.

Because of the limitations of available tests for hereditary colon cancer, testing is not recommended for the general population. However, individuals in families at high risk may consider testing. Genetic counselors can help individuals make decisions regarding testing.

Section 38.4

Heredity and Skin Cancer

"Learning About Skin Cancer," National Human Genome Research Institute, 2004; available online at http://www.genome.gov.

Skin cancer is the most common type of cancer in the United States. An estimated 40 to 50 percent of Americans who live to age 65 will have skin cancer at least once. The most common skin cancer is basal cell carcinoma, which accounts for more than 90 percent of all skin cancers in the United States.

The most virulent form of skin cancer is melanoma. In some parts of the world, especially in Western countries, the number of people who develop melanoma is increasing faster than any other cancer. In the United States, for example, the number of new cases of melanoma has more than doubled in the past 20 years.

What are the most common forms of skin cancer?

Three types of skin cancer are the most common:

- **Basal cell carcinoma** is a slow-growing cancer that seldom spreads to other parts of the body. Basal cells, which are round, form the layer just underneath the epidermis, or outer layer of the skin.

- **Squamous cell carcinoma** spreads more often than basal cell carcinoma, but still is considered rare. Squamous cells, which are flat, make up most of the epidermis.

- **Melanoma** is the most serious type of skin cancer. It occurs when melanocytes, the pigment cells in the lower part of the epidermis, become malignant, meaning that they start dividing uncontrollably. If melanoma spreads to the lymph nodes it may also reach other parts of the body, such as the liver, lungs or brain. In such cases, the disease is called metastatic melanoma.

What are the symptoms of skin cancer?

The most commonly noticed symptom of skin cancer is a change on the skin, especially a new growth or a sore that doesn't heal. Both basal and squamous cell cancers are found mainly on areas of the skin that are exposed to the sun—the head, face, neck, hands and arms. However, skin cancer can occur anywhere.

For melanoma, the first sign often is a change in the size, shape, color or feel of an existing mole. Melanomas can vary greatly in the way they look, but generally show one or more of the ABCD features:

- Their shape may be **A**symmetrical.

- Their **B**orders may be ragged or otherwise irregular.

- Their **C**olor may be uneven, with shades of black and brown.

- Their **D**iameter may change in size.

What do we know about the causes and heredity of skin cancer?

Ultraviolet (UV) radiation from the sun is the main cause of skin cancer, although artificial sources of UV radiation, such as sunlamps and tanning booths, also play a role. UV radiation can damage the DNA, or genetic information, in skin cells, creating misspellings in their genetic code and, as a result, alter the function of those cells.

Cancers generally are caused by a combination of environmental and genetic factors. With skin cancer, the environment plays a greater role, but individuals can be born with a genetic disposition toward or vulnerability to getting cancer. The risk is greatest for people who have light-colored skin that freckles easily—often those who also have red or blond hair and blue or light-colored eyes—although anyone can get skin cancer.

Skin cancer is related to lifetime exposure to UV radiation, therefore, most skin cancers appear after age 50. However, the sun's damaging effects begin at an early age. People who live in areas that get high levels of UV radiation from the sun are more likely to get skin cancer. For example, the highest rates of skin cancer are found in South Africa and Australia, areas that receive high amounts of UV radiation.

About 10 percent of all patients with melanoma have family members who also have had the disease. Research suggests that a mutation in the *CDKN2* gene on chromosome 9 plays a role in this form of melanoma. Studies have also implicated genes on chromosomes 1 and 12 in cases of familial melanoma.

Can I do anything to prevent or test for skin cancer?

When it comes to skin cancer, prevention is your best line of defense. Protection should start early in childhood and continue throughout life. Suggested protections include:

- Whenever possible, avoid exposure to the midday sun.

- Wear protective clothing—for example, long sleeves and broad-rimmed hats.

- Use sunscreen lotions with an SPF factor of at least 15.

- If a family member has had melanoma, have your doctor check for early warning signs regularly.

How is skin cancer treated?

Melanoma can be cured if it is diagnosed and treated when the tumor has not deeply invaded the skin. However, if a melanoma is not removed in its early stages, cancer cells may grow downward from the skin surface. When a melanoma becomes thick and deep, the disease often spreads to other parts of the body and is difficult to control.

Surgery is the standard treatment for melanoma, as well as other skin cancers. However, if the cancer has spread to other parts of the body, doctors may use other treatments, such as chemotherapy, immunotherapy, radiation therapy or a combination of these methods.

Section 38.5

Heredity and Prostate Cancer

"Learning About Prostate Cancer," National Human Genome Research
Institute, 2004; available online at http://www.genome.gov.

What do we know about prostate cancer?

Prostate cancer is the most common cancer in American men. It
is a slow-growing, potentially lethal disease usually found in men over
the age of 50. Although cases of the disease have been reported in all
age groups, more than 80 percent of all prostate cancers occur in men
over the age of 65.

According to the National Cancer Institute, doctors diagnosed
198,100 new cases of prostate cancer in 2001, and about 31,500 men
died from the disease. That means about 19 out of every 100 men
born today will be diagnosed with prostate cancer, and four of every 100 men will die from the disease, or about one death every 16
minutes.

Age is the most important risk factor for contracting prostate
cancer. Others are race, family history and environment. The incidence of prostate cancer is 40 percent higher for African American
men than for white men, and the number who will die is double
that of white men.

Is there a hereditary risk for prostate cancer?

Heredity—currently under intense research at the National Human Genome Research Institute (NHGRI)—also increases risk. Risk
for families where a father or brother has had prostate cancer is increased by twofold. Hereditary prostate cancer accounts for about one
in every 10 cases of the disease.

Environmental factors likely account for the prostate cancers found
in men with no family history. Environmental factors also contribute
to the incidence of prostate cancer in men with a family history. Environmental factors can include geographic location, a high-fat diet,
high caloric intake, and a sedentary lifestyle.

What is the prostate?

The prostate is a small, walnut-sized and shaped gland deeply imbedded in the center of the pelvis where it produces a milky fluid that carries sperm during ejaculation. Wrapped around the urethra (the tube that carries urine out of the body), it sits just below the bladder and is known more for the problems it causes than the function it serves.

It was thought to protect against urinary tract infection (the word prostate is from the Greek word for protector). But the prostate is not necessary for normal sexual function nor is it clear that it has a direct influence on preventing urinary tract infection.

How is prostate cancer diagnosed and treated?

Symptoms of prostate cancer develop along with the gradual enlargement of the gland, often affecting urinary and sexual function. An enlarged prostate can squeeze the urethra and block the outflow of urine, causing frequent, small urination, difficulty beginning urination or even an inability to urinate. The flow of urine can stop and start, be weak, or create pain or a burning sensation. Erection may be painful and there can be blood in the urine or semen. Referred pain can occur in the back, hips, or upper thighs.

Diagnosis is based on symptoms, family history, rectal exam to feel for any enlargement or unusual lumps in the prostate, and the level of prostate specific antigen (PSA) in the blood. PSA is an enzyme secreted by the prostate that can be detected in the blood. If the level of PSA in the blood is abnormally elevated, it can indicate the presence of prostate cancer.

Treatment depends on the point of diagnosis and the severity of the disease. Small clusters of early stage, prostate cancer can be found in millions of men in an apparently harmless, latent form. It's not unusual for physicians to take a wait and watch approach to these early cancers, and monitor the progression of the disease with regular PSA levels and physical examinations. Often the disease can be managed this way for years, as long as progression remains slow. Surgery may be another treatment choice if the tumor is contained and the patient is healthy enough to tolerate the operation.

If the prostate is enlarged and there is a palpable mass, surgery may be indicated to remove as much of the prostate, tumor and surrounding lymph tissue as possible to check for metastasis (spread of the cancer cells). Although surgery can cause nerve damage that impairs sexual function, improved surgical techniques have reduced that risk and surgeons are now better able to preserve sexual function.

Radiation therapy is sometimes used after surgery or instead of surgery, and is targeted directly at the tumor to destroy cancer cells. It also is used in later stages of the disease to relieve pain.

In more advanced forms of the disease, hormonal therapy, with either surgical or other medical intervention, suppresses the activity of male hormones (androgens) that fuel tumor growth. It can be effective for many years, holding the disease at bay, but eventually that effectiveness may subside. Side effects from hormonal therapy can be significant, and include impotence, decreased sexual desire, reduced muscle mass, and tenderness or enlargement of breast tissue.

Chemotherapy has become a more common treatment with the recent development of sophisticated oral medications that are free of the side effects associated with previous chemotherapy regimes such as vomiting, hair loss and fatigue. Chemotherapy can stabilize the disease and inhibit growth. It is used in men who have undergone surgery, but whose disease may recur; who have had surgery and/or radiation, have a detectable PSA level but no cancer spread; or in men with metastatic disease where hormone suppression has ceased to be effective.

Chapter 39

Genital and Urinary Tract Defects

There are many birth defects that involve the genitals and urinary tract. These defects can affect the kidneys (organs that filter wastes from the blood and form urine), ureters (tubes leading from the kidneys to the bladder), bladder (sac that holds urine), urethra (the tube that drains urine out of the body from the bladder), and the male and female genitals. For boys, the genitals include the penis, prostate gland, and testes. For girls, the genitals include the vagina, uterus, fallopian tubes, and ovaries.

Abnormalities of the genitals and urinary tract are among the most common birth defects, affecting as many as one in ten babies. Some of these abnormalities are minor problems that may cause no symptoms (such as having two ureters leading from one kidney to the bladder), and go undiagnosed unless the child has an x-ray, ultrasound examination, or surgery for a related or unrelated problem. Other abnormalities can cause problems such as urinary tract infections, blockages, pain, and kidney damage, or failure.

What is the cause of genital and urinary tract defects?

A few genital and urinary tract defects or disorders are inherited from parents who have the disorder or carry the gene for it. Specific

417

causes of most of these conditions are unknown, however. Genetics and environmental factors presumably play various roles during development of these organs. A family with an affected child should consult a genetic counselor, geneticist, or a physician who is familiar with genetic disorders. These experts can discuss what is known about the cause of the specific defect and what the risks may be that the defect or disorder will occur again in subsequent offspring.

How are urinary tract defects diagnosed?

Many urinary tract defects can be diagnosed before or after birth with an ultrasound examination, which uses sound waves to examine internal organs of the fetus. After birth, ultrasound and/or a number of other tests may be recommended to provide more information on how well the kidneys and other urinary tract structures are functioning.

What are the most common urinary tract defects?

Some of the most common urinary tract defects include: renal agenesis, hydronephrosis, polycystic kidney disease, multicystic kidneys, low urinary tract obstruction, bladder exstrophy and epispadias, hypospadias, and ambiguous genitals.

What is renal agenesis?

Renal agenesis is the absence of one or both kidneys. About one in 4,000 babies is born with neither kidney (bilateral renal agenesis). Tragically, about one-third of these babies are stillborn and the rest die in the first days of life. There is no treatment that can save them.

Babies with bilateral renal agenesis often have birth defects affecting other organs, such as the heart and lungs. A fetus that has no kidneys cannot produce urine, a major part of the amniotic fluid that is crucial for normal fetal lung expansion and development. Therefore, most of these deaths result from underdeveloped lungs. Lack of amniotic fluid also contributes to the abnormal facial features and limb defects seen in these babies.

Up to 20 times as many babies (about one in 550) are born with a single kidney (unilateral renal agenesis). These babies often can live normal lives, although they may be at increased risk for kidney infections, kidney stones, high blood pressure, and kidney failure. Some affected babies, however, have other birth defects involving the urinary tract, genitals, or other organs. These children may face a variety of health problems, depending upon the specific birth defects involved.

What is hydronephrosis?

Hydronephrosis involves swelling of one or both kidneys, with accumulation of urine that cannot flow out of the kidney(s) because of a blockage somewhere in the urinary tract. Significant hydronephrosis is diagnosed in about one in 500 pregnancies during a prenatal ultrasound examination.

The blockage that causes hydronephrosis often is caused by a flap of tissue near where urine empties from the bladder (posterior urethral valves). In severe cases, the fetus's bladder becomes swollen with urine, and the urine backs up and may damage or destroy the kidneys. When hydronephrosis is diagnosed before birth, the doctor will monitor the fetus with repeated ultrasound examinations to see if the condition is worsening. Some babies with severe hydronephrosis are sick at birth, with breathing problems, urinary tract infections, and kidney failure. Once these problems have been treated, the urinary blockage can be surgically corrected (although some kidney damage may remain). Many mild cases of hydronephrosis resolve without surgery.

Occasionally, hydronephrosis can become life-threatening before birth. In such cases, a small tube called a shunt may be inserted into the fetus's bladder to drain urine into the amniotic fluid until birth, when the blockage can be repaired. Prenatal treatment of these obstructions has been the most successful form of fetal surgery to date.

Urinary blockages also commonly occur where the ureter connects to the kidney (uretero-pelvic junction obstruction). This condition varies in severity, with some cases causing kidney failure in newborns and infants, and others improving without treatment. Surgery often is recommended in the first year or two of life to relieve the obstruction and prevent further kidney damage, urinary tract infections, and pain.

What is polycystic kidney disease?

Polycystic kidney disease (PKD) is an inherited disorder that results in the growth of numerous cysts in the kidneys, reduced kidney function and, often, kidney failure. There are two main forms of the disorder: autosomal dominant and autosomal recessive PKD. Besides kidney failure, both forms can cause frequent urinary tract infections, pain, high blood pressure, and other problems.

Autosomal dominant PKD is one of the most common genetic disorders, affecting between one in 200 and one in 1,000 individuals of all ages. It most often is inherited from a parent who has the disease, although up to one-quarter of cases occur in individuals without a family history of the disease. Symptoms usually begin between the ages of 30 and 40, although children can sometimes be affected.

Autosomal recessive PKD is a rare form of the disease that affects children, with cysts sometimes developing before birth. About one in 10,000 to one in 40,000 babies are born with the disorder. Severely affected babies die in the first days of life, while others with a milder version may live into their teens or twenties. This form of PKD is inherited when both parents (who are unaffected) pass along the gene for the disorder to their child.

Drug treatment can control PKD-related problems such as high blood pressure and urinary tract infections. If kidney failure develops, the patient is treated regularly with a procedure called dialysis that does the kidney's job to cleanse the blood and sometimes treated with a kidney transplant.

Kidney cysts are a feature of certain other disorders. These include multicystic kidneys, which affect about one in 4,000 babies. This disorder, which varies greatly in severity, can cause death in the newborn period when both kidneys are affected. It is believed that multicystic kidneys result from an obstruction in the urinary tract during the early stages of development. Babies with only one affected kidney may have few consequences, such as urinary tract infections. While the affected kidney often does not function (and, in some cases, may need to be removed), an affected child can live a normal life with one healthy kidney.

Kidney cysts also can be a feature of a number of genetic syndromes. In many cases, such cysts cause few or no problems.

What are bladder exstrophy and epispadias?

Bladder exstrophy is a malformation of the bladder in which the bladder is turned inside out and located on the outside of the abdomen. In addition, the skin on the lower abdomen does not form properly, the pelvic bones are widely spaced, and there may be genital abnormalities. Bladder exstrophy, which occurs in about one in 30,000 births, affects boys about five times more often than girls.

Epispadias is a related defect involving the urethra and genitals. It often accompanies bladder exstrophy, but may occur by itself. In boys, the urethra often is short and split, with an opening on the upper surface of the penis. The penis itself appears short and flat. In girls, the clitoris may be split, and the urinary opening also is abnormally placed. Up to half of children with epispadias have bladder control problems.

Bladder exstrophy and epispadias can be repaired surgically. Many affected children require a number of surgeries over the first several years of life to achieve bladder control and normal-appearing genitals. In children with bladder exstrophy, the first surgery usually is performed within 48 hours of birth to close the bladder and replace it in the pelvis, close the abdominal wall and bring the pelvic bones into their correct position. Genital repair often is done during this procedure in girls, but repair of the penis usually is done at between the ages of one and two years. Additional surgery to control urine leakage may be done around three years of age. Studies show that about 85 percent of affected children can control their bladders following these surgeries.

What is hypospadias?

Hypospadias is a common birth defect of the penis that affects nearly one percent of baby boys. The urethra does not extend to the tip of the penis; instead, the opening of the urethra is located somewhere along the underside of the penis.

Hypospadias generally is diagnosed during the newborn examination in the hospital nursery. Affected boys should not be circumcised because the foreskin (which is removed by circumcision) may be needed to help surgically repair the defect. Surgery, which extends the urethra to the tip of the penis, usually is performed between the ages of 9 and 15 months. Without surgery, most affected boys would have to urinate sitting down and, as adults, would suffer pain during intercourse.

What are ambiguous genitals?

Babies who are born with ambiguous genitals have external genital organs that do not appear clearly male or female, or have features of both. For example, a girl may be born with a large clitoris that resembles a penis, or a boy may have testicles with female-like external genitals. An estimated one in 1,000 to one in 2,000 babies are affected.

There are many causes of ambiguous genitals, including chromosomal and genetic disorders, hormonal disturbances, enzyme deficiencies, and unexplained abnormalities of the fetal tissues that are destined to become the genitals. The most common cause of ambiguous genitals is an inherited disorder called congenital adrenal hyperplasia (CAH) which, in severe forms, also can disturb kidney function and may cause death. CAH involves an enzyme deficiency that causes the adrenal glands to produce excess amounts of male hormones (androgens). The excess androgens cause the clitoris of a girl with CAH to grow too large, resembling a penis. The disorder, which can be diagnosed with blood tests, requires lifelong treatment with the missing hormones. Affected girls may require surgery to correct the appearance of their genitals. (CAH can be diagnosed before birth with a prenatal test called chorionic villus sampling, allowing for prenatal drug treatment that sometimes can prevent genital defects.)

Another common cause of ambiguous genitals is androgen insensitivity syndrome. Affected babies have male chromosomes (XY) but, due to genetic defects, their cells do not respond or respond incompletely to androgens (male hormones). Babies with complete androgen insensitivity have testes (which usually remain inside the abdomen) and female external genitals, although they do not have a uterus or ovaries. These children are almost always raised as girls and have a completely normal female appearance, although they need treatment with hormones to undergo pubertal changes. Babies with partial androgen sensitivity have cells that partially respond to androgens and often have ambiguous external genitals.

A number of chromosomal abnormalities also can result in ambiguous genitals. These include gonadal dysgenesis, in which the baby has normal male chromosomes (XY), with either female internal and external genital organs, or ambiguous external genitals and some combination of male and female internal organs.

When a child is born with ambiguous genitals, various diagnostic studies need to be done in an attempt to define the baby's gender. These will include physical examination, blood tests (including chromosomal analysis and measurement of the levels of various hormones), urine tests and, sometimes, ultrasound examination or surgery to look at the internal organs. A team of medical specialists will use these tests to help determine whether the baby is developing more like a male or female, and may recommend assigning a gender for the baby. They may then recommend hormone therapy or reconstructive surgery on the genitals. Doctors often recommended that a boy with a very underdeveloped penis and other genital ambiguities undergo reconstructive surgery and be raised as a girl. More recently, in such cases, doctors are somewhat more likely to suggest that the parents raise the child as a girl, but to hold off on surgery to see how the child is developing—and, very importantly, whether the child feels more like a boy or girl. These situations can be extremely difficult for the child and family, so ongoing psychological counseling is strongly recommended.

References

Bernstein, J. The kidneys and the urinary tract, in: Rudolph A.M. et al (eds.), *Rudolph's Pediatrics, 20th edition*. Stamford, CT, Appleton & Lange, 1996, pages 1347–1405.

Fausto-Sterling, A. The five sexes revisited. *The Sciences*, July/August 2000, pages 19–23.

Hendricks, M. Into the hands of babes. *Johns Hopkins Magazine*, September 2000, pages 12–17.

National Institute of Diabetes and Digestive and Kidney Diseases. Polycystic Kidney Disease. NIH Publication No. 96-4008, 1998.

Thomas, D.F.M. *Urological Disease in the Fetus and Infant: Diagnosis and Management*. Oxford, England, Butterworth Heinemann, 1997.

Chapter 40

Diabetes and Genetics

Extraordinary Research Opportunities: The Genetics of Diabetes

Both type 1 and type 2 diabetes are complex genetic diseases that result from interactions between multiple genes and environmental factors. The identification and understanding of the many genetic determinants of both forms of diabetes and the complications that they share are of critical importance to conquering this disease. With greater understanding of the genetic causes of diabetes will come the ability to identify those individuals who are at highest risk, and to identify new targets for action to prevent the disease or at least stop it in its tracks.

Identification of genetic variations that predispose an individual to diabetes and its complications may reveal new molecular pathways that will provide targets for the development of candidate drugs. Once researchers know the series of cascading events that result in full-blown

Thic chapter contains excerpts from "Extraordinary Research Opportunities: The Genetics of Diabetes," from *Conquering Diabetes: Highlights of Program Efforts, Research Advances and Opportunities: A Scientific Progress Report on the Diabetes Research Working Group's Strategic Plan*, 2002; excerpts from "The Pima Indians: Genetic Research," from *The Pima Indians: Pathfinders for Health*, National Institute of Diabetes and Digestive and Kidney Diseases (NIDDK), May 2002; and excerpts from "Gene Variants May Increase Susceptibility to Type 2 Diabetes," a National Institutes of Health News Release dated March 11, 2004.

diabetes or its complications, they will be able to devise and deliver interventions at various points along this continuum. In the future, knowledge of an individual's genetic makeup may also help physicians tailor therapies or prevention measures with great specificity to individual patients in order to maximize benefits and minimize unwanted side effects. While the absolute prevention of diabetes is the ultimate goal, the ability to delay the onset of diabetes by even a few years would have enormous benefits because the severity of diabetes complications correlates with duration of disease. Thus, the potential of genetic tests to identify high risk patients, who could benefit most from intervention, assumes added importance with the recent demonstration of success in delaying onset of type 2 diabetes in clinical trials. Finally, because diabetes appears to result from an interaction of genetic susceptibility with environmental factors, a better understanding of the genetics of diabetes could help to isolate the environmental influences and point the way to avoiding or minimizing their effects.

Genetics of Type 1 Diabetes

Type 1 diabetes usually strikes in childhood or young adulthood but can affect an individual at any age. It is an "autoimmune disease," in which the body attacks its own tissue. Type 1 diabetes is characterized by the immune system's destruction of insulin-producing beta cells, which are contained in clusters, called islets, within the pancreas. Without insulin, the body cannot regulate glucose metabolism—a condition that can rapidly cause death.

Researchers have yet to determine the precise factors that cause the immune system, which normally protects the body from harmful bacteria and viruses, to initiate this misguided attack on its own insulin-producing cells. However, many studies have suggested that an environmental exposure of some sort may trigger this autoimmune disease process in individuals who have an underlying genetic susceptibility to develop type 1 diabetes. Multiple genes are believed to be involved in this susceptibility and to interact with each other and with the environment to initiate the cascade that leads to the development of type 1 diabetes.

Scientists have already identified variations within genes of the major histocompatibility complex (MHC) that are major contributors to type 1 diabetes. The MHC genes are key to the immune system's ability to differentiate between what is "foreign" to the body compared to what is "self." Research has shown that the strongest genetic predisposition to type 1 diabetes is conferred by two common genetic variations of MHC molecules known as human leukocyte antigens (HLA, a subset of the human MHC genes). About 85 to 90 percent of individuals with type 1 diabetes are positive for HLA types known as *DR3-DQ2* or *DR4-DQ8*. People who have those HLA types are also much more likely to develop diabetes than are persons with other forms of HLA. Conversely, some HLA types have been identified that appear to reduce the risk of developing type 1 diabetes. With this knowledge, it is already possible to identify individuals at increased risk for type 1 diabetes, and these genetic tests have already been incorporated into ongoing clinical trials for diabetes prevention and clinical research to identify environmental triggers of the disease. The identification of other genes contributing to disease risk would greatly increase our ability to predict who will develop type 1 diabetes. It may eventually enable the introduction of prevention strategies in those at risk before an autoimmune attack is launched, while it can effectively be arrested or mitigated.

Genetics of Type 2 Diabetes and Obesity

As with type 1 diabetes, susceptibility to type 2 diabetes and obesity is determined by both genetic and environmental factors. For type 1 diabetes, we have identified a major disease gene (HLA) but we know relatively little about environmental factors involved in development of disease. In contrast, for type 2 diabetes, we know that environmental factors such as diet and activity are risk factors but we know much less about the specific genes involved in disease susceptibility.

We have gathered clues on the genes that may be involved by studying rare syndromes that have diabetes as a key feature of the disease (see Table 40.1) but which develop because of defects in a single gene. Over ten years ago, the first gene to be directly linked to diabetes, the insulin receptor gene, was identified. Mutations in this gene were responsible for the development of several syndromes: leprechaunism, type A insulin resistance and Rabson-Mendenhall syndrome. More recently, five genes have been identified that, when mutated, can lead to the development of maturity onset diabetes of the young (MODY). MODY occurs when there is defective glucose-stimulated insulin secretion from the beta cell. Four of the MODY genes, HNF-4 alpha (*MODY1*), HNF-1alpha (*MODY3*), IPF-1 (*MODY4*) and HNF-1beta (*MODY5*), are transcription factors that are important for the development of the beta cell. *MODY2* is the glucokinase gene, which is the beta cell's glucose sensor. Mutation of a novel gene required for beta cell function has been identified as the cause of another diabetic syndrome, Wolfram Syndrome. Several different mutations in mitochondrial DNA have been shown to lead to diabetes that is often associated with deafness. Finally, three mutant genes responsible for lipoatrophic diabetes have been identified; these genes may help to elucidate the role of the fat cell in the development of diabetes.

As demonstrated by these monogenic syndromes, there are many different pathways that lead to the development of diabetes. The spectrum of clinical presentations of type 2 diabetes—and the close association of the disease with other conditions such as obesity, high blood pressure, and lipid abnormalities—add to the complexity of defining the causative genes. Characterization of specific subgroups of people with the disease is important for genetic analysis. For example, if a gene were predominantly responsible for the early onset of type 2 diabetes, then the effects of that gene would be easier to observe in a study that focused on type 2 diabetes in children. Its effects could be diluted in a study that looked at all ages. While these considerations make it particularly challenging to identify the genetic variations or mutations that predispose to type 2 diabetes, it is nonetheless critically important to meet this challenge, given the huge and increasing health burden type 2 diabetes imposes on the American people and its disproportionately heavy burden on minority populations.

Table 40.1. Genes Causing Monogenic Forms of Diabetes

Gene/Protein	Syndrome	Year Identified
Insulin Receptor	Leprechaunism	1988
	Type A Insulin Resistance	1989
	Rabson-Mendenhall	1990
tRNALeu	MELAS Syndrome	1991
HNF-4alpha (MODY 1)	MODY	1996
Glucokinase (MODY 2)	MODY	1992
HNF-1alpha (MODY 3)	MODY	1996
IPF-1 (PDX) (MODY 4)	MODY	1999
HNF-1beta (MODY 5)	MODY	1999
Wolframin	Wolfram Syndrome	1998
Lamin A/C	Dunnigan Lipoatrophy	2000
Seipin	Berardinelli-Seip	2001
Scurfin	X-linked Neonatal Diabetes	2001
AGPAT2	Berardinelli-Seip	2002
ALMS1	Alstrom Syndrome	2002

Genetics of the Complications of Diabetes

Genes are a critical factor not only in the onset of type 1 and type 2 diabetes but also in the onset and progression of the complications that result from both forms of the disease. For example, previous studies have suggested a familial clustering of diabetic kidney disease.

Because the complications of diabetes do not appear in all patients, nor with the same severity, researchers believe that some diabetes patients carry gene variants that make them more susceptible to certain complications than other patients. For example, it is known that diabetes patients from minority groups are more prone to certain complications than non-minorities with diabetes.

The Pima Indians: Genetic Research and Diabetes

Why do so many Pima Indians have diabetes? The question is simple, but the answers are not. They are part of a very complex puzzle that National Institute of Health (NIH) researchers are trying to decode through genetic research.

With the help of the Pima Indians, NIH scientists have already learned that type 2 diabetes develops when a person's body doesn't use insulin effectively. They know that other genes probably influence some people's bodies to burn energy at a slow rate, and/or to want to eat more, making it more likely that they will become overweight. If it were not for families of Pima Indian volunteers and technology developed in the last 10 years, it would not be possible to search for the genetic causes of so complex a disease as diabetes, according to Dr. Clifton Bogardus of the National Institute of Diabetes and Digestive and Kidney Diseases (NIDDK).

"We got into this work because of Pima families," Dr. Bogardus says. "NIDDK scientists, including Drs. Bennett, Knowler, and Pettitt, have studied well over 90 percent of the people on the reservation at least once. We know the families, and DNA has been collected from them routinely since the mid 1980s."

Shortly after that, other scientists began to develop ways of creating maps that show where genes are located on chromosomes in cells. They learned how to cut a fragment of DNA, and find its code. Because fragments of DNA will naturally attach to complementary fragments like a zipper, scientists learned how to identify unfamiliar pieces of DNA by using familiar fragments that were electronically labeled. If the labeled DNA found a match, scientists were able to use x-ray film to make a "picture" of the unfamiliar DNA fragment.

When researchers have volunteers from large families of several generations whose medical and genetic history is well known to them, blood samples from those volunteers are extremely valuable in learning about a disease. Using laboratory techniques, they can separate the volunteers' DNA from their blood, and compare DNA from family members who have disease and those who do not.

The researchers look for a piece of DNA shared only by members of a family who have disease. When they find the same genetic variation in many people with disease, that variation is called a marker. Because a marker and a gene that helps cause disease are often inherited together, researchers can then use that marker like a signpost to search for the sought-after gene itself.

Because diabetes is such a complex disease, Dr. Bogardus and his staff are attempting to narrow their search by first looking for the genetic causes of physical conditions that can lead to diabetes, such as the genes that influence a person's cells to secrete less and respond less to insulin that is needed to regulate blood sugar.

In 1993, they identified a gene called *FABP2* that may contribute to insulin resistance. This gene makes an intestinal fatty acid binding protein using one of two amino acids. When the gene makes the protein with threonine, one of those amino acids, the body seems to absorb more fatty acids from the fat in meals. NIH scientists think that could lead to a higher level of certain fats and fatty acids in the blood, which could contribute to insulin resistance.

Gene Variants May Increase Susceptibility to Type 2 Diabetes

International research teams studying two distinct populations have found variants in a gene that may predispose people to type 2 diabetes, the most common form of the disease. The researchers, who collaborated extensively in their work, report their findings in companion articles in the April 2004 issue of *Diabetes*.

Homing in on a wide stretch of chromosome 20 flagged by earlier studies as a likely location for a type 2 diabetes susceptibility gene, the teams identified four genetic variants, called single nucleotide polymorphisms (SNPs), which are strongly associated with type 2 diabetes in Finnish and Ashkenazi Jewish populations.

All four SNPs cluster in the regulatory region of a single gene, hepatocyte nuclear factor 4 alpha (*HNF4A*), a transcription factor that acts as a "master switch" regulating the expression of hundreds of other genes. *HNF4A* turns genes on and off in many tissues, including the liver and pancreas. In the beta cells of the pancreas, it influences the secretion of insulin in response to glucose.

"It's a nice coalescence of findings," said Dr. Francis S. Collins, Director of the National Human Genome Research Institute (NHGRI) and senior author of the article describing the Finnish study results. "What we found is a common variation in this gene. If you have this variation, it appears to raise your risk of type 2 diabetes about 30 percent. The variation isn't going to cause diabetes unless you have it in combination with other yet-to-be-identified genetic susceptibility factors, together with certain environmental influences such as obesity and lack of physical exercise."

Translating the discovery into a treatment that benefits people with diabetes or those at risk is still years away. "We need to learn much more about this gene and how to modulate its function," Dr. Collins cautioned.

The Finland-United States Investigation of NIDDM [non-insulin dependent diabetes mellitus] Genetics (FUSION) examined polymorphisms in 793 Finnish adults diagnosed with typical type 2 diabetes (formerly known as adult-onset or non-insulin dependent diabetes) and 413 non-diabetic controls. The researchers identified a total of 10 SNPs within and near the *HNF4A* gene that are associated with type 2 diabetes in the Finnish population. The most significant results were found in a region of DNA (called the "promoter") that regulates the gene's expression in the insulin-secreting cells of the pancreas. Individuals who inherited the risk variant tended to have higher levels of blood glucose at fasting and 2 hours after a glucose challenge.

The other international team of researchers studied 100 SNPs in 275 Ashkenazi Jewish adults in Israel with type 2 diabetes and 342 non-diabetic controls. They found diabetes-related associations for SNPs in the same region of *HNF4A*.

An NIH-funded study in the February 27, 2004, issue of *Science* suggests how polymorphisms in the *HNF4A* promoter might confer susceptibility to type 2 diabetes. In that work, Dr. Richard A. Young of the Whitehead Institute for Biomedical Research in Boston and coworkers examined the genes regulated by several HNF transcription factors. They found *HNF4A* to be a highly active transcription factor, regulating a surprising number of beta cell and liver cell genes in humans. A misstep in the binding site for other transcription factors in the *HNF4A* promoter, they conclude, could result in "misregulation of *HNF4A* expression and thus its downstream targets, leading to beta cell malfunction and diabetes."

For years, scientists have known that single-gene mutations, most affecting beta cell function, contribute to rare forms of diabetes, including the six types of maturity onset diabetes of the young or MODY. Such mutations account for about 2 to 3 percent of all diabetes cases. A mutation in the coding region of *HNF4A* causes MODY type 1, a rare form of diabetes that begins before age 25 in people of normal weight.

Unlike MODY, however, type 2 diabetes usually begins after age 40 in overweight, inactive people and is more common in those with a family history of diabetes. In the United States, type 2 diabetes disproportionately affects African Americans, Hispanic/Latino Americans, and American Indians. Affecting about 17 million people nationwide, this form of diabetes accounts for 90 to 95 percent of all diabetes cases in the U.S. Its prevalence has been steadily rising in the past 30 years, and it is increasingly being seen in younger people, even in children. Hallmarks of the disease are insulin resistance—the inability of target tissues to respond to insulin—and a gradual failure of beta cells to produce enough insulin.

Scientists have come a long way in understanding the basis for diseases arising from single-gene mutations. Understanding the genetic basis of the more common, polygenic diseases such as diabetes has been much more difficult.

Chapter 41

Genetic Factors in Obesity

Obesity and Genetics: What We Know, What We Don't Know and What It Means

Rising rates of obesity seem to be a consequence of modern life, with access to large amounts of palatable, high-calorie food and limited need for physical activity. However, this environment of plenty affects different people in different ways. Some are able to maintain a reasonable balance between energy input and energy expenditure. Others have a chronic imbalance that favors energy input, which expresses itself as overweight and obesity. What accounts for these differences between individuals?

What We Know

- Biological relatives tend to resemble each other in many ways, including body weight. Individuals with a family history of obesity may be predisposed to gain weight and interventions that prevent obesity are especially important.

- In an environment made constant for food intake and physical activity, individuals respond differently. Some people store more energy as fat in an environment of excess; others lose less fat in

"Obesity and Genetics: What We Know, What We Don't Know and What It Means," and "Obesity," from *Public Health Perspectives*, Genomics and Disease Prevention, Centers for Disease Control (CDC), February 2004.

an environment of scarcity. The different responses are largely due to genetic variation between individuals.

• Fat stores are regulated over long periods of time by complex systems that involve input and feedback from fatty tissues, the brain and endocrine glands like the pancreas and the thyroid. Overweight and obesity can result from only a very small positive energy input imbalance over a long period of time.

• Rarely, people have mutations in single genes that result in severe obesity that starts in infancy. Studying these individuals is providing insight into the complex biological pathways that regulate the balance between energy input and energy expenditure.

• Obese individuals have genetic similarities that may shed light on the biological differences that predispose to gain weight. This knowledge may be useful in preventing or treating obesity in predisposed people.

• Pharmaceutical companies are using genetic approaches (pharmacogenomics) to develop new drug strategies to treat obesity.

• The tendency to store energy in the form of fat is believed to result from thousands of years of evolution in an environment characterized by tenuous food supplies. In other words, those who could store energy in times of plenty, were more likely to survive periods of famine and to pass this tendency to their offspring.

What We Don't Know

• Why are biological relatives more similar in body weight? What genes are associated with this observation? Are the same genetic associations seen in every family? How do these genes affect energy metabolism and regulation?

• Why are interventions based on diet and exercise more effective for some people than others? What are the biological differences between these high and low responders? How do we use these insights to tailor interventions to specific needs?

• What elements of energy regulation feedback systems are different in individuals? How do these differences affect energy metabolism and regulation?

- Do additional obesity syndromes exist that are caused by mutations in single genes? If so, what are they? What are the natural history, management strategy, and outcome for affected individuals?

- How do genetic variations that are shared by obese people affect gene expression and function? How do genetic variation and environmental factors interact to produce obesity? What are the biological features associated with the tendency to gain weight? What environmental factors are helpful in countering these tendencies?

- Will pharmacologic approaches benefit most people affected with obesity? Will these drugs be accessible to most people?

- How can thousands of years of evolutionary pressure be countered? Can specific factors in the modern environment (other than the obvious) be identified and controlled to more effectively counter these tendencies?

What It Means

1. For people who are genetically predisposed to gain weight, preventing obesity is the best course. Predisposed persons may require individualized interventions and greater support to be successful in maintaining a healthy weight.

2. Obesity is a chronic lifelong condition that is the result of an environment of caloric abundance and relative physical inactivity modulated by a susceptible genotype. For those who are predisposed, preventing weight gain is the best course of action.

3. Genes are not destiny. Obesity can be prevented or can be managed in many cases with a combination of diet, physical activity, and medication.

4. Drugs that will aid in losing weight or maintaining a healthy weight are being developed and are expected to be available in the next few years.

5. People who are affected with overweight and obesity are often victims of stigmatization and discrimination. It is time to stop blaming the victim. Many obesity researchers believe that people who struggle with their weight are pushing against thousands of years of evolution that has selected for storing energy as fat in times of plenty for use in times of scarcity. It is time to recognize

their struggle, understand their challenges, and support their need for lifelong efforts to achieve better health.

Single Gene Disorders That Have Obesity as a Primary Feature

A relatively small proportion of obesity in the population can be explained by mutations in single genes. However, significant understanding of how fat stores are regulated has been gained from studying the biology and clinical presentations of these rare individuals and families and the animal models of these conditions.

These conditions exhibit autosomal recessive, autosomal dominant, or X-linked patterns of inheritance. Information on the genes, the clinical findings and, when available, the treatment interventions, are provided via links to the Online Mendelian Inheritance in Man (OMIM) database.[1] Although these conditions occur rarely in human populations, they are important in helping understand the complex systems that regulate energy intake and expenditure in humans.

Table 41.1. Single Gene Mutations That Have Obesity as a Primary Feature

Gene Product	Gene (OMIM #)	Mode of Inheritance
Leptin	*LEP* (164160)	Autosomal Recessive
Leptin Receptor	*LEPR* (601007)	Autosomal Recessive
Proopiomelanocortin	*POMC1* (176830)	Autosomal Recessive
Human Homolog of Drosophila Single-Minded 1	*SIM1* (603128)	Likely Autosomal Dominant
Prohormone Convertase 1	*PC1* (162150)	Autosomal Recessive
Melanocortin-4 Receptor	*MC4R* (155541)	Autosomal Dominant

Reference

1. Online Mendelian Inheritance in Man, OMIM™. McKusick-Nathans Institute for Genetic Medicine, Johns Hopkins University (Baltimore, MD) and National Center for Biotechnology Information, National Library of Medicine (Bethesda, MD), 2000, http://www.ncbi.nlm.nih.gov/omim.

Chapter 42

Multiple Genetic and Environmental Factors Influence Heart Disorders

Chapter Contents

Section 42.1—Congenital Cardiovascular Defects 438
Section 42.2—Familial Dilated Cardiomyopathy 450
Section 42.3—Genetics Linked with Sudden
   Cardiac Death 456

Section 42.1

Congenital Cardiovascular Defects

What Is a Congenital Cardiovascular Defect?

Congenital means inborn or existing at birth. Among the terms you may hear are congenital heart defect, congenital heart disease and congenital cardiovascular disease. The word defect is more accurate than disease. A congenital cardiovascular defect occurs when the heart or blood vessels near the heart don't develop normally before birth.

What Causes Congenital Cardiovascular Defects?

Congenital cardiovascular defects are present in about one percent of live births. They're the most common congenital malformations in newborns. In most cases scientists don't know why they occur. Sometimes a viral infection causes serious problems. German measles (rubella) is an example. If a woman contracts German measles while pregnant, it can interfere with how her baby's heart develops or produce other malformations. Other viral diseases also may cause congenital defects.

Heredity sometimes plays a role in congenital cardiovascular defects. More than one child in a family may have a congenital cardiovascular defect, but this rarely occurs. Certain conditions affecting multiple organs, such as Down's syndrome, can involve the heart, too. Some prescription drugs and over-the-counter medicines, as well as alcohol and street drugs, may increase the risk of having a baby with a heart defect. Researchers are studying other factors.

What Are the Types of Congenital Defects?

Most heart defects either obstruct blood flow in the heart or vessels near it, or cause blood to flow through the heart in an abnormal pattern. Rarely defects occur in which only one ventricle (single ventricle) is present, or both the pulmonary artery and aorta arise from the same ventricle (double outlet ventricle). A third rare defect occurs when the right or left side of the heart is incompletely formed—hypoplastic heart.

The following defects are described in this section: (For information on congenital defects in Spanish, see the website, www.american heart.org/Spanish/index.html).

- Aortic stenosis (AS)
- Atrial septal defect (ASD)
- Atrioventricular (A-V) canal defect
- Bicuspid aortic valve
- Coarctation of the aorta (Coarct)
- Ebstein's anomaly
- Eisenmenger's complex
- Hypoplastic left heart syndrome
- Patent ductus arteriosus (PDA)
- Pulmonary stenosis (PS)
- Pulmonary atresia
- Subaortic stenosis
- Tetralogy of Fallot
- Total anomalous pulmonary venous (P-V) connection
- Transposition of the great arteries
- Tricuspid atresia
- Truncus arteriosus
- Ventricular septal defect (VSD)

Patent Ductus Arteriosus (PDA)

This defect (PA'tent DUK'tus ar-te"re-O'sis) allows blood to mix between the pulmonary artery and the aorta. Before birth an open passageway (the ductus arteriosus) exists between these two blood vessels. Normally this closes within a few hours of birth. When this doesn't happen, some blood that should flow through the aorta and on to nourish the body returns to the lungs. A ductus that doesn't close is quite common in premature infants but rather rare in full-term babies.

If the ductus arteriosus is large, a child may tire quickly, grow slowly, catch pneumonia easily, and breathe rapidly. In some children symptoms may not occur until after the first weeks or months of life. If the ductus arteriosus is small, the child seems well. If surgery is needed, the surgeon can close the ductus arteriosus by tying it, without opening the heart. If there's no other defect, this restores the circulation to normal.

Obstruction Defects

An obstruction is a narrowing that partly or completely blocks the flow of blood. Obstructions called stenoses (sten-O'seez) can occur in heart valves, arteries, or veins.

The three most common forms are pulmonary stenosis, aortic stenosis, and coarctation of the aorta. Related but less common forms include bicuspid aortic valve, subaortic stenosis, and Ebstein's anomaly.

Pulmonary stenosis (PUL'mo-nair-e sten-O'sis) **(PS):** The pulmonary or pulmonic valve is between the right ventricle and the pulmonary artery. It opens to allow blood to flow from the right ventricle to the lungs. A defective pulmonary valve that doesn't open properly is called stenotic (sten-OT'ik). This forces the right ventricle to pump harder than normal to overcome the obstruction.

If the stenosis is severe, especially in babies, some cyanosis (si"ah-NO'sis) (blueness) may occur. Older children usually have no symptoms. Treatment is needed when the pressure in the right ventricle is higher than normal. In most children the obstruction can be relieved by a procedure called balloon valvuloplasty (VAL'vu-lo-plas-te). Others may need open-heart surgery. Surgery usually opens the valve satisfactorily. The outlook after balloon valvuloplasty or surgery is favorable, but follow-up is required to determine if heart function returns to normal.

People with pulmonary stenosis, before and after treatment, are at risk for getting an infection of the valve (endocarditis). To help prevent this, they'll need to take antibiotics before certain dental and surgical procedures.

Aortic stenosis (a-OR'tik sten-O'sis) **(AS):** The aortic valve, between the left ventricle and the aorta, is narrowed. The heart has difficulty pumping blood to the body. Aortic stenosis occurs when the aortic valve didn't form properly. A normal valve has three leaflets (cusps) but a stenotic (sten-OT'ik) valve may have only one cusp (unicuspid) or two cusps (bicuspid), which are thick and stiff. (See bicuspid aortic valve following.)

Sometimes stenosis is severe and symptoms occur in infancy. Otherwise, most children with aortic stenosis have no symptoms. Some children may have chest pain, unusual tiring, dizziness, or fainting. The need for surgery depends on how bad the stenosis is. In children, a surgeon may be able to enlarge the valve opening. Surgery may improve the stenosis, but the valve remains deformed. Eventually the valve may need to be replaced with an artificial one.

Balloon valvuloplasty (VAL'vu-lo-plas-te) has been used in some children with aortic stenosis. The long-term results of this procedure are still being studied. Children with aortic stenosis need lifelong medical follow-up. Even mild stenosis may worsen over time, and surgical relief of a blockage is sometimes incomplete. Check with your pediatric cardiologist about limiting some kinds of exercise.

People with aortic stenosis, before and after treatment, are at risk for getting an infection of the valve (endocarditis). To help prevent this, they'll need to take antibiotics before certain dental and surgical procedures.

Coarctation (ko"ark-TA'shun) **of the aorta (Coarct):** The aorta is pinched or constricted. This obstructs blood flow to the lower body and increases blood pressure above the constriction. Usually there are no symptoms at birth, but they can develop as early as a baby's first week. A baby may develop congestive heart failure or high blood pressure that requires early surgery. Otherwise, surgery usually can be delayed. A child with a severe coarctation should have surgery in early childhood. This prevents problems such as developing high blood pressure as an adult.

The outlook after surgery is favorable, but long-term follow-up is required. Rarely, coarctation of the aorta may recur. Some of these cases can be treated by balloon angioplasty. The long-term results are still being studied. Also, blood pressure may stay high even when the aorta's narrowing has been repaired.

People with coarctation of the aorta, before and after treatment, are at risk for getting an infection within the aorta or the heart valves (endocarditis). To help prevent this, they'll need to take antibiotics before certain dental and surgical procedures.

Bicuspid aortic (bi-KUS'pid a-OR'tik) **valve:** The normal aortic valve has three flaps (cusps) that open and close. A bicuspid valve has only two flaps. There may be no symptoms in childhood, but by adulthood (often middle age or older), the valve can become stenotic (sten-OT'ik) (narrowed), making it harder for blood to pass through it, or regurgitant (allowing blood to leak backward through it). Treatment depends on how well the valve works.

People with bicuspid aortic valve, before and after treatment, are at risk for getting an infection within the aorta or the heart valves (endocarditis). To help prevent this, they'll need to take antibiotics before certain dental and surgical procedures.

Subaortic stenosis (sub"a-OR'tik sten-O'sis): Stenosis means constriction or narrowing. Subaortic means below the aorta. Subaortic stenosis refers to a narrowing of the left ventricle just below the aortic valve, which blood passes through to go into the aorta. This stenosis limits the flow of blood out of the left ventricle. This condition may be congenital or may be due to a particular form of cardiomyopathy (kar"de-o-mi-OP'ah-the) known as idiopathic hypertrophic (hi"per-TRO'fik) subaortic stenosis (IHSS). Treatment depends on the cause and the severity of the narrowing. It can include drugs or surgery.

People with subaortic stenosis, before and after treatment, are at risk for getting an infection within the aorta or the heart valves (endocarditis). To help prevent this, they'll need to take antibiotics before certain dental and surgical procedures.

Ebstein's anomaly (ah-NOM'ah-lee): This is a congenital downward displacement of the tricuspid valve (located between the heart's upper and lower chambers on the right side) into the heart's right bottom chamber (or right ventricle). It's usually associated with an atrial septal defect (see following).

People with Ebstein's anomaly, before and after treatment, are at risk for getting an infection within the heart valve (endocarditis). To help prevent this, they'll need to take antibiotics before certain dental and surgical procedures.

Septal Defects

Some congenital cardiovascular defects let blood flow between the heart's right and left chambers. This happens when a baby is born with an opening between the wall (septum) that separates the right and left sides of the heart. This defect is sometimes called a hole in the heart.

The two most common types of this defect are atrial septal defect and ventricular septal defect. Two variations are Eisenmenger's complex and atrioventricular canal defect.

Atrial septal (A'tre-al SEP'tal) **defect (ASD):** An opening exists between the heart's two upper chambers. This lets some blood from the left atrium (blood that's already been to the lungs) return via the hole to the right atrium instead of flowing through the left ventricle, out the aorta and to the body. Many children with ASD have few, if any, symptoms. Closing the atrial defect by open-heart surgery in childhood can prevent serious problems later in life.

Ventricular septal (ven-TRIK'u-ler SEP'tal) **defect (VSD):** An opening exists between the heart's two lower chambers. Some blood that's returned from the lungs and been pumped into the left ventricle flows to the right ventricle through the hole instead of being pumped into the aorta. Because the heart has to pump extra blood and is over-worked, it may enlarge.

If the opening is small, it doesn't strain the heart. In that case, the only abnormal finding is a loud murmur. But if the opening is large, open-heart surgery is recommended to close the hole and prevent se-rious problems. Some babies with a large ventricular septal defect don't grow normally and may become undernourished. Babies with VSD may develop severe symptoms or high blood pressure in their lungs. Repairing a ventricular septal defect with surgery usually re-stores normal blood circulation. The long-term outlook is good, but long-term follow-up is required.

People with a ventricular septal defect are at risk for getting an infection of the heart's walls or valves (endocarditis). To help prevent this, they'll need to take antibiotics before certain dental and surgi-cal procedures. After a VSD has been successfully fixed with surgery, antibiotics should no longer be needed.

Eisenmenger's complex: This is a ventricular septal defect coupled with pulmonary high blood pressure, the passage of blood from the right side of the heart to the left (right to left shunt), an enlarged right ventricle and a latent or clearly visible bluish discoloration of the skin called cyanosis (si"ah-NO'sis). It may also include a malpositioned aorta that receives ejected blood from both the right and left ventricles (an overriding aorta).

People with Eisenmenger's complex, before and after treatment, are at risk for getting an infection within the aorta or the heart valves (endocarditis). To help prevent this, they'll need to take antibiotics before certain dental and surgical procedures.

Atrioventricular (A'tre-o-ven-TRIK'u-ler) **(A-V) canal defect (also called endocardial cushion defect or atrioventricular septal defect):** A large hole in the center of the heart exists where the wall between the upper chambers joins the wall between the lower chambers. Also, the tricuspid and mitral valves that normally separate the heart's upper and lower chambers aren't formed as individual valves. Instead, a single large valve forms that crosses the defect. The large opening in the center of the heart lets oxygen-rich (red) blood from the heart's left side—blood that's just gone through the lungs— pass into the heart's right side. There, the oxygen-rich blood, along with venous (bluish) blood from the body, is sent back to the lungs. The heart must pump an extra amount of blood and may enlarge. Most babies with an atrioventricular canal don't grow normally and may become undernourished. Because of the large amount of blood flowing to the lungs, high blood pressure may occur there and damage the blood vessels.

In some babies the common valve between the upper and lower chambers doesn't close properly. This lets blood leak backward from the heart's lower chambers to the upper ones. This leak, called regurgitation or insufficiency, can occur on the right side, left side or both sides of the heart. With a valve leak, the heart pumps an extra amount of blood, becomes overworked and enlarges.

In babies with severe symptoms or high blood pressure in the lungs, surgery usually must be done in infancy. The surgeon closes the large hole with one or two patches and divides the single valve between the heart's upper and lower chambers to make two separate valves. Surgical repair of an atrioventricular canal usually restores the blood circulation to normal. However, the reconstructed valve may not work normally.

Rarely, the defect may be too complex to repair in infancy. In this case, the surgeon may do a procedure called pulmonary artery banding to reduce the blood flow and high pressure in the lungs. When a child is older, the band is removed and corrective surgery is done. More medical or surgical treatment is sometimes needed.

People with atrioventricular canal defect, before and after treatment, are at risk for getting an infection within the heart's walls or valves (endocarditis). To help prevent this, they'll need to take antibiotics before certain dental and surgical procedures.

Cyanotic Defects

Another type of heart defect is congenital cyanotic (si"ah-NOT'ik) heart defects. In these defects, blood pumped to the body contains less oxygen than normal. This causes a condition called cyanosis (si"ah-NO'sis), a blue discoloration of the skin. Infants with cyanosis are often called blue babies.

Examples of cyanotic defects are tetralogy of Fallot, transposition of the great arteries, tricuspid atresia, pulmonary atresia, truncus arteriosus and total anomalous pulmonary venous connection.

Tetralogy of Fallot (TE'TRAL'o-je of fal-O') has four components. The two major ones are a large hole, or ventricular septal defect, that lets blood pass from the right to the left ventricle without going through the lungs; and a narrowing (stenosis) at or just beneath the pulmonary valve. This narrowing partially blocks the blood flow from the heart's right side to the lungs. The other two components are: the right ventricle is more muscular than normal; and the aorta lies directly over the ventricular septal defect.

This results in cyanosis (blueness), which may appear soon after birth, in infancy or later in childhood. These blue babies may have sudden episodes of severe cyanosis with rapid breathing. They may even become unconscious. During exercise, older children may become short of breath and faint. These symptoms occur because not enough blood flows to the lungs to supply the child's body with oxygen.

Some infants with severe tetralogy of Fallot may need an operation to give temporary relief by increasing blood flow to the lungs with a shunt. This is done by making a connection between the aorta and the pulmonary artery. Then some blood from the aorta flows into the lungs to get more oxygen. This reduces the cyanosis and allows the child to grow and develop until the problem can be fixed when they are older.

Most children with tetralogy of Fallot have open-heart surgery before school age. The operation involves closing the ventricular septal defect and removing the obstructing muscle. After surgery the long-term outlook varies, depending largely on how severe the defects were before surgery. Lifelong medical follow-up is needed.

People with tetralogy of Fallot, before and after treatment, are at risk for getting an infection within the aorta or the heart valves (endocarditis). To help prevent this, they'll need to take antibiotics before certain dental and surgical procedures.

Transposition of the great arteries: The positions of the pulmonary artery and the aorta are reversed. The aorta is connected to the right ventricle, so most of the blood returning to the heart from the body is pumped back out without first going to the lungs. The pulmonary artery is connected to the left ventricle, so most of the blood returning from the lungs goes back to the lungs again.

Infants born with transposition survive only if they have one or more connections that let oxygen-rich blood reach the body. One such connection may be a hole between the two atria, called atrial septal defect, or between the two ventricles, called ventricular (ven-TRIK'u-ler) septal defect. Another may be a vessel connecting the pulmonary artery with the aorta, called patent ductus arteriosus (PA'tent DUK'tus ar-te"re-O'sis). Most babies with transposition of the great arteries are extremely blue (cyanotic) (si"ah-NOT'ik) soon after birth because these connections are inadequate.

To improve the body's oxygen supply, a special procedure called balloon atrial septostomy (sep-TOS'to-me) is used. Two general types of surgery may be used to help fix the transposition. One is a venous switch or intra-atrial baffle procedure that creates a tunnel inside the atria. Another is an arterial switch. After surgery, the long-term outlook varies quite a bit. It depends largely on how severe the defects were before surgery. Lifelong follow-up is needed.

People with transposition of the great arteries, before and after treatment, are at risk for getting an infection on the heart's walls or valves (endocarditis). To help prevent this, they'll need to take antibiotics before certain dental and surgical procedures.

Tricuspid atresia (tri-KUS'pid ah-TRE'zhuh): In this condition, there's no tricuspid valve. That means no blood can flow from the right atrium to the right ventricle. As a result, the right ventricle is small and not fully developed. The child's survival depends on there being an opening in the wall between the atria called an atrial septal defect and usually an opening in the wall between the two ventricles called a ventricular (ven-TRIK'u-ler) septal defect. Because the circulation is abnormal, the blood can't get enough oxygen, and the child looks blue (cyanotic) (si"ah-NOT'ik).

Often a surgical shunting procedure is needed to increase blood flow to the lungs. This reduces the cyanosis. Some children with tricuspid atresia have too much blood flowing to the lungs. They may need a procedure (pulmonary artery banding) to reduce blood flow to the lungs. Other children with tricuspid atresia may have a more functional repair (Fontan procedure). Children with tricuspid atresia require lifelong follow-up by a cardiologist.

People with tricuspid atresia, before and after treatment, are at risk for getting an infection of the valves (endocarditis). To help prevent this, they'll need to take antibiotics before certain dental and surgical procedures.

Pulmonary atresia (PUL'mo-nair-e ah-TRE'zhuh): No pulmonary valve exists, so blood can't flow from the right ventricle into the pulmonary artery and on to the lungs. The right ventricle acts as a blind pouch that may stay small and not well developed. The tricuspid valve is often poorly developed, too.

An opening in the atrial septum lets blood exit the right atrium, so venous (bluish) blood mixes with the oxygen-rich (red) blood in the left atrium. The left ventricle pumps this mixture of oxygen-poor blood into the aorta and out to the body. The baby appears blue (cyanotic) (si"ah-NOT'ik) because there's less oxygen in the blood circulating through the arteries. The only source of lung blood flow is the patent ductus arteriosus (PA'tent DUK'tus ar-te"re-O'sis) (PDA), an open passageway between the pulmonary artery and the aorta. If the PDA narrows or closes, the lung blood flow is reduced to critically low levels. This can cause very severe cyanosis.

Early treatment often includes using a drug to keep the PDA from closing. A surgeon can create a shunt between the aorta and the pulmonary artery to help increase blood flow to the lungs. A more complete repair depends on the size of the pulmonary artery and right ventricle. If they're very small, it may not be possible to correct the defect with surgery. In cases where the pulmonary artery and right ventricle are a more normal size, open-heart surgery may produce a good improvement in how the heart works.

If the right ventricle stays too small to be a good pumping chamber, the surgeon can compensate by connecting the right atrium directly to the pulmonary artery. The atrial defect also can be closed to relieve the cyanosis. This is called a Fontan procedure. Children with tricuspid atresia require lifelong follow-up by a cardiologist.

People with pulmonary atresia, before and after treatment, are at risk for getting an infection on the heart's walls or valves (endocarditis). To help prevent this, they'll need to take antibiotics before certain dental and surgical procedures.

Truncus arteriosus (TRUN'kus ar-te"re-O'sis): This is a complex malformation where only one artery arises from the heart and forms the aorta and pulmonary artery. Surgery for this condition usually is required early in life. It includes closing a large ventricular (ven-TRIK'u-ler) septal defect within the heart, detaching the pulmonary arteries from the large common artery, and connecting the pulmonary arteries to the right ventricle with a tube graft. Children with truncus arteriosus need lifelong follow-up to see how well the heart is working.

People with truncus arteriosus, before and after treatment, are at risk for getting an infection on the heart's walls or valves (endocarditis). To help prevent this, they'll need to take antibiotics before certain dental and surgical procedures.

Total anomalous pulmonary venous (ah-NOM'ah-lus PUL'mo-nair-e VE'nus) **(P-V) connection:** The pulmonary veins that bring oxygen-rich (red) blood from the lungs back to the heart aren't connected to the left atrium. Instead, the pulmonary veins drain through abnormal connections to the right atrium.

In the right atrium, oxygen-rich (red) blood from the pulmonary veins mixes with venous (bluish) blood from the body. Part of this mixture passes through the atrial septum (atrial septal defect) into the left atrium. From there it goes into the left ventricle, to the aorta and out to the body. The rest of the poorly oxygenated mixture flows through the right ventricle, into the pulmonary artery and on to the lungs. The blood passing through the aorta to the body doesn't have enough oxygen, which causes the child to look blue (cyanotic) (si"ah-NOT'ik).

This defect must be surgically repaired in early infancy. The pulmonary veins are reconnected to the left atrium and the atrial septal defect is closed. When surgical repair is done in early infancy, the long-term outlook is very good. Still, lifelong follow-up is needed to make sure that any remaining problems, such as an obstruction in the pulmonary veins or irregularities in heart rhythm, are treated properly. It's important to make certain that a blockage doesn't develop in the pulmonary veins or where they're attached to the left atrium. Heart rhythm irregularities (arrhythmias) also may occur at any time after surgery.

Hypoplastic Left Heart Syndrome

In hypoplastic (hi"po-PLAS'tik) left heart syndrome, the left side of the heart is underdeveloped—including the aorta, aortic valve, left ventricle and mitral valve. Blood returning from the lungs must flow through an opening in the wall between the atria, called an atrial septal defect. The right ventricle pumps the blood into the pulmonary artery, and blood reaches the aorta through a patent ductus arteriosus (PA'tent DUK'tus ar-te"re-O'sis). (See previous.)

The baby often seems normal at birth, but will come to medical attention within a few days as the ductus closes. Babies with this syndrome become ashen, have rapid and difficult breathing, and have difficulty feeding. This heart defect is usually fatal within the first days or months of life without treatment.

This defect isn't correctable, but some babies can be treated with a series of operations or with a heart transplant. Until an operation is performed, the ductus is kept open by intravenous (IV) medication.

Because these operations are complex and different for each patient, you need to discuss all the medical and surgical options with your child's doctor. Your doctor will help you decide which is best for your baby.

If you and your child's doctor choose surgery, it will be done in several stages. The first stage, called the Norwood procedure, allows the right ventricle to pump blood to both the lungs and the body. It must be performed soon after birth. The final stage(s) has many names including bi-directional Glenn, Fontan operation, and lateral tunnel. These operations create a connection between the veins returning blue blood to the heart and the pulmonary artery. The overall goal is to allow the right ventricle to pump only oxygenated blood to the body and to prevent or reduce mixing of the red and blue blood. Some infants require several intermediate operations to achieve the final goal.

Some doctors will recommend a heart transplant to treat this problem. Although it provides the infant with a heart that has normal structure, the infant will require lifelong medications to prevent rejection. Many other problems related to transplants can develop. You should discuss these with your doctor.

Children with hypoplastic left heart syndrome require lifelong follow-up by a cardiologist for repeated checks of how their heart is working. Virtually all the children will require heart medicines.

People with hypoplastic left heart syndrome, before and after treatment, are at risk for getting an infection on the heart's inner lining or valves (endocarditis). To help prevent this, they'll need to take antibiotics before certain dental and surgical procedures.

Good dental hygiene also lowers the risk of endocarditis. For more information about dental hygiene and preventing endocarditis, ask your pediatric cardiologist.

(For more information on children and heart disease, see the American Heart Association Web site www.americanheart.org/children. For information on congenital heart defects in Spanish, see www.american heart.org/Spanish/index.html.)

Section 42.2

Familial Dilated Cardiomyopathy

"Familial Dilated Cardiomyopathy," by Lisa Ku, MS; Jennie Feiger, MS, MA; Matthew Taylor, MD; Luisa Mestroni, MD; on behalf of the Familial Cardiomyopathy Registry, *Circulation,* vol. 108, i. 17, October 28, 2003, pp. e118–e121. © 2003 American Heart Association, Inc. and Lippincott Williams and Wilkins; reprinted with permission.

Cardiomyopathies are diseases of the heart muscle that render the heart unable to properly pump enough blood to the body. In the dilated form of cardiomyopathy (called dilated cardiomyopathy or DCM), the heart is enlarged (Figure 42.1).

As the heart enlarges, it becomes less effective in pumping blood, which then leads to symptoms of heart failure and irregular heart rhythms (arrhythmias). It is estimated that approximately one out of every 2,500 persons has DCM, although the disease is probably even more common. DCM affects both men and women and can affect both adults and children. As with other types of cardiomyopathies, DCM is a chronic disease without a known cure. However, the treatments currently available can significantly improve its course.

What Are the Clinical Signs of DCM?

DCM is usually detected by signs of heart failure, the common symptoms of which are shortness of breath, swelling of the ankles and legs, and fatigue. Age of onset and severity of symptoms can vary in affected individuals. Occasionally, some DCM patients may have signs of muscle weakness or dystrophy. Finally, some individuals with DCM may not have any clinical symptoms or signs, and can only be identified by diagnostic testing.

How Is DCM Diagnosed?

Echocardiography, an ultrasound test that produces images of the heart, is often the best way to identify DCM. An echocardiogram would be able to show enlargement of the left ventricle of the heart and reduced pumping ability in individuals with DCM. Other recommended screening tests are a physical examination and a standard electro-cardiogram (ECG). Occasionally, more invasive testing, such as a biopsy of the heart or a coronary angiogram, may be necessary to distinguish DCM from other forms of heart disease.

Treatment for DCM

The treatment of DCM involves management of the patient's heart failure, arrhythmia, and problems with the natural electrical signal that makes the heart beat (conduction defects). The treatment of heart failure is based on administering medications such as angiotensin-converting enzyme (ACE) inhibitors, beta-blocking agents, diuretics, and digoxin. Management of more advanced heart failure may consist of synchronization of contraction of the right and left ventricles by means of a biventricular pacemaker, or heart transplantation. An arrhythmia can be managed with an implantable cardioverter-defibrillator to stop life threatening rhythm disturbances via an electrical shock. Conduction defects may require a pacemaker to maintain a normal heart rate.

Origin of DCM: Importance of Genetic Factors

There are many possible causes of dilatation and dysfunction of the heart, such as coronary artery disease, infection, and excessive use of alcohol. In cases where the cause of DCM is unknown, the condition is called idiopathic dilated cardiomyopathy. About one-third to one-half of patients with idiopathic DCM have a family history of the disease in one or more relatives. These patients are considered to have familial dilated cardiomyopathy. Familial DCM is caused by defective genes that affect the function of the heart muscle. Several familial DCM genes are currently known, whereas others are still under investigation.

Familial Dilated Cardiomyopathy

Many individuals with DCM do not even consider that they may have an inherited form of the condition until they begin to analyze their family history. Familial DCM is clinically and diagnostically the same as other forms of DCM, so careful attention to family history is essential. It is important to recognize that if a person with DCM has just one affected relative, this could suggest a diagnosis of familial DCM.

Occasionally, familial DCM is not limited to problems with the pumping function of the heart. Additional complications may also be present, such as conduction defects that cause low heart rate and loss of consciousness, arrhythmia that causes irregular heartbeats and potentially sudden unexpected death, or conditions involving other muscles in the body that cause muscle weakness. It is important to consider these other features of familial DCM when evaluating your family history.

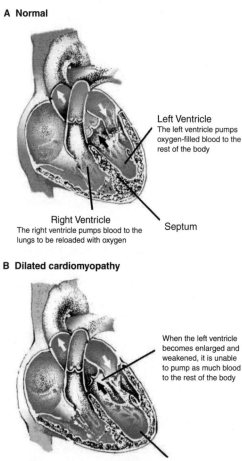

A Normal

Left Ventricle
The left ventricle pumps
oxygen-filled blood to the
rest of the body

Right Ventricle
The right ventricle pumps blood to the
lungs to be reloaded with oxygen

Septum

B Dilated cardiomyopathy

When the left ventricle
becomes enlarged and
weakened, it is unable
to pump as much blood
to the rest of the body

Enlarged Ventricle

Figure 42.1. Normal (A) and DCM (B) hearts. DCM occurs as a result of enlargement of the left ventricle. Inefficient pumping of the blood can cause heart failure, and DCM may be complicated by arrhythmia, sudden death, and possibly the need for a heart transplant.

What Is Being Done to Identify Family Members at Risk?

If a person is suspected to have a familial DCM, his/her relatives could be at risk for DCM. A detailed family tree (called a pedigree) provides important clues about whether familial DCM is present in a family. Among affected relatives, symptoms can be quite variable. For example, age of onset of symptoms can be anywhere from infancy to the 70s, even within the same family. Your physician or a genetic counselor can help construct your pedigree and analyze it for inheritance patterns. Most of the time, familial DCM follows an autosomal dominant inheritance pattern, although other patterns, such as recessive and sex-linked, have been reported as well. In autosomal dominant inheritance, men and women are equally affected, and first-degree relatives (parents, siblings, and children) of a patient with DCM have a 50% chance of inheriting familial DCM. Often, several generations are affected (Figure 42.2).

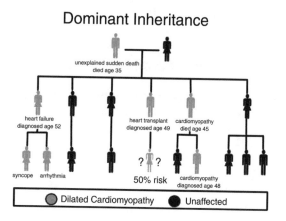

Dominant Inheritance

unexplained sudden death
died age 35

heart failure
diagnosed age 52

heart transplant
diagnosed age 49

cardiomyopathy
died age 45

syncope   arrhythmia

? ?
50% risk

cardiomyopathy
diagnosed age 48

Dilated Cardiomyopathy   Unaffected

Figure 42.2. Example of a family history with autosomal dominant transmission, the most common mode of inheritance for familial DCM. Both men and women are affected, and multiple generations are involved. Detailed evaluations, including echocardiograms, of relatives at risk can help determine affected or unaffected status. The woman indicated in gray in the third generation has not been evaluated yet. As she has an affected parent, she has a 50% risk of inheriting the condition (and equally a 50% risk of not inheriting the condition).

453

Family members, especially first degree relatives, might benefit from screening for DCM. Screening tests are the same as those for diagnosing DCM (physical examination, ECG, echocardiogram). Family screening frequently detects relatives with asymptomatic mild heart disease. In these cases, early diagnosis and treatment to prevent or delay the progression of heart failure (with ACE inhibitors and/or beta-blocking agents) and arrhythmia may be indicated. In the beginning stages of this disease, early diagnosis and treatment can potentially save lives and preserve quality of life.

If the screening results are normal, it does not necessarily mean that the family members are free of DCM, particularly if these relatives are young. It is often worthwhile for relatives to be screened every 2 to 3 years. Talk to your doctor about appropriate recommendations for you and your family.

Genetic testing may also be an option to identify family members at risk. More than 10 genes have been identified in familial DCM. Currently, genetic tests are available for a small subset of these genes. Research is ongoing to identify more genes and to develop genetic tests. If a gene mutation is identified in a person who has familial DCM, then his/her relatives could undergo genetic testing to determine if they are predisposed to DCM.

Important Clues In Your Family History

Ask your relatives about these symptoms to help determine if there is an inherited form of DCM in your family.

- History of DCM
- History of heart failure and its symptoms:
  - Shortness of breath
  - Fluid retention/swelling of ankles and legs
  - Fatigue/tiredness
- Unexplained sudden death/cardiac arrest (some people will mistakenly call sudden death a heart attack, which is caused by coronary artery disease, when it might really be caused by DCM)
- Muscle problems (cramps, stiffness, history of muscular dystrophy)
- Heart rhythm or conduction problems, including those that require implantation of a defibrillator or pacemaker
- Palpitations (fluttering or awareness of heartbeat)

- Syncope (loss of consciousness)
- Young age of onset in any of the above

Genetic Counseling for Familial DCM

Genetic counselors are health professionals who can help provide risk information about familial DCM to patients and their families. They can explain the role of heredity in developing DCM. They can analyze your family history, select appropriate genetic tests, and interpret genetic test results. They can also help you manage the challenges of having or being at risk for a genetic disorder. To find a genetic counselor near you, contact the National Society of Genetic Counselors at 610-872-1192.

References

1. Mestroni L, Maisch B, McKenna WJ, et al. Guidelines for the study of familial dilated cardiomyopathies. *Eur Heart J.* 1999;20:93–102.

Additional Resources

American Heart Association
Website: http://www.americanheart.org

American Heart Association
Circulation journal: cardiology patient page
Website: http://www.circ.ahajournals.org/collected/patient.shtml

National Society of Genetic Counselors
Website: http://www.nsgc.org

University of Colorado Cardiovascular Institute
University of Colorado Health Sciences Center
Website: http://www.uchsc.edu/cvi

Section 42.3

Genetics Linked with Sudden Cardiac Death

Recent studies have found that a person's family history of sudden cardiac death may increase that person's risk of sudden cardiac death from causes such as coronary artery disease. According to an article published in the May 22, 2001 issue of *Circulation,* a family history of sudden cardiac death remained an independent predictor of sudden cardiac death even after other cardiovascular risk factors had been taken into account. The authors pointed out that sudden cardiac death is probably attributable in most cases to atherosclerosis (hardening of the arteries), the formation of potentially fatal blood clots or a heart attack—all of which have been associated with genetics.

Sudden cardiac death is the leading type of death in the world's industrialized countries. It claims about one American life every minute and approximately 250,000 American lives every year. Although sudden cardiac death often strikes without warning, the event rarely takes place in the absence of advanced heart disease unless other factors (for example, recreational drug use or other heart conditions) are present. Two or more major arteries were found to be narrowed in 90 percent of people who died a sudden cardiac death.

Younger people who do not have advanced heart disease may still have a condition that puts them at risk of sudden cardiac death. These conditions include the following:

- **Hypertrophic cardiomyopathy:** A condition in which the heart's ability to pump blood is weakened because of enlargement, thickening or stiffening of the heart.

- **Wolff-Parkinson-White syndrome:** A condition in which abnormal electrical pathways between the heart's chambers cause the ventricles to receive abnormal signals, prompting a rapid and irregular heart beat.

- **Long Q-T syndrome:** A disorder of the heart's electrical system that may lead to a rapid heartbeat in times of stress, fear or anger, and could lead to sudden cardiac death.

More rarely, other conditions known to cause sudden cardiac death in some cases include the following:

- **Congenital heart disease:** Certain types of congenital heart disease or heart defects.

- **Embolism:** The blockage of a blood vessel by a foreign substance, such as a blood clot.

- **Kawasaki Disease:** A disease, usually seen in young children, which affects blood vessels and heart muscle.

- **Severe aortic stenosis:** Narrowing of the aortic valve of the heart.

- **Coronary artery spasm:** An abnormal constriction of the muscle fibers in a coronary artery.

About HeartCenterOnline

HeartCenterOnline is a cardiovascular specialized health care website providing tools to help patients and their families better understand the complex nature of heart-related conditions, treatments, and preventive care. The website includes a library of physician-edited patient education information, interactive health-tracking tools, and an online cardiovascular community for patients, their families and other site visitors.

HeartCenterOnline
One South Ocean Boulevard, Suite 201
Boca Raton, FL 33432
Website: http://www.heartcenteronline.com

Chapter 43

Genetics and High Blood Pressure

Genetics of Hypertension

The most comprehensive genome-wide analysis for the genetic causes of hypertension ever conducted shows that this health threat to 50 million Americans has diverse and subtle genetic roots.

Five papers and two editorials published together in the February edition of the *American Journal of Hypertension* highlight a series of areas in the genome but no "silver bullet" gene with large effects across all populations.

Findings come from an unusual collaborative alliance called the Family Blood Pressure Program (FBPP) made up of four research networks based at the University of Michigan, the Pacific Health Research Institute (Stanford University), the University of Utah and The University of Texas (UT) Health Science Center at Houston. The FBPP is funded by a five-year $48.6 million grant from the National Heart, Lung and Blood Institute (NHLBI) of the National Institutes of Health.

"The Family Blood Pressure Program has identified regions of the genome that house hypertension susceptibility genes that have small or moderate effects," said Eric Boerwinkle, Ph.D., director of the Family Blood Pressure Program and director of the Human Genetics Center at the UT School of Public Health at Houston.

"We also found there are no common genes with large effects that influence risk for hypertension. That's something we previously had assumed, but this study provides definitive confirmation. It's the largest study by far in terms of sample size at 6,250 individuals and the most racially diverse," said Boerwinkle, who is also director of the Research Center for Human Genetics at the Institute of Molecular Medicine for the Prevention of Human Diseases and holds a faculty appointment at the UT Graduate School of Biomedical Sciences at Houston.

Findings are consistent with evidence that hypertension springs from a complex blend of causes—genetics (multiple genes), demographics and behavioral factors. Family studies have long established that genetics account for 30 to 50 percent of blood pressure variation in a population.

An accompanying editorial in the journal describes the papers "as a progress report on what is undoubtedly the largest frontal assault ever directed at the genetics of a common disease."

Such common diseases as hypertension, diabetes, cardiovascular disease and cancer have a genetic aspect but are not caused solely by genetic variation. This makes pinpointing genetic causes more difficult than in diseases that are caused strictly by genetic factors.

Hypertension is a major risk factor for stroke, renal failure and cardiovascular disease, all among the most common causes of death and illness in the United States.

Network members conducted genome-wide linkage scans for genetic variations that contribute to hypertension among groups of relatives in geographically diverse populations of African Americans, non-Hispanic Caucasians, and people of Japanese or Chinese ancestry. They then conducted a meta-analysis of all four studies that encompassed 6,250 individuals.

Among African Americans, portions of chromosomes 1 and 2 were found likely to harbor susceptibility genes for hypertension. Among persons of Japanese or Chinese ancestry, a portion of chromosome 10 was most significant. Results for non-Hispanic Caucasians showed several genetic areas with possible small effects but none as statistically significant as the leading areas among African American and Asian populations. Across populations, small effects were noted in portions of a variety of chromosomes including 1, 2, 5, 9, 10, and 14.

Boerwinkle said FBPP research networks are following up on these results in a variety of ways. Association studies of candidate genes are being conducted to narrow down areas identified by the linkage study. One network is subjecting the FBPP data, which today includes more than 14,000 individuals, to complex statistical analyses both to clarify the implicated regions and to identify new areas of the genome housing hypertension susceptibility genes.

Another strategy is to subdivide populations and more closely examine smaller groups that share common characteristics. Because age, gender, diet, obesity, tobacco use and other factors contribute to hypertension, it's likely that genes interact with these factors to affect a person's risk, Boerwinkle said. FBPP networks are analyzing these specific sub-samples—for example, looking at the genetics of hypertensive smokers or of lean people who have hypertension. Boerwinkle's group also is making a concerted effort to identify a gene on chromosome 2, an area that has provided convincing and consistent evidence for a hypertension gene.

"Given the public health impact of hypertension, it's crucial to identify the genes involved," Boerwinkle said. The complexity of hypertension's causes—genes interacting with other genes or genes interacting with other risk factors—holds promise for highly customized treatment, such as:

- Knowledge of the genes involved could be used to identify people most at risk for hypertension and to prescribe healthy lifestyles that would prevent it.

- New and better treatments could focus on the underlying molecular causes of the disease, rather than on the symptoms.

- Medication could be tailored to the individual based on her genetic makeup. Presently, the dozens of medications available for hypertension vary in their effectiveness from person to person. Genetic differences are one suspected cause.

The American Journal of Hypertension is a forum of scientific inquiry of the highest standards in the fields of hypertension and related cardiovascular disease. It is the journal of the American Society of Hypertension, the largest U.S. organization devoted exclusively to hypertension and related cardiovascular disease.

About the Family Blood Pressure Program

A family connection for hypertension has been noted by physicians and scientists for decades. Family studies estimate that about 30 to 50 percent of blood pressure variation in a population is attributable to genetic variation. However, hypertension is not a Mendelian genetic disorder—one that is strictly caused by genetic variation.

In 1995, the National Heart, Lung and Blood Institute of the National Institutes of Health in the U.S. Department of Health and Human Services funded research in the genetics of hypertension with 20 separate grants to four research networks. The four networks were drawn to cooperate as the degree of difficulty in pinpointing the genetics of hypertension became clear. Multiple genes are involved, since blood pressure control involves the body's cardiovascular, renal, endocrine and neurological systems. Behavioral and demographic factors also are important.

By April 1998 the networks agreed to pool data, resources and talents in what is now called the Family Blood Pressure Program, with Roger Williams, M.D., founder of the University of Utah School of Medicine's Cardiovascular Genetics Research Clinic, as its first director. After Williams perished in a plane crash in September 1998, Eric Boerwinkle, Ph.D., of The University of Texas Health Science Center at Houston, became program director.

In 1999, the four networks submitted a unified application for renewed funding. The NHLBI funded the program in 2000 for a total of $48.6 million over five years.

The networks pursue their original unique research aims while collaborating intensively in a variety of ways, Boerwinkle said. Research findings are shared in advance of publication. A pooled database facilitates validation of research. And coordination of research plays to the individual strengths of the networks while avoiding duplication.

In addition to the genetics of hypertension, the networks are analyzing the genetics of diseases related to hypertension: stroke, cardiovascular disease and renal failure.

Information on the FBPP is available at http://www.bloodpressure genetics.org.

—by Scott Merville, Public Affairs

Chapter 44

Hereditary Factors in Allergy and Asthma

Chapter Contents

Section 44.1—Genetic Risk for Allergy and Asthma 464
Section 44.2—Scientists Identify Genes That Regulate
　　　　　　　Allergic Response to Diesel Fumes 466

Section 44.1

Genetic Risk for Allergy and Asthma

As pediatricians and family physicians battle the rising incidence of asthma and allergies among their patients, ongoing research at the Cincinnati Children's Division of Allergy and Immunology is revealing new knowledge about the genetic components of the disease, how humans are affected, and what new treatments and preventive measures might be possible.

A new study led by Gurjit Khurana Hershey, MD, PhD, reinforces previous findings that allergies and asthma are largely genetic disorders that also can be influenced by environment. The study found that the presence of two common genetic polymorphisms of the IL-4 receptor α gene contributes to the development of asthma. These polymorphisms are very common and occur in 20 to 40 percent of the population. Thus, physicians are likely to have patients who have these polymorphisms. Some of these individuals may already have asthma, while others are at risk of developing it, even if they are not yet symptomatic.

The IL-4Rα gene is known to be associated with asthma. IL-4Rα is part of the receptor for the products of both the IL-4 and IL-13 genes, thus it is critical for the action of IL-4 and IL-13. These two genes have been proven essential in the development of allergies in human and animal studies; IL-4 is also essential for T-cell differentiation. "The IL-4Rα gene itself has eight known polymorphisms, and two of them occur commonly, in 20 to 40 percent of the population. We wanted to determine the effect those common polymorphisms might have on asthma and allergy," Dr. Hershey explains.

Two Gene Variations Important

In the laboratory, researchers created four variations on IL-4Rα: the wild type, or the gene as it occurs normally; one with the polymorphism

R576; another with the polymorphism V75; and a fourth with a combination of the two, V75R576. When cells expressing each of the four types were exposed to IL-4, the cells with both polymorphisms produced a response three times higher than the other types of cells. "From these findings, we hypothesized that people with both polymorphisms are much more likely to have asthma and allergies," Dr. Hershey says.

Strikingly, the laboratory study also revealed that both polymorphisms must be present to increase the risk; either one alone is not as strong as both variations appearing together. "There is something different about the receptor itself when both polymorphisms are present," Dr. Hershey explains.

These findings were confirmed in a study of 200 asthmatic individuals and 65 nonatopic individuals in a control group. Genotyping revealed that the V75R576 combined polymorphism was significantly associated with atopic asthma in the group of patients with asthma. As in the laboratory, the combination was more strongly associated with asthma than either variation by itself.

This study is part of the comprehensive approach to asthma and allergy research which has merited Cincinnati Children's millions of dollars in funding from the National Institutes of Health and other agencies. Researchers are studying not only the molecular and genetic bases of asthma, but also the role of mediators, and employing mouse models to gain a better understanding of how the disease functions.

Identifying Multiple Asthma Genes

"We are working to find the combination of genes that produces asthma. In patients with asthma, we're using DNA chip arrays to determine which genes are turned on so that we can identify other genes we should be studying," Dr. Hershey says.

Currently, Dr. Hershey is conducting extensive studies focused on gene and environment interactions in the development of childhood allergies and asthma. "The question we're asking is, can we genotype you as an infant and predict that you'll get allergies? If we can make that prediction, then we should be able to intervene," she says.

"We're planning additional studies to determine if we can prevent or change the course of allergies or asthma before children with the genetic predisposition show any symptoms. We've shown that if you have two copies of the IL-4Rα polymorphisms, you're more likely to get severe asthma. I believe that a genetic test for asthma will be developed in the next 10 years. Physicians will be able to better customize their treatment if they know their patient is genetically predisposed to develop severe asthma."

This study was published in *The Journal of Immunology* (169[3]: 1604–1610, 2002 August 1) and was supported by grants from the National Institutes of Health and the March of Dimes.

Section 44.2

Scientists Identify Genes That Regulate Allergic Response to Diesel Fumes

From a new release of the National Institute of Allergy and Infectious Diseases (NIAID) and National Institutes of Health (NIH) dated January 8, 2004.

The risk of developing respiratory allergies from exposure to diesel emissions depends largely on genetics, according to a study funded by the National Institute of Allergy and Infectious Diseases (NIAID), part of the National Institutes of Health (NIH). Given their findings, researchers estimate that up to 50 percent of the United States population could be in jeopardy of experiencing health problems related to air pollution. The study is published in the January 10, 2004 issue of the British journal *The Lancet*.

"This important study adds to previous data that suggest how modern environmental factors interact with the body's defenses to produce airway diseases considered rare before the advent of industrialized society," says Anthony S. Fauci, M.D., director of NIAID.

"The knowledge provided by this work will help us identify people who are susceptible to the deleterious effects of diesel emissions on the clinical course of asthma and hay fever," says Kenneth Adams, Ph.D., who oversees asthma research funded by NIAID. "It will also help accelerate development of drugs to treat and prevent these diseases."

This study also received support from the National Institute of Environmental Health Sciences, another NIH component.

The authors of the study examined how a family of antioxidant-related genes—*GSTM1*, *GSTT1* and *GSTP1*—reacts to diesel exhaust particles, a common air pollutant. The body generates antioxidants to detoxify harmful particles and limit the corresponding allergic reaction.

Researchers sampled the DNA of volunteers who are allergic to ragweed to find which forms of the genes they had. The participants were then given doses of ragweed through the nose, followed by either a placebo or quantities of diesel exhaust particles equivalent to breathing the air in Los Angeles, California, for 40 hours.

The mix of ragweed and diesel exhaust triggered greater allergic responses than ragweed alone. Additionally, the diesel particles caused volunteers who lacked the antioxidant-producing form of the *GSTM1* gene to have significantly greater allergic responses, compared to the other participants. Up to 50 percent of the U.S. population does not have this form of the *GSTM1* gene. Within the group that lacked *GSTM1*, those who had a particular variant of the *GSTP1* gene experienced even greater allergic reactions. Researchers estimate that 15 to 20 percent of the U.S. population falls into this category.

"Diesel emissions can trigger allergic symptoms, but the genetic factors involved in the process are quite complex," says David Diaz-Sanchez, Ph.D., assistant professor in the Division of Immunology and Allergy at the University of California Los Angeles, who co-authored the study with scientists from the University of Southern California. "Our findings suggest that people who lack the genes to make key antioxidants may have difficulty fighting the harmful effects of air pollution."

Dr. Diaz-Sanchez says that he and the other researchers will work to find other genes involved in pollution-related health problems such as asthma, lung cancer and heart disease, with the goal of discovering possible treatments and preventions. "We are focused on investigating ways we can overcome this genetic deficiency," he says. "This may be accomplished by either giving people drugs that replace the role of the genes or by boosting the body's natural defenses."

NIAID is a component of the National Institutes of Health (NIH), which is an agency of the Department of Health and Human Services. NIAID supports basic and applied research to prevent, diagnose and treat infectious and immune-mediated illnesses, including HIV/AIDS and other sexually transmitted diseases, illness from potential agents of bioterrorism, tuberculosis, malaria, autoimmune disorders, asthma and allergies.

Reference: F Gilliland et al. Effect of glutathione-S-transferase M1 and P1 genotypes on xenobiotic enhancement of allergic responses: randomized, placebo-controlled crossover study. *The Lancet* 363 (9403): 119–25 (2004).

Chapter 45

Heredity and Parkinson Disease

What Do We Know about Heredity and Parkinson Disease?

Parkinson disease is a chronic and progressive disorder of the nervous system that causes tremors and muscular rigidity. It affects about 500,000 to one million people throughout the United States.

There are several types of Parkinson disease. The two most prevalent are early-onset and late-onset. Early-onset Parkinson begins before age 50 and accounts for between 5 and 10 percent of all cases. Late-onset Parkinson starts at age 50 or older and accounts for most cases of the disease.

For many years, researchers debated whether genes or the environment caused Parkinson. Scientists have linked susceptibility to early-onset Parkinson to variations in genes on two chromosomes: 4 and 6. Most significant were variations in the *Parkin* gene on chromosome 6, frequently found in families with early-onset Parkinson. However, researchers continued to think that environmental factors were primarily responsible for late-onset Parkinson.

Genes Linked to Early- and Late-Onset Parkinson

Research from Duke University Medical Center (November 2001) indicates that heredity plays a part in late-onset Parkinson as well as early-onset. The Duke study, funded in part the National Institutes

---

"Learning about Parkinson's Disease," National Human Genome Research Institute, February 2004. Available online at http://www.genome.gov/10001217.

of Health (NIH), conducted genetic analyses of blood samples from 174 families with Parkinson disease.

The study turned up strong evidence that several genes may influence the development of late-onset Parkinson. The *Parkin* gene mutation on chromosome 6 (previously linked to early onset Parkinson Disease) was also detected in families with late-onset Parkinson. But the strongest linkage to late-onset Parkinson occurred on chromosome 17, near the Tau gene. This gene has previously been shown to be involved in other degenerative diseases of the nervous system. In addition, variations in genes on chromosomes 5, 8 and 9 were also linked to Parkinson.

Genes and Environment Most Likely Cause Parkinson

Inheriting a mutation in a Parkinson-linked gene does not mean that an individual will develop the disease. In some illnesses, such as Huntington disease, a single defective gene causes the disease in everyone who inherits it. But in Parkinson disease, inherited mutations, perhaps in several genes, convey susceptibility. Some people who inherit mutations will get the disease, but others won't.

What Determines Who Gets Parkinson Disease?

Scientists believe that environmental factors trigger the disease in people with a genetic susceptibility. Researchers don't know which environmental factors, but they speculate that pesticide exposure, head injury, or hormonal therapy may be triggers.

Is There a Test for Hereditary Parkinson Disease?

Researchers have made great advances in finding genetic linkages to Parkinson disease. But there is still no widely available genetic test for the disease.

Chapter 46

Genes and the Development of Alzheimer's Disease

Introduction

Scientists do not yet fully understand what causes Alzheimer's disease (AD). However, the more they learn about AD, the more they become aware of the important function genes play in the development of this devastating disease.

Genes

All living things are made up of basic units called cells, which are so tiny that you can only see them through the lens of a strong microscope. Most of the billions of cells in the human body have one nucleus that acts as a control center, housing our 46 chromosomes. A chromosome is a thread-like structure found in the cell's nucleus, which can carry hundreds, sometimes thousands, of genes. In humans, a set of 23 chromosomes is inherited from each parent. The genetic material on these 23 chromosomes is collectively referred to as the human genome. Through research, scientists now believe the human genome is made up of about 30,000 genes. Genes direct almost every aspect of the construction, operation, and repair of all living things. For example, genes contain information that determines eye and hair color and other traits inherited from our parents. In addition, genes ensure that we have two hands and can use them to do things, like play the piano.

"Alzheimer's Disease Genetics Fact Sheet," Alzheimer's Disease Education and Referral Center (ADEAR), NIH Pub. No. 03-4012, February 2003.

Genes alone are not all-powerful. Most genes can do little until spurred on by other substances. Although they are necessary in their own right, genes basically wait inside the cell's nucleus for other molecules to come along and read their messages. These messages provide the cell with instructions for building a specific protein.

Proteins are an important building block in all cells. Bones and teeth, muscles and blood, for example, are formed from different proteins. They help our bodies grow, work properly, and stay healthy. Amino acids are the building blocks of proteins. A gene provides the code, or blueprint, for the type and order of amino acids needed to build a specific protein. Sometimes a genetic mutation (or defect) can occur, leading to the production of a faulty protein. In addition to gene mutations, the environment (the food we eat, the air we breath, or chemicals we are exposed to) can affect the production of a protein by interrupting the translation of the genetic message. Faulty proteins can cause cell malfunction, disease, and death.

Scientists are studying genes to learn more about the proteins they make and what these proteins actually do in the body. They also hope to discover what illnesses are caused when genes don't work right.

The Genetics of Alzheimer's Disease

Diseases such as cystic fibrosis, muscular dystrophy, and Huntington disease are single-gene disorders. If a person inherits the gene that causes one of these disorders, he or she will usually get the disease. AD, on the other hand, is not caused by a single gene. More than one gene mutation can cause AD, and genes on multiple chromosomes are involved.

The two basic types of AD are familial and sporadic. Familial AD (FAD) is a rare form of AD, affecting less than ten percent of AD patients. All FAD is early-onset, meaning the disease develops before age 65. It is caused by gene mutations on chromosomes 1, 14, and 21. Even if one of these mutated genes is inherited from a parent, the person will almost always develop early-onset AD. This inheritance pattern is referred to as autosomal dominant inheritance. In other words, all offspring in the same generation have a 50/50 chance of developing FAD if one of their parents had it.

ApoE in Sporadic Alzheimer's Disease

The majority of AD cases are sporadic, meaning they have no known cause. Because this type of AD usually develops after age 65, it often is referred to as late-onset AD. Sporadic AD shows no obvious inheritance pattern; however, in some families, clusters of cases have been seen. Although a specific gene has not been identified as the cause of sporadic AD, genetics does appear to play a role in the development of this form of AD. Researchers have identified an increased risk of developing sporadic AD related to the apolipoprotein E (apoE) gene found on chromosome 19. This gene codes for a protein that helps carry cholesterol in the bloodstream. ApoE comes in several different forms, or alleles, but three occur most frequently: apoE2 (E2), apoE3 (E3), and apoE4 (E4).

People inherit one apoE allele from each parent. Having one or two copies of the E4 allele increases a person's risk of getting AD. That is, having the E4 allele is a risk factor for AD, but it does not mean that AD is certain. Some people with two copies of the E4 allele (the highest risk group) do not develop the disease while others with no E4s do. The rarer E2 allele appears to be associated with a lower risk of AD. The E3 allele is the most common form found in the general population and may play a neutral role in AD. The exact degree of risk of AD for any given person cannot be determined based on apoE status.

ApoE Testing in Research or Diagnosis

A blood test is available that can identify which apoE alleles a person has. However, because the apoE4 gene is only a risk factor for AD, this blood test cannot tell whether a person will develop AD or not. Instead of a yes or no answer, the best information a person can get from this genetic test for apoE is maybe or maybe not. Although some people want to know whether they will get AD later in life, this type of prediction is not yet possible. In fact, some researchers believe that screening measures may never be able to predict AD with 100 percent accuracy.

In a research setting, apoE testing may be used to identify study volunteers who may be at a higher risk of getting AD. In this way, researchers can look for early brain changes in some patients. This test also helps researchers compare the effectiveness of treatments for patients with different apoE profiles. Most researchers believe that the apoE test is useful for studying AD risk in large groups of people but not for determining one person's individual risk. Predictive screening in otherwise healthy people will be useful if an accurate/reliable test is developed and effective ways to treat or prevent AD are available.

In diagnosing AD, apoE testing is not a common practice. The only definite way to diagnose AD is by viewing a sample of a person's brain tissue under a microscope to determine if there are plaques and tangles present. This is usually done after the person dies. However, through a complete medical evaluation (including a medical history, laboratory tests, neuropsychological tests, and brain scans), doctors can diagnose AD correctly up to 90 percent of the time. Doctors look to rule out other diseases and disorders that can cause the same symptoms of Alzheimer's disease. If no cause is identified, a person is said to have "probable" or "possible" AD. In some cases, apoE testing may be used in combination with these other medical test to strengthen a suspected case of AD.

Concerns about Confidentiality

ApoE testing, and indeed all genetic testing, raises ethical, legal, and social questions for which we have few answers. Generally, confidentiality laws protect apoE information gathered for research purposes. On the other hand, information obtained in apoE testing may not remain confidential if it becomes part of a person's medical records. Thereafter, employers, insurance companies, and other health care organizations could find out this information, and discrimination could result. For example, employment opportunities or insurance premiums could be affected.

Genetic Counseling

Depending on the study, research volunteers may have the opportunity, during genetic counseling, to learn the results of their apoE testing. The meaning of these results is complex. Since the results of apoE testing can be hard to understand, and more importantly, devastating to those tested, the National Institute on Aging (NIA) and the Alzheimer's Association recommend that research volunteers and their families receive genetic counseling before and after testing.

People who learn through testing that they have an increased risk of getting AD may experience emotional distress and depression about the future because there is not yet an effective way to prevent or cure the disease. Through counseling, families can learn about the genetics of AD, the tests themselves, and possible meanings of the results. Due to privacy, emotional, and health care issues, the primary goal of genetic counseling is to help people with AD and their families explore and cope with the consequences of such knowledge.

Experts still do not know how limited information about AD risk can benefit people. Among the issues are privacy and confidentiality policies related to genetic information and AD, and the small number of genetic counselors now trained in neurodegenerative disorders. In addition, little is known about how stigma associated with an increased risk for AD may affect people's families and their lives.

Research Questions

Learning more about the role of apoE in the development of AD may help scientists identify who would benefit from prevention and treatment efforts. Age, still the most important known risk factor for AD, continues to be associated with the disease even when no known genetic factors are present. Research focusing on advancing age may help explain the role that other genes play in most AD cases. Scores of AD researchers are studying the genetics of AD. In addition, researchers, ethicists, and health care providers are developing policies about the appropriate use of genetic testing and counseling for AD.

Recent research suggests that certain alleles of other as yet unidentified genes also may increase risk in late-onset cases. The NIA has launched a major initiative focused on discovering remaining genetic risk factors for late-onset AD. Together with commercial researchers, geneticists from the NIA's Alzheimer's Disease Centers are working to create a genetic sampling of families affected by multiple cases of late-onset AD. Researchers are seeking large families with more then one living relative with late-onset AD. Families interested in participating in this study can contact the National Cell Repository for Alzheimer's Disease at 800-526-2839. Information may also be requested through their website, www.iupui.edu/~medgen/research/alz/alzheimer.html

For More Information

Accurate, current information about AD and its risk factors is important to patients and their families, health professionals, and the public. The Alzheimer's Disease Education and Referral (ADEAR) Center is a service of the NIA and is funded by the federal government. The ADEAR Center offers information and publications about diagnosis, treatment, patient care, caregiver needs, long-term care, education and training, and research related to AD. Staff respond to telephone, e-mail, and written requests and make referrals to local and national resources.

ADEAR Center
P.O. Box 8250
Silver Spring, MD 20907-8250
Toll-Free: 800-438-4380
Fax: 301-495-3334
Website: http://www.alzheimers.org
E-mail: adear@alzheimers.org

For the free fact sheet, "Genetic Counseling: Valuable Information for You and Your Family," write, fax, or e-mail the National Society for Genetic Counselors (NSGC). Their address is: NSGC, Executive Office, 233 Canterbury Drive, Wallingford, PA 19086-6617; Fax: 610-872-1192; Website: http://www.nsgc.org. The NSGC does not provide information about specific genetic disorders.

Additional Internet information about AD and genetics is available from the National Human Genome Research Institute (NHGRI), part of the National Institutes of Health. Visit the NHGRI website at http://www.genome.gov.

The National Library of Medicine (NLM) National Center for Biotechnology Information (NCBI) has produced a gene map of the human genome, which can be viewed at www.ncbi.nlm.nih.gov/science96. It features information about the relationship between Alzheimer's disease and genes on chromosomes 1 and 14. The NCBI also maintains the "Online Mendelian Inheritance in Man Database," a catalog of human genes and genetic disorders, including Alzheimer's disease, which can be viewed at www3.ncbi.nlm.nih.gov:80/Omim/searchomim.html.

Chapter 47

Mental Illness: Evidence of a Genetic Component

Chapter Contents

Section 47.1—Family History of Mental Illness 478
Section 47.2—Hunting for Genes Associated with
        Mental Illnesses 481

Section 47.1

Family History of Mental Illness

A mental illness is a disease that causes mild to severe disturbances in thought and/or behavior, resulting in an inability to cope with the ordinary demands and routines or life. There are more than 200 classified forms of mental illness. Some of the more common disorders are depression, bipolar disorder, dementia, schizophrenia and anxiety disorders. Symptoms may include changes in mood, personality, personal habits and/or social withdrawal. With proper care and treatment many individuals learn to cope or recover from a mental illness or emotional disorder.

Mental illness is inherited in a multifactorial pattern (caused by the interaction of various genetic and environmental factors). Causes may include a reaction to environmental stresses, genetic factors, biochemical imbalances, or a combination of these. Because genetic factors are involved, when one family member is affected, other close relatives may be at increased risk.

Unipolar Disorder and Bipolar Disorder

In any given one-year period, 9.5 percent of the population, or about 18.8 million American adults, suffer from a depressive illness. This includes major depressive disorder, manic depression and dysthymia, a milder, longer-lasting form of depression.

More than 2 million American adults, or about one percent of the population age 18 and older in any given year, have bipolar disorder. Bipolar disorder, also known as manic depression, is an illness involving one or more episodes of serious mania and depression. The illness causes a person's mood to swing from excessively "high" to irritable, sad and/or hopeless, with periods of a normal mood in between.

With any type of mood disorder in a family, there can be up to a 20–25 percent recurrence risk for first degree relatives of affected individuals. Specifically, recurrence risks for first degree relatives (children, parents, siblings) are 10–20 percent for individuals with unipolar depression (two to four times the population risk) and 5–10 percent for first degree relatives of individuals with bipolar disorder (up to ten times the population risk for manic depression, some sources state a risk as high as 25 percent). Relatives of individuals who were diagnosed with depression earlier in life are at a greater risk than relatives of individuals who were diagnosed later in life. In families with both unipolar depression and bipolar disorder, the genetic risks are increased.

Schizophrenia

Schizophrenia is a serious disorder which affects how a person thinks, feels, and acts. Someone with schizophrenia may have difficulty distinguishing between what is real and what is imaginary; may be unresponsive or withdrawn; and may have difficulty expressing normal emotions in social situations. Contrary to public perception, schizophrenia is not split personality or multiple personality. The vast majority of people with schizophrenia are not violent and do not pose a danger to others. Schizophrenia is not caused by childhood experiences, poor parenting or lack of willpower, nor are the symptoms identical for each person.

There are several types of schizophrenia including paranoid schizophrenia (a person feels extremely suspicious, persecuted, or grandiose, or experiences a combination of these emotions), disorganized schizophrenia (a person is often incoherent in speech and thought, but may not have delusions), catatonic schizophrenia (a person is withdrawn, mute, negative and often assumes very unusual body positions), residual schizophrenia (a person is no longer experiencing delusions or hallucinations, but has no motivation or interest in life) and schizo-affective disorder (a person has symptoms of both schizophrenia and a major mood disorder such as depression).

Schizophrenia affects one percent of the general population. The risks to first degree relatives (parents, offspring and siblings) range from 9–15 percent. The risk to second degree relatives (grandchildren, aunts, uncles) is approximately three percent and the risk to third degree relatives (first cousins) is one to two percent. Quoted risks may be higher depending upon the number of affected relatives. In some families the risk may be as high as 50 percent.

Attention Deficit Disorder/Attention Deficit Hyperactivity Disorder

Young people with attention deficit/hyperactivity disorder typically are overactive, unable to pay attention, and impulsive. They also tend to be accident prone. Children or adolescents with attention deficit/hyperactivity disorder may not do well in school or even fail, despite normal or above-normal intelligence. Attention deficit/hyperactivity disorder is sometimes referred to as ADHD.

First degree relatives of affected individuals have a five to six fold increased risk over the general population to develop the condition. The risk for second degree relatives is approximately one to two percent. Family members of affected individuals are also at an increased risk for personality disorders, substance abuse, depression, anxiety, and learning disabilities.

Substance Abuse

There have been many studies which indicate an increased risk for substance abuse and/or dependence among close relatives of substance abusers. Alcohol, marijuana, cocaine, tranquilizer and sedative use as well as other drugs have been studied, and an inherited predisposition for abuse has been demonstrated. For instance, the risk for first-degree relatives of individuals with alcoholism is three times the population risk to develop alcoholism and two times the population risk to develop abusive behavior of other drugs. In family histories with multiple affected family members the risk may be higher.

Resources

Further information regarding these and other forms of mental illness is available through the following organizations.

National Institute of Mental Health
Toll-Free: 800-421-4211
Website: http://www.nimh.nih.gov

National Mental Health Association
Toll-Free: 800-969-6642
Website: http://www.nmha.org

Section 47.2

Hunting for Genes Associated with Mental Illnesses

"Gene Hunting," National Institute of Mental Health (NIMH), NIH Pub. No. 01-4600, 2001, updated July 2002.

Many years of research have demonstrated that vulnerability to mental illnesses—such as schizophrenia, bipolar disorder, early-onset depression, anxiety disorders, autism, and attention deficit hyperactivity disorder—has a genetic component. It is now clear that these disorders are not due to a single defective gene, but to the joint effects of many genes acting together with nongenetic factors.[1,2,3] Despite the daunting complexity, progress is being made. Researchers are hunting genes because they are likely to be a vital key to deciphering what goes wrong in the brain in mental illness.

Detecting multiple genes, each contributing only a small effect, requires large sample sizes and powerful technologies that can associate genetic variations with disease [4,5,6] and thereby pinpoint candidate genes from among the many genes that are expressed in the human brain. And even after human disease vulnerability genes are found, sophisticated tools will be needed to find out what activates them, what brain components they code for, and how they affect behavior. The prospect of acquiring such molecular knowledge holds great hope for the engineering of new therapies.

Linkage studies are often based on the identification of large, densely affected families so that the inheritance patterns of known sections of DNA (called "markers") can be compared to the family's transmission of the disorder.[7] If a known marker can be correlated with the presence or absence of the disorder, this finding narrows the location of the suspect gene.

Linkage-disequilibrium studies in isolated populations capitalize on the likelihood that the susceptibility genes for a particular disorder probably came from one or a few founding members.[8] Whether the isolation is geographic or cultural, there are fewer individuals in the community's genealogies and therefore fewer variations of the disease genes within the population. This limited variation makes the search easier. In addition, the groups of markers that surround each of these susceptibility genes are likely to have the same limited variation, which further simplifies identification.

Association studies depend on the investigator hypothesizing that a specific gene or genes may influence the disorder. In this type of study, the investigator examines whether those people with the disorder have a different version of the gene than those without the disorder among related or unrelated individuals.[9]

Evidence suggests that unaffected family members may share with their ill relatives genes that predispose for milder, but qualitatively similar behavioral characteristics. For example, some relatives of people with schizophrenia or autism may exhibit subtle cognitive problems.[10,11] Family members may also share biological anomalies that could be clues to the underlying genetic component of the illness. For example, they may share telltale chemical signatures in cells of implicated brain circuits. National Institute of Mental Health (NIMH)-supported investigators are studying such families to characterize these behavioral and biological traits, in hopes of tracing the variations in the genetic blueprint that contribute to illness.

Some gene variants are likely to turn on too much or too little—or in the wrong place. This could interfere with the way brain cells work. It may also affect how cells migrate to other parts of the brain and connect with one another during early development. NIMH has mounted an effort to vastly expand the set of available tools for discovering the molecular mistakes that produce mental illness.

A vital resource for doing this, now under development, will be a shared scientific infrastructure called the Brain Molecular Anatomy Project (BMAP). The goals of this multidisciplinary effort are to catalog the genes that are active in various parts of the brain at different developmental stages, and to make this information readily available to investigators on a web-based map.

The mouse's brain is a major initial focus of BMAP. A web-based digital mouse brain atlas will offer 3-D and 2-D views of this biological blueprint, covering different strains and ages of animals. In addition to advancing basic knowledge, the BMAP database promises to enhance clinical science, providing new leads for studying gene expression in post-mortem tissue, for the identification of candidate genes, and enhanced capacity to screen for individuals who might be at risk for developing brain disorders.

A related set of developing tools also centers on the mouse: identifying the neural basis of complex behaviors.[12] The mouse has become a critical model in studying human disease because scientists have access to many inbred strains, each expressing distinctive physiological and behavioral characteristics. Researchers can now insert, knock out, or mutate mouse genes, quickly breed a generation that expresses the change, and then see how it affects behavior. When illness-linked genes are discovered, they will be inserted and expressed in mice to find out what they do at the molecular, cellular and behavioral levels. Researchers will be able to track a wiring abnormality, a cell migration abnormality, or other anomaly that may lead to symptoms in humans.

References

1. Risch NJ. Linkage strategies for genetically complex traits: I. multilocus models. *American Journal of Human Genetics*, 1990; 46(2): 222–8.

2. Craddock N, Khodel V, VanEerdewegh P, et al. Mathematical limits of multilocus models: the genetic transmission of bipolar disorder. *American Journal of Human Genetics*, 1995; 57(3): 690–702.

3. Risch NJ, Spiker D, Lotspeich L, et al. A genomic screen of autism: evidence for a multilocus etiology. *American Journal of Human Genetics*, 1999; 65(2): 493–507.

4. Lander ES. The new genomics: global views of biology. *Science*, 1996; 274(5287): 536–9.

5. Chakravarti A. Population genetics-making sense out of sequence. *Nature Genetics*, 1999; 21(1 Suppl): 56–60.

6. Risch NJ. Searching for genetic determinants in the new millennium. *Nature*, 2000; 405(6788): 847–56.

7. Ott J. *Analysis of human genetic linkage, third edition*. Baltimore, MD: Johns Hopkins University Press, 1999.

8. Jorde LB. Linkage disequilbrium as a gene-mapping tool. *American Journal of Human Genetics*, 1995; 56(1): 11–4.

9. Spielman RS, Ewens WJ. A sibship test for linkage in the presence of association: the sib transmission/disequilbrium test. *American Journal of Human Genetics*, 1998; 62(2): 450–8.

10.   Faraone SV, Siedman LJ, Kremen WS, et al. Neuropsychologi-
       cal functioning among the nonpsychotic relatives of schizo-
       phrenic patients: a 4-year follow-up study. *Journal of
       Abnormal Psychology*, 1999; 108(1): 176–81.

11.   Folstein SE, Santangelo SL, Gilman SE, et al. Predictors of
       cognitive test patterns in autism families. *Journal of Child
       Psychology and Psychiatry*, 1999; 40(7): 1117–28.

12.   Tarantino LM, Bucan M. Dissection of behavior and psychiat-
       ric disorders using the mouse as a model. *Human Molecular
       Genetics*, 2000; 9(6): 953–65.

Chapter 48

Addiction and Genetics

Chapter Contents

Section 48.1—The Genetics of Alcoholism 486
Section 48.2—Gene Linked to Drug Addiction 493
Section 48.3—Is There an Inherited Vulnerability
          to Nicotine Addiction? 495

Section 48.1

The Genetics of Alcoholism

Alcohol Alert, No. 60, National Institute on Alcohol Abuse
and Alcoholism, July 2003.

Research has shown conclusively that familial transmission of alcoholism risk is at least in part genetic and not just the result of family environment.[1] The task of current science is to identify what a person inherits that increases vulnerability to alcoholism and how inherited factors interact with the environment to cause disease. This information will provide the basis for identifying people at risk and for developing behavioral and pharmacologic approaches to prevent and treat alcohol problems. The advances being made now are built on the discovery 50 years ago of the role in inheritance of DNA, the genetic material in cells that serves as a blueprint for the proteins that direct life processes. Alcoholism research, like other fields, is capitalizing on the scientific spinoffs of this milestone, among them the Human Genome Project and related efforts to sequence the genomes, the complete DNA sequences, of selected animals.

A Complex Genetic Disease

Studies in recent years have confirmed that identical twins, who share the same genes, are about twice as likely as fraternal twins, who share on average 50 percent of their genes, to resemble each other in terms of the presence of alcoholism. Recent research also reports that 50 to 60 percent of the risk for alcoholism is genetically determined, for both men and women.[2-5] Genes alone do not preordain that someone will be alcoholic; features in the environment along with gene-environment interactions account for the remainder of the risk.

Research suggests that many genes play a role in shaping alcoholism risk. Like diabetes and heart disease, alcoholism is considered genetically complex, distinguishing it from genetic diseases, such as cystic fibrosis, that result primarily from the action of one or two copies of a single gene and in which the environment plays a much smaller role, if any. The methods used to search for genes in complex diseases have to account for the fact that the effects of any one gene may be subtle and a different array of genes underlies risk in different people.

Scientists have bred lines of mice and rats that manifest specific and separate alcohol-related traits or phenotypes, such as sensitivity to alcohol's intoxicating and sedative effects, the development of tolerance, the susceptibility to withdrawal symptoms, and alcohol-related organ damage.[6,7] Risk for alcoholism in humans reflects the mix and magnitude of these and other phenotypes, shaped by underlying genes, in interaction with an environment in which alcohol is available. Genetic research on alcoholism seeks to tease apart the genetic underpinnings of these phenotypes and how they contribute to risk.

One well-characterized relationship between genes and alcoholism is the result of variation in the liver enzymes that metabolize (break down) alcohol. By speeding up the metabolism of alcohol to a toxic intermediate, acetaldehyde, or slowing down the conversion of acetaldehyde to acetate, genetic variants in the enzymes alcohol dehydrogenase (ADH) or aldehyde dehydrogenase (ALDH) raise the level of acetaldehyde after drinking, causing symptoms that include flushing, nausea, and rapid heartbeat. The genes for these enzymes and the alleles, or gene variants, that alter alcohol metabolism have been identified. Genes associated with flushing are more common among Asian populations than other ethnic groups, and the rates of drinking and alcoholism are correspondingly lower among Asian populations.[8,9]

Genes, Behavior, and the Brain

Addiction is based in the brain. It involves memory, motivation, and emotional state. The processes involved in these aspects of brain function have thus been logical targets for the search for genes that underlie risk for alcoholism. Much of the information on potential alcohol-related genes has come from research on animals. Research has demonstrated a similarity in the mechanisms of many brain functions across species as well as an overlap between the genomes of animal—seven invertebrates—and humans.

One approach to identifying alcohol-related genes is to start with an aspect of brain chemistry on which alcohol is thought to have an impact, and work forward, identifying and manipulating the underlying genes and ultimately determining whether the presence or absence of different forms, or alleles, of a gene influence alcoholism risk. For example, genetic technology now permits scientists to delete or inactivate specific genes, or alternatively, to increase the expression of specific genes, and watch the effects in living animals. Because genes act in the context of many other genes, interpretation of these studies can be difficult. If one gene is disabled, for example, others may compensate for the loss of function. Alternatively, the loss of a single gene throughout development may be harmful or lethal. Nonetheless, these techniques can provide important clues to function. These approaches have been used to study how altering the expression of genes encoding the receptors (or their subunits) for neurotransmitters and intracellular messenger molecules alters the response to alcohol.[10]

Scientists also have an increasing array of methods for locating alcohol-related genes and gene locations and only then determining how the genes function, an approach known as reverse genetics. Quantitative trait loci (QTL) analysis seeks to identify stretches of DNA along chromosomes that influence traits, like alcohol sensitivity, that vary along a spectrum (height is another quantitative trait). QTLs have been identified for alcohol sensitivity, alcohol preference, and withdrawal severity.[11] Ultimately, the goal is to identify and determine which candidate genes within the QTLs are responsible for the observed trait. Among the candidate genes already known to lie near alcohol-related QTLs are several that encode neurotransmitter receptors and neurotransmitters themselves. One of these, neuropeptide Y (NPY), lies within a QTL for alcohol preference in rats. NPY is a small protein molecule that is abundant in the brain and has been shown to influence the response to alcohol.[12]

Scientists also can scan the genome to identify genes whose activity differs among animals that respond differently to alcohol. The methods used are designed to measure the amount of messenger RNA which, as the first intermediary in the process by which DNA is translated into protein, is a reflection of gene expression. The advantage of this approach is its power to survey the activities of thousands of genes, some of which might not otherwise have been identified as candidates for involvement in alcohol-related behavior. Recent work in rats identified a gene that is differentially expressed in brain regions of alcohol-preferring rats and alcohol-nonpreferring rats. The gene is within an already identified QTL for alcohol preference and codes for alpha-synuclein, a protein that has been shown to regulate dopamine transmission.[13]

Genetic Studies in Humans

Knowledge gained from animal studies has assisted scientists in identifying the genes underlying brain chemistry in humans. Much research suggests that genes affecting the activity of the neurotransmitters serotonin and GABA (gamma-aminobutyric acid) are likely candidates for involvement in alcoholism risk. A recent preliminary study looked at five genes related to these two neurotransmitters in a group of men who had been followed over a 15-year period.[14] The men who had particular variants of genes for a serotonin transporter and for one type of GABA receptor showed lower response to alcohol at age 20 and were more likely to have met the criteria for alcoholism. Another study found that college students with a particular variant of the serotonin transporter gene consumed more alcohol per occasion, more often drank expressly to become inebriated, and engaged more frequently in binge drinking than students with another variant of the gene.[15] The relationships between neurotransmitter genes and alcoholism are complex, however; not all studies have shown a connection between alcoholism risk and these genes.

Individual variation in response to stressors such as pain is genetically influenced and helps shape susceptibility to psychiatric diseases, including alcoholism. Scientists recently found that a common genetic variation in an enzyme (catechol-O-methyltransferase) that metabolizes the neurotransmitters dopamine and norepinephrine results in a less efficient form of the enzyme and increased pain susceptibility.[16] Scientists in another study found that the same genetic variant influences anxiety in women. In this study, women who had the enzyme variant scored higher on measures of anxiety and exhibited an electroencephalogram (EEG) pattern associated with anxiety disorders and alcoholism.[17]

The drug naltrexone has been shown to help some, but not all, alcohol-dependent patients reduce their drinking. Preliminary results from a recent study showed that alcoholic patients with different variations in the gene for a receptor on which naltrexone is known to act (the mu-opioid receptor) responded differently to treatment with the drug.[18] This work demonstrates how genetic typing may in the future be helpful in tailoring treatment for alcoholism to each individual.

The National Institute on Alcohol Abuse and Alcoholism's (NIAAA) Collaborative Study on the Genetics of Alcoholism (COGA) is searching for alcohol-related genes through studies of families with multiple generations of alcoholism. Using existing markers—known variations in the DNA sequence that serve as signposts along the length of a chromosome—and observing to what extent specific markers are inherited along with alcoholism risk, they have found "hotspots" for alcoholism risk on five chromosomes and a protective area on one chromosome near the location of genes for alcohol dehydrogenase.[19] They have also examined patterns of brain waves measured by electroencephalogram. EEGs measure differences in electrical potential across the brain caused by synchronized firing of many neurons. Brain wave patterns are characteristic to individuals and are shaped genetically—they are quantitative genetic traits, varying along a spectrum among individuals. COGA researchers have found that reduced amplitude of one wave that characteristically occurs after a stimulus correlates with alcohol dependence, and they have identified chromosomal regions that appear to affect this P300 wave amplitude.[20] Recently, COGA researchers found that the shape of a characteristic brain wave measured in the frequency stretch between 13 and 25 cycles per second (the "beta" wave) reflected gene variations at a specific chromosomal site containing genes for one type of GABA receptor.[21] They suggest that this site is in or near a previously identified QTL for alcoholism risk. Thus, brain wave patterns reflect underlying genetic variation in a receptor for a neurotransmitter known to be involved in the brain's response to alcohol. Findings of this type promise to help researchers identify markers of alcoholism risk and ultimately, suggest ways to reduce the risk or to treat the disease pharmacologically.

Genetics Research—A Commentary by NIAAA Director, Ting-Kai Li, M.D.

Even from the first drink, individuals differ substantially in their response to alcohol. Genetics research is helping us understand how genes shape the metabolic and behavioral response to alcohol and what makes one person more vulnerable to addiction than another. An understanding of the genetic underpinnings of alcoholism can help us identify those at risk and, in the long term, provide the foundation for tailoring prevention and treatment according to the particular physiology of each individual.

References

1. National Institute on Alcohol Abuse and Alcoholism (NIAAA). The Genetics of Alcoholism. *Alcohol Alert* No. 18. Rockville, MD: NIAAA, 1992.

2. Heath, A.C.; Bucholz, K.K.; Madden, P.A.F.; et al. Genetic and environmental contributions to alcohol dependence risk in a national twin sample: Consistency of findings in women and men. *Psychological Medicine* 27:1381–1396, 1997.

3. Heath, A.C., and Martin, N.G. Genetic influences on alcohol consumption patterns and problem drinking: Results from the Australian NH&MRC twin panel follow-up survey. *Annals of the New York Academy of Sciences* 708:72–85, 1994.

4. Kendler, K.S.; Neale, M.C.; Heath, A.C.; et al. A twin-family study of alcoholism in women. *American Journal of Psychiatry* 151:707–715, 1994.

5. Prescott, C.A., and Kendler, K.S. Genetic and environmental contributions to alcohol abuse and dependence in a population-based sample of male twins. *American Journal of Psychiatry* 156: 34–40, 1999.

6. Crabbe, J.C. Alcohol and genetics: New models. *American Journal of Medical Genetics (Neuropsychiatric Genetics)* 114:969–974, 2002.

7. Tabakoff, B., and Hoffman, P.L. Animal models in alcohol research. *Alcohol Research & Health* 24(2):77–84, 2000.

8. Li, T.K. Pharmacogenetics of responses to alcohol and genes that influence alcohol drinking. *Journal of Studies on Alcohol* 61:5–12, 2000.

9. Makimoto, K. Drinking patterns and drinking problems among Asian-Americans and Pacific Islanders. *Alcohol Health & Research World* 22(4):270–275, 1998.

10. Bowers, B.J. Applications of transgenic and knockout mice in alcohol research. *Alcohol Research & Health* 24(3):175–184, 2000.

11. Crabbe, J.C.; Phillips, T.J.; Buck, K.J.; et al. Identifying genes for alcohol and drug sensitivity: Recent progress and future directions. *Trends in Neurosciences* 22(4):173–179, 1999.

12. Pandey, S.C.; Carr, L.G.; Heilig, M.; et al. Neuropeptide Y and alcoholism: Genetic, molecular, and pharmacological evidence. *Alcoholism: Clinical and Experimental Research* 27:149–154, 2003.

13. Liang, T.; Spence, J.; Liu, L.; et al. a-Synuclein maps to a quantitative trait locus for alcohol preference and is differentially expressed in alcohol-preferring and -nonpreferring rats. *Proceedings of the National Academy of Sciences of the U.S.A.* 100(8): 4690–4695, 2003.

14. Schuckit, M.A.; Mazzanti, C.; Smith, T.L.; et al. Selective genotyping for the role of 5-HT_{2A}, 5-HT_{2C}, and $GABA_{a6}$, receptors and the serotonin transporter in the level of response to alcohol: A pilot study. *Biological Psychiatry* 45: 647–651, 1999.

15. Herman, A.I.; Philbeck, J.W.; Vasilopoulos, N.L.; and Depetrillo, P.B. Serotonin transporter promoter polymorphism and differences in alcohol consumption behaviour in a college student population. *Alcohol and Alcoholism* 38: 446–449, 2003.

16. Zubieta, J.-K.; Heitzeg, M.M.; Smith, Y.R.; et al. COMT val[158]met genotype affects μ-opioid neurotransmitter responses to a pain stressor. *Science* 299:1240–1243, 2003.

17. Enoch, M.A.; Xu, K.; Ferro, E.; et al. Genetic origins of anxiety in women: A role for a functional catechol-O-methyltransferase polymorphism. *Psychiatric Genetics* 13(1):33–41, 2003.

18. Oslin, D.W.; Berrettini, W.; Kranzler, H.R.; et al. A functional polymorphism of the μ-opioid receptor gene is associated with naltrexone response in alcohol-dependent patients. *Neuropsychopharmacology* 28:1546–1552, 2003.

19. Edenberg, H.J. The collaborative study on the genetics of alcoholism: An update. *Alcohol Research & Health* 26(3):214–217, 2002.

20. Begleiter, H.; Porjesz, B.; Reich, T.; et al. Quantitative trait loci analysis of human event-related brain potentials: P3 voltage. *Electroencephalography and Clinical Neurophysiology* 103(3):244–250, 1998.

21. Porjesz, B.; Almasy, L.; Edenberg, H.J.; et al. Linkage disequilibrium between the beta frequency of the human EEG and a $GABA_A$ receptor gene locus. *Proceedings of the National Academy of Sciences of the U.S.A.* 99:3729–3733, 2002.

Section 48.2

Gene Linked to Drug Addiction

Howard Hughes Medical Institute (HHMI) investigators at Duke University Medical Center have linked a gene previously shown to play a role in learning and memory to the early manifestations of drug addiction in the brain. Although scientists had previously speculated that similar brain processes underlie aspects of learning and addiction, the current study in mice is the first to identify a direct molecular link between the two.

The findings suggest new genetic approaches for assessing an individual's susceptibility to drug addiction. They also illuminate the complex series of molecular events that underlie addiction, the researchers said, and ultimately may lead to new therapeutic methods to interfere with that process, thereby curbing the cravings common to addiction.

The Duke-based study, which examined genes involved in the brain's response to cocaine, appeared in the February 19, 2004, issue of *Neuron*. The work was supported by the National Institutes of Health, the Zaffaroni Foundation and the Wellcome Trust.

"There has been the idea that brain changes in response to psychostimulants may be similar to those critical for learning and memory," said Marc G. Caron, Ph.D., an HHMI investigator at Duke. "Now, for the first time, we have found a molecule that links drug-induced plasticity in one part of the brain to a mechanism that underlies learning and memory in another brain region." Caron is also interim director of the Center for Models of Human Disease, part of Duke's Institute for Genome Sciences and Policy, and James B. Duke professor of cell biology.

Previous work by other researchers revealed that exposure to cocaine triggers changes in a brain region called the striatum—a reward center that also plays a fundamental role in movement and emotional responses. Cocaine leads to a sharp increase in communication among nerve cells in the striatum that use dopamine as their chemical messenger. This brain chemical surge is responsible for the feeling of pleasure, or high, that leads drug users to crave more.

"Drugs essentially hijack the brain's natural reward system," thereby leading to addiction, explained Wei-Dong Yao, Ph.D., an HHMI fellow at Duke and first author of the new study.

The study sought to identify genes involved in the brain's heightened response after drug use. The researchers compared the activity of more than 36,000 genes in the striatum of mice that had "supersensitivity" to cocaine due to a genetic defect or prior cocaine exposure, with the gene activity in the same brain region of normal mice. The genetic screen revealed six genes with consistently increased or decreased activity in super-sensitive versus normal mice, the team reported.

The protein encoded by one of the genes—known as postsynaptic density-95 or PSD-95—dropped by half in the brains of super-sensitive mice, the researchers found. The protein had never before been linked to addiction, Caron said, but had been shown by Seth Grant, a member of the research team at the Wellcome Trust Sanger Institute, to play a role in learning. Mice lacking PSD-95 take longer than normal mice to learn their way around a maze. In other words, mice with normal amounts of PSD-95 appear less likely to become addicted and more likely to learn.

Two of the other five genes had earlier been suggested to play a role in addiction. The function of the remaining three genes is not known, Caron said, and will be the focus of further investigation.

Among the mice more responsive to the effects of cocaine, the decline in PSD-95 occurred only in the striatum, while levels of the protein in other brain regions remained unaffected. In normal mice, the protein shift occurred after three injections of cocaine and lasted for more than two months.

The researchers also measured the activity of nerve cells in brain slices from the different groups of mice. Neurons in the brains of super-sensitive mice exhibited a greater response to electrical stimulation than did the nerve cells of control mice. Neurons from mice lacking a functional copy of PSD-95 showed a similar increase in activity, the team reported.

Mice deficient in PSD-95 also became more hyperactive than normal mice following cocaine injection, further linking the protein to the drug's brain effects. However, the deficient mice failed to gain further sensitivity upon repeated cocaine exposure, as mice typically do.

"Drug abuse is a complex disorder and will therefore be influenced by multiple genes," Caron noted. "PSD-95 represents one cog in the wheel."

The brain protein likely plays a role in addiction to other drugs—including nicotine, alcohol, morphine and heroine—because they all exert effects through dopamine, Caron added. Natural variation in brain levels of PSD-95 might lead to differences in individual susceptibility to drugs of abuse, he suggested. The gene might therefore represent a useful marker for measuring such differences.

The researchers will next examine the effects of PSD-95 on the addictive behavior of mice, Caron said. For example, they will test whether PSD-95-deficient mice self-administer greater amounts of cocaine than do normal mice.

Other study investigators at Duke include Raul Gainetdinov, M.D., Tatyana Sotnikova, Ph.D., Michel Cyr, Ph.D., Jean-Martin Beaulieu, Ph.D. and Gonzalo Torres, Ph.D. Margaret Arbuckle, Ph.D., of the University of Edinburgh also contributed to the research.

Section 48.3

Is There an Inherited Vulnerability to Nicotine Addiction?

"Evidence Builds That Genes Influence Cigarette Smoking," by Patrick Zickler, *NIDA NOTES*, Volume 15, Number 2, National Institute on Drug Abuse (NIDA), August, 2000.

More than one in four Americans older than 17 regularly smokes cigarettes despite increasing public awareness of tobacco's severe health risks. Some start younger than others and, among those who try to quit, some are more successful than others. National Institute on Drug Abuse (NIDA)-supported scientists are finding increasing evidence that these differences may be due in part to an inherited vulnerability to nicotine addiction.

A Medical College of Virginia study involving 949 female twin pairs found genetic factors to be more influential than environmental factors in smoking initiation and nicotine dependence. Likewise, a St. Louis University study of 3,356 male twin pairs found genetic factors to be more influential for dependence on nicotine and alcohol.

At the St. Louis University Health Sciences Center, Dr. William True and Dr. Hong Xian interviewed male twin pairs to assess genetic influences on smoking. In twin studies, researchers compare patterns of tobacco use in fraternal and identical twin pairs, who typically are exposed to common environmental influences. If genes play a role in determining tobacco use, identical twins—who share the same genes—will be more similar in their use of tobacco than fraternal twins, who share roughly half of their genes. The St. Louis University researchers found that among the 3,356 twin pairs studied, genetic factors make a stronger contribution to nicotine dependence (61 percent) than do environmental factors (39 percent) and also play a more prominent role (55 percent) than environmental factors (45 percent) in alcohol dependence. In another study, Dr. Kenneth Kendler and his colleagues at the Medical College of Virginia in Richmond interviewed 949 female twin pairs and found that genetic factors play a more important role (78 percent) than do environmental factors (22 percent) in smoking initiation and in nicotine dependence (72 percent vs. 28 percent).

"These studies emphasize the importance of understanding the role of genetic influences in smoking," says Dr. Jaylan Turkkan, chief of NIDA's Behavioral Sciences Research Branch. "The more we understand about vulnerabilities, risks, and possible protective factors, the better able we will be to tailor treatments that help people stop smoking."

Other NIDA-supported scientists are studying genes that are polymorphic—that is, in different individuals the same gene has slight variations called alleles—and have found that individuals with one type of allele are more likely to begin smoking or to have greater success quitting than are individuals with another type. For example, researchers at the University of Toronto have found that different alleles in a gene that helps regulate nicotine metabolism may protect some smokers from becoming dependent on nicotine.

Dr. Caryn Lerman, principal investigator of the NIDA-supported Transdisciplinary Tobacco Use Research Center at Georgetown University in Washington, D.C., and her colleagues studied two genes, designated *SLC6A3* and *DRD2*, that may influence smoking behavior by affecting the action of the brain chemical dopamine. In a study involving 289 smokers and 233 nonsmokers (42 percent male, 58 percent female, average age 43), the researchers found that smokers were less likely to have an allele designated *SLC6A3-9* (46.7 percent) than were nonsmokers (55.8 percent). The likelihood of smoking was even lower if the individual had both the *SLC6A3-9* allele and the *DRD2-A2* allele. In addition, Dr. Lerman observed that smokers with the *SLC6A3-9* allele were more likely to have started smoking later and to have had longer periods of smoking cessation than those without the allele. These findings imply that the allele may impart a protective effect. Therefore, Dr. Lerman suggests, smokers without the *SLC6A3-9* allele may be better able to quit smoking if their treatment incorporates a medication such as bupropion that acts on the brain's dopamine pathway. This hypothesis is currently being tested in a randomized trial.

Dr. Lerman and her colleagues also studied a polymorphism in a gene, designated *5-HTTLPR*, that helps regulate the brain chemical serotonin to determine the gene's possible role in smoking. The polymorphism has two alleles, one designated the short, or S, allele, the other the long, or L allele. In previous studies the S allele has been linked to neuroticism—an anxiety-related personality trait. Dr. Lerman and her colleagues studied 185 smokers (46 percent male, 54 percent female, and average age 45) to investigate the possible relationship between genetically influenced neuroticism and smoking behavior. They found that neuroticism was associated with increased nicotine dependence, smoking for stimulation, and smoking to relieve negative mood in the group of smokers who had the S allele. Among smokers with the L allele, neuroticism was not associated with these smoking patterns. "Anxious persons tend to smoke more and have more difficulty quitting," Dr. Lerman says. The new findings suggest that among smokers with neuroticism, determining the *5-HTTLPR* genotype may help identify who will be more responsive to a particular type of treatment. "Once validated, these results may lead to targeted pharmacotherapy for smoking cessation," says Dr. Lerman.

"This area of research represents our first small steps along a very complicated path to understanding the role that genes play in drug abuse," notes Dr. Harold Gordon of NIDA's Clinical Neurobiology Branch. "Many genes interact with each other and with other biological and environmental factors. Defining these interactions and understanding their influence on nicotine addiction will be crucial to development of treatments for smoking and for other addictions."

Sources

Kendler, K., et al. A population-based twin study in women of smoking initiation and nicotine dependence. *Psychological Medicine* 29(2): 299–308, 1999.

Lerman, C., et al. Evidence suggesting the role of specific genetic factors in cigarette smoking. *Health Psychology* 18(1):14–20, 1999.

Lerman, C., et al. Interacting effects of the serotonin transporter gene and neuroticism in smoking practices and nicotine dependence. *Molecular Psychiatry* 5:189–192, 2000.

True, W.R., et al. Common genetic vulnerability for nicotine and alcohol dependence in men. *Archives of General Psychiatry* 56(7):655–661, 1999.

Part Five

Genetics and Family Matters

Chapter 49

Genetic Counseling

If you and your partner are newly pregnant, you may be amazed at the number and variety of prenatal tests available to you. Blood tests, urine tests, monthly medical exams, diet questionnaires, and family history forms crowd your schedule and your desk, but each of these helps to assess the health of you and your baby—and to predict any potential health risks.

Unlike your parents, you may also have the option of genetic testing. These tests identify the likelihood of passing certain genetic diseases or disorders (those caused by a defect in the genes, the tiny, DNA-containing units of heredity that determine the characteristics and functioning of the entire body) to your children. Some of the more familiar genetic disorders are Down syndrome, cystic fibrosis, sickle cell anemia, and Tay-Sachs disease (a fatal disease affecting the central nervous system). If your history suggests that genetic testing would be helpful, you may be referred to a genetic counselor. Or you might decide to seek out genetic counseling yourself.

What do genetic counselors do, and how can they help your family-to-be?

This information was provided by KidsHealth, one of the largest resources online for medically reviewed health information written for parents, kids, and teens. For more articles like this one, visit www.KidsHealth.org, or www.TeensHealth.org. © 2002 The Nemours Center for Children's Health Media, a division of The Nemours Foundation.

What Is Genetic Counseling?

Genetic counseling is the process of evaluating family history and medical records, ordering genetic tests, evaluating the results of this investigation, and helping parents understand and reach decisions about what to do next.

Genetic tests are done by analyzing small samples of blood or body tissues. They determine whether you, your partner, or your baby carry genes for certain inherited disorders.

Genes are made up of DNA molecules, which are the simplest building blocks of heredity. They are grouped together in specific patterns within a person's chromosomes, forming the unique "blueprint" for every physical and biological characteristic of that person.

Humans have 46 chromosomes, arranged in pairs in every living cell of our bodies. When the egg and sperm join at conception, half of each chromosomal pair is inherited from each parent. This newly formed combination of chromosomes then copies itself again and again during fetal growth and development, passing identical genetic information to each new cell in the growing fetus. Current science suggests that human chromosomes carry about 30,000 genes. An error in just one gene (and in some instances, even the alteration of a single piece of DNA) can sometimes be the cause for a serious medical condition.

Some diseases, such as Huntington's disease (a degenerative nerve disease) and Marfan syndrome (a connective tissue disorder), can be inherited from just one parent. Most disorders cannot occur unless both the mother and father pass along the gene. Some of these are cystic fibrosis, sickle cell anemia, and Tay-Sachs disease. Other diseases, such as Down syndrome, are not inherited. In general, they result from an error (mutation) in the cell division process during conception or fetal development. Still others, such as achondroplasia (the most common form of dwarfism), may either be inherited or the result of a genetic mutation.

Genetic tests don't yield easy-to-understand results. They can reveal the presence, absence, or malformation of genes or chromosomes. Deciphering what these complex tests mean is where a genetic counselor comes in.

Who Are Genetic Counselors?

Genetic counselors are professionals who have completed a master's program in medical genetics and counseling skills. They then pass a certification exam administered by the American Board of

Genetic Counseling. This profession has existed officially only since 1971, when the first class of master's degree genetic counselors graduated from Sarah Lawrence College. (Interestingly, your counselor will probably be a "she." According to a January 2000 survey by the National Society of Genetic Counselors, 94% of genetic counselors are female.)

Genetic counselors can help identify and interpret the risks of an inherited disorder, explain inheritance patterns, suggest testing, and lay out possible scenarios. (They refer you to a doctor or a laboratory for the actual tests.) They will explain the meaning of the medical science involved. They also provide support and address any emotional issues often raised by the results of the genetic testing.

Who Should See One?

Most couples planning a pregnancy or who are expecting do not need genetic counseling. About 3% of babies are born with birth defects each year, according to the U.S. Centers for Disease Control and Prevention—and of the malformations that do occur, the most common are also among the most treatable. Cleft palate and clubfoot, two of the more common birth defects, can be surgically repaired, as can many heart malformations.

The best time to seek genetic counseling is before becoming pregnant, when a counselor can help assess your risk factors. But even after you become pregnant, a meeting with a genetic counselor can still be helpful. Robert Resta, a genetic counselor, cites the example of babies born diagnosed with spina bifida before birth. Recent research suggests that delivering a baby with spina bifida via cesarean section (avoiding the trauma of travel through the birth canal) can minimize damage to the baby's spine—and perhaps reduce the likelihood that the child will need a wheelchair.

You should consider genetic counseling if any of the following risk factors apply to you:

- If a standard prenatal screening test (such as the alpha fetoprotein test) yields an abnormal result.

- If an amniocentesis yields an unexpected result (such as a chromosomal defect in the unborn baby).

- If either parent or a close relative has an inherited disease or birth defect.

- If either parent already has children with birth defects or genetic disorders.

- If the mother-to-be has had two or more miscarriages or babies that died in infancy.

- If the mother-to-be will be 35 or older when the baby is born. (Chances of having a child with Down syndrome increase with the mother's age: a 35-year-old woman has a one in 350 chance of conceiving a child with Down syndrome. This chance increases to one in 110 by age 40 and one in 30 by age 45.)

- If parents are concerned about genetic defects that occur frequently in their ethnic or racial group. (African-American couples are most at risk for having a child with sickle cell anemia; Jewish couples of central or eastern European descent may be carriers of Tay-Sachs disease; couples of Italian, Greek, or Middle Eastern descent may carry the gene for thalassemia, a red blood cell disorder.)

What to Expect During a Visit With a Genetic Counselor

Before you meet with a genetic counselor in person, you will be asked to gather information about your family history. The counselor will want to know of any relatives with genetic disorders, multiple miscarriages, and early or unexplained deaths. The counselor will also want to look over your medical records, including any ultrasounds, prenatal test results, past pregnancies, and medications or you may have taken before or during pregnancy.

If more tests are necessary, the counselor will help you set up those appointments and track the paperwork. When results come in, the counselor will call you with the news. Often, counselor will encourage you to come in for a discussion.

The counselor will study your records before meeting with you so you can make the best use of your time together. During your session, he or she will go over any gaps or potential problem areas in your family or medical history. The counselor can then help you understand the inheritance patterns of any potential disorders and help assess your chances of having a child with those disorders.

He or she will distinguish between risks that every pregnancy faces and risks that you personally face. Even if you discover you have a particular problem gene, science cannot always predict the severity of the related disease. For instance, a child with cystic fibrosis can have debilitating lung problems—or, less commonly, milder respiratory symptoms.

After Counseling

You and your family will have to decide what to do next. Genetic counselors help you adjust to the difficulties and uncertainties you face and understand your options.

If you've learned prior to conception that you and/or your partner is at high risk for having a child with a severe or fatal defect, your options might include:

- pre-implantation diagnosis, which occurs when eggs that have been fertilized in vitro (in a laboratory, outside of the womb) are tested for defects at the 8-cell (blastocyst) stage—and only nonaffected blastocysts are implanted in the uterus to establish a pregnancy

- using donor sperm or donor eggs

- adoption

If you've received a prenatal diagnosis of a severe or fatal defect, your options might include:

- preparing yourself for the challenges you'll face when you have your baby

- fetal surgery to repair the defect before birth (Surgery can only be used to treat some defects, such as spina bifida or congenital diaphragmatic hernia, a hole in the diaphragm that can cause severely underdeveloped lungs. Most defects cannot be surgically repaired.)

- ending the pregnancy

For some families, knowing that they will have an infant with a severe or fatal genetic condition seems too much to bear. Other families are able to adapt to the news—and to the birth—remarkably well.

Genetic counselors can share the experiences they've had with other families in your situation. But they will not suggest a particular course of action. A good genetic counselor understands that what is right for one family may not be right for another.

Genetic counselors can, however, refer you to specialists for further help. For instance, many babies with Down syndrome are born with heart defects. Your counselor might encourage you to meet with a cardiologist to discuss heart surgery, and a neonatologist to discuss the care of a post-operative newborn. Genetic counselors can also refer you to social workers, support groups, or mental health professionals to help you adjust to and prepare for your complex new reality.

Finding a Genetic Counselor

Working with a genetic counselor can be reassuring and informative, especially if you or your partner have known risk factors. Talk to your doctor if you feel you would benefit from genetic counseling. Many doctors have a list of local genetic counselors with whom they work. You can also contact the National Society for Genetic Counselors for more information.

—Reviewed by Linda Nicholson, MS, MC,

Chapter 50

Genetic Testing

What is genetic testing?

Genetic testing is a type of medical test that identifies changes in chromosomes, genes, or proteins. Most of the time, testing is used to find changes that are associated with inherited disorders. The results of a genetic test can confirm or rule out a suspected genetic condition or help determine a person's chance of developing or passing on a genetic disorder. Several hundred genetic tests are currently in use, and more are being developed.

Genetic testing is voluntary. Because testing has both benefits and limitations, the decision about whether to be tested is a personal and complex one. A genetic counselor can help by providing information about the pros and cons of the test and discussing the social and emotional aspects of testing.

What are the uses of genetic testing?

Genetic testing can provide information about a person's genes and chromosomes throughout life. Available types of testing include:

Newborn screening: Newborn screening is used just after birth to identify genetic disorders that can be treated early in life. The

"Genetic Testing," from *Genetics Home Reference: Your Guide to Understanding Genetic Conditions,* a service of the U.S. National Library of Medicine, March 2004; available online at http://ghr.nlm.nih.gov.

routine testing of infants for certain disorders is the most widespread use of genetic testing—millions of babies are tested each year in the United States. All states currently test infants for phenylketonuria (a genetic disorder that causes mental retardation if left untreated) and hypothyroidism (a disorder of the thyroid gland). Some states also test for other genetic disorders.

Diagnostic testing: Diagnostic testing is used to diagnose or rule out a particular genetic or chromosomal condition. It is usually offered to people who have signs of a particular disorder. This type of testing can be performed at any time during a person's life, but is not available for all genetic conditions. The results of a diagnostic test can influence a person's choices about health care and the management of symptoms.

Carrier testing: Carrier testing is used to identify people who carry one copy of a gene mutation that, when present in two copies, causes a genetic disorder. This type of testing is offered to individuals who have a family history of a genetic disorder and to people in ethnic groups with an increased risk of specific genetic conditions. If both parents are tested, the test can provide information about a couple's risk of having a child with a genetic condition.

Prenatal testing: Prenatal testing is used to detect changes in a fetus's genes or chromosomes before birth. This type of testing is offered to couples with an increased risk of having a baby with a genetic or chromosomal disorder. In some cases, prenatal testing can lessen a couple's uncertainty or help them make decisions about a pregnancy. It cannot identify all possible inherited disorders and birth defects, however.

Predictive and presymptomatic testing: These types of testing are used to detect gene mutations associated with disorders that appear later in life. Predictive testing can identify mutations that increase a person's risk of developing disorders with a genetic basis, such as certain types of cancer. Presymptomatic testing can determine whether a person will develop a genetic disorder, such as Huntington disease (an inherited brain disorder that appears during midlife), before any symptoms appear. The results of predictive and presymptomatic testing can help people make decisions about medical care.

Forensic testing: Forensic testing uses DNA sequences to identify an individual for legal purposes. Unlike the tests described above, forensic testing is not used to detect gene mutations associated with disease. This type of testing can identify crime or catastrophe victims, rule out or implicate a crime suspect, or establish biological relationships between people (for example, paternity).

How is genetic testing done?

Once a person decides to proceed with genetic testing, a medical geneticist, genetic counselor, primary care doctor, or specialist can order the test. Genetic testing is often done as part of a genetic consultation.

Genetic tests are performed on a sample of blood, hair, skin, amniotic fluid (the fluid that surrounds a fetus during pregnancy), or other tissue. For example, a procedure called a buccal smear uses a small brush or cotton swab to collect a sample of cells from the inside surface of the cheek. The sample is sent to a laboratory where technicians look for specific changes in chromosomes, DNA, or proteins, depending on the suspected disorder. The laboratory reports the test results in writing to a person's doctor or genetic counselor.

Newborn screening tests are done on a small blood sample, which is taken by pricking the baby's heel. Unlike other types of genetic testing, a parent will usually only receive the result if it is positive. If the test result is positive, additional testing is needed to determine whether the baby has a genetic disorder.

Before a person has a genetic test, it is important that he or she understands the testing procedure, the benefits and limitations of the test, and the possible consequences of the test results. The process of educating a person about the test and obtaining permission is called informed consent.

What is the cost of genetic testing, and how long does it take to get the results?

The cost of genetic testing can range from under $100 to more than $2,000, depending on the nature and complexity of the test. The cost increases if more than one test is necessary or if multiple family members must be tested to obtain a meaningful result. For newborn screening, costs vary by state. Some states cover part of the total cost, but most charge a fee of $15 to $60 per infant.

From the date that a sample is taken, it may take a few weeks to several months to receive the test results. Results for prenatal testing are usually available more quickly because time is an important consideration in making decisions about a pregnancy. The doctor or genetic counselor who orders a particular test can provide specific information about the cost and time frame associated with that test.

Will health insurance cover the costs of genetic testing?

In many cases, health insurance plans will cover the costs of genetic testing when it is recommended by a person's doctor. Health insurance providers have different policies about which tests are covered, however. A person interested in submitting the costs of testing may wish to contact his or her insurance company beforehand to ask about coverage.

Some people may choose not to use their insurance to pay for testing because the results of a genetic test can affect a person's health insurance coverage. Instead, they may opt to pay out-of-pocket for the test. People considering genetic testing may want to find out more about their state's privacy protection laws before they ask their insurance company to cover the costs.

What are the benefits of genetic testing?

Genetic testing has potential benefits whether the results are positive or negative for a gene mutation. Test results can provide a sense of relief from uncertainty and help people make informed decisions about managing their health care. For example, a negative result can eliminate the need for unnecessary checkups and screening tests in some cases. A positive result can direct a person toward available prevention, monitoring, and treatment options. Some test results can also help people make decisions about having children. Newborn screening can identify genetic disorders early in life so treatment can be started as early as possible.

What are the risks and limitations of genetic testing?

The physical risks associated with most genetic tests are very small, particularly for those tests that require only a blood sample or buccal smear (a procedure that samples cells from the inside surface of the cheek). The procedures used for prenatal testing carry a small but real risk of losing the pregnancy (miscarriage) because they require a sample of amniotic fluid or tissue from around the fetus.

Many of the risks associated with genetic testing involve the emotional, social, or financial consequences of the test results. People may feel angry, depressed, anxious, or guilty about their results. In some cases, genetic testing creates tension within a family because the results can reveal information about other family members in addition to the person who is tested. The possibility of genetic discrimination in employment or insurance is also a concern.

Genetic testing can provide only limited information about an inherited condition. The test often can't determine if a person will show symptoms of a disorder, how severe the symptoms will be, or whether the disorder will progress over time. Another major limitation is the lack of treatment strategies for many genetic disorders once they are diagnosed.

A genetics professional can explain in detail the benefits, risks, and limitations of a particular test. It is important that any person who is considering genetic testing understand and weigh these factors before making a decision.

What is genetic discrimination?

Genetic discrimination occurs when people are treated differently by their employer or insurance company because they have a gene mutation that causes or increases the risk of an inherited disorder. People who undergo genetic testing may be at risk for genetic discrimination.

The results of a genetic test are normally included in a person's medical records. When a person applies for life, disability, or health insurance, the insurance company may ask to look at these records before making a decision about coverage. An employer may also have the right to look at an employee's medical records. As a result, genetic test results could affect a person's insurance coverage or employment. People making decisions about genetic testing should be aware that when test results are placed in their medical records, the results might not be kept private.

Fear of discrimination is a common concern among people considering genetic testing. Several laws at the federal and state levels help protect people against genetic discrimination; however, genetic testing is a fast-growing field and these laws don't cover every situation.

How does genetic testing in a research setting differ from clinical genetic testing?

The main differences between clinical genetic testing and research testing are the purpose of the test and who receives the results. The goals of research testing include finding unknown genes, learning how genes work, and advancing our understanding of genetic conditions. The results of testing done as part of a research study are usually not available to patients or their healthcare providers. Clinical testing, on the other hand, is done to find out about an inherited disorder in an individual patient or family. People receive the results of a clinical test and can use them to help them make decisions about medical care or reproductive issues.

It is important for people considering genetic testing to know whether the test is available on a clinical or research basis. Clinical and research testing both involve a process of informed consent in which patients learn about the testing procedure, the risks and benefits of the test, and the potential consequences of testing.

Chapter 51

Evaluating Gene Tests

Considerations for evaluating gene testing include test quality, the potential usefulness of the information the test provides, available preventive or treatment options, and social issues.

Test Quality

The analytical validity of a test can be determined by its:

- *Sensitivity:* Test detects the mutations it was designed to detect.

- *Specificity:* Test detects only those mutations it was designed to detect (for example, it does not flag other DNA sequence variations, some of which may be normal variation).

Clinical Utility

What practical information can this test provide? What is the probability that a person who has or will get a disease will test positively? There is a need to consider test results in the context of mutation variability, gene penetrance, and gene expressivity.

"Evaluating Gene Tests: Some Considerations," Human Genome Project Information, Oak Ridge National Laboratory, 1998. Reviewed and updated by David A. Cooke, M.D., July 2004.

Mutation Variability (Heterogeneity)

Many different mutations can cause the same disease. Mutations can be in the same or different genes. Mutation tests often test for only the most common mutations.

Example: Cystic fibrosis (CF) is linked to more than 900 mutations (most are rare) in *CFTR* gene. Current tests are for about 25 common mutations.

It is important to consider the proportion of people with clinically significant disease that are detected by the test (clinical sensitivity). CF is much more common in some ethnic groups than others. In some groups, just one or two mutations account for nearly all CF cases. Both can have a large effect on test reliability. For example, one particular mutation causes 75% of all CF cases in Caucasians of northern European descent, so a test for this mutation gives much more reliable results in this group than for other racial groups. Overall, CF tests pick up 90% of CF mutations in whites, 50% in African Americans and Hispanics, and 30% in Asian Americans.

Gene Penetrance

Gene penetrance relates to the probability of getting the disease when mutation is present. Incomplete penetrance means that an individual with a mutation may never get the disease.

Examples: *BRCA1* and *BRCA2* genes (associated with a rare form of breast cancer) and *ApoE* gene (modifies risk of Alzheimer's disease) are associated with varying levels of penetrance.

Possible reasons for incomplete penetrance: Some mutations work together with other (unknown) mutations or with environmental factors.

Some mutations are completely penetrant—an individual with the mutation always gets the disease. Examples are Huntington disease and familial adenomatous polyposis (FAP)—a rare, inherited colon cancer that accounts for about 1% of all colorectal cancers.

Gene Expressivity

Gene expressivity impacts the range of disease severity from a mutation. Severity can vary widely for some diseases, and few specific mutations have been correlated with the severity of their expression in an individual.

Example: Severity of cystic fibrosis ranges from mild bronchial symptoms and male sterility to severe lung, pancreatic, and intestinal difficulties (usually fatal by 30 years of age). The most common mutation in Caucasians has been associated with pancreatic insufficiency, but few other correlations have been made of disease gene mutations and their particular expression.

Available Treatment Options

Few treatments or preventive strategies exist for patients testing positive for most gene tests. Unfortunately, knowledge of a gene mutation alone is insufficient information for researchers trying to devise intervention strategies. Researchers must first understand the normal function of the disease-associated gene(s) and determine how the mutation disrupts that function.

Some exceptions exist, such as that for FAP. Experts recommend that even children at high risk be screened for mutations in the *APC* gene associated with FAP, because they can be monitored more frequently for growths and effective preventive surgical options can be chosen. Left untreated, FAP causes death at an average age of 42.

Social Issues

Genetic information is personal, powerful, potentially predictive, pedigree sensitive (affects families as well as individuals), permanent, and prejudicial.

Education: Education on implications of testing and results is critical, yet only 2000 specially trained genetic counselors are currently available in the U.S., and training programs are not increasing their rolls. Most people will need to rely on primary-care physicians to explain results. This poses a great challenge for physicians, many of whom are not trained in molecular genetics. Many commercially available gene tests are still controversial in the scientific community, where their interpretation is debated.

Psychological issues: Psychological issues related to gene testing include fear of unknown, coping with uncertainty, guilt, shame, survivor guilt, and family dynamics.

Discrimination risk: The results of gene testing can lead to discrimination by employers, insurers, commercial institutions, schools, army, and others.

Ethical issues: Privacy and confidentiality, fairness in use of information, commercialization/patents, social concepts of health and disease, and reproductive rights are among the ethical issues to consider when evaluating gene testing.

Chapter 52

Prenatal Testing

Prenatal Tests

Every parent-to-be spends happy hours envisioning a healthy baby. But these daydreams are often accompanied by moments of worry— what if the baby has a serious or untreatable health problem? What would I do? Would it be my fault?

Concerns like these are completely natural, and some may be exaggerated by news stories about genetics and genetic testing, which promises that someday parents may be able to pick only "desirable" traits in their unborn children. With all the medical information available, you may feel as though you have to undergo a battery of prenatal tests to make sure your baby is healthy.

Prenatal tests can serve a useful function in terms of identifying, and sometimes treating, health problems that could endanger both you and your unborn child. However, they have limitations. As an expecting parent, you should take the time to educate yourself about these tests and to think about what you would do if a health problem is detected.

Why Are Prenatal Tests Performed?

Prenatal tests do several different things. They can identify:

This information was provided by KidsHealth, one of the largest resources online for medically reviewed health information written for parents, kids, and teens. For more articles like this one, visit www.KidsHealth.org, or www.TeensHealth.org. © 2000 The Nemours Center for Children's Health Media, a division of The Nemours Foundation.

- treatable health problems in the mother that can affect the baby's health

- characteristics of the fetus, including size, sex, age, and placement in the uterus

- the chance that a baby has certain congenital, genetic, or chromosomal problems

- certain types of fetal abnormalities, including heart problems

The last two items on this list may seem the same, but there's a key difference. Some prenatal tests are screening tests and only reveal the possibility of a problem existing—they don't provide a definitive diagnosis. Other prenatal tests are diagnostic in nature, which means they can determine with a fair degree of certainty whether a fetus has a specific problem. Many women whose screening tests reveal the possibility of an abnormality have healthy babies, but in the interest of making the more specific determination, the screening test may be followed by a more invasive—and riskier—diagnostic test.

The issue of prenatal testing is further complicated by the fact that approximately 250 birth defects can be diagnosed in an unborn fetus—many more than can be treated or cured. This raises the question of what a parent will do once a defect or problem is detected.

What Do Prenatal Tests Find?

Among other things, routine prenatal tests can determine key things about the mother's health including her blood type, whether she suffers from gestational diabetes, her immunity to certain diseases, and whether she has a sexually transmitted disease (STD) or cervical cancer. All of these conditions can affect the health of the fetus.

Prenatal tests also can determine things about the fetus' health including whether it's one of the 2% to 3% of babies in the United States that the American College of Obstetricians and Gynecologists (ACOG) says have major congenital birth defects. There are different categories of defects screened by prenatal tests, including:

Dominant Gene Disorders

In dominant gene disorders, there's a 50/50 chance a child will inherit the gene from the affected parent and have the disorder. Dominant gene disorders include:

- achondroplasia, a rare abnormality of the skeleton causing shorter-than-normal arms and legs

- Huntington disease, a disease of the nervous system that causes neurologic deterioration affecting people in their 30s and 40s

Recessive Gene Disorders

Because there are so many genes in each cell, everyone carries some abnormal recessive genes, but most people don't have a defect because the normal gene overrules the abnormal one. But if a fetus has a pair of abnormal recessive genes (one from each parent), the child will have the disorder. It's more likely for this to happen in children born to certain ethnic groups or to parents who are blood relatives. Recessive gene disorders include:

- cystic fibrosis (most common among people of northern European descent), a disease that causes the respiratory system to produce thick mucus that clogs the lungs

- sickle cell disease (most common among people of African descent), a disease where red blood cells form a "sickle" shape, rather than the typical donut shape, get caught in blood vessels, and cut off oxygen to tissues

- Tay-Sachs disease (most common among people of European [Ashkenazi] Jewish descent), a disorder causing mental retardation, blindness, seizures, and death

- beta thalassemia (most common among people of Mediterranean descent), a disorder causing anemia

X-Linked Disorders

These disorders are determined by genes on the X chromosome of the pair of chromosomes that determine sex. These disorders are much more common in boys because the pair of sex chromosomes in males contains only one X chromosome (the other is a Y chromosome). If the disease gene is present on the one X chromosome, the X-linked disease shows up because there's no other paired gene to overrule the disease gene. Hemophilia is one such X linked disorder; people who have it lack a crucial clotting agent in their blood.

Chromosomal Disorders

Some chromosomal disorders are inherited, but most are caused by a sporadic error in the genetics of the egg or sperm. The chance of a child having these disorders increases with the age of the mother. For example, according to the ACOG, one in 1,667 live babies born to 20-year-olds have Down syndrome; that number changes to one in 378 for 35-year-olds and one in 106 for 40-year-olds. Down syndrome causes mental retardation and physical defects.

Multifactorial Disorders

This final category includes disorders that are caused by a mix of genetic and environmental factors. The frequency of these disorders varies from country to country; some can be detected during pregnancy. Multifactorial disorders include neural tube defects, which occur when the tube enclosing the spinal cord doesn't form properly. Neural tube defects include spina bifida and anencephaly. Spina bifida is also called "open spine" and occurs when the lower part of the neural tube doesn't close during embryo development, leaving the spinal cord and nerve bundles exposed. Anencephaly occurs when the brain and head don't develop properly, with the top half of the brain being completely absent. Neural tube defects have been associated with inadequate intake of folic acid during the early part of pregnancy, among other factors.

Other multifactorial disorders include:

- congenital heart defects
- club foot
- cleft lip and palate
- hip dislocations

Who Has Prenatal Tests?

Certain prenatal tests are considered routine—that is, almost all pregnant women receiving prenatal care get these tests. Others are recommended only for certain women, especially those who have what are known as high-risk pregnancies. George Macones, MD, the director of maternal/fetal medicine and director of obstetrics for the University of Pennsylvania Health System in Philadelphia, typically recommends nonroutine tests to women who:

- are age 35 or older

- have had a premature baby

- have had a baby with a birth defect—especially heart or genetic problems

- have high blood pressure, diabetes, lupus, asthma, or a seizure disorder

- have or whose partner has an ethnic background where genetic disorders are common

- have or whose partner has a family history of mental retardation

Dr. Macones is also careful to point out that although he recommends these tests, ultimately it's up to the mother if she wants to have them. "I spend a lot of time talking to parents before the mother undergoes, for example, amniocentesis," he says. "Patients need to be educated before they make decisions."

In addition to talking to their obstetricians, women who have a family history of genetic problems in their families (or whose partners do) may want to consult with a genetic counselor who can help them construct a family tree going back as far as three generations.

To decide which tests are right for you, it's important to carefully discuss with your doctor what these tests are supposed to measure, how reliable they are, the potential risks, and your options and plans if the results indicate a disorder or defect.

Routine Prenatal Tests

On your first visit to the doctor for prenatal care, you'll undergo certain tests regardless of your age or genetic background.

- *Blood tests* determine your blood type and Rh factor. If your blood is Rh negative and your partner's is Rh positive, you may develop antibodies that prove dangerous to your fetus. This can be treated through a course of injections. Blood tests also measure the level of iron in your blood and check for hepatitis B, syphilis, and HIV. You'll also be tested to see whether you're immune to rubella (German measles).

- *Urine tests* check for kidney infections and signs of gestational diabetes and pregnancy-induced high blood pressure (which can cause a specific protein to show in the urine).

521

- *Cervical tests* check for STDs (such as chlamydia and gonorrhea), cervical cancer, and group B streptococcus infection. Group B streptococcus, which are bacteria that are not transmitted sexually, can cause serious infections in newborns.

Around the 16th to 18th week of pregnancy, most women will have a maternal blood screening test performed. Also known as a "triple-marker" test, it measures the levels of a protein produced by the fetus and two pregnancy-produced hormones in the mother's blood. This test can reveal the chances that a mother is carrying a fetus with neural tube defects or Down syndrome.

It's at this point that most women will also have their first ultrasound test, which helps the doctor identify the position of the baby and its gender as well as helping to detect Down syndrome, other chromosome abnormalities, structural defects such as spina bifida and anencephaly, and inherited metabolic disorders.

Around the 24th week of pregnancy, an additional screening for gestational diabetes may be performed.

Chart of Prenatal Tests

This chart includes some tests that are now performed almost routinely in the United States and those that are performed only in high-risk pregnancies or if the doctor suspects an abnormality in the fetus.

Chorionic Villus Sampling (CVS)

Why Is This Test Performed? Chorionic villi are microscopic finger-like projections that make up the placenta. They develop from the same fertilized egg as the fetus and reflect the fetal genetic makeup. This newer alternative to amniocentesis removes some of the chorionic villi and tests them for chromosomal abnormalities, such as Down syndrome. Its advantage over amniocentesis is that it can be performed earlier, allowing more time for expectant parents to receive counseling and make decisions.

Should I Have This Test? If you are older than age 35, have a family history of genetic disorders (or a partner who does), or have a previous child with a birth defect, your doctor may recommend this test for you. ACOG says this test carries between a 0.5% and 1% risk of miscarriage. It may cause intrauterine growth retardation, prematurity, or early labor. Other risks include infection and spotting or bleeding (this is more common in the transcervical test).

When Should I Have This Test? 10 to 12 weeks

How Is the Test Performed? This test is performed in one of two ways:

- *Transcervical:* Using ultrasound as a guide, a thin tube is passed from the vagina into the cervix. Gentle suction removes a sample of tissue from the chorionic villi. No anesthetic is used, although some women do experience a pinch and cramping.

- *Transabdominal:* A needle is inserted through the abdominal wall—this minimizes chances of intrauterine infection, and in women whose uterus is tipped, reduces the chance of miscarriage. After the sample is taken, the doctor will check the fetal heart rate. You should rest for a couple hours afterward.

When Are the Results Available? Less than one week for Down syndrome or about two weeks for a thorough analysis

Maternal Blood Screening

Why Is This Test Performed? Doctors use this to test the mother's blood only for alpha-fetoprotein (AFP). AFP is the protein produced by the fetus, and it appears in varying amounts in the mother's blood and the amniotic fluid at different times during pregnancy. A certain level in the mother's blood is considered normal, but higher or lower levels may indicate a problem. This test has been expanded, however, to include two pregnancy hormones called estriol and human chorionic gonadotropin (HCG), which is why it's now sometimes referred to as a "triple screen." This test calculates a woman's individual risk of birth defects based on the levels of the three (or more) substances plus her age, weight, race, and whether she has diabetes requiring insulin treatment. It's important to note that this screening test determines risk only—it doesn't diagnose a condition.

Should I Have This Test? All women are offered this test. Remember that this is a screening, not a definite test—it indicates whether a woman is likely to be carrying an affected fetus. It's also not foolproof—spina bifida may go undetected, and some women with high levels have been found to be carrying a healthy baby. Further testing is recommended to confirm a positive result.

When Should I Have This Test? 16 to 18 weeks

How Is the Test Performed? Blood is drawn from the mother.

When Are the Results Available? Three to five days, although it may take up to a week or two.

Amniocentesis

Why Is This Test Performed? This test is used most often to detect Down syndrome and other chromosome abnormalities, structural defects such as spina bifida and anencephaly, and inherited metabolic disorders. Other common birth defects, such as heart disorders and cleft lip and palate, can't be determined using this test. Late in the pregnancy, this test can reveal if a baby's lungs are strong enough to allow the baby to breathe normally after birth, which can help the doctor make decisions about inducing labor.

Should I Have This Test? If you are older than age 35, have a family history of genetic disorders (or a partner who does), or have a previous child with a birth defect, your doctor may recommend this test for you. This test can be very accurate—close to 100%—but only certain disorders can be detected. According to the Centers for Disease Control and Prevention (CDC), the rate of miscarriage with this procedure is between one in 400 and one in 200. The procedure also carries a lower risk of uterine infection (less than one in 1,000), which can cause miscarriage.

When Should I Have This Test? 16 to 18 weeks

How Is the Test Performed? A needle is inserted through the abdominal wall into the uterus, removing some of the amniotic fluid. A local anesthetic may be used. Some women report they experience cramping when the needle enters the uterus or pressure while the doctor retrieves the sample. The doctor will check the fetus' heartbeat after the procedure to make sure it's normal. Most doctors recommend rest for a couple hours after the procedure. One ounce of fluid is withdrawn and sent to a lab for testing. The cells in the fluid are grown in a special culture and then analyzed. The specific tests conducted depend on personal and family medical history.

When Are the Results Available? Up to one month (with the possibility that the lab will ask for a repeat), but tests of lung maturity are available immediately

Ultrasound

Why Is This Test Performed? In this test, sound waves are bounced off the baby's bones and tissues to construct an image showing the baby's shape and position in the uterus. Ultrasounds were once used only in high-risk pregnancies but have become so common that they are often part of routine prenatal care. In addition to showing the fetus' age, rate of growth, position, movement, breathing, and heart rate, it shows the number of fetuses and the amount of amniotic fluid in the uterus. The test is used most often to detect Down syndrome and other chromosome abnormalities, structural defects such as spina bifida and anencephaly, and inherited metabolic disorders. Congenital heart defects, gastrointestinal and kidney malformations, and cleft lip or palate may also be determined. Ultrasound can indicate the position of the placenta in late pregnancy (which may be blocking the baby's way out of the uterus). They can be used to detect pregnancies outside the uterus and they can guide other tests by showing placement of the fetus.

Should I Have This Test? Most women have this test. You may want to ask your doctor about ultrasound. Find out if it's the most appropriate test for you and discuss the risks and benefits. There are no proven side effects of ultrasound to the mother or fetus, although it's still being studied.

When Should I Have This Test? 16 to 18 weeks (it can be done earlier and later if necessary, especially if your doctor wants to monitor fetal growth)

How Is the Test Performed? Women need to have a full bladder for a transabdominal ultrasound to be performed in the early months—you may be asked to drink a lot of water and not urinate. You'll lie on an examining table, and your abdomen will be coated with a special ultrasound gel. A technician will pass a transducer back and forth over your abdomen, while a computer translates the waves into an image called a sonogram. You may want to ask to have the picture interpreted for you, even in late pregnancy—it often doesn't look like a baby to the untrained eye. Sometimes, if the radiologist isn't getting a good enough image from the ultrasound, he or she will determine that a transvaginal ultrasound is necessary. This is especially common in early pregnancy. For this procedure, your bladder should be empty. Instead of a transducer being moved over your abdomen, the high-frequency waves will be emitted by a probe called an endovaginal transducer, which is placed in your vagina. This technique often provides improved images of the uterus and ovaries. A radiologist, who is a physician experienced in obstetric ultrasound, will analyze the images and send a signed report with his or her interpretation to your doctor.

When Are the Results Available? Immediately (but a full evaluation may take up to one week)

Glucose Screening

Why Is This Test Performed? Glucose screening checks for gestational diabetes, a short-term form of diabetes that develops in some women during pregnancy. Gestational diabetes occurs in 1% to 3% of pregnancies and can cause health problems for the baby.

Should I Have This Test? Most women have this test at 24 weeks, but if you've had high sugar in two routine urine tests, your doctor may order it earlier.

When Should I Have This Test? 24 weeks

How Is the Test Performed? Blood is drawn after you've consumed a sugary drink. If the reading is high, you'll have a glucose-tolerance test, which means you'll drink a glucose solution on an empty stomach and have your blood drawn once every hour for three hours.

When Are the Results Available? Immediately.

Nonstress Test

Why Is This Test Performed? If you've gone beyond your due date, this test uses external fetal monitoring to determine fetal movement. This test is used mostly in high-risk pregnancies or when the doctor is uncertain of fetal movement. The nonstress test can help a doctor make sure that the baby is receiving enough oxygen and that the nervous system is responding. A nonresponsive baby doesn't necessarily mean that the baby is in danger.

Should I Have This Test? Your doctor may recommend this if you have a high-risk pregnancy or if you have a low-risk pregnancy and you're past your due date.

When Should I Have This Test? One week after due date.

How Is the Test Performed? The doctor will measure the response of the fetus' heart rate to each movement the fetus makes as reported by the mother or observed by the doctor on an ultrasound screen. If the fetus doesn't move during the test, he may be asleep and the doctor may use a buzzer to wake him.

When Are the Results Available? Immediately.

Contraction Stress Test

Why Is This Test Performed? This test stimulates the uterus with Pitocin, a synthetic form of oxytocin (a hormone secreted during childbirth), and determines the effect of contractions on fetal heart rate. It's usually recommended when a nonstress test indicates a problem and can determine whether the baby's heart rate remains stable during contractions.

Should I Have This Test? This test is usually ordered if the nonstress test indicates a problem. It does have a high false-positive rate, though, and can cause labor to be induced prematurely.

When Should I Have This Test? After 40 weeks.

How Is the Test Performed? Mild contractions are brought on either by injections of Pitocin or by squeezing the mother's nipples (which causes oxytocin to be secreted). The fetus' heart rate is then monitored.

When Are the Results Available? Immediately.

Percutaneous Umbilical Vein Sampling (PUVS)

Why Is This Test Performed? This test obtains fetal blood by guiding a needle into the umbilical vein. It's primarily used in addition to ultrasound and amniocentesis if your doctor needs to quickly check your baby's chromosomes for defects or disorders or if your doctor is concerned that your baby may be anemic. The advantage to this test is its speed. There are situations (such as when a fetus shows signs of distress) in which it's helpful to know whether the fetus has a fatal chromosomal defect. If the fetus is suspected to be anemic, this test is the only way to confirm this, and it also allows transfusion while the needle is in place.

Should I Have This Test? This test is used late in a pregnancy after an abnormality has been noted on an ultrasound, when amniocentesis results are not conclusive, if the fetus may have Rh disease, or if you've been exposed to an infectious disease that could potentially affect fetal development.

When Should I Have This Test? Between 18 and 36 weeks.

How Is the Test Performed? A fine needle is passed through your abdomen and uterus into the fetal vein in the umbilical cord and blood is withdrawn for testing.

When Are the Results Available? Three days.

Talking to Your Doctor about Prenatal Tests

Prenatal tests can be stressful, and because many aren't definitive, even a negative result may not ease any anxiety you may be experiencing. Because many women who have abnormal tests end up having healthy babies and because many of the problems that are detected cannot be treated, some women decide to forgo some of the testing.

One important thing to consider is what you will do in the event that a birth defect is discovered. Implicit in much of this testing is that you can make a decision to terminate the pregnancy based on the results. Your obstetrician or a genetic counselor can help you establish priorities, give you facts, and discuss your options.

It's important to remember that tests are offered to women—they are not mandatory. You should feel free to ask your doctor why he or she is ordering a certain test, what the risks and benefits of the test are, and most importantly, what the results will—and won't—tell you.

"The women who are most stressed about tests are the women who don't understand what the results are going to be like," Dr. Macones says. "It's important that doctors educate the patient—if not right in the office, then by giving her literature about each type of test."

If you think that your doctor isn't answering your questions adequately, you should say so. You don't have to accept the answer "I do this test on all of my patients." Questions to ask include:

- How much will the test cost? Will it be covered by insurance?

- What do I need to do to prepare?

- How long before I get the results? How accurate is this test?

- What are you looking to get from these test results? What do you hope to learn?

- Is the procedure painful? Is it dangerous to me or the fetus? Do the potential benefits outweigh the risks?

- What could happen if I don't undergo this test?

Preventing Birth Defects

The best thing that mothers-to-be can do to avoid birth defects is to make sure they take care of their bodies during pregnancy by:

- not smoking (and avoiding second-hand smoke)

- avoiding alcohol

- eating a healthy diet and taking prenatal vitamins

- getting exercise and plenty of rest

- getting prenatal care

Dr. Macones also points out that there are women who should talk to their doctor before becoming pregnant (including women with diabetes and seizure disorders) to obtain genetic counseling.

Chapter 53

Newborn Screening Tests

What You Need to Know

All states screen newborns for certain metabolic birth defects. (Metabolic refers to chemical changes that take place within living cells.) These conditions cannot be seen in the newborn, but can cause physical problems, mental retardation and, in some cases, death.

Fortunately, most babies receive a clean bill of health when tested. When test results show that the baby has a birth defect, early diagnosis and treatment can make the difference between lifelong disabilities and healthy development.

The March of Dimes recommends that all newborns be screened for at least nine metabolic disorders and for hearing loss.

The disorders are:

- Phenylketonuria (PKU)
- Congenital hypothyroidism
- Congenital adrenal hyperplasia (CAH)
- Biotinidase deficiency
- Maple syrup urine disease
- Galactosemia

- Homocystinuria

- Sickle cell anemia

- Medium chain acyl-CoA dehydrogenase deficiency (MCAD)

Do not be overly alarmed if test results come back abnormal. The initial screening tests give only preliminary information that must be followed up by more precise testing.

Testing the Newborn for Metabolic Birth Defects

What do the tests look for?

The conditions most commonly screened for are:

- **PKU (phenylketonuria):** Babies with this disorder cannot process a substance called phenylalanine that is found in almost all food. Without treatment, phenylalanine builds up in the bloodstream and causes brain damage and mental retardation. When PKU is detected early, mental retardation can be prevented by feeding the child a special diet. All states and U.S. territories screen for PKU.

- **Hypothyroidism:** Babies with this disorder have a hormone deficiency that slows growth and brain development. If it is detected in time, a baby can be treated with oral doses of the hormone to permit normal development. All states and U.S. territories screen for hypothyroidism.

- **Galactosemia:** Babies with this disorder cannot convert galactose, a sugar present in milk, into glucose, a sugar that the body uses as an energy source. Galactosemia can cause death in infancy, or blindness and mental retardation. The treatment for the condition is to eliminate milk and all other dairy products from the baby's diet.

- **Sickle Cell Anemia:** This inherited blood disease causes bouts of pain; damage to vital organs such as the lungs, kidneys and brain; and, sometimes serious infections and death in childhood. Early treatment can prevent some of the complications of sickle cell anemia.

- **Congenital Adrenal Hyperplasia (CAH):** Babies who have this group of disorders are deficient in certain hormones. CAH affects genital development and, in severe cases, can disturb kidney function and cause death. Lifelong treatment with the missing hormones suppresses the disease.

- **Hearing Loss:** Early detection of hearing loss allows the baby to be fitted with hearing aids before six months of age. This early intervention helps prevent serious speech and language problems.

How are the tests done?

Most of the tests use a blood specimen taken before the baby leaves the hospital. The baby's heel is pricked to obtain a few drops of blood for laboratory analysis. The same blood sample can be used to screen for a number of disorders.

Usually, the baby's blood sample is sent to a state public health laboratory for testing. The health care provider responsible for the infant's care receives the results.

Hearing loss tests measure how a baby responds to sounds. The tests use either a tiny, soft earphone or microphone that is placed in the baby's ear. If these tests show abnormal results, the baby may need more extensive testing to see if he or she has hearing loss.

What should I do if my baby is diagnosed with one of the conditions?

Your baby may need treatment at a specialized pediatric center. It is essential for your child's healthy development to follow the recommendations of his or her doctor.

For More Information

Find out which tests are routinely done in your state by asking your health care provider or state health department. You can also visit the website of the National Newborn Screening and Genetics Resource Center at http://genes-r-us.uthscsa.edu.

Chapter 54

A Guide for Parents of Children with Chronic Conditions

What is a chronic condition?

All children will likely have many different health problems during infancy and childhood, but for most children these problems are relatively mild and intermittent, and do not interfere with their daily life and development. For some children, however, chronic health conditions affect their everyday lives throughout their childhood.

We'll define a chronic health condition as a health problem that lasts over three months, affects your child's normal activities, and requires lots of hospitalizations and/or home health care and/or extensive medical care.

Chronic condition is an "umbrella" term. Children with chronic illnesses may be ill or well at any given time, but they are always living with their condition. Some examples of chronic conditions include (but are not limited to):

- Asthma (the most common)

- Diabetes

"Children with Chronic Conditions," written and compiled by Jennifer Laundy, M.D. and Lina Boujaoude, M.D., with contributions from Kyla Boyse, R.N. Edited and updated by Kyla Boyse, R.N. Reviewed by Richard Solomon, M.D. Reprinted with permission from, *Your Child: Development and Behavior Resources*, http://www.med.umich.edu/1libr/yourchild/, a website of the University of Michigan Health System. Copyright © 2004 Regents of the University of Michigan. All websites listed in this chapter were verified and accessed in July 2004.

- Cerebral palsy

- Sickle cell anemia

- Cystic fibrosis

- Cancer

- AIDS

- Epilepsy

- Spina bifida

- Congenital heart problems

Even though these are very different illnesses, kids and families dealing with any chronic condition have a lot in common. Learning to live with a chronic condition can be very challenging for a child, for parents, and for siblings and friends. Read on for more information, support and resources.

How common are chronic conditions?

About 15% to 18% of children in the United States have a chronic health condition (based on the definition we're using). It's hard to estimate, though, because it really depends on how you define "chronic condition."

How might a chronic illness affect my child?

Children with chronic illnesses are more likely than other children to experience frequent doctor and hospital visits. Some of their treatments may be scary or painful. Hospital stays can be frightening and lonely.

Children with chronic illnesses will feel "different" than other children. Their activities may be limited, and, in many cases, their families must change how they live to accommodate the child.

How do kids adjust to and cope with chronic illnesses?

The way children react to diagnosis with a chronic illness depends on several factors, including the child's personality, the specific illness, and their family. One big factor is the child's developmental stage. Kids' understandings of illness and their coping strategies change as they grow older.

Here's some information about how kids adjust at different stages:

Infants and Toddlers: Infants and toddlers are beginning to develop trust and an overall sense of security. They generally have very little understanding of their illness. They experience pain, restriction of motion, and separation from parents as challenges to developing trust and security. Parents can help by being present for painful procedures, staying with their children (when possible) during hospitalizations, and holding, soothing, and interacting with their baby as much as possible.

Preschool Children: Preschool children are beginning to develop a sense of independence. They may understand what it means to get sick, but they may not understand the cause and effect nature of illness. For example, they may believe that throwing up causes them to get sick, rather than the other way around. Being in the hospital or adjusting to medication schedules can challenge the child's developing independence. The child may try to counter lack of control over their world by challenging limits set by parents. Parents can help by being firm with things the child does not have a choice over (never ask "Do you want to take your medicine now?" unless there's really a choice—almost all children will say "NO!"), but by offering choices over flexible aspects of treatment. (For example, "Which to you want to take first, the pink medicine or the purple?" or "Do you want to sit on my lap while you have your blood drawn, or in the chair with me holding your hand?")

Some tips for helping young children learn to cope with stress are available in a document produced by the University of New Hampshire Cooperative Extension. It is available online at http://ceinfo.unh .edu/Family/Documents/famfoc14.pdf.

Early School-aged Children: Children at this age are developing a sense of mastery over their environment. They can describe reasons for illness, but these reasons may not be entirely logical. Children this age often have "magical thinking." They may believe they caused an illness by thinking bad thoughts, by hitting their brother, or by not eating their vegetables. Children also begin to sense that they are different from their peers. Parents can help by allowing children to help in management of their illness (with close adult supervision). They should also reassure their children that the illness is not their fault.

Older School-aged Children: As children grow older they are more capable of understanding their illness and its treatment, but they should not be expected to react as adults do. They may feel left out when they miss school or activities with their peers. Parents may feel the need to protect their children by restricting them from activities with other children. This is a natural reaction, but it can interfere with the child's independence and sense of mastery. To the extent allowed by the child's doctors, parents should help the child to participate in school or other activities.

Information can be empowering, and reading what other kids have to say can make a kid feel less alone. Kidshealth.org has a special section of kid-friendly information on all kinds of health and illness topics (http://www.kidshealth.org/kid).

Adolescents: Teens begin to develop their own identity separate from their family. Self-image becomes extremely important during the teenage years. That can be a problem when the teen's appearance is altered by illness or medication. Teens are also beginning to develop a real independence from their families. Parents who have been very involved in their teen's care for many years may find it difficult to let go of their role as primary caregiver.

Many teens will go through times of denial of their illness when they may neglect to take medications, follow special diets, or check blood sugars. In addition, the adolescent's body is rapidly changing, which may change the symptoms of the illness or the doses of medications needed. It is important to help teens to gain control of their disease management. Keep in mind also that even with chronic illness, teens are teens. Don't forget to talk about issues facing all teens: independence, college planning, sexuality, substance abuse, etc.

There are some great websites just for teens:

- Encourage Online (http://www.encourageonline.org) is a place for teens living with chronic illness and their family and friends to talk, connect, and have fun with others who understand.

- Teenshealth.org (http://www.teenshealth.org) has information for teens on all kinds of health and illness topics.

- Teens share their stories and experiences on Chronic Illness Resources for Teens (http://www.dartmouth.edu/dms/koop/resources/chronic_illness/chronic.shtml).

What effects can I expect my child's chronic condition to have on our family?

Chronic illness doesn't just affect the person with the condition. The whole family must come to terms with the illness, make major changes in schedules and priorities, and somehow manage to remain a family.

Parents may struggle with their own feelings about the child's illness while trying to keep up a brave front for the child. It is normal to feel a sense of grief or loss for the way you imagined your child's life would be (without any chronic condition). Divorce is somewhat more common in families with seriously ill children, mainly because of the great stress of parenting an ill child. While your child will need at least one parent with them during times of acute illness or hospitalization, it is important for you to find at least short times now and then to spend alone together with your partner.

Siblings of the ill child may feel left out, and later may feel guilty at any bad feelings they have toward their sick brother or sister. While less time will be available to spend with the other children in the family, parents need to let them know that they are still special and important. You can't just assume that they know this. If you can carve out just 10–15 minutes a day to really focus on each sibling, it will go a long way.

- A Sibling's Site (http://asiblingssite.com) is run just for siblings by a teen whose brother is chronically ill. It has a bulletin board.

Caregiver burnout and stresses on relationships in the family can become overwhelming. Sometimes counseling can help everyone in the family make the adjustment more smoothly. Find out when your family should seek help and what kinds of help are out there from the American Association for Marriage and Family Therapy (A web document is available at http://www.aamft.org/families/Consumer_Updates/ChronicIllness.asp or you can contact American Association for Marriage and Family Therapy, 112 South Alfred Street, Alexandria, VA 22314-3061; Phone: 703-838-9808; Fax: 703-838-9805; Website: http://www.aamft.org.)

The most successful families tend to be those who are able to move on from seeing the illness as an intrusion toward working together as a team to face the new responsibilities of managing a long-term illness. They build on their family's strengths to cope with the new stress. For more information on coping with family stress, check out the series of publications from the University of Minnesota Extension Service, available online at http://www.extension.umn.edu/distribution/familydevelopment/components/familystress.html.

What can our family do to cope better, and to help our child cope better with the chronic illness?

Stay involved and give information: Discuss with your child (at their age level) what their illness is all about, and what will happen to them in the hospital. When you don't do this, kids may imagine the worst.

Plan for procedures: Unexpected stress is more difficult to cope with than anticipated stress. Some procedures can cause physical and psychological distress. Some children do better with several days to prepare, while others worry themselves sick. Good communication and flexibility are essential.

Give them choices: Some tasks for children with chronic illness must be done no matter what. Others are more flexible. Know what tasks are mandatory (scheduled medications, specific diets) and which are open for discussion ("as-needed" medicines, choice of foods within a given diet). Conflict may arise when a child tries to assert independence. As preschoolers, and even older kids, test adults' limits, there is natural conflict with adults' demands. Children with chronic illness, more than other kids, need chances to make choices—to have control over any part of their lives they can control.

Support their friendships and activities with peers: Illness often interferes with routines and activities. For children and teens, a particularly devastating consequence can be the weakening or loss of friendships. Friends can grow apart as a result of these changes. Keeping kids involved with their peers and making extra efforts to maintain those connections can go a long way in helping a kid cope with an illness. Helping your child to find new ways to make and maintain new relationships is critical during this time.

You may also need to help your child find ways to cope with teasing from peers. A helpful article is "Easing the Teasing: How Parents Can Help Their Children," *ERIC Digests*, July 1999. It available online at http://www.ericfacility.net/ericdigests/ed431555.html.

Children need to feel like they belong: Their peer relationships are an important arena for them to do this. Try to help your child find interests and activities that provide opportunities to connect with other kids with similar illnesses. Give them opportunities to spend time with friends. Teens need to be exposed to other caring adults they can trust. Contact with these adults should be encouraged in order to help shape the direction of their lives and provide stability. Most major hospitals and clinics can help you find support groups for parents, families, and for children affected by the illness.

Special camps can also provide opportunities for belonging:

- To learn more about camps specifically designed for kids with chronic conditions, the Federation for Children with Special

Needs has a summer camp listing, updated each year, which includes useful information on selecting a camp. Contact them at: Federation for Children with Special Needs, 1135 Tremont Street, Suite 420, Boston, MA 02120; Phone: 617-236-7210; Toll-Free in Massachusetts: 800-331-0688; Fax: 617-572-2094; Website: http://www.fcsn.org.

- National Dissemination Center for Children with Disabilities has a great summer camp resource online at http://www.nichcy.org/pubs/genresc/camps.pdf, or contact them at: National Dissemination Center for Children with Disabilities; P.O. Box 1492; Washington, DC 20013-1492; Toll-Free: 800-695-0285 (Voice/TTY); Website: www.nichcy.org.

- The Hole in the Wall Gang Camps are free of charge. They have camps in Florida, Connecticut, New York, Ireland, and France. For more information contact: The Association of Hole in the Wall Camps, One Century Tower, 265 Church St., #503, New Haven, CT 06510; Phone: 203-562-1203; Fax: 203-562-1207; Website: www.holeinthewallcamps.org; E-mail info@holeinthewallcamps.org.

- Your local children's hospital may also have listings of camps near you for kids with chronic conditions.

Once you've found the perfect camp, find out what you can do to get ready by reading "Sending Your Child with Special Needs to Camp" by KidsHealth.org and available online at http://www.kidshealth.org/parent/system/ill/sending_child_camp.html.

Be hopeful: Coping with a chronic illness can be discouraging and scary. It is incredibly important to stay hopeful. Don't ignore your worries or your negative feelings—they need to be recognized and addressed. But it's not helpful to dwell on them. If you try to find the positive side of things and keep your eye on the potential positive outcomes, you will be teaching your child a valuable lesson, and maintaining your ability to cope as well.

Listen: Be available so your child can talk about the problems they are facing. Ask them how it's going, and listen to the answer. Listen to their troubles and help them find solutions to their problems. Be able to recognize the warning signs of depression. If your child talks about suicide, take it seriously. Allow your child to express his or her fears; validate your child's feelings. There's nothing worse than feeling scared and confused and not being able to talk about it. Find out more about depression in children and adolescents with chronic illnesses by reading "Depression in Children and Adolescents with a Chronic Disease," by the New York University School of Medicine's Child Study Center. It is available online at http://www.aboutourkids.org/aboutour/articles/depres_chronic_disease.html.

Be flexible: To help your child adapt to their illness, you will need to both recognize their limitations and help them to continue with life as usual, whenever possible.

Have fun together as a family: You can expect the whole family to be under increased stress. Maintaining your commitment to your family and getting support from each other may be harder during times of stress, but it is also even more important. Spend time together that is not focused on the illness. To carve out time for family activities you may need to schedule family time, including one-on-one time for parents and parent-child "dates," as well as whole family activities.

Involve the whole family and even an extended support network: Allow each family member to help in any way that they are willing and able. Seek support and help from people outside your immediate family, such as through your extended family, school, religious community, neighborhood, or children's hospital. People you know will generally be very pleased if they can help, such as bringing over a meal, having your other children over to play, or even just lending a listening ear. Often folks don't know exactly what you need—so don't wait for them to offer it. If someone gives you a generic offer of help, tell them what you need specifically, and ask if they can do it for you. You'll be surprised at how glad people are to be able to do what's needed for your family.

Teach coping skills: Parents need to help children learn new ways to cope with the special challenges of an illness. Discussing with teens how their illness is affecting them and finding ways to help solve problems or cope with the feelings is very helpful. They can learn to build on their strengths and can even develop pride in their abilities to meet the challenges. You can do a lot to help your child cope with the stress that comes with a chronic illness. For additional suggestions read "Helping Children Cope with Stress," by Karen DeBord, Ph.D., Child Development Specialist, North Carolina Cooperative Extension Service, available online at http://www.ces.ncsu.edu/depts/fcs/human/pubs/copestress.html.

Don't let your kids hear more than you intend: If your conversations are private have them away from your children. Kids hear more than you may think; don't assume they are sleeping when their eyes are closed.

Coordinate with your child's school: When your child with special health needs goes to school, good communication between your family and school is very important. The Center for Children with Special Needs (at the Children's Hospital and Regional Medical Center, Seattle, WA) has developed a handout titled "When Your Child with Special Health Needs Goes to School" that includes a checklist to help parents prepare for school and a place to keep track of important phone numbers. It is available online at http://www.cshcn.org/resources/return-to-school _pl.htm (it is also available in Spanish, Russian, and Vietnamese).

Take care of yourself and stick to your family routine: Caregivers/parents need to take good care of themselves—otherwise, they won't be able to give good care. Talk with other parents who have children with special health care needs, carve out time to do something you enjoy, get support, find someone to listen to you vent, take breaks, spend time with your partner, and learn to deal positively with your stress. If you can keep your family routine as normal as possible, that will help, too. For additional information, read:

- "Keeping Family Routine when a Child is Seriously Ill," University of Michigan Health System; available online at http:// www.med.umich.edu/1libr/pa/pa_familytr_hhg.htm

- "Replace Stress with Peace," by H. Wallace Goddard, Extension Family and Child Development Specialist, Department of Family and Child Development, Auburn University; available online at http://www.humsci.auburn.edu/parent/stress/index.html.

Make use of respite care: Everyone needs a break once in a while—especially the parents of kids with special needs. Respite care is short-term, specialized childcare. Respite care services can help keep family caregivers from getting burned out. To find out more, check out these resources on respite care:

- "Respite Care," by Debby Ingram, Research Associate, Family Support Project, "Strengthening American Families Through National and Grassroots Support." Available from The ARC, http://www.thearc.org/faqs/respite.html.

- "Respite Care," a publication from NICHCY (http://www.nichcy.org/ pubs/outprint/nd12txt.htm), has more information, but the list of resources may be somewhat out of date. Use NICHCY's state resource pages (http://www.nichcy.org/states.htm) to locate your state's vocational rehabilitation, and parent training and information center to find out whether any of these can help with finding respite care.

- The ARCH National Respite Network and Resource Center (800 Eastowne Drive, Suite 105, Chapel Hill, NC 27514; Phone: 919-490-5577; Fax: 919-490-4905; Website: http://www.archrespite.org) has a National Respite Locator Service (http://www.respite locator.org/index.htm) and State Respite Coalition listings (http://www.archrespite.org/coalitions.htm).

- You may want to use childcare services to give yourself a break. "Choosing Quality Childcare for a Child with Special Needs" by ChildCareAware (http://www.childcareaware.org/en/tools/pubs/ pdf/102e.pdf) will help answer your questions.

- The benefits of inclusive education programs are discussed in an article produced by the National Association for the Education of Young Children titled "The Benefits of an Inclusive Education: Making It Work," available online at http://www.naeyc.org/ resources/eyly/1996/07.htm

Remember your other children: Siblings will need extra attention, and may need counseling; they can experience jealousy, anger, and depression. It's important that you address their fears, concerns, and grief, and make sure they don't feel pushed aside. A document titled "Siblings of Kids with Special Needs" is available from the University of Michigan Health System at http://www.med.umich.edu/1libr/ yourchild/specneed.htm.

Stay organized: Getting organized will lower the overall stress level in your family. One helpful tip is to keep all of your child's information in one place. A care notebook can become a lifesaver. Write everything down—don't count on your memory. If you have it all in writing, you can relax more. Keep a running list of questions, so that you will remember what to ask at medical visits.

Be aware of the risks unique to your child's illness: It's important to be very familiar with your child's illness, no matter how scary it is. If children feel like they know more than you, they will feel responsible for protecting you. Read as much as you can about your child's illness. The more knowledge you have, the more likely you will be able to obtain the best care for your child. If you want more information about your child's chronic illness or health condition ask your county public health nurses, or the child's health care provider. Keep a written list of questions that come up, so you can ask at each medical visit. Don't hesitate to call your child's doctor with your questions or concerns.

In addition, there are many national organizations for specific health conditions, and many of the resources mentioned in this chapter can help you find information specific to your family's needs. You can also research online and learn more about your specific health, illness and medical procedure questions. Some helpful resources are:

- University of Michigan Health System Health Topics A-Z: http://www.med.umich.edu/1libr/1libr.htm

- Kidshealth.org: http://www.kidshealth.org/parent

- The illustrated MedlinePlus medical encyclopedia: http://www.nlm.nih.gov/medlineplus/encyclopedia.html

- The Medem Network: http://www.medem.com

What are some other sources of information and support for kids and families living with a chronic illness?

More information sources for further reading include:

- "Pain and Your Child or Teen" (http://www.med.umich.edu/1libr/yourchild/pain.htm)

- "Pediatric Hypnotherapy: Hypnosis Helping Kids" (http://www.med.umich.edu/1libr/yourchild/hypnosis.htm)

- "A Look at Biofeedback" (http://www.med.umich.edu/1libr/yourchild/biofeed.htm)

- "How to Care for a Seriously Ill Child: Suggestions for Parents" (http://kidshealth.org/parent/system/ill/seriously_ill.html)

- "National Network for Child Care: Caring for Children with Special Needs" (http://www.ces.ncsu.edu/depts/fcs/human/pubs/nc11.html)

- The National Dissemination Center for Children with Disabilities (NICHCY) has online information (including Spanish language information) about various disabilities and illnesses, as well as general information about special needs youth (birth to age 22). You can also call 800-695-0285, visit http://www.nichcy.org, or E-mail nichcy@aed.org with any specific questions. They can help you locate your local state resources.

- "Moving on with Life," by the National Cancer Institute (http://www.nci.nih.gov/CancerInformation/youngpeople/Page9) is a helpful section of a brochure for families with kids who have cancer. It talks about how to support your child, and how to deal with siblings, family, and friends.

- "Youth Living with Chronic Illness" by the Myalgic Encephalo-myelitis Association of Ontario (http://www.meao-cfs.on.ca/pdf/a-y-broc.pdf) is a Canadian brochure for kids and parents that gives a nice overview of the issues, talks about society's myths and values, and offers specific messages for kids, friends, parents, and teachers.

- Friends and siblings of your child with chronic illness may want to read "When Someone You Know Has a Chronic Illness," written just for kids by KidsHealth.org (http://www.kidshealth.org/kid/feeling/thought/someone_chronic.html).

- "Supporting Students with Asthma" (http://www.ericfacility.net/ericdigests/ed438339.html) is a news digest that draws on research to discuss how schools can help support kids who have asthma.

- A list of books for kids about disabilities and illnesses and other resources related to sibling issues is available from The Arc at http://www.thearc.org/siblingsupport/resourcespage.htm.

- A list of books for kids about going to the hospital is available from the University of Michigan Health System at http://www.med.umich.edu/1libr/pa/pa_blhospit_pep.htm.

- Books for parents:

  When Your Child Has a Disability: The Complete Sourcebook of Daily and Medical Care, Revised Edition, by Mark Batshaw (Published by Paul H. Brookes, 2001). This useful book covers a wide range of medical and educational issues, as well as daily and long-term care requirements of specific disabilities. It discusses parent concerns like behavior, medication, and potential complications and also addresses issues such as prematurity, early intervention, legal rights, attention-deficit/hyperactivity disorder, learning disabilities, genetic syndromes, and changes in health.

Coping With Your Child's Chronic Illness, by Alesia T. Barrett Singer (Robert D. Reed Publishers, 1999). This book is a good introduction and general guide to coping for parents of a newly diagnosed child.

Whole Parent, Whole Child: A Parent's Guide to Raising a Child With a Chronic Illness, by Patricia M. Moynihan and Broatch Haig (Chronimed Publishing, 1989). This book helps you answer the questions: "What kind of parent am I now? What kind of parent do I want to be? How can I help my child with a chronic illness lead the fullest life possible?" This book aims to help you keep your perspective, and will remind you that you are not alone.

Organizations that can help include:

- **Asthmabusters** (http://www.asthmabusters.org) is an online club from the American Lung Association for kids aged 7–14 with asthma.

- **Brave Kids** (http://www.bravekids.org) is an online community for kids with special needs and their families.

- **Cystic Fibrosis Foundation** (6931 Arlington Road, Bethesda, MD 20814; Toll-Free: 800-FIGHT-CF; Phone: 301-951-4422; Fax: 301-951-6378; Website: http://www.cff.org; E-mail: info@cff.org) funds research and provides information.

- **Juvenile Diabetes Research Foundation International** (120 Wall Street, New York, NY 10005-4001; Toll-Free: 800-533-CURE; Fax: 212-785-9595; Website: http://www.jdrf.org; E-mail: info@jdrf.org) funds research and has some useful information on their site.

- **National Easter Seal Society** (230 West Monroe Street, Suite 1800, Chicago, IL 60606; Phone: 312-551-7147; TTD: 312-726-4258; Fax: 312-726-1494; Website: http://www.easterseals.com) offers services for people with disabilities and special needs and their families. They have local chapters.

- **Our-Kids** (http://www.our-kids.org) is devoted to raising children with special needs. They provide information and support for kids with special needs and their caregivers.

- **PACER** (Parent Advocacy Coalition for Educational Rights, 8161 Normandale Blvd., Minneapolis, MN 55437; Phone: 952-838-9000; TTY: 952-838-0190; Fax: 952-838-0199; Website: http://www.pacer.org; E-mail: pacer@pacer.org) works for better opportunities and quality of life for kids and teens with disabilities and their families through parents helping parents.

- **The Starbright Foundation** (1850 Sawtelle Blvd., Suite 450, Los Angeles, CA 90025, Toll Free: (800) 315-2580; Phone: 310-479-1212; Fax: 310-479-1235; Website: http://www.starbright.org) is dedicated to the development of projects that empower seriously ill children to combat the medical and emotional challenges they face on a daily basis. They have developed free CD-ROMs for kids with diabetes, asthma, and cystic fibrosis and their families.

Chapter 55

Special Education Services for Children with Disabilities

Introduction

Every year, under the federal law known as the Individuals with Disabilities Education Act (IDEA), millions of children with disabilities receive special services designed to meet their unique needs. For infants and toddlers with disabilities, from birth through age two, and their families, special services are provided through an early intervention system. For school-aged children and youth (aged three through 21), special education and related services are provided through the school system. These services can be very important in helping children and youth with disabilities develop, learn, and succeed in school and other settings.

Who Is Eligible for Services?

Under the IDEA, states are responsible for meeting the special needs of eligible children with disabilities. To find out if a child is eligible for services, he or she must first receive a full and individual initial evaluation. This evaluation is free. Two purposes of the evaluation are:

- to see if the child has a disability, as defined by IDEA, and

- to learn in more detail what his or her special needs are.

"General Information about Disabilities," Document GR3, National Dissemination Center for Children with Disabilities (NICHCY), 2002. Additional information is available online at http://www.nichcy.org.

Infants and Toddlers, Birth through Two

Under the IDEA, "infants and toddlers with disabilities" are defined as children from birth through age two who need early intervention services because they:

- Are experiencing developmental delays, as measured by appropriate diagnostic instruments and procedures, in one or more of the following areas:

  - cognitive development.

  - physical development, including vision and hearing.

  - communication development.

  - social or emotional development.

  - adaptive development; or

- Have a diagnosed physical or mental condition that has a high probability of resulting in developmental delay.

The term may also include, if a state chooses, children from birth through age two who are at risk of having substantial developmental delays if early intervention services are not provided. (34 *Code of Federal Regulations* §303.16)

Children Aged Three through Nine

It is important to know that, under IDEA, states and local educational agencies (LEAs) are allowed to use the term "developmental delay" with children aged three through nine, rather than one of the disability categories previously listed. This means that, if they choose, states and LEAs do not have to say that a child has a specific disability. For children aged three through nine, a state and LEA may choose to include as an eligible "child with a disability" a child who is experiencing developmental delays in one or more of the following areas:

- physical development,

- cognitive development,

- communication development,

- social or emotional development, or

- adaptive development

and who, because of the developmental delays, needs special education and related services.

"Developmental delays" are defined by the state and must be measured by appropriate diagnostic instruments and procedures.

Children and Youth Aged Three through 21

The IDEA lists 13 different disability categories under which three through 21-year-olds may be eligible for services. For a child to be eligible for services, the disability must affect the child's educational performance. The disability categories listed in IDEA are:

- autism,
- deaf-blindness,
- deafness,
- emotional disturbance,
- hearing impairment,
- mental retardation,
- multiple disabilities,
- orthopedic impairment,
- other health impairment,
- specific learning disability,
- speech or language impairment
- traumatic brain injury, or
- visual impairment (including blindness).

Under IDEA, a child may not be identified as a "child with a disability" just because he or she speaks a language other than English and does not speak or understand English well. A child may not be identified as having a disability just because he or she has not had enough instruction in math or reading.

How Does IDEA Define the 13 Disability Categories?

The IDEA provides definitions of the 13 disability categories listed above. These federal definitions guide how states define who is eligible for a free appropriate public education under IDEA. The definitions of disability terms are as follows:

Autism: Autism means a developmental disability significantly affecting verbal and nonverbal communication and social interaction, generally evident before age three, that adversely affects educational performance. Characteristics often associated with autism are engaging in repetitive activities and stereotyped movements, resistance to changes in daily routines or the environment, and unusual responses to sensory experiences. The term autism does not apply if the child's educational performance is adversely affected primarily because the child has emotional disturbance.

A child who shows the characteristics of autism after age three could be diagnosed as having autism if the criteria above are satisfied.

Deaf-Blindness: Deaf-blindness means concomitant [simultaneous] hearing and visual impairments, the combination of which causes such severe communication and other developmental and educational needs that they cannot be accommodated in special education programs solely for children with deafness or children with blindness.

Deafness: Deafness means a hearing impairment so severe that a child is impaired in processing linguistic information through hearing, with or without amplification, that adversely affects a child's educational performance.

Emotional Disturbance: Emotional disturbance means a condition exhibiting one or more of the following characteristics over a long period of time and to a marked degree that adversely affects a child's educational performance:

- An inability to learn that cannot be explained by intellectual, sensory, or health factors.

- An inability to build or maintain satisfactory interpersonal relationships with peers and teachers.

- Inappropriate types of behavior or feelings under normal circumstances.

- A general pervasive mood of unhappiness or depression.

- A tendency to develop physical symptoms or fears associated with personal or school problems.

The term includes schizophrenia. The term does not apply to children who are socially maladjusted, unless it is determined that they have an emotional disturbance.

Hearing Impairment: Hearing impairment means an impairment in hearing, whether permanent or fluctuating, that adversely affects a child's educational performance but is not included under the definition of "deafness."

Mental Retardation: Mental retardation means significantly subaverage general intellectual functioning, existing concurrently [at the same time] with deficits in adaptive behavior and manifested during the developmental period, that adversely affects a child's educational performance.

Multiple Disabilities: Multiple disabilities means concomitant [simultaneous] impairments (such as mental retardation-blindness, mental retardation-orthopedic impairment, etc.), the combination of which causes such severe educational needs that they cannot be accommodated in a special education program solely for one of the impairments. The term does not include deaf-blindness.

Orthopedic Impairment: Orthopedic impairment means a severe orthopedic impairment that adversely affects a child's educational performance. The term includes impairments caused by a congenital anomaly (e.g., clubfoot, absence of some member, etc.), impairments caused by disease (e.g., poliomyelitis, bone tuberculosis, etc.), and impairments from other causes (e.g., cerebral palsy, amputations, and fractures or burns that cause contractures).

Other Health Impairment: Other health impairment means having limited strength, vitality, or alertness, including a heightened alertness to environmental stimuli, that results in limited alertness with respect to the educational environment, that:

- is due to chronic or acute health problems such as asthma, attention deficit disorder or attention deficit hyperactivity disorder, diabetes, epilepsy, a heart condition, hemophilia, lead poisoning, leukemia, nephritis, rheumatic fever, and sickle cell anemia; and

- adversely affects a child's educational performance.

Specific Learning Disability: Specific learning disability means a disorder in one or more of the basic psychological processes involved in understanding or in using language, spoken or written, that may manifest itself in an imperfect ability to listen, think, speak, read, write, spell, or to do mathematical calculations. The term includes such conditions as perceptual disabilities, brain injury, minimal brain dysfunction, dyslexia, and developmental aphasia. The term does not include learning problems that are primarily the result of visual, hearing, or motor disabilities; of mental retardation; of emotional disturbance; or of environmental, cultural, or economic disadvantage.

Speech or Language Impairment: Speech of language impairment means a communication disorder such as stuttering, impaired articulation, a language impairment, or a voice impairment that adversely affects a child's educational performance.

Traumatic Brain Injury: Traumatic brain injury means an acquired injury to the brain caused by an external physical force, resulting in total or partial functional disability or psychosocial impairment, or both, that adversely affects a child's educational performance. The term applies to open or closed head injuries resulting in impairments in one or more areas, such as cognition; language; memory; attention; reasoning; abstract thinking; judgment; problem-solving; sensory, perceptual, and motor abilities; psychosocial behavior; physical functions; information processing; and speech. The term does not include brain injuries that are congenital or degenerative, or brain injuries induced by birth trauma.

Visual Impairment Including Blindness: Visual impairment including blindness means an impairment in vision that, even with correction, adversely affects a child's educational performance. The term includes both partial sight and blindness.

Finding Out More about Disabilities

IDEA's definitions of disability terms help states, schools, service providers, and parents decide if a child is eligible for early intervention or special education and related services. Beyond these definitions, there is a great deal of information available about specific disabilities, including disabilities not listed in IDEA. NICHCY [National Dissemination Center for Children with Disabilities] would be pleased to help you find that information, beginning with:

- our disability fact sheets (available online at www.nichcy.org/ disabinf.asp) and other publications on the disabilities listed in IDEA;

- contact information for many organizations that focus their work on a particular disability. These groups have a lot of information to share.

More about Services

Special services are available to eligible children with disabilities and can do much to help children develop and learn. For infants and toddlers aged birth through two, services are provided through an early intervention system. This system may be run by the Health Department in the state, or another department such as Education. If you are a parent and you would like to find out more about early intervention in your state, including how to have your child evaluated at no cost to you, try any of these suggestions:

• ask your child's pediatrician to put you in touch with the early intervention system in your community or region;

• contact the pediatrics branch in a local hospital and ask where you should call to find out about early intervention services in your area;

• call NICHCY and ask for the contact information for early intervention in your state. The state office will refer you to the contact person or agency in your area.

For children and youth ages three through 21, special education and related services are provided through the public school system. Probably the best way to find out about these services is to call your local public school. The school should be able to tell you about special education policies in your area or refer you to a district or county office for this information. If you are a parent who thinks your child may need special education and related services, be sure to ask how to have your child evaluated under IDEA for eligibility. Often there are materials available to tell parents and others more about local and state policies for special education and related services.

There is a lot to know about early intervention, about special education and related services, and about the rights of children with disabilities under the IDEA, our nation's special education law. NICHCY offers many publications, all of which are available on our website, www.nichcy.org, or by contacting us directly. We can also tell you about materials available from other groups.

Other Sources of Information for Parents

There are many sources of information about services for children with disabilities. Within your community, you may wish to contact:

- the Child Find Coordinator for your district or county (IDEA requires that states conduct Child Find activities to identify, locate, and evaluate infants, toddlers, children, and youth with disabilities aged birth through 21)

- the principal of your child's school

- the Special Education Director of your child's school district or local school

Any of these individuals should be able to answer specific questions about how to obtain special education and related services, or early intervention services, for your child.

In addition, every state has a Parent Training and Information (PTI) center, which is an excellent source of information. The PTI can:

- help you learn about early intervention and special education services

- tell you about what the IDEA requires

- connect you with disability groups and parent groups in the community or state

To find out how to contact your state's PTI, look at the NICHCY "State Resource Sheet" for your state (available at http://www .nichcy.org/states.htm or by calling NICHCY directly, 800-695-0285). You'll find the PTI listed there, as well as many other information resources, such as community parent resource centers, disability-specific organizations, and state agencies serving children with disabilities.

Chapter 56

Genetics Privacy and Legislation

Federal Policy History

No federal legislation has been passed relating to genetic discrimination in individual insurance coverage or to genetic discrimination in the workplace. Several bills were introduced during the last decade. Some of these bills attempted to amend existing civil rights and labor laws, while others stood alone. The primary public concerns are that:

1. Insurers will use genetic information to deny, limit, or cancel insurance policies

2. Employers will use genetic information against existing workers or to screen potential employees

Because DNA samples can be held indefinitely, there is the added threat that samples will be used for purposes other than those for which they were gathered.

Executive Order Protecting Federal Employees

On February 8, 2000, U.S. President Clinton signed an Executive Order (EO) prohibiting every federal department and agency from using genetic information in any hiring or promotion action. This

Excerpted from "Genetics Privacy and Legislation," Human Genome Project Information, Oak Ridge National Laboratory (www.ornl.gov), December 2003.

Executive Order, endorsed by the American Medical Association, the American College of Medical Genetics, the National Society of Genetic Counselors, and the Genetic Alliance:

- Prohibits federal employers from requiring or requesting genetic tests as a condition of being hired or receiving benefits. Employers cannot request or require employees to undergo genetic tests in order to evaluate an employee's ability to perform his or her job.

- Prohibits federal employers from using protected genetic information to classify employees in a manner that deprives them of advancement opportunities. Employers cannot deny employees promotions or overseas posts because of a genetic predisposition for certain illnesses.

- Provides strong privacy protections to any genetic information used for medical treatment and research. Under the EO, obtaining or disclosing genetic information about employees or potential employees is prohibited, except when it is necessary to provide medical treatment to employees, ensure workplace health and safety, or provide occupational and health researchers access to data. In every case where genetic information about employees is obtained, it will be subject to all federal and state privacy protections.

State Policy History

States have a patchwork of genetic-information nondiscrimination laws, none of them comprehensive. Existing state laws differ in coverage, protections afforded, and enforcement schemes. Some of the first state laws enacted to address this issue prohibited discrimination against individuals with specific genetic traits or disorders. Other state laws regulate both the use of genetic testing in employment decisions and the disclosure of genetic test results. These state laws generally prohibit employers from requiring workers and applicants to undergo genetic testing as a condition of employment. Some states permit genetic testing when it is requested by the worker or applicant for the purpose of investigating a compensation claim or determining the worker's susceptibility to potentially toxic chemicals in the workplace. These statutes often require the worker to provide informed written consent for such testing, contain specific restrictions governing disclosure, and prevent the employer from taking adverse action against the employee.

Existing Federal Anti-Discrimination Laws and How They Apply to Genetics

Although no specific federal genetic nondiscrimination legislation has been enacted, some believe that parts of existing nondiscrimination laws could be interpreted to include genetic discrimination. Here is a brief overview of these laws and how they apply to genetics.

Americans with Disabilities Act of 1990 (ADA)

The most likely current source of protection against genetic discrimination in the workplace is provided by laws prohibiting discrimination based on disability. Title I of the Americans with Disabilities Act (ADA), enforced by the Equal Employment Opportunity Commission (EEOC), and similar disability-based antidiscrimination laws such as the Rehabilitation Act of 1973 do not explicitly address genetic information, but they provide some protections against disability-related genetic discrimination in the workplace.

- Prohibits discrimination against a person who is regarded as having a disability.

- Protects individuals with symptomatic genetic disabilities the same as individuals with other disabilities.

- Does not protect against discrimination based on unexpressed genetic conditions.

- Does not protect potential workers from requirements or requests to provide genetic information to their employers after a conditional offer of employment has been extended but before they begin work. (Note: This is a heightened concern because genetic samples can be stored.)

- Does not protect workers from requirements to provide medical information that is job related and consistent with business necessity.

In March 1995, the EEOC issued an interpretation of the ADA. The guidance, however, is limited in scope and legal effect. It is policy guidance that does not have the same legal binding effect on a court as a statute or regulation and has not been tested in court. According to the interpretation:

- Entities that discriminate on the basis of genetic predisposition are regarding the individuals as having impairments, and such individuals are covered by the ADA.

- Unaffected carriers of recessive and X-linked disorders and individuals with late-onset genetic disorders who may be identified through genetic testing or family history as being at high risk of developing the disease are not covered by the ADA.

Health Insurance Portability and Accountability Act of 1996 (HIPAA)

The Health Insurance Portability and Accountability Act (HIPAA) applies to employer-based and commercially issued group health insurance only. HIPAA is the only federal law that directly addresses the issue of genetic discrimination. There is no similar law applying to private individuals seeking health insurance in the individual market.

- Prohibits group health plans from using any health status-related factor, including genetic information, as a basis for denying or limiting eligibility for coverage or for charging an individual more for coverage.

- Limits exclusions for preexisting conditions in group health plans to 12 months and prohibits such exclusions if the individual has been covered previously for that condition for 12 months or more.

- States explicitly that genetic information in the absence of a current diagnosis of illness shall not be considered a preexisting condition.

- Doesn't prohibit employers from refusing to offer health coverage as part of their benefits packages.

HIPAA National Standards to Protect Patients' Personal Medical Records, December 2002

This regulation would protect medical records and other personal health information maintained by health care providers, hospitals, health plans and health insurers, and health care clearinghouses. The regulation was mandated when Congress failed to pass comprehensive privacy legislation (as required by HIPAA) by 1999. The new standards: limit the nonconsensual use and release of private health information; give patients new rights to access their medical records and to know who else has accessed them; restrict most disclosure of health information to the minimum needed for the intended purpose; establish new criminal and civil sanctions for improper use or disclosure; and establish new requirements for access to records by researchers and others. They are not specific to genetics, rather they are sweeping regulations governing all personal health information.

Title VII of the Civil Rights Act of 1964

An argument could be made that genetic discrimination based on racially or ethnically linked genetic disorders constitutes unlawful race or ethnicity discrimination.

- Protection is available only where an employer engages in discrimination based on a genetic trait that is substantially related to a particular race or ethnic group.

- A strong relationship between race or national origin has been established for only a few diseases.

Recommendations for Future Legislation

Workplace Discrimination

Based on previous recommendations from the National Action Plan on Breast Cancer (NAPBC) and the NIH-DOE [National Institutes of Health; Department of Energy] Working Group on the Ethical, Legal, and Social Implications (ELSI) of human genome research, in a 1998 report the Clinton Administration announced recommendations for future legislation to ensure that discoveries made possible by the Human Genome Project are used to improve health and not to discriminate against workers or their families. These recommendations are:

- Employers should not require or request that employees or potential employees take a genetic test or provide genetic information as a condition of employment or benefits.

- Employers should not use genetic information to discriminate against, limit, segregate, or classify employees in a way that would deprive them of employment opportunities.

- Employers should not obtain or disclose genetic information about employees or potential employees under most circumstances.

Genetic testing and the use of genetic information by employers should be permitted in the following situations to ensure workplace safety and health and to preserve research opportunities. However, in all cases where genetic information about employees is obtained, the information should be maintained in medical files that are kept separate from personnel files, treated as confidential medical records, and protected by applicable state and federal laws.

- An employer should be permitted to monitor employees for the effects of a particular substance found in the workplace to which continued exposure could cause genetic damage under certain circumstances. Informed consent and assurance of confidentiality should be required. In addition, employers may use the results only to identify and control adverse conditions in the workplace and to take action necessary to prevent significant risk of substantial harm to the employee or others.

- The statutory authority of a federal agency or contractor to promulgate regulations, enforce workplace safety and health laws, or conduct occupational or other health research should not be limited.

- An employer should be able to disclose genetic information for research and other purposes with the written, informed consent of the individual.

These recommendations should apply to public and private-sector employers, unions, and labor-management groups that conduct joint apprenticeship and other training programs. Employment agencies and licensing agencies that issue licenses, certificates, and other credentials required to engage in various professions and occupations also should be covered.

Individuals who believe they have been subjected to workplace discrimination based on genetic information should be able to file a charge with the Equal Employment Opportunity Commission, Department of Labor, or other appropriate federal agency for investigation and resolution. The designated agency should be authorized to bring lawsuits in the federal courts to resolve issues that would not settle amicably. The courts should have the authority to halt the violations and order relief, such as hiring, promotion, back pay, and compensatory and punitive damages to the individual. Alternatively, an individual should be able to elect to bring a private lawsuit in federal or state court to obtain the same type of relief plus reasonable costs and attorney's fees. To enforce these protections, the designated enforcement agency must be given sufficient additional resources to investigate and prosecute allegations of discrimination.

Insurance Discrimination

In 1995, the NIH-DOE Joint Working Group on Ethical, Legal, and Social Implications of Human Genome Research (ELSI Working Group) and the National Action Plan on Breast Cancer (NAPBC) developed and published the following recommendations for state and federal policy makers to protect against genetic discrimination (*Science*, vol. 270, Oct. 20, 1995):

Definitions

- "Genetic information" is information about genes, gene products, or inherited characteristics that may derive from the individual or a family member.

- "Insurance provider" means an insurance company, employer, or any other entity providing a plan of health insurance or health benefits, including group and individual health plans whether fully insured or self-funded.

Recommendations

- Insurance providers should be prohibited from using genetic information or an individual's request for genetic services to deny or limit any coverage or establish eligibility, continuation, enrollment, or contribution requirements.

- Insurance providers should be prohibited from establishing differential rates or premium payments based on genetic information or an individual's request for genetic services.

- Insurance providers should be prohibited from requesting or requiring collection or disclosure of genetic information. Insurance providers and other holders of genetic information should be prohibited from releasing genetic information without the individual's prior written authorization. Written authorization should be required for each disclosure and include to whom the disclosure would be made.

Why Legislation Is Needed Now

1. Based on genetic information, employers may try to avoid hiring workers they believe are likely to take sick leave, resign, or retire early for health reasons (creating extra costs in recruiting and training new staff), file for workers' compensation, or use healthcare benefits excessively.

2. Some employers may seek to use genetic tests to discriminate against workers—even those who do not and may never show signs of disease—because the employers fear the cost consequences.

3. The economic incentive to discriminate based on genetic information is likely to increase as genetic research advances and the costs of genetic testing decrease.

4. Genetic predisposition or conditions can lead to workplace discrimination, even in cases where workers are healthy and unlikely to develop disease or where the genetic condition has no effect on the ability to perform work.

5. Given the substantial gaps in state and federal protections against employment discrimination based on genetic information, comprehensive federal legislation is needed to ensure that advances in genetic technology and research are used to address the health needs of the nation—and not to deny individuals employment opportunities and benefits. Federal legislation would establish minimum protections that could be supplemented by state laws.

6. Insurers can still use genetic information in the individual market in decisions about coverage, enrollment, and premiums.

7. Insurers can still require individuals to take genetic tests.

8. Individuals are not protected from the disclosure of genetic information to insurers, plan sponsors (employers), and medical information bureaus, without their consent.

9. Penalties in HIPAA for discrimination and disclosure violations should be strengthened in order to ensure individuals of the protections afforded by the legislation.

Cases of Genetic Discrimination

Although no genetic-employment discrimination case has been brought before U.S. federal or state courts, in 2001 the Equal Employment Opportunity Commission (EEOC) settled the first lawsuit alleging this type of discrimination.

EEOC filed a suit against the Burlington Northern Santa Fe (BNSF) Railroad for secretly testing its employees for a rare genetic condition that causes carpal tunnel syndrome as one of its many symptoms. BNSF claimed that the testing was a way of determining whether the high incidence of repetitive-stress injuries among its employees was work-related. Besides testing for this rare problem, company-paid doctors also were instructed to screen for several other medical conditions such as diabetes and alcoholism. BNSF employees examined by company doctors were not told that they were being genetically tested. One employee who refused testing was threatened with possible termination.

On behalf of BNSF employees, EEOC argued that the tests were unlawful under the Americans with Disabilities Act because they were not job-related, and any condition of employment based on such tests would be cause for illegal discrimination based on disability. The lawsuit was settled quickly with BNSF agreeing to everything sought by EEOC.

Besides the BNSF case, the Council for Responsible Genetics claims that hundreds of genetic-discrimination cases have been documented and describes select cases in its "Genetic Discrimination Position Paper" (PDF available online at http://www.gene-watch.org/educational/genetic_discrimination.pdf). In one case, genetic testing indicated that a young boy had fragile X syndrome, an inherited form of mental retardation. The insurance company for the boy's family dropped his health coverage, claiming the syndrome was a preexisting condition. In another case, a social worker lost her job within a week of mentioning that her mother had died of Huntington disease and that she had a 50% chance of developing it.

Despite claims of hundreds of genetic-discrimination incidents, an article from the January 2003 issue of the *European Journal of Human Genetics* reports a real need for a comprehensive investigation of these claims. The article warns that many studies rely on unverified, subjective accounts from individuals who believe they have been unfairly subjected to genetic discrimination by employers or insurance companies. Rarely are these subjective accounts assessed objectively to determine whether actions taken by employers and insurers were truly based on genetic factors or other legitimate concerns.

Chapter 57

Genetic Discrimination in Health Insurance

More than a decade of research on the human genome has yielded a wealth of information. Scientists have mapped and sequenced the genome, identified individual genes or sets of genes that are associated with diseases ranging from Alzheimer's to diabetes and certain forms of cancer, and developed genetic tests to determine an individual's predisposition for some of these diseases. Developments and discoveries like these—and others likely to come in the years ahead—offer hope that many deadly illnesses can be diagnosed, treated and perhaps even cured both earlier and with better results than is now possible.

By learning more about their genetic makeup and susceptibility to certain diseases, people now have more choices, and potentially more control, when dealing with their health and future. Genetic information may lead people to ask their physicians to screen them regularly for certain diseases, to take preventive measures earlier in life, or even to rethink their reproductive plans and choices.

But genetic information can also be misused. It can be used to discriminate against people in health insurance and employment. People known to carry a gene that increases their likelihood of developing cancer, for example, may get turned down for health insurance. Without health insurance, it may be impossible for some people to get treatment for a disease that could be fatal. This may lead some people to decide against genetic testing for fear of what the results might show,

National Human Genome Research Institute (www.genome.gov), March 2004.

567

and who might find out about them. It also could lead some people to decline participation in biomedical research such as studies of gene mutations associated with certain diseases that examine the history of families prone to those maladies.

Each of us probably has half a dozen or more genetic mutations that place us at risk for some disease. That does not mean that we will develop the disease, only that we are more likely to get it than people who do not have the same genetic mutations we do. As our knowledge of the human genome increases, more and more people will likely be identified as carriers of mutations associated with a greater risk of certain diseases. That means that virtually all people are potential victims of genetic discrimination in health insurance.

Public Concerns

As a result, Americans have become concerned about the possible misuse of genetic information, especially in health insurance and employment. A *Time* magazine/Cable News Network (CNN) poll, published in June 2000, found that 75 percent of those surveyed would not want their insurance company to have information about their genetic code. A 1998 survey released by the National Center for Genome Resources (NCGR) found that 85 percent of those polled think employers should not have access to information about their employees' genetic conditions, risks or predispositions.

People have reason to be concerned. Employer-sponsored health insurance plans in the private sector cover more than half of all Americans. Numerous reports in the news media and from expert groups have already uncovered instances where people were denied health insurance or coverage for particular conditions based on genetic information. In one case, a young boy, who had inherited an altered gene from his mother making him susceptible to a potentially fatal heart condition, was denied coverage by a health insurer when the boy's father lost his job and group coverage, and then tried to buy new insurance.

In 1993, the Ethical, Legal and Social Implications (ELSI) Working Group of the Human Genome Project issued a report titled "Genetic Information and Health Insurance" (this report can be found online at www.genome.gov/10001750). The report recommended that people be eligible for health insurance no matter what is known about their past, present or future health status. Two years later, the ELSI Working Group and the National Action Plan on Breast Cancer (NAPBC) jointly developed guidelines to assist federal and state agencies in preventing genetic discrimination in health insurance.

Further, the ELSI Working Group and NAPBC recommended that health insurers be prohibited from using genetic information or an individual's request for genetic services to deny or limit health insurance coverage, establish differential rates or have access to an individual's genetic information without that individual's written authorization. Written authorization, the groups said, should be required for each separate disclosure and should specify the recipient of the disclosed information.

Next, the National Human Genome Research Institute (NHGRI) and the United States Department of Energy, acting through the ELSI Working Group, cosponsored a series of workshops in the mid-1990s on genetic discrimination in health insurance and the workplace. The findings and recommendations of the workshop participants were published in *Science: (Genetic Information and the Workplace: Legislative Approaches and Policy Challenges)* magazine, the monthly journal of the American Association for the Advancement of Science.

Legislative Protections

Those recommendations, and earlier ones issued by the ELSI Working Group and NAPBC led, in part, to new legislation and policies at both the federal and state levels. The Health Insurance Portability and Accountability Act (HIPAA) of 1996 provided the first federal protections against genetic discrimination in health insurance. The act prohibited health insurers from excluding individuals from group coverage due to past or present medical problems, including genetic predisposition to certain diseases. It limited exclusions from group plans for preexisting conditions to 12 months and prohibited such exclusions for people who had been covered previously for that condition for 12 months or more. And the law specifically stated that genetic information in the absence of a current diagnosis of illness did not constitute a preexisting condition.

On the other hand, HIPAA did not prohibit health insurers from charging a higher rate to individuals based on their genetic makeup, prevent insurers from collecting genetic information or limit the disclosure of genetic information about individuals to insurers. Nor did it prevent insurers from requiring applicants to undergo genetic testing.

The next step in addressing the issue of genetic discrimination was taken by President Bill Clinton. The President had earlier supported proposed legislation that would have banned all health plans—group or individual—from denying coverage or raising premiums on the basis of genetic information. When the legislation failed to pass Congress,

President Clinton issued an Executive Order in February 2000 prohibiting agencies of the federal government from obtaining genetic information about their employees or job applicants and from using genetic information in hiring and promotion decisions. In announcing the order, President Clinton said, "We must not allow advances in genetics to become the basis of discrimination against any individual or any group. We must never allow these discoveries to change the basic belief upon which our government, our society, and our system of ethics is founded—that all of us are created equal, entitled to equal treatment under the law."

Both before and since that Executive Order, a number of bills have been introduced into Congress to further deal with genetic discrimination in health insurance and employment. Nine bills were introduced in the 106th Congress (1999–2001) and four in the 107th Congress (2001–03). Meanwhile, 41 states have enacted legislation related to genetic discrimination in health insurance and 31 states have adopted laws regarding genetic discrimination in the workplace. The state laws regarding health insurance conform to HIPAA.

There continues to be a high degree of interest in these topics in state legislatures. More than one hundred bills were introduced in state legislatures in 2000 alone. Some would inaugurate protection from genetic discrimination while others would modify or clarify existing legislation.

Chapter 58

Planning for the Future
for People with Special Needs

This is the first generation of persons with special needs who will typically survive their parents. Therefore, planning is no longer an option, it is a very significant part of your loved one's future. When should a family begin planning? Yesterday. Whether the person with special needs is four of forty years old, it is imperative that families create a plan. A parent never knows when they will no longer be here to care for their loved one. According to the U.S. census of 1991–92, there are now over 10,000,000 persons with developmental disabilities. Less than 20% of these families have done any planning.

The purpose of this text is to educate families on the issues needed to be addressed in the planning process, and to provide them with a simple method on how to proceed whether they create a plan on their own or with professional guidance. In addition, options will be provided to enable families to decide which is the best method that makes the process simple and easy to complete.

As families begin their plan they should first identify the people who can assist in the planning process. In addition to family members, it could include, the person with a disability, an attorney, a financial advisor, caseworkers, medical practitioners, teachers, therapists, anyone involved in providing services, and a lifetime assistance planner to act as a "team" advisor to make sure that all parts of the plan are coordinated and complete.

Excerpted from "Futures and Special Needs Planning for Persons with a Disability," and reprinted with permission from the National Down Syndrome Society, http://www.ndss.org. © 2004 National Down Syndrome Society. All rights reserved.

There are four key issues to be addressed in planning for the future. The first, lifestyle planning is where the family puts in writing what they want for the future of their loved one. This information is recorded in a document called the, "Letter of Intent." Although not a legal document, it is as important as the will and "Special Need Trust." Lifestyle issues require decisions regarding where the person will live, continued educational programs, employment, social activities, religion affiliation, medical care, behavior management, advocacy and/or guardianship, trustees, and final arrangements. In addition, detailed instructions are provided for assisting the person with the typical activities of daily living such as bathing, dressing, feeding, and toileting. Perhaps the person has a special way of communicating that only the immediate family members know and understand. It is important that this information be included. In addition, discuss the person in different social settings such as; home, school, day care center, etc. Prior to providing details regarding the assistance your loved one requires, it is also important to inform others of what the person can do for themselves. Their self-esteem, ego, or personal satisfaction in accomplishing a task is important. Great care and attention should be given to this matter as it can plan an important role in the person's peace of mind.

Legal planning enables the family to state their wishes as to the distribution of their assets and appoint executors to settle their estate. In conjunction with this, a trust is usually executed to provide professional money management, appoint successor trustees and guardians, maintain government benefits, and protect the assets left for the individual. It is important to note that not all assets pass by your will. Life insurance, annuities, IRAs and 401(k)s pass by beneficiary designation in the policies or plans themselves. It is, therefore, important to check how each asset in your estate will be transferred after your death.

The "Irrevocable Special Needs Trust" is the most commonly used document to provide supplemental funds for the exclusive benefit of the person with special needs. When properly drafted, the assets are not considered in the name of the person, so they will not cause the loss of SSI (supplemental security income) and health care benefits. In addition, these funds are not exposed to repayment of Medicaid benefits. This trust has proven invaluable to families regardless of the size of their estate or the amount of assets they are leaving for the person. This trust enables you to appoint a trustee to manage these funds in the future after your death or inability to perform this function.

Financial needs planning is used to determine the supplemental needs of the person. First a monthly budget is established based on today's needs while projecting for the future. Then by using a reasonable rate of return on principal, the family calculates how much money is needed projected into the future using an inflation factor. Once this is completed the family then identifies the resources to be used to fund the trust. This may include stocks, mutual funds, IRAs, 401(k)s, real estate, home, life insurance, etc. Professional management for investing the assets may be done by the trustee, or the trustee may elect to hire advisors.

Government entitlements are for many persons the only or primary source if income and benefits. The cash and health care benefits are received through SSI, SSA (Social Security Administration), SSDI (Social Security disability insurance), Medicaid, and/or Medicare. A basic understanding of federal and state entitlement programs is essential in order to be sure that the person gets all that they are eligible to receive. It is important to make sure that assets received from family members through gifts and inheritance or a settlement from litigation does not result in the ineligibility and termination of government benefits or the government claiming reimbursement for benefits provided from assets received by the person. This is accomplished by making provisions through legal documents, beneficiary changes, and notification of family that the person with special need should not be named as a direct beneficiary. The "Special Needs Trust" should be named to receive these assets in order to avoid the loss of benefits or reimbursement for those already received.

It is evident that each of these issues is interrelated and requires they be coordinated in the planning process. Those persons who provide advice in one particular area should be made cognizant of what others are doing. This emphasizes the importance of an organized plan.

The result of completing a comprehensive plan provides: lifetime supervision and care; maintaining government benefits; provide supplementary funds to help ensure a comfortable lifestyle; provide management of funds; provide dignified final arrangements; and avoid family conflict.

In order to prepare a plan in a simple step-by-step procedure without feeling overwhelmed by the process it is important that families commit to following ten life planning steps. If these steps are followed, the family will create a directive that addresses the lifestyle and care needs of the person. It is important to note that you work on one step at a time and no more than an hour or two each evening. By doing this, you will have time to review each step, think about what you want and not feel pressured or overwhelmed. A professional special needs planner can assist you through the entire process or work on a limited consulting basis as you develop your plan.

Step 1—Prepare a Life Plan

Decide what you want for the future regarding residential need, employment, education, social activities, and general lifestyle.

Step 2—Prepare Informational and Lifestyle Directives

Put your hopes, desire, instructions, and goals for your loved one in a written "Letter of Intent." Include information regarding care providers and assistance, attending physicians, dentists, medicine, functioning abilities, types of activities enjoyed, daily living skills, diet, monitoring medication, and rights and values. Videotape interacting with the person at home, work, school, communicating, and assisting with daily activities and needs.

Step 3—Decide on Supervision

Guardianship and conservatorship are legal appointments requiring court ordered mandates. Individuals or institutions manage the estate of the people judged incapable (not necessarily incompetent) of caring for their own affairs. Guardians and conservators are also responsible for the care and decisions made on behalf of people who are unable to care for themselves. Legal guardianship may not be appropriate for the person if they are able to perform most tasks for themselves, are gainfully employed, and are living, to some degree, independently. Legal counsel, care providers, and physicians should be consulted for guidance. An alternative to guardianship would be a "Durable Legal and Medical Power of Attorney." The person with special needs would need to be able to understand and sign a legal document. This would provide others with the authority to make legal and medical decisions on behalf of the person, if and when they are unable.

Step 4—Determine the Cost

Make a list of current and anticipated monthly expenses. When this amount has been calculated, decide on a reasonable return on investments, and estimate how much you will need to provide enough funds to support the person's lifestyle. Government entitlements and the effects of inflation should be included.

Step 5—Identify Resources to Fund Plan

Resources include government benefits, family assistance, inheritances, savings, life insurance, pensions, real estate, and investments.

Most families do not have the available assets to fund the trust immediately, but designate specific assets through their will and beneficiary designations.

Step 6—Prepare Legal Documents

Choose a qualified attorney to prepare the necessary documents which may include: wills, trusts, guardianship, conservatorship, and power of attorney.

Step 7—Consider Creating a "Special Needs Trust"

The "Special Needs Trust" holds assets for the benefit of persons with special needs and uses the income to provide for their supplemental needs. When drafted properly, assets are not considered in the person's name so as not to jeopardize government entitlements including cash and health care benefits. In addition, it can avoid repayment of health care provided by the government. Trustees are appointed to manage the trust and successor trustees are also named.

Step 8—Put All Documents in a Binder

Place all pertinent information in a binder and let those who will take over the care and supervision of the individual know where to find it. Copies of legal documents should be placed in the binder. Original documents should be in a safe fireproof location.

Step 9—Hold a Meeting

Give relevant copies of documents and instructions to family and care providers. Review everyone's responsibility and make sure they understand and agree.

Step 10—Review the Plan

As the person with special needs grows and changes, needs will change. It is for this reason that each year the plan should be reviewed. If necessary, make changes in the "Letter of Intent" and consult with an attorney if legal documents need to be modified.

Once families make a commitment to prepare a plan for their loved one, by following this process, they can complete it in a very short time. With this information, families learn why it is important and how they can accomplish this endeavor. What greater gift to give a person with a disability than the continuing love and guidance of his or her parents through a comprehensive plan that takes effect when Mom and Dad are no longer able to provide care.

—by Barton Y. Stevens, ChLAP
(Chartered Lifetime Assistance Planner)

Part Six

Genetic Research

Chapter 59

The Human Genome Project

What was the Human Genome Project and why has it been important?

The Human Genome Project was an international research effort to determine the sequence of the human genome and identify the genes that it contains. The Project was coordinated by the National Institutes of Health and the U.S. Department of Energy. Additional contributors included universities across the United States and international partners in the United Kingdom, France, Germany, Japan, and China. The Human Genome Project formally began in 1990 and was completed in 2003, two years ahead of its original schedule.

The work of the Human Genome Project has allowed researchers to begin to understand the blueprint for building a person. As researchers learn more about the functions of genes and proteins, this knowledge will have a major impact in the fields of medicine, biotechnology, and the life sciences.

What were the goals of the Human Genome Project?

The main goals of the Human Genome Project were to provide a complete and accurate sequence of the three billion DNA base pairs

Excerpted from "The Human Genome Project and Genomic Research," *Genetics Home Reference: Your Guide to Understanding Genetic Conditions*, a service of the U.S. National Library of Medicine, March 2004. The complete text, including links to additional information, is available online through the *Genetics Home Reference* website at, http://ghr.nlm.nih.gov.

that make up the human genome and to find all 30,000 to 40,000 human genes. The Project also aimed to sequence the genomes of several other organisms that are important to medical research, such as the mouse and the fruit fly.

In addition to sequencing DNA, the Human Genome Project sought to develop new tools to obtain and analyze the data and to make this information widely available. Also, because advances in genetics have consequences for individuals and society, the Human Genome Project committed to exploring the consequences of genomic research through its Ethical, Legal, and Social Implications (ELSI) program.

What did the Human Genome Project accomplish?

In April 2003, researchers announced that the Human Genome Project had completed a high-quality sequence of essentially the entire human genome. This sequence closed the gaps from a working draft of the genome, which was published in 2001. It also identified the locations of many human genes and provided information about their structure and organization. The Project made the sequence of the human genome and tools to analyze the data freely available via the internet.

In addition to the human genome, the Human Genome Project sequenced the genomes of several other organisms, including brewers' yeast, the roundworm, and the fruit fly. In 2002, researchers announced that they had also completed a working draft of the mouse genome. By studying the similarities and differences between human genes and those of other organisms, researchers can discover the functions of particular genes and identify which genes are critical for life.

What were some of the ethical, legal, and social implications addressed by the Human Genome Project?

The Ethical, Legal, and Social Implications (ELSI) program was founded in 1990 as an integral part of the Human Genome Project. The mission of the ELSI program was to identify and address issues raised by genomic research that would affect individuals, families, and society. A percentage of the Human Genome Project budget at the National Institutes of Health and the U.S. Department of Energy was devoted to ELSI research.

The ELSI program focused on the possible consequences of genomic research in four main areas:

- Privacy and fairness in the use of genetic information, including the potential for genetic discrimination in employment and insurance.

- The integration of new genetic technologies, such as genetic testing, into the practice of clinical medicine.

- Ethical issues surrounding the design and conduct of genetic research with people, including the process of informed consent.

- The education of healthcare professionals, policy makers, students, and the public about genetics and the complex issues that result from genomic research.

What are the next steps in genomic research?

Discovering the sequence of the human genome was only the first step in understanding how the instructions coded in DNA lead to a functioning human being. The next stage of genomic research will begin to derive meaningful knowledge from the DNA sequence. Research studies that build on the work of the Human Genome Project are under way worldwide.

The objectives of continued genomic research include the following:

- Determine the function of genes and the elements that regulate genes throughout the genome.

- Find variations in the DNA sequence among people and determine their significance. These variations may one day provide information about a person's disease risk and response to certain medications.

- Discover the 3-dimensional structures of proteins and identify their functions.

- Explore how DNA and proteins interact with one another and with the environment to create complex living systems.

- Develop and apply genome-based strategies for the early detection, diagnosis, and treatment of disease.

- Sequence the genomes of other organisms, such as the rat, cow, and chimpanzee, in order to compare similar genes between species.

- Develop new technologies to study genes and DNA on a large scale and store genomic data efficiently.

- Continue to explore the ethical, legal, and social issues raised by genomic research.

What is pharmacogenomics?

Pharmacogenomics is the study of how genes affect a person's response to drugs. This relatively new field combines pharmacology (the science of drugs) and genomics (the study of genes and their functions) to develop effective, safe medications and doses that will be tailored to a person's genetic makeup.

Many drugs that are currently available are "one size fits all," but they don't work the same way for everyone. It can be difficult to predict who will benefit from a medication, who will not respond at all, and who will experience negative side effects (called adverse drug reactions). Adverse drug reactions are a significant cause of hospitalizations and deaths in the United States. With the knowledge gained from the Human Genome Project, researchers are learning how inherited differences in genes affect the body's response to medications. These genetic differences will be used to predict whether a medication will be effective for a particular person and to help prevent adverse drug reactions.

The field of pharmacogenomics is still in its infancy. Its use is currently quite limited, but new approaches are under study in clinical trials. In the future, pharmacogenomics will allow the development of tailored drugs to treat a wide range of health problems, including cardiovascular disease, Alzheimer disease, cancer, HIV/AIDS, and asthma.

Chapter 60

Beyond Genes: Scientists Venture Deeper into the Human Genome

The National Human Genome Research Institute (NHGRI) today announced the first grants in a three-year, $36 million scientific reconnaissance mission aimed at discovering all parts of the human genome that are crucial to biological function.

In recent years, researchers have made tremendous progress in sequencing the genomes of humans and other organisms. Scientists use DNA sequence data to help find genes, which are the parts of the genome that code for proteins. However, the protein-encoding component of DNA comprises just a small fraction of the genome, accounting for roughly 1.5 percent of the genetic material of humans and other mammals. There is compelling evidence that other parts of the genome must have important functions, but at present there is only very limited information available about how these other parts work.

"The Human Genome Project has provided us with a wonderful foundation, but obviously having the human genomic sequence is not enough. We must keep on exploring this newfound wealth of knowledge if we are to realize the full potential of genome research to improve human health," said NHGRI Director Francis S. Collins, M.D., Ph.D., who led the public effort to sequence all three billion base pairs in human DNA.

Excerpted from "Beyond Genes: Scientists Venture Deeper into the Human Genome," National Human Genome Research Institute, October 2003. The complete text, including grant recipient names and related links, is available online at http://www.genome.gov/11009066.

"Our experimental and computational methods are still primitive when it comes to identifying functional elements that are not involved in protein coding. That has to change. So, with NHGRI's support, research teams around the world are embarking on a daunting mission: to build a comprehensive 'parts list' of the human genome by identifying and precisely locating all functional elements in our DNA sequence," Dr. Collins said.

The new effort, which is called the ENCyclopedia Of DNA Elements (ENCODE) project, will be carried out by an international consortium made up of scientists in government, industry, and academia. A major aspect of this initiative is a three-year pilot project in which research groups will work cooperatively to test efficient, high-throughput methods for identifying, locating, and fully analyzing all of the functional elements contained in a set of DNA target regions that covers approximately 30 megabases, or about one percent, of the human genome. If the pilot effort proves successful, the project will be expanded to cover the entire genome.

"The ultimate goal of the ENCODE project is to create a reference work that will help researchers fully utilize the human sequence to gain a deeper understanding of human biology, as well as to develop new strategies for preventing and treating disease," said Elise A. Feingold, Ph.D., the NHGRI program director in charge of the ENCODE project. "Following the model established by the Human Genome Project, data generated by ENCODE researchers will be collected and stored in databases, and will be rapidly and freely available to the entire scientific community.

The ENCODE pilot effort is being implemented by a consortium because the wide range of technologies that need to be tested and developed is well beyond the scope of any single scientific team. The DNA target regions were selected to provide a good cross section of different types of genome sequence and to encourage researchers to look for functional elements beyond genes, transcription-factor binding sites, and others that are already fairly well characterized.

"Each member of the consortium will look at all the target regions. Researchers won't be able to come in and just focus on their favorite area of the genome," Dr. Feingold said. "By working together in a highly cooperative manner, we fully expect this consortium to lay the groundwork for a future, large-scale effort."

In addition to studying the human genome itself, another prominent component of the ENCODE project will be the comparison of genomic sequences from many different animals. "Multi-species comparisons enable us to zero in on DNA sequences that have been highly conserved throughout evolution, which is a strong indicator that these sequences reflect functionally important regions of the human genome," said NHGRI Scientific Director Eric D. Green, M.D., Ph.D., whose team recently published a pioneering study in the journal *Nature* that compared genomic sequences among 13 vertebrate species.

In the first year of the ENCODE project, NHGRI awarded approximately $10.5 million in funds to researchers who will study the large-scale application of existing technologies for determining functional elements. Ultimately, approximately $28 million is expected to be allocated to this part of the effort over three years.

A number of other groups will participate in the ENCODE consortium, including those headed by NHGRI's Dr. Green, who will spearhead the comparative sequencing efforts for this project; the University of California, Santa Cruz's David Haussler, Ph.D., who will coordinate the database for all sequence-related data; NHGRI's Andreas D. Baxevanis, Ph.D., who will coordinate the database for other data types; and Children's Hospital Oakland Research Institute's Pieter de Jong, Ph.D., who will lead the team that will create the clone resources needed to support the comparative sequencing. Furthermore, the ENCODE project is open to other investigators willing to participate within the criteria and guidelines established for the consortium.

Simultaneously, NHGRI awarded $2.6 million in first-year funding to researchers for a second component of the ENCODE project: to develop new or improved technologies for finding functional elements in genomic DNA. Further technology development is critical to the long-term goal of the project because scientists currently do not have all of the necessary tools to complete the encyclopedia for the entire human genome in a rapid, efficient, and cost-effective manner. Approximately $7.8 million will be allocated to this part of the effort over three years.

For more information about NHGRI's ENCODE project, go to http://www.genome.gov/10005107. Additional information about NHGRI can be found at its website, http://www.genome.gov.

Chapter 61

Recently Developed Medical Technologies

Polymerase Chain Reaction (PCR)

What is PCR?

Sometimes called "molecular photocopying," the polymerase chain reaction (PCR) is a fast and inexpensive technique used to "amplify," copy, small segments of DNA. Because significant amounts of a sample of DNA are necessary for molecular and genetic analyses, studies of isolated pieces of DNA are nearly impossible without PCR amplification.

Often heralded as one of the most important scientific advances in molecular biology, PCR revolutionized the study of DNA to such an extent that its creator, Kary B. Mullis, was awarded the Nobel Prize for Chemistry in 1993.

What is PCR used for?

Once amplified, the DNA produced by PCR can be used in many different laboratory procedures. For example, most mapping techniques in the Human Genome Project (HGP) rely on PCR.

This chapter contains "Polymerase Chain Reaction (PCR)," February 2004; "Fluorescence in Situ Hybridization (FISH)," January 2004; "Spectral Karyotyping," reviewed May 2004; "DNA Chip Technology," reviewed May 2004; "DNA Microarray Technology," reviewed May 2004; and "Nanomedicine," March 2004; all produced by the National Human Genome Research Institute (NHGRI) and available online through the NHGRI website at http://www.genome.gov.

PCR is also valuable in a number of newly emerging laboratory and clinical techniques, including DNA fingerprinting, detection of bacteria or viruses (particularly AIDS), and diagnosis of genetic disorders.

How does PCR work?

To amplify a segment of DNA using PCR, the sample is first heated so the DNA denatures, or separates into two pieces of single-stranded DNA. Next, an enzyme called "Taq polymerase" synthesizes, builds, two new strands of DNA, using the original strands as templates. This process results in the duplication of the original DNA, with each of the new molecules containing one old and one new strand of DNA. Then each of these strands can be used to create two new copies, and so on, and so on. The cycle of denaturing and synthesizing new DNA is repeated as many as 30 or 40 times, leading to more than one billion exact copies of the original DNA segment.

The entire cycling process of PCR is automated and can be completed in just a few hours. It is directed by a machine called a thermocycler, which is programmed to alter the temperature of the reaction every few minutes to allow DNA denaturing and synthesis.

Fluorescence in Situ Hybridization (FISH)

What is FISH?

FISH provides researchers with a way to visualize and map the genetic material in an individual's cells, including specific genes or portions of genes. This is important for understanding a variety of chromosomal abnormalities and other genetic mutations. Unlike most other techniques used to study chromosomes, FISH does not have to be performed on cells that are actively dividing. This makes it a very versatile procedure.

How does FISH work?

FISH is useful, for example, to help a researcher identify where a particular gene falls within an individual's chromosomes. The first step is to prepare short sequences of single-stranded DNA that match a portion of the gene the researcher is looking for. These are called probes. The next step is to label these probes by attaching one of a number of colors of fluorescent dye.

DNA is composed of two strands of complementary molecules that bind to each other like chemical magnets. Since the researchers' probes are single-stranded, they are able to bind to the complementary strand of DNA, wherever it may reside on a person's chromosomes. When a probe binds to a chromosome, its fluorescent tag provides a way for researchers to see its location.

What is FISH used for?

Scientists use three different types of FISH probes, each of which has a different application:

Locus specific probes bind to a particular region of a chromosome. This type of probe is useful when scientists have isolated a small portion of a gene and want to determine on which chromosome the gene is located.

Alphoid or **centromeric repeat probes** are generated from repetitive sequences found in the middle of each chromosome. Researchers use these probes to determine whether an individual has the correct number of chromosomes. These probes can also be used in combination with "locus specific probes" to determine whether an individual is missing genetic material from a particular chromosome.

Whole chromosome probes are actually collections of smaller probes, each of which binds to a different sequence along the length of a given chromosome. Using multiple probes labeled with a mixture of different fluorescent dyes, scientists are able to label each chromosome in its own unique color. The resulting full-color map of the chromosome is known as a spectral karyotype. Whole chromosome probes are particularly useful for examining chromosomal abnormalities, for example, when a piece of one chromosome is attached to the end of another chromosome.

Spectral Karyotyping

What is SKY?

Spectral karyotyping (SKY) is a laboratory technique that allows scientists to visualize all of the human chromosomes at one time by "painting" each pair of chromosomes in a different fluorescent color.

What is SKY used for?

Many diseases are associated with particular chromosomal abnormalities. For example, chromosomes in cancer cells frequently exhibit aberrations called translocations, in which a piece of one chromosome breaks off and attaches to the end of another chromosome. Identifying such chromosomal abnormalities and determining their role in disease is an important step in developing new methods for diagnosing many genetic disorders.

Traditional karyotyping allows scientists to view the full set of human chromosomes in black and white, a technique that is useful for observing the number, size and shape of the chromosomes. Interpreting these karyotypes, however, requires an expert, who might need hours to examine a single chromosome. By using SKY, even non-experts can easily see instances where a chromosome, painted in one color, has a small piece of a different chromosome, painted in another color, attached to it.

How does SKY work?

SKY involves the preparation of a large collection of short sequences of single-stranded DNA called probes. Each of the individual probes in this DNA library is complementary to a unique region of one chromosome—together, all of the probes make up a collection of DNA that is complementary to all of the chromosomes within the human genome.

Each probe is labeled with a fluorescent color that is designated for a specific chromosome. For example, probes that are complementary to chromosome 1 are labeled with yellow molecules, while those that are complementary to chromosome 2 are labeled with red molecules, and so on.

When these probes are mixed with the chromosomes from a human cell, the probes hybridize, bind, to the DNA in the chromosomes. As they hybridize, the fluorescent probes essentially paint the full set of chromosomes in a rainbow of colors. Scientists can then use computers to analyze the painted chromosomes to determine whether any of them exhibits translocations or other structural abnormalities.

DNA Chip Technology

What is a DNA microchip?

Scientists know that a mutation, or alteration, in a particular gene's DNA often results in a certain disease. However, it can be very difficult to develop a test to detect these mutations, because most large genes have many regions where mutations can occur. For example, researchers believe that mutations in the genes *BRCA1* and *BRCA2* cause as many as 60 percent of all cases of hereditary breast and ovarian cancers. But there is not one specific mutation responsible for all of these cases. Researchers have already discovered over 800 different mutations in *BRCA1* alone.

The DNA microchip is a revolutionary new tool used to identify mutations in genes like *BRCA1* and *BRCA2*. The chip, which consists of a small glass plate encased in plastic, is manufactured somewhat like a computer microchip. On the surface, each chip contains thousands of short, synthetic, single-stranded DNA sequences, which together, add up to the normal gene in question.

What is a DNA microchip used for?

Because chip technology is still relatively new, it is currently only a research tool. Scientists hope to be able to use it to conduct large-scale population studies—for example, to determine how often individuals with a particular mutation actually develop breast cancer.

As we gain more insight into the mutations that underlie various diseases, researchers will likely produce new chips to help assess individual risks for developing different cancers as well as heart disease, diabetes and other diseases.

How does a DNA microchip work?

To determine whether an individual possesses a mutation for *BRCA1* or *BRCA2*, a scientist first obtains a sample of DNA from the patient's blood as well as a control sample—one that does not contain a mutation in either gene.

The researcher then denatures the DNA in the samples—a process that separates the two complementary strands of DNA into single-stranded molecules. The next step is to cut the long strands of DNA into smaller, more manageable fragments and then to label each fragment by attaching a fluorescent dye. The individual's DNA is labeled with green dye and the control, or normal, DNA is labeled with red dye. Both sets of labeled DNA are then inserted into the chip and allowed to hybridize, or bind, to the synthetic *BRCA1* or *BRCA2* DNA on the chip. If the individual does not have a mutation for the gene, both the red and green samples will bind to the sequences on the chip.

591

If the individual does possess a mutation, the individual's DNA will not bind properly in the region where the mutation is located. The scientist can then examine this area more closely to confirm that a mutation is present.

DNA Microarray Technology

What is DNA microarray technology?

Although all of the cells in the human body contain identical genetic material, the same genes are not active in every cell. Studying which genes are active and which are inactive in different cell types helps scientists to understand both how these cells function normally and how they are affected when various genes do not perform properly. In the past, scientists have only been able to conduct these genetic analyses on a few genes at once. With the development of DNA microarray technology, however, scientists can now examine how active thousands of genes are at any given time.

What is DNA microarray technology used for?

Microarray technology will help researchers to learn more about many different diseases, including heart disease, mental illness, and infectious diseases, to name only a few. One intense area of microarray research at the National Institutes of Health (NIH) is the study of cancer. In the past, scientists have classified different types of cancers based on the organs in which the tumors develop. With the help of microarray technology, however, they will be able to further classify these types of cancers based on the patterns of gene activity in the tumor cells. Researchers will then be able to design treatment strategies targeted directly to each specific type of cancer. Additionally, by examining the differences in gene activity between untreated and treated tumor cells—for example those that are radiated or oxygen-starved—scientists will understand exactly how different therapies affect tumors and be able to develop more effective treatments.

How does DNA microarray technology work?

DNA microarrays are created by robotic machines that arrange minuscule amounts of hundreds or thousands of gene sequences on a single microscope slide. Researchers have a database of over 40,000 gene sequences that they can use for this purpose. When a gene is activated, cellular machinery begins to copy certain segments of that gene. The resulting product is known as messenger RNA (mRNA), which is the body's template for creating proteins. The mRNA produced by the cell is complementary, and therefore will bind to the original portion of the DNA strand from which it was copied.

To determine which genes are turned on and which are turned off in a given cell, a researcher must first collect the messenger RNA molecules present in that cell. The researcher then labels each mRNA molecule by attaching a fluorescent dye. Next, the researcher places the labeled mRNA onto a DNA microarray slide. The messenger RNA that was present in the cell will then hybridize, or bind, to its complementary DNA on the microarray, leaving its fluorescent tag. A researcher must then use a special scanner to measure the fluorescent areas on the microarray.

If a particular gene is very active, it produces many molecules of messenger RNA, which hybridize to the DNA on the microarray and generate a very bright fluorescent area. Genes that are somewhat active produce fewer mRNAs, which results in dimmer fluorescent spots. If there is no fluorescence, none of the messenger molecules have hybridized to the DNA, indicating that the gene is inactive. Researchers frequently use this technique to examine the activity of various genes at different times.

Nanomedicine

What if doctors had tiny tools that could search out and destroy the very first cancer cells of a tumor developing in the body? What if a cell's broken part could be removed and replaced with a functioning miniature biological machine? Or what if molecule-sized pumps could be implanted in sick people to deliver life-saving medicines precisely where they are needed? These scenarios may sound unbelievable, but they are the ultimate goals of nanomedicine, a cutting-edge area of biomedical research that seeks to use nanotechnology tools to improve human health.

What is a nanometer?

A lot of things are small in today's high-tech world of biomedical tools and therapies. But when it comes to nanomedicine, researchers are talking very, very small. A nanometer is one-billionth of a meter, too small even to be seen with a conventional lab microscope.

What is nanotechnology?

Nanotechnology is the broad scientific field that encompasses nanomedicine. It involves the creation and use of materials and devices at the level of molecules and atoms, which are the parts of matter that combine to make molecules. Non-medical applications of nanotechnology now under development include tiny semiconductor chips made out of strings of single molecules and miniature computers made out of DNA, the material of our genes. Federally supported research in this area, conducted under the rubric of the National Nanotechnology Initiative, is ongoing with coordinated support from several agencies.

What is being done to advance nanomedicine?

For hundreds of years, microscopes have offered scientists a window inside cells. Researchers have used ever more powerful visualization tools to extensively categorize the parts and sub-parts of cells in vivid detail. Yet, what scientists have not been able to do is to exhaustively inventory cells, cell parts, and molecules within cell parts to answer questions such as, "How many?" "How big?" and "How fast?" Obtaining thorough, reliable measures of quantity is the vital first step of nanomedicine.

As part of the National Institutes of Health (NIH) Roadmap for Medical Research (http://nihroadmap.nih.gov), the NIH will establish a handful of nanomedicine centers. These centers will be staffed by a highly interdisciplinary scientific crew including biologists, physicians, mathematicians, engineers and computer scientists. Research conducted over the first few years will be spent gathering extensive information about how molecular machines are built. A key activity during this time will be the development of a new kind of vocabulary, or lexicon, to define biological parts and processes in engineering terms.

Once researchers have completely catalogued the interactions between and within molecules, they can begin to look for patterns and a higher order of connectedness than is possible to identify with current experimental methods. Mapping these networks and understanding how they change over time will be a crucial step toward helping scientists understand nature's rules of biological design. Understanding these rules will, in many years' time, enable researchers to use this information to address biological issues in unhealthy cells.

The availability of innovative, body-friendly nanotools will help scientists figure out how to build synthetic biological devices, such as miniature, implantable pumps for drug delivery or tiny sensors to scan for the presence of infectious agents or metabolic imbalances that could spell trouble for the body.

Chapter 62

Single Nucleotide Polymorphisms (SNPs)

Wouldn't it be wonderful if you knew exactly what measures you could take to stave off, or even prevent, the onset of disease? Wouldn't it be a relief to know that you are not allergic to the drugs your doctor just prescribed? Wouldn't it be a comfort to know that the treatment regimen you are undergoing has a good chance of success because it was designed just for you? With the recent harvest of more than one million SNPs, biomedical researchers now believe that such exciting medical advances are not that far away.

What Are SNPs and How Are They Found?

A single nucleotide polymorphism, or SNP (pronounced "snip"), is a small genetic change, or variation, that can occur within a person's DNA sequence. The genetic code is specified by the four nucleotide "letters" A (adenine), C (cytosine), T (thymine), and G (guanine). SNP variation occurs when a single nucleotide, such as an A, replaces one of the other three nucleotide letters—C, G, or T.

An example of a SNP is the alteration of the DNA segment AAGGTTA to ATGGTTA, where the second "A" in the first snippet is replaced with a "T." On average, SNPs occur in the human population more than one percent of the time. Because only about three to five percent of a person's DNA sequence codes for the production of

"SNPs: Variations on a Theme," from *A Science Primer: Just the Facts: A Basic Introduction to the Science Underlying NCBI Resources*, National Center for Biotechnology Information (NCBI), revised March 2004.

proteins, most SNPs are found outside of "coding sequences." SNPs found within a coding sequence are of particular interest to researchers because they are more likely to alter the biological function of a protein. Because of the recent advances in technology, coupled with the unique ability of these genetic variations to facilitate gene identification, there has been a recent flurry of SNP discovery and detection.

Although many SNPs do not produce physical changes in people, scientists believe that other SNPs may predispose a person to disease and even influence their response to a drug regimen.

Needles in a Haystack

Finding single nucleotide changes in the human genome seems like a daunting prospect, but over the last 20 years, biomedical researchers have developed a number of techniques that make it possible to do just that. Each technique uses a different method to compare selected regions of a DNA sequence obtained from multiple individuals who share a common trait. In each test, the result shows a physical difference in the DNA samples only when a SNP is detected in one individual and not in the other.

Many common diseases in humans are not caused by a genetic variation within a single gene but are influenced by complex interactions among multiple genes as well as environmental and lifestyle factors. Although both environmental and lifestyle factors add tremendously to the uncertainty of developing a disease, it is currently difficult to measure and evaluate their overall effect on a disease process. Therefore, we refer here mainly to a person's genetic predisposition, or the potential of an individual to develop a disease based on genes and hereditary factors.

Genetic factors may also confer susceptibility or resistance to a disease and determine the severity or progression of disease. Because we do not yet know all of the factors involved in these intricate pathways, researchers have found it difficult to develop screening tests for most diseases and disorders. By studying stretches of DNA that have been found to harbor a SNP associated with a disease trait, researchers may begin to reveal relevant genes associated with a disease. Defining and understanding the role of genetic factors in disease will also allow researchers to better evaluate the role non-genetic factors—such as behavior, diet, lifestyle, and physical activity—have on disease.

Because genetic factors also affect a person's response to a drug therapy, DNA polymorphisms such as SNPs will be useful in helping researchers determine and understand why individuals differ in their abilities to absorb or clear certain drugs, as well as to determine why an individual may experience an adverse side effect to a particular drug. Therefore, the recent discovery of SNPs promises to revolutionize not only the process of disease detection but the practice of preventative and curative medicine.

SNPs and Disease Diagnosis

It will only be a matter of time before physicians can screen patients for susceptibility to a disease by analyzing their DNA for specific SNP profiles.

Each person's genetic material contains a unique SNP pattern that is made up of many different genetic variations. Researchers have found that most SNPs are not responsible for a disease state. Instead, they serve as biological markers for pinpointing a disease on the human genome map, because they are usually located near a gene found to be associated with a certain disease. Occasionally, a SNP may actually cause a disease and, therefore, can be used to search for and isolate the disease-causing gene.

To create a genetic test that will screen for a disease in which the disease-causing gene has already been identified, scientists collect blood samples from a group of individuals affected by the disease and analyze their DNA for SNP patterns. Next, researchers compare these patterns to patterns obtained by analyzing the DNA from a group of individuals unaffected by the disease. This type of comparison, called an "association study," can detect differences between the SNP patterns of the two groups, thereby indicating which pattern is most likely associated with the disease-causing gene. Eventually, SNP profiles that are characteristic of a variety of diseases will be established. Then, it will only be a matter of time before physicians can screen individuals for susceptibility to a disease just by analyzing their DNA samples for specific SNP patterns.

SNPs and Drug Development

Using SNPs to study the genetics of drug response will help in the creation of "personalized" medicine.

As mentioned earlier, SNPs may also be associated with the absorbance and clearance of therapeutic agents. Currently, there is no simple way to determine how a patient will respond to a particular medication. A treatment proven effective in one patient may be ineffective in others. Worse yet, some patients may experience an adverse immunologic reaction to a particular drug. Today, pharmaceutical companies are limited to developing agents to which the "average" patient will respond. As a result, many drugs that might benefit a small number of patients never make it to market.

In the future, the most appropriate drug for an individual could be determined in advance of treatment by analyzing a patient's SNP profile. The ability to target a drug to those individuals most likely to benefit, referred to as "personalized medicine," would allow pharmaceutical companies to bring many more drugs to market and allow doctors to prescribe individualized therapies specific to a patient's needs.

Snps and NCBI

Most SNPs are not responsible for a disease state. Instead, they serve as biological markers for pinpointing a disease on the human genome map.

Because SNPs occur frequently throughout the genome and tend to be relatively stable genetically, they serve as excellent biological markers. Biological markers are segments of DNA with an identifiable physical location that can be easily tracked and used for constructing a chromosome map that shows the position of known genes, or other markers, relative to each other. These maps allow researchers to study and pinpoint traits resulting from the interaction of more than one gene. NCBI plays a major role in facilitating the identification and cataloging of SNPs through its creation and maintenance of the public SNP database (dbSNP). This powerful genetic tool may be accessed by the biomedical community worldwide and is intended to stimulate many areas of biological research, including the identification of the genetic components of disease.

Chapter 63

Novel Mechanism Preserves Y Chromosome Genes

A detailed analysis of the completed sequence of the human Y chromosome—the chromosome that distinguishes males from females—has uncovered a novel mechanism by which it maintains its genetic integrity. The study is published in *Nature* (June 2003).

All other chromosomes occur in pairs and preserve genetic integrity by exchanging information with matching genes on the homologous chromosome, a process called "crossing over." But the Y chromosome lacks that option, being the only chromosome that is unpaired. Instead, the Y appears to exchange genes between the two arms that make up the chromosome itself.

This phenomenon, called gene conversion—the non-reciprocal transfer of genetic information from one DNA molecule to another—has been previously observed on a small scale over long evolutionary timescales between repeated sequences on the same chromosome, but not at the dramatic frequency apparently employed by the Y chromosome.

A research team, led by David C. Page, M.D., a Howard Hughes Medical Institute investigator at the Whitehead Institute for Biomedical Research in Cambridge, Massachusetts; Richard K. Wilson, Ph.D., director of the Genome Sequencing Center at Washington University School of Medicine in St. Louis; and Robert H. Waterston, M.D., Ph.D., formerly of Washington University's sequencing center and now at the University of Washington, Seattle, discovered that many of the

"Researchers Discover Use of Novel Mechanism Preserves Y Chromosome Genes," a press release from *NIH News*, National Institutes of Health and the National Human Genome Research Institute (NHGRI), June 28, 2003.

sequences of chemical units—called bases or base pairs—that carry genetic information on the Y chromosome are arranged as palindromes. Palindromes are phrases or sentences that read the same backward or forward, such as "Madam, I'm Adam."

In the case of the Y, the palindromes are not just "junk" DNA; these strings of bases contain functioning genes important for male fertility. The team found that most of the sequence pairs are greater than 99.97 percent identical. The extensive use of gene conversion appears to play a role in the ability of the Y chromosome to edit out genetic mistakes and maintain the integrity of the relatively few genes it carries.

"This analysis of the Y chromosome could not have been done without the highly accurate sequence data produced by the Human Genome Project and made freely available to researchers everywhere in the world," said Francis S. Collins, M.D., Ph.D., director of the National Human Genome Research Institute (NHGRI), which, along with the U.S. Department of Energy, led the Human Genome Project in the United States. "Unless the human sequence had been finished to the highest level of accuracy—less than one mistake in every 10,000 bases, the Y chromosome researchers would not have been able to identify the Y's unusual genetic structure and the novel mechanism for maintaining its integrity. Of all the human chromosomes, this was probably the most challenging to assemble correctly, and could never have been done without the painstaking map-based approach adopted by the International Human Genome Sequencing Consortium."

In a separate paper in the same issue of *Nature*, the team confirmed its findings by comparing similar regions of the Y chromosome in humans to the Y chromosomes of chimpanzees, bonobos (the pygmy chimpanzee) and gorillas. The comparison demonstrated that the same phenomenon of gene conversion appeared to be at work more than five million years ago, when humans and the non-human primates diverged from each other.

"The comparison between human and non-human primate chromosomes confirming the finding shows the power of comparative genomics," Dr. Collins said. "Without the ability to compare the genetic material across species, it would have been difficult for the team to test their hypothesis." NHGRI now funds a number of genome sequencing projects on model organisms, including the dog, the chimp, the chicken and the honeybee. The mouse, rat and fruit fly sequencing projects are essentially completed—except, ironically, for the Y chromosome of each of those species, which are still under construction.

The sequencing work on the Y chromosome was carried out at the Genome Sequencing Center at the Washington University School of Medicine as part of the Human Genome Project, which receives substantial funding from NHGRI. The Human Genome Project officially began in October 1990 and was completed in April 2003; sequencing the rough draft of the human genome sequence cost an estimated $300 million. The entire project, including genetic mapping, technology development, the study of model organisms, and the ethical, legal and social implications (ELSI) program was initially projected to take 15 years, but was completed more than two years early at a cost that was $400 million less than expected.

Chapter 64

Gene Discovery Opens Door to Further Research in Inherited Neurological Disorders

Scientists at the National Human Genome Research Institute (NHGRI) and at the National Institute of Neurological Disorders and Stroke (NINDS) have identified the gene responsible for two related, inherited neurological disorders, and have, for the first time, directly implicated this gene and its enzyme product in a human genetic disease.

The discovery supports further investigation of this gene family for additional neurological disease genes, research that may shed light on a range of disorders, including carpal tunnel syndrome, which affects the hands and the wrists, and the fatal degenerative disease amyotrophic lateral sclerosis (ALS), also known as Lou Gehrig's disease.

NHGRI and NINDS scientists, working together at the National Institutes of Health (NIH), found the gene responsible for Charcot-Marie-Tooth (CMT) disease type 2D and distal spinal muscular atrophy (dSMA) type V. The gene, called *GARS*—the glycyl tRNA synthetase gene—is located on chromosome 7 and encodes, or provides the instructions to make, one of the aminoacyl tRNA synthetases, a family of enzymes vital to the cell's ability to build proteins.

"The identification of the defective gene on chromosome 7 responsible for a type of Charcot-Marie-Tooth disease provides another vivid example of how the recently completed human genome sequence is accelerating studies in human genetics," said Francis S. Collins, M.D., Ph.D., director of NHGRI. "With this discovery, we now know that the

An *NIH News Release*, National Institutes of Health and the National Human Genome Research Institute (NHGRI), April 2003, reviewed January 2004.

GARS gene—whose function is so fundamental to biological processes—can be mutated in a fashion that results in a highly discrete neurological disease."

The study, a collaboration between the laboratories of Eric Green, M.D., Ph.D., at NHGRI, Kenneth Fischbeck, M.D., at NINDS, and Lev Goldfarb, M.D., also at NINDS, was published in the May 2003 issue of the *American Journal of Human Genetics*. Lead author Anthony Antonellis, a graduate student in Dr. Green's laboratory, directed the project.

The scientists identified four disease-related mutations and speculate that a mutated copy of *GARS* leads to a reduction in the activity of the gene's enzyme product. More research into why this disruption produces the specific symptoms of CMT type 2D and dSMA type V will be necessary.

"Identifying this chromosome 7 disease gene at this particular time was especially gratifying in light of the recent completion of a finished sequence of this chromosome," said Dr. Green, who is the Scientific Director of NHGRI and chief of its Genome Technology Branch. Dr. Green also directs the NIH Intramural Sequencing Center. His laboratory has been involved in mapping and sequencing chromosome 7 as part of the Human Genome Project.

"This discovery is another piece of a jigsaw puzzle picture of how peripheral nerve diseases and motor neuron diseases happen," said Dr. Fischbeck, chief of the Neurogenetics Branch at NINDS. Dr. Fischbeck's laboratory studies hereditary motor neuron diseases and peripheral neuropathies. "It provides a more complete view of the mechanism of these diseases. This will hopefully lead to new treatment approaches. The more complete the picture, the more we know how to intervene."

Charcot-Marie-Tooth disease, named after the three physicians who first reported it in 1886, is a group of genetic diseases that causes muscle weakness and wasting, or atrophy, in the feet, legs, hands, and forearms, as well as diminished sensation in the limbs. CMT disease affects the peripheral nerves—the nerves that travel to the muscles of the limbs—and is therefore known as a peripheral neuropathy. Estimated to affect one in 2,500 individuals, it is the most common inherited neurological disorder.

Some forms of CMT disease are autosomal dominant, meaning that a person needs to inherit only one defective copy of the responsible gene to acquire the disease. Other forms are autosomal recessive, meaning both copies of the gene must be defective to result in illness. There is also a form of CMT that is X-linked, meaning that the responsible gene is located on the X chromosome, one of the two sex chromosomes.

In most cases, CMT disease begins with mild symptoms, typically foot and ankle weakness and fatigue. As atrophy progresses, the patient develops a distinct walk, a consequence of muscle weakness in the front of the leg: the feet slap with each step and the body may sway from side to side. Eventually the toes and the fingers curl due to weakness and atrophy in the small muscles of the feet and the hands. Writing and other functions of the hands become difficult. The sensory loss that accompanies the atrophy diminishes the patient's ability to distinguish between hot and cold and affects the patient's sense of touch.

People with CMT disease usually begin to experience symptoms in adolescence or early adulthood. There is no cure for the disease, but there are treatment options, including physical therapy and bracing. Life expectancy is usually normal.

CMT disease can be divided into two classes, depending on where the dysfunction occurs in the peripheral nerves. In CMT type 1, the peripheral nerves' axons—the part of the nerve cell that transmits electrical signals to the muscles—lose their protective outer coverings, their myelin sheaths. This disrupts the axons' function. In CMT type 2, the axons' responses are diminished due to a defect within the axons themselves.

CMT type 2, the less common of the two classes, can be further separated into at least six subtypes, caused by defects in different genes. The *GARS* gene is implicated in CMT type 2D, a form of CMT that primarily affects the hands and the forearms. CMT type 2D is inherited in an autosomal dominant fashion.

Spinal muscular atrophy (SMA) refers to a group of genetic diseases more diverse than those of CMT. SMA is characterized by weakness and wasting of the muscles of the limbs, but the types vary greatly in severity. Most common are autosomal recessive childhood-onset forms that may be fatal. Other types of SMA are inherited in an autosomal dominant fashion. All types of SMA are due to the degeneration of nerve cells within the spinal cord, as opposed to degeneration of the peripheral nerves.

Distal spinal muscular atrophy (dSMA) disease is a type of SMA that affects the hands and the feet. The *GARS* gene is implicated in dSMA type V. Its symptoms of muscle weakness and atrophy in the hands and the forearms mirror those of CMT type 2D, except that people with dSMA type V do not experience sensory loss. dSMA type V is also an autosomal dominant genetic disorder, like CMT type 2D.

Even though the *GARS* gene is implicated in only two specific types of CMT and SMA, this discovery will guide researchers in studying other forms of these diseases, as well as other neurological disorders. Because carpal tunnel syndrome affects the hands and the forearms, scientists may now investigate whether the *GARS* gene plays some role in this disorder. And two defective forms of the gene implicated in Lou Gehrig's disease are known to interact with a *GARS* family member.

Ultimately, the *GARS* gene and its family may provide a rich new resource for scientists investigating inherited and non-inherited neurological diseases.

"The next step is to explore what it is about motor nerve cells that make them particularly vulnerable to mutations in these genes," said Dr. Fischbeck.

Chapter 65

Researchers Identify Gene for Premature Aging Disorder

A team led by the National Human Genome Research Institute (NHGRI) announced the discovery of the genetic basis of a disorder that causes the most dramatic form of premature aging, a finding that promises to shed new light on the rare disease, as well as on normal human aging.

In their study, published in the journal *Nature* [April 2003], researchers identified the genetic mutations responsible for Hutchinson-Gilford progeria syndrome (HGPS), commonly referred to as progeria. Derived from the Greek word for old age, "geras," progeria is estimated to affect one in eight million newborns worldwide. There currently are no diagnostic tests or treatments for the progressive, fatal disorder.

Francis S. Collins, M.D., Ph.D., director of the NHGRI and leader of the research team, said, "This genetic discovery represents the first piece in solving the tragic puzzle of progeria. Without such information, we in the medical community were at loss about where to focus our efforts to help these children and their families. Now, we finally know where to begin."

Dr. Collins added, "The implications of our work may extend far beyond progeria to each and every human being. What we learn about the molecular basis of this model of premature aging may provide us with a better understanding of what occurs in the body as we all grow older."

An *NIH News Release*, National Institutes of Health and the National Human Genome Research Institute (NHGRI), April 2003.

In addition to NHGRI, the multi-institution research team included scientists from the Progeria Research Foundation; the New York State Institute for Basic Research in Developmental Disabilities in Staten Island, N.Y.; the University of Michigan in Ann Arbor; and Brown University in Providence, R.I.

W. Ted Brown, M.D., Ph.D., co-author of the study and chairman of the Department of Human Genetics at the Institute for Basic Research, said, "Many people consider progeria to be the most dramatic example of a genetic disease that clearly resembles accelerated aging. The children appear to have an aging rate that is five to ten times what is normal." Dr. Brown is widely regarded as the world's leading clinical expert on progeria.

Children with progeria usually appear normal at birth. However, within a year, their growth rate slows and their appearance begins to change. Affected children typically become bald with aged-looking skin and pinched noses. They often suffer from symptoms typically seen in elderly people, especially severe cardiovascular disease. Death occurs on average at age 13, usually from heart attack or stroke.

Leslie Gordon, M.D., Ph.D., medical director of the Progeria Research Foundation (PRF) and executive director of the PRF Genetics Consortium, said, "Isolating this gene is just the beginning. It is our goal to find treatments and possibly a cure for this rare, life-threatening disease that robs children of their adulthood. The Progeria Research Foundation will continue to lead the fight against progeria."

In 2001, PRF co-hosted a workshop with various institutes and centers of the National Institutes of Health (NIH), including the National Institute on Aging and the Office of Rare Diseases. The workshop brought together leading scientists from around the world to identify promising areas of research in progeria. This partnership eventually led to funding for progeria research and the formation of the PRF Genetics Consortium, a group of 20 scientists whose common goal is to find the genetic cause of progeria and to develop ways of treating the disease. Six of those scientists are co-authors of the study to be published in *Nature*.

Dr. Collins commended the collaborative efforts, saying, "The Progeria Research Foundation's commitment and cooperation played a key role in the hunt for the disease gene. They brought the urgent need to find this gene to the attention of the biomedical research community."

Dr. Collins, as leader of the Human Genome Project, announced the successful completion of the international project's effort to sequence the three billion letters that make up the human genetic instruction book. "Free and unrestricted access to the human genome sequence is greatly speeding the pace of disease gene discovery. Finding the gene for progeria would have been impossible without the tools provided by the Human Genome Project," said Dr. Collins, who still spends some of his time in a small research lab at the National Institutes of Health (NIH). "This was a particularly challenging project for the gene hunters, since there are no families in whom the disease has recurred, and geneticists generally depend on such families to track the responsible gene. This was a detective story with very few clues."

Taking advantage of an array of genomic technologies—from whole-genome scans to high-throughput sequencing of targeted DNA regions—researchers determined the most common cause of progeria is a single-letter "misspelling" in a gene on chromosome 1 that codes for lamin A, a protein that is a key component of the membrane surrounding the cell's nucleus. Specifically, the researchers found that 18 out of 20 children with classic progeria harbored exactly the same misspelling in the lamin A (*LMNA*) gene, a substitution of just a single DNA base—a change from cytosine (C) to thymine (T)—among the gene's 25,000 base pairs. In addition, one of the remaining progeria patients had a different single base substitution—guanine (G) to adenine (A)—just two bases upstream. In every instance, the parents were found to be normal indicating that the misspelling was a new, or "de novo," mutation in the child.

At first glance, the point substitution in the *LMNA* gene would appear to have no effect on the production of lamin A protein. "Initially, we could hardly believe that such a small substitution was the culprit. How could these bland-looking mutations lead to such terrible consequences in the body?" said NHGRI's Maria Eriksson, Ph.D., a post-doctoral fellow in Dr. Collins' lab and the first author of the study.

However, when Dr. Eriksson conducted laboratory tests on cells from progeria patients, she found that the minute change in the *LMNA* gene's DNA sequence dramatically changed the way in which the sequence was spliced by the cell's protein-making machinery. The end result was the production of an abnormal lamin A protein that is missing a stretch of 50 amino acids near one of its ends.

To determine what effect abnormal lamin A has upon cells, the NHGRI-led team used fluorescent antibodies to track lamin A in skin cells taken from progeria patients known to have the common misspelling, as well as skin cells taken from unaffected people. The studies showed that about half of the cells from the progeria patients had misshapen nuclear membranes, compared with less than one percent of the cells from the unaffected controls.

"We suspect that this instability of the nuclear membrane may pose major problems for tissues subjected to intense physical stress—tissues such as those found in the cardiovascular and musculoskeletal systems, which are so severely affected in progeria," said Dr. Eriksson, noting that nuclear instability ultimately may lead to widespread death of cells.

Researchers hope to move their new findings into the clinic almost immediately with the development of a genetic test for progeria. Such a test will help doctors diagnose or rule out progeria in young children much earlier than their current method of looking at outward physical changes.

The new findings also may have implications for the treatment of progeria, with the newfound understanding of progeria's molecular roots pointing to possible therapeutic approaches. For example, researchers plan to explore the possibility that statins and/or other drugs known to inhibit a step in protein processing, known as farnesylation, might reduce the production of abnormal lamin A in progeria patients. Another avenue for identifying possible therapies involves screening large libraries of chemical molecules with the hope of finding a compound that can reverse the nuclear membrane irregularities seen in the cells of progeria patients.

"It is impossible to predict how soon our findings will translate into treatments for children suffering from progeria. We and other researchers across the nation will be working hard to find ways of helping them. Unfortunately, as we have witnessed with other genetic discoveries, the road from the lab to the clinic is not always swift or smooth," Dr. Collins said.

More also remains to be done to determine what role the *LMNA* gene may play in the normal aging process. "Aging clearly has a strong genetic component. Discovery of this key genetic mutation that causes progeria may lead to a much clearer understanding of what causes aging in us all. Eventually, this information may lead to improvements in health care for our aging population," said Dr. Brown.

Researchers plan to look at the *LMNA* genes of people who are exceptionally long-lived to see if there are any variants of the gene associated with longevity. Other studies might focus on determining whether repeated damage to the *LMNA* gene over the course of a lifetime may influence the rates at which people age.

"Our hypothesis is that *LMNA* may help us solve some of the great mysteries of aging," Dr. Collins said. "However, it will probably take more than one genetic key to unlock the secrets to a biological process as complex as aging. There are probably a host of other genes related to aging still waiting to be discovered."

Another interesting footnote to the recent findings is that different mutations in other regions of the *LMNA* gene previously have been shown to be responsible for a half-dozen other rare, genetic disorders. Those disorders are: Emery-Dreifuss muscular dystrophy type 2; limb girdle muscular dystrophy type 1B; Charcot-Marie-Tooth disorder type 2B1; the Dunnigan type of familial partial lipodystrophy; mandibuloacral dysplasia; and a familial form of dilated cardiomyopathy.

Prior to coming to NIH to lead the Human Genome Project in 1993, Dr. Collins had established a reputation as a relentless gene hunter using an approach that he named "positional cloning." In contrast to previous methods for finding genes, positional cloning enabled scientists to identify disease genes without knowing in advance what the functional abnormality underlying the disease might be. Dr. Collins' lab, together with collaborators, applied the new approach in 1989 in their successful quest for the long-sought gene responsible for cystic fibrosis. Other major discoveries soon followed, including identification of the genes for neurofibromatosis; Huntington's disease; multiple endocrine neoplasia type 1; one type of adult acute leukemia; and Alagille syndrome.

Chapter 66

Behavioral Genetics

Toward Behavioral Genomics

The genetics of behavior offers more opportunity for media sensationalism than any other branch of current science. Frequent news reports claim that researchers have discovered the "gene for" such traits as aggression, intelligence, criminality, homosexuality, feminine intuition, and even bad luck. Such reports tend to suggest, usually incorrectly, that there is a direct correspondence between carrying a mutation in the gene and manifesting the trait or disorder. Rarely is it mentioned that traits involving behavior are likely to have a more complex genetic basis. This is probably because most journalists—in common with most educated laypeople (and some biologists)—tend to have a straightforward, single-gene view of genetics. But single genes do not determine most human behaviors. Only certain rare disorders such as Huntington's disease have a simple mode of transmission in which a specific mutation confers the certainty of developing the disorder. Most types of behavior have no such clear-cut pattern and depend on interplay between environmental factors and multiple genes. Genes in such multiple-gene systems are called quantitative trait loci

---

This chapter begins with text reprinted with permission from "Toward Behavioral Genomics," by Peter McGuffin, Brien Riley, and Robert Plomin, *SCIENCE*, Volume 291, Issue 5507, 1232-1249, February 16, 2001. Copyright 2001 American Association for the Advancement of Science. Additional material is also reprinted from *SCIENCE*: "Rethinking Behavior Genetics" by Dean Hamer, *SCIENCE*, Volume 298, Issue 5591, 71-72, October 4, 2002.

(QTLs), because they are likely to result in continuous (quantitative) distributions of phenotypes that underlie susceptibility to common disorders.

Although in many ways behavior presents geneticists with the same challenges as other complex physiological and medical traits, behavior is unique in that it is the product of our most complicated organ, the brain. Most valuable for behavioral genetics will be the sequencing of multiple human genomes and identification of the several million DNA base pairs that differ among us. These DNA variations are responsible for the ubiquitous genetic influences on individual differences in behavioral dimensions and disorders. The most solid genetic findings about individual differences in human behavior come from quantitative genetic research such as twin and adoption studies that consistently converge on the conclusion that genetic variation makes a substantial contribution to phenotypic variation for all behavioral domains. The best-studied areas are psychopathology, personality, and cognitive abilities and disabilities, all of which have been assessed by recent model-fitting. There are two striking findings. The first is that nearly all behaviors that have been studied show moderate to high heritability—usually, to a somewhat greater degree than do many common physical diseases.[1] Second, although environment plays a role, its contribution tends to be of the nonshared type, that is, environmental factors make people different from, rather than similar to, their relatives.

Such quantitative approaches, however, can no longer be seen as ends in themselves, and the information and techniques generated by the human genome sequence will be valuable in locating and identifying genes involved in behavior. Although some genes that have major effects on behavior have been identified (see Table 66.1), progress so far has been slow, partly because genes with effects large enough to be readily detectable by linkage are probably rare. For example, a recent genome scan in schizophrenia in almost 200 families effectively excluded a gene having a large effect from most of the genome.[2] A further issue is the definition of phenotypes. Modern methods allow reliable diagnosis of disorders such as schizophrenia but there are several competing diagnostic schemes, raising the question of which one is "most valid" for genetic research.[3]

It has long been known that a complementary approach, allelic association, can detect genes that account for as little as 1% of the variance in a trait.[4] Until recently this approach was hampered by the lack of sufficiently detailed marker maps. Now, with the human genome sequence available, association studies should be able to locate

Table 66.1. Current Understanding of the Genetic Basis of Selected Behavioral Disorders and Traits[2]

Behavioral trait	Pattern of inheritance	Gene mapping
Huntington's disease	Rare autosomal dominant dynamic mutation	Gene identified (huntingtin) with unstable trinucleotide repeat.
Early onset (familial) Alzheimer's disease	Rare autosomal dominant	Three distinct genes identified (presenilins 1 and 2, and amyloid precursor protein).
Fragile X mental retardation	Nonstandard X-linked dynamic mutation	Two genes identified (*FMR1* and *2*), both with unstable trinucleotide repeats.
Late onset Alzheimer's disease	Common complex	Increased risk with apolipoprotein e4 allele.
Attention deficit, hyperactivity disorder	Common complex	Three contributory loci in the dopamine system, *DRD4, DAT1* and *DRD5*; *DRD4* best replicated, others less certain.
Dyslexia	Common complex	Two contributory loci suggested on chromosomes 6 and 15; findings replicated.
Schizophrenia	Common complex	Numerous reported linkages including chromosomes 1, 5, 6, 10, 13, 15, and 22 but no consensus; a few promising candidate genes include $5\text{-}HT_{2A}$ and *CHRNA7*.
Aggression	Common complex	Mutation reported in X-linked *MAOA* gene in one family; no evidence of broader relevance.
Male homosexuality	Common complex	Linkage reported at X-linked marker locus in sib pairs; not replicated.

QTLs with the aid of a greatly improved map based on hundreds of thousands of single-nucleotide polymorphisms (SNPs) and new methods of very high-throughput genotyping, as discussed by Peltonen and McKusick.[5] Another new benefit is that much of the hard work of positional cloning has been replaced by cloning by computer. Thus, gene sequences, and even polymorphisms can be identified by searching appropriate computer databases.

Identifying QTLs is one thing, but understanding their effects will take much more time. Functional genomics and proteomics,[6] where the focus is on gene products, their structure and expression, can be generally viewed as bottom-up strategies. But there are other levels of analysis at which we can understand how genes work. A top-down approach highlights the behavior of the whole organism. For example, we can ask how the effects of specific genes unfold in behavioral development and how they interact and correlate with experience. This top-down, behavioral genomic level of analysis[7] will complement the current functional approaches in the human species. Furthermore, genome sequences of other organisms will be especially important because of the great similarity of genes and gene organization between, for example, mouse and man.[8]

Ultimately, the human genome sequence will revolutionize psychology and psychiatry. The most important impact will be on understanding the neurobiological basis of individual differences and achieving a better grasp of the etiology of diseases. The latter, in turn, should lead to the discovery of new and more specific drug treatments. The use of genomics as a path to drug discovery holds considerable potential.[9] It is also probable that DNA testing will be used to predict which patients will respond to different drugs or be susceptible to particular side effects.[10] However, there are two built-in limitations to this DNA revolution. The first is that all behavior involves gene-environment interplay. The second is the unsolved question of the distribution of effect sizes of QTLs; some may involve effects so small or so complicated that they will never be detected.

The probabilistic rather than deterministic influence of genes on behavior means that some of the ethical specters raised by the advent of behavioral genomics probably have little substance. For example, it has sometimes been suggested that geneticization is likely to increase the stigma of mental disorders. To the contrary, far from increasing the stigma, advances in genetics have the opposite effect. As a case in point, it is now perfectly acceptable for an ex-president of the United States and his family to acknowledge that he has Alzheimer's disease, a disorder for which much progress has been made in understanding its basis at a molecular level. In the recent past this might have been called "going senile" and would have been seen as somehow morally reprehensible. We predict that this is the start of a trend and that identifying genes involved in behavioral disorders will do much to improve public perception and tolerance of behavioral disorders.

References

1. R. Plomin, M. J. Owen, P. McGuffin, *Science* 264, 1733 (1994).

2. N. M. Williams et al., Hum. Mol. *Genet.* 8, 1729 (1999).

3. P. McGuffin, A. Farmer, *Am. J. Med. Genet.* (*Neuropsychiatric Genetics*) 105, 39 (2001) (published online 29 Dec. 2000).

4. J. H. Edwards, *Ann. Hum. Genet.* 29, 77 (1965).

5. L. Peltonen, V. A. McKusick, *Science* 291, 1224 (2001).

6. A. Pandey, M. Mann, *Nature* 405, 837 (2000).

7. R. Plomin, J. C. Crabbe, *Psychol. Bull.* 126, 806 (2000).

8. J. Battey, E. Jordan, D. Cox, W. Dove, Nature Genet. 21, 73 (1999).

9. A. D. Roses, *Nature* 405, 857 (2000).

10. M. J. Arranz et al., *Lancet* 355, 1615 (2000).

11. R. Plomin, J. DeFries, G.1 McClearn, P. McGuffin, *Behavioral Genetics* (Freeman, New York, ed. 4, 2001).

The authors are at the Social, Genetic and Developmental Psychiatry Research Centre, Institute of Psychiatry, Kings College London, De Crespigny Park, London SE5 8AF, UK.

Rethinking Behavior Genetics

The first 100 years spent studying the genetics of behavior were straightforward. The aim was to determine the extent to which individual differences in the way people think, feel, and behave are due to variations in their genetic makeup. The basic approaches, first described by Sir Francis Galton in the late 1800s, were to compare identical and fraternal twins, other family members, and adoptees that had been raised together or apart.

The results were consistently striking, albeit slow to be accepted. Genes were shown to influence virtually every aspect of human personality, temperament, cognitive style, and psychiatric disorder. The effects of heredity were substantial, typically representing 30 to 70% of total variation, and highly replicable across societies and cultures. The long reach of genes extended from a friendly disposition to xenophobia, from bipolar disease to bedwetting, from getting married to keeping a job. About the only characteristics that seemed not to be at least partially heritable were purely learned traits such as the particular language one spoke or the religion one believed in.[1]

The second century of behavior genetics has gotten off to a less satisfying start. The current aim is to identify the specific genes that contribute to individual differences and determine what they do in the brain. The approach is to search for DNA sequence variations that correlate with behavioral and personality traits, either by tracking anonymous markers close to the genes of interest in family members (linkage analysis) or by directly comparing the coding and regulatory sequences of candidate genes (association analysis).

The results have been disappointing and inconsistent. Large and well-funded linkage studies of the major psychiatric disorders including schizophrenia, alcoholism, Tourette syndrome, and bipolar disorder have come up empty-handed; not a single new gene has been conclusively identified. Most candidate gene findings have failed consistent replication, and even those that have been verified account for only a small fraction of total variation. Meanwhile, the statisticians who are supposed to be guiding and evaluating the research are unable to agree on how to design experiments or to interpret the results; their advice has proven as faddish (and useful) as the Hula-Hoop.

What's the problem? It's not the basic premise of linkage and candidate gene analysis; these approaches have identified dozens of genes involved in inherited diseases. Nor is it the lack of DNA sequence information; virtually the entire code of the human genome is now known. The real culprit is the assumption that the rich complexity of human thought and emotion can be reduced to a simple, linear relation between individual genes and behaviors. This oversimplified model, which underlies most current research in behavior genetics, ignores the critical importance of the brain, the environment, and gene expression networks.

Three publications in *Science* show how measuring brain activity, environmental variables, and subtle alterations in gene expression can strengthen behavior genetics research. Hariri et al.[2] examined the influence of the serotonin transporter gene in the response of the amygdala to a fearful stimulus. There is a frequent DNA sequence variation in the control region of the human serotonin transporter gene that influences the expression levels of this protein and thereby the amount of synaptic serotonin, a potent modulator of emotional responses. When the polymorphism was discovered, it was found to be associated with abnormal levels of anxiety as assessed by self-report questionnaires.[3] Although this finding has been replicated in numerous subsequent studies and verified in mice lacking the serotonin transporter gene, the effect of this gene on subjective measures of personality is modest, typically accounting for only a few percent of total variance.[4]

Hariri and colleagues predicted that the gene would have a larger effect on directly measured brain activity. To test this idea, they performed functional nuclear magnetic resonance imaging on normal subjects as they performed either an emotional task—matching the affect of angry or afraid faces to a target face—or a sensorimotor control task. As expected, subjects with the poorly transcribed, high-anxiety serotonin transporter genotype showed a larger response of the amygdala to the emotional task than did the subjects with the highly transcribed, low-anxiety genotype; there was no difference between the two genotypes on the control task. Importantly, the difference between the two genotype groups was nearly fivefold, accounting for 20% of total variance—an effect size nearly 10-fold higher than in typical experiments using subjective behavioral or personality measures as the outcome. This is precisely as expected from viewing the brain as the obligatory intermediate between genotype and behavior.

Technical advances in noninvasive functional neuroimaging will rapidly make this type of analysis both more routine and more powerful.[5,6] Besides increasing signal size and thereby decreasing statistical noise, the main advantage of directly studying the brain will be to focus attention on those behaviors that have a dedicated brain circuit to begin with. It should be obvious that the heritability of some complex traits, like sexual orientation[7] and language acquisition,[8] is probably the direct result of evolutionarily selected genetic programs whereas others, like getting divorced or cigarette smoking, are more likely to involve an unrelated set of characteristics that happen to be amalgamated by culture. All too often, though, the decision of what to study is driven by socio-medical politics rather than biological logic.

The study by Caspi et al.[9] also analyzed a promoter region polymorphism, in this case for the gene encoding monoamine oxidase A

(*MAOA*), an enzyme that breaks down the neurotransmitters seroto-nin, dopamine, and norepinephrine. Although the *MAOA* gene had previously been implicated in aggression and impulse control in both humans and rodents,[10] this transcriptional variant had not been as-sociated with personality traits.[11] Caspi et al. hypothesized that the effect of the gene would be more readily revealed if the environment were explicitly taken into account.

Their study group was a large birth cohort, representative of the male population of New Zealand, whose development had been carefully followed for 26 years. The environmental variable of in-terest was childhood maltreatment, and the outcome was a com-posite measure of antisocial behavior. Although the *MAOA* genotype by itself failed to predict antisocial behavior, there was a signifi-cant interaction with childhood history; individuals with both a low-activity genotype and previous maltreatment were by far the most likely to have committed a violent crime and to be diagnosed with conduct disorder. Over 85% of the males who had both "bad genes" and a "bad environment" developed some form of antisocial behavior by the time they were 26. It will now be crucial to repeat this intriguing finding on other populations with documented de-velopmental histories.

The serotonin transporter and *MAOA* stories nicely illustrate how changes in regulatory rather than coding sequences can influence brain function and behavior. Such variations in gene expression probably play a predominant role in many types of individual differences, but this has been difficult to prove in humans because we are so genetically outbred. Yan and colleagues[12] devised an elegant solution to this problem. They measured the expression of different alleles in a single person who was heterozygous for the locus in question, thus avoiding the problems of extraneous differences in genetic background or other factors. Remark-ably, even though most of the variations they studied were random single-nucleotide substitutions far from the promoter region, almost half of them were associated with detectable changes in messenger RNA levels. A few of the genes they studied are expressed in the brain, and many more will soon follow.

Although the Hariri, Caspi, and Yan reports provide tantalizing glimpses of how the study of complex traits can be improve, they are still at the primitive stage of examining single genes. This isn't how the brain works. Human behaviors, and the brain circuits that produce them, are undoubtedly the product of intricate networks involving hundreds to thousands of genes working in concert with multiple developmental and environmental events. Further advances in the field will require the development of techniques, such as microarray analysis, that measure the activity of many different genes simultaneously. Only then will the gene hunters have a shot at achieving the promises held out by the past century of classical behavior genetics research.

References

1. D. H. Hamer, P. Copeland, *Living With Our Genes* (Doubleday, New York, 1998).

2. A. R. Hariri et al., *Science* 297, 400 (2002).

3. K. P. Lesch et al., *Science* 274, 1527 (1996).

4. D. L Murphy et al., *Brain Res. Bull* 56, 487 (2001).

5. S. Y. Bookheimer et al., *N. Engl. J. Med.* 343, 450 (2000).

6. M. F. Egan et al., *Proc. Natl. Acad. Sci.* U.S.A. 98, 6917 (2001).

7. D. H. Hamer et al., *Science* 261, 321 (1993).

8. C. S. Lai et al., *Nature* 413, 519 (2001).

9. A. Caspi et al., *Science* 297, 851 (2002).

10. J. C. Shih, R. F. Thompson, *Am. J. Hum. Genet.* 65, 593 (1999).

11. S. Z. Sabol et al., *Hum. Genet.* 103, 273 (1998).

12. H. Yan et al., *Science* 291, 1143 (2002).

The author is at the Laboratory of Biochemistry, National Cancer Institute, National Institutes of Health, Bethesda, MD 20892, USA.

Chapter 67

The Promise of Pharmacogenomics

Adverse Drug Reaction. These three simple words convey little of the horror of a severe negative reaction to a prescribed drug. But such negative reactions can nonetheless occur. A 1998 study of hospitalized patients published in the *Journal of the American Medical Association* reported that in 1994, adverse drug reactions accounted for more than 2.2 million serious cases and over 100,000 deaths, making adverse drug reactions (ADRs) one of the leading causes of hospitalization and death in the United States. Currently, there is no simple way to determine whether people will respond well, badly, or not at all to a medication: therefore, pharmaceutical companies are limited to developing drugs using a "one size fits all" system. This system allows for the development of drugs to which the "average" patient will respond. But, as the statistics above show, one size does not fit all, sometimes with devastating results. What is needed is a way to solve the problem of ADRs before they happen. The solution is in sight though, and it is called pharmacogenomics.

What Is Pharmacogenomics?

The way a person responds to a drug (this includes both positive and negative reactions) is a complex trait that is influenced by many different genes. Without knowing all of the genes involved in drug response, scientists have found it difficult to develop genetic tests that

"One Size Does Not Fit All: The Promise of Pharmacogenomics," National Center for Biotechnology Information (NCBI), revised March 2004.

623

could predict a person's response to a particular drug. Once scientists discovered that people's genes show small variations (or changes) in their nucleotide (DNA base) content, all of that changed—genetic testing for predicting drug response is now possible. Pharmacogenomics is a science that examines the inherited variations in genes that dictate drug response and explores the ways these variations can be used to predict whether a patient will have a good response to a drug, a bad response to a drug, or no response at all.

The Difference between Pharmacogenomics and Pharmacogenetics

* Pharmacogenomics refers to the general study of all of the many different genes that determine drug behavior.

* Pharmacogenetics refers to the study of inherited differences (variation) in drug metabolism and response.

The distinction between the two terms is considered arbitrary, however, and now the two terms are used interchangeably.

How Will Gene Variation Be Used in Predicting Drug Response?

Right now, there is a race to catalog as many of the genetic variations found within the human genome as possible. These variations, or SNPs (pronounced "snips"), as they are commonly called, can be used as a diagnostic tool to predict a person's drug response. For SNPs to be used in this way, a person's DNA must be examined (sequenced) for the presence of specific SNPs. (DNA sequencing is the determination of the order of nucleotides (the base sequence) in a DNA molecule.) The problem is, however, that traditional gene sequencing technology is very slow and expensive and has therefore impeded the widespread use of SNPs as a diagnostic tool. DNA microarrays (or DNA chips) are an evolving technology that should make it possible for doctors to examine their patients for the presence of specific SNPs quickly and affordably. A single microarray can now be used to screen 100,000 SNPs found in a patient's genome in a matter of hours. As DNA microarray technology is developed further, SNP screening in the doctor's office to determine a patient's response to a drug, prior to drug prescription, will be commonplace.

How Will Drug Development and Testing Benefit from Pharmacogenomics?

SNP screenings will benefit drug development and testing because pharmaceutical companies could exclude from clinical trials those people whose pharmacogenomic screening would show that the drug being tested would be harmful or ineffective for them. Excluding these people will increase the chance that a drug will show itself useful to a particular population group and will thus increase the chance that the same drug will make it into the marketplace. Pre-screening clinical trial subjects should also allow the clinical trials to be smaller, faster, and therefore less expensive; therefore, the consumer could benefit in reduced drug costs. Finally, the ability to assess an individual's reaction to a drug before it is prescribed will increase a physician's confidence in prescribing the drug and the patient's confidence in taking the drug, which in turn should encourage the development of new drugs tested in a like manner.

What Is NCBI'S Role in Pharmacogenomics?

The explosion in both SNP and microarray data generated from the human genome project has necessitated the development of a means of cataloging and annotating (briefly describing) these data so that scientists can more easily access and use it for their research. The National Center for Biotechnology Information (NCBI), always on the forefront of bioinformatics research, has developed database repositories for both SNP (dbSNP; online at http://www.ncbi.nlm .nih.gov/snp) and microarray GEO (Gene Expression Omnibus; online at http://www.ncbi.nlm.nih.gov/geo) data. These databases include descriptive information about the data within the sites and links to NCBI and external information resources. Access to these data and information resources will allow scientists to more easily interpret data that will be used not only to help determine drug response but to study disease susceptibility and conduct basic research in population genetics.

The Promise of Pharmacogenomics

Right now, in doctors' offices all over the world, patients are given medications that either don't work or have bad side effects. Often, a patient must return to their doctor over and over again until the doctor can find a drug that is right for them. Pharmacogenomics offers a very appealing alternative. Imagine a day when you go into your doctor's office and, after a simple and rapid test of your DNA, your doctor changes her/his mind about a drug considered for you because your genetic test indicates that you could suffer a severe negative reaction to the medication. However, upon further examination of your test results, your doctor finds that you would benefit greatly from a new drug on the market, and that there would be little likelihood that you would react negatively to it. A day like this will be coming to your doctor's office soon, brought to you by pharmacogenomics.

Chapter 68

Gene Therapy

What is gene therapy?

Genes, which are carried on chromosomes, are the basic physical and functional units of heredity. Genes are specific sequences of bases that encode instructions on how to make proteins. Although genes get a lot of attention, it's the proteins that perform most life functions and even make up the majority of cellular structures. When genes are altered so that the encoded proteins are unable to carry out their normal functions, genetic disorders can result.

Gene therapy is a technique for correcting defective genes responsible for disease development. Researchers may use one of several approaches for correcting faulty genes:

- A normal gene may be inserted into a nonspecific location within the genome to replace a nonfunctional gene. This approach is most common.

- An abnormal gene could be swapped for a normal gene through homologous recombination.

- The abnormal gene could be repaired through selective reverse mutation, which returns the gene to its normal function.

- The regulation (the degree to which a gene is turned on or off) of a particular gene could be altered.

Human Genome Project Information, Oak Ridge National Laboratory, December 2003. For additional information visit http://www.doegenomes.org or http://www.ornl.gov.

How does gene therapy work?

In most gene therapy studies, a "normal" gene is inserted into the genome to replace an "abnormal," disease-causing gene. A carrier molecule called a vector must be used to deliver the therapeutic gene to the patient's target cells. Currently, the most common vector is a virus that has been genetically altered to carry normal human DNA. Viruses have evolved a way of encapsulating and delivering their genes to human cells in a pathogenic manner. Scientists have tried to take advantage of this capability and manipulate the virus genome to remove disease-causing genes and insert therapeutic genes.

Target cells such as the patient's liver or lung cells are infected with the viral vector. The vector then unloads its genetic material containing the therapeutic human gene into the target cell. The generation of a functional protein product from the therapeutic gene restores the target cell to a normal state.

Some of the different types of viruses used as gene therapy vectors:

- **Retroviruses:** A class of viruses that can create double-stranded DNA copies of their RNA genomes. These copies of its genome can be integrated into the chromosomes of host cells. Human immunodeficiency virus (HIV) is a retrovirus.

- **Adenoviruses:** A class of viruses with double-stranded DNA genomes that cause respiratory, intestinal, and eye infections in humans. The virus that causes the common cold is an adenovirus.

- **Adeno-associated viruses:** A class of small, single-stranded DNA viruses that can insert their genetic material at a specific site on chromosome 19.

- **Herpes simplex viruses:** A class of double-stranded DNA viruses that infect a particular cell type, neurons. Herpes simplex virus type 1 is a common human pathogen that causes cold sores.

Besides virus-mediated gene-delivery systems, there are several non-viral options for gene delivery. The simplest method is the direct introduction of therapeutic DNA into target cells. This approach is limited in its application because it can be used only with certain tissues and requires large amounts of DNA.

Another non-viral approach involves the creation of an artificial lipid sphere with an aqueous core. This liposome, which carries the therapeutic DNA, is capable of passing the DNA through the target cell's membrane.

Therapeutic DNA also can get inside target cells by chemically linking the DNA to a molecule that will bind to special cell receptors. Once bound to these receptors, the therapeutic DNA constructs are engulfed by the cell membrane and passed into the interior of the target cell. This delivery system tends to be less effective than other options.

Researchers also are experimenting with introducing a 47th (artificial human) chromosome into target cells. This chromosome would exist autonomously alongside the standard 46—not affecting their workings or causing any mutations. It would be a large vector capable of carrying substantial amounts of genetic code, and scientists anticipate that, because of its construction and autonomy, the body's immune systems would not attack it. A problem with this potential method is the difficulty in delivering such a large molecule to the nucleus of a target cell.

What is the current status of gene therapy research?

The Food and Drug Administration (FDA) has not yet approved any human gene therapy product for sale. Current gene therapy is experimental and has not proven very successful in clinical trials. Little progress has been made since the first gene therapy clinical trial began in 1990. In 1999, gene therapy suffered a major setback with the death of 18-year-old Jesse Gelsinger. Jesse was participating in a gene therapy trial for ornithine transcarboxylase deficiency (OTCD). He died from multiple organ failures four days after starting the treatment. His death is believed to have been triggered by a severe immune response to the adenovirus carrier.

Another major blow came in January 2003, when the FDA placed a temporary halt on all gene therapy trials using retroviral vectors in blood stem cells. FDA took this action after it learned that a second child treated in a French gene therapy trial had developed a leukemia-like condition. Both this child and another who had developed a similar condition in August 2002 had been successfully treated by gene therapy for X-linked severe combined immunodeficiency disease (X-SCID), also known as "bubble baby syndrome."

FDA's Biological Response Modifiers Advisory Committee (BRMAC) met at the end of February 2003 to discuss possible measures that could allow a number of retroviral gene therapy trials for treatment of life-threatening diseases to proceed with appropriate safeguards. FDA has yet to make a decision based on the discussions and advice of the BRMAC meeting.

What factors have kept gene therapy from becoming an effective treatment for genetic disease?

- **Short-lived nature of gene therapy:** Before gene therapy can become a permanent cure for any condition, the therapeutic DNA introduced into target cells must remain functional and the cells containing the therapeutic DNA must be long-lived and stable. Problems with integrating therapeutic DNA into the genome and the rapidly dividing nature of many cells prevent gene therapy from achieving any long-term benefits. Patients will have to undergo multiple rounds of gene therapy.

- **Immune response:** Anytime a foreign object is introduced into human tissues, the immune system is designed to attack the invader. The risk of stimulating the immune system in a way that reduces gene therapy effectiveness is always a potential risk. Furthermore, the immune system's enhanced response to invaders it has seen before makes it difficult for gene therapy to be repeated in patients.

- **Problems with viral vectors:** Viruses, while the carrier of choice in most gene therapy studies, present a variety of potential problems to the patient—toxicity, immune and inflammatory responses, and gene control and targeting issues. In addition, there is always the fear that the viral vector, once inside the patient, may recover its ability to cause disease.

- **Multigene disorders:** Conditions or disorders that arise from mutations in a single gene are the best candidates for gene therapy. Unfortunately, some the most commonly occurring disorders, such as heart disease, high blood pressure, Alzheimer's disease, arthritis, and diabetes, are caused by the combined effects of variations in many genes. Multigene or multifactorial disorders such as these would be especially difficult to treat effectively using gene therapy.

What are some recent developments in gene therapy research?

- University of California, Los Angeles, research team gets genes into the brain using liposomes coated in a polymer call polyethylene glycol (PEG). The transfer of genes into the brain is a significant achievement because viral vectors are too big to get across the "blood-brain barrier." This method has potential for treating Parkinson's disease. For more information see "Undercover genes slip into the brain" at www.NewScientist.com (March 20, 2003).

- RNA interference or gene silencing may be a new way to treat Huntington disease. Short pieces of double-stranded RNA (short, interfering RNAs or siRNAs) are used by cells to degrade RNA of a particular sequence. If a siRNA is designed to match the RNA copied from a faulty gene, then the abnormal protein product of that gene will not be produced. For more information see "Gene therapy may switch off Huntington's" at www.NewScientist.com (March 13, 2003).

- New gene therapy approach repairs errors in messenger RNA derived from defective genes. Technique has potential to treat the blood disorder thalassemia, cystic fibrosis, and some cancers. For more information see "Subtle gene therapy tackles blood disorder" at www.NewScientist.com (October 11, 2002).

- Gene therapy for treating children with X-SCID (sever combined immunodeficiency) or the "bubble boy" disease is stopped in France when the treatment causes leukemia in one of the patients. For more information see "'Miracle' gene therapy trial halted" at www.NewScientist.com (October 3, 2002).

- Researchers at Case Western Reserve University and Copernicus Therapeutics are able to create tiny liposomes 25 nanometers across that can carry therapeutic DNA through pores in the nuclear membrane. For more information see "DNA nanoballs boost gene therapy" at www.NewScientist.com (May 12, 2002).

- Sickle cell is successfully treated in mice. For more information see "Murine Gene Therapy Corrects Symptoms of Sickle Cell Disease" from March 18, 2002, issue of *The Scientist*.

What are some of the ethical considerations for using gene therapy?

- What is normal and what is a disability or disorder, and who decides?

- Are disabilities diseases? Do they need to be cured or prevented?

- Does searching for a cure demean the lives of individuals presently affected by disabilities?

- Is somatic gene therapy (which is done in the adult cells of persons known to have the disease) more or less ethical than germline gene therapy (which is done in egg and sperm cells and prevents the trait from being passed on to further generations)? In cases of somatic gene therapy, the procedure may have to be repeated in future generations.

- Preliminary attempts at gene therapy are exorbitantly expensive. Who will have access to these therapies? Who will pay for their use?

Part Seven

Additional Help and Information

Chapter 69

Glossary of Genetic Terms

additive genetic effects: When the combined effects of alleles at different loci are equal to the sum of their individual effects.[1]

adenine (A): A nitrogenous base, one member of the base pair AT (adenine-thymine).[1]

affected relative pair: Individuals related by blood, each of whom is affected with the same trait. Examples are affected sibling, cousin, and avuncular pairs.[1]

allele: Alternative form of a genetic locus; a single allele for each locus is inherited from each parent (for example, at a locus for eye color the allele might result in blue or brown eyes).[1]

allogeneic: Variation in alleles among members of the same species.[1]

amino acid: Any of a class of 20 molecules that are combined to form proteins in living things. The sequence of amino acids in a protein and hence protein function are determined by the genetic code.[1]

Terms in this glossary were excerpted from "Dictionary of Genetic Terms," *Genomics and Its Impact on Medicine and Society: A 2001 Primer*, Oak Ridge National Laboratory, updated January 2004, (marked 1); "Talking Glossary of Genetic Terms," National Human Genome Research Institute, reviewed March 2004, (marked 2); and "More Information: Glossary," National Center for Biotechnology Information, July 2000, (marked 3).

anticipation: Each generation of offspring has increased severity of a genetic disorder; for example, a grandchild may have earlier onset and more severe symptoms than the parent, who had earlier onset than the grandparent.[1]

antisense: Nucleic acid that has a sequence exactly opposite to an mRNA molecule made by the body; binds to the mRNA molecule to prevent a protein from being made.[1]

autoradiography: A technique that uses X-ray film to visualize radioactively labeled molecules or fragments of molecules; used in analyzing length and number of DNA fragments after they are separated by gel electrophoresis.[1]

autosomal dominant: A gene on one of the non-sex chromosomes that is always expressed, even if only one copy is present. The chance of passing the gene to offspring is 50% for each pregnancy.[1]

autosome: A chromosome not involved in sex determination. The diploid human genome consists of a total of 46 chromosomes: 22 pairs of autosomes, and 1 pair of sex chromosomes (the X and Y chromosomes).[1]

avuncular relationship: The genetic relationship between nieces and nephews and their aunts and uncles.[1]

base: One of the molecules that form DNA and RNA molecules.[1]

base pair: Two bases which form a "rung of the DNA ladder." A DNA nucleotide is made of a molecule of sugar, a molecule of phosphoric acid, and a molecule called a base. The bases are the "letters" that spell out the genetic code. In DNA, the code letters are A, T, G, and C, which stand for the chemicals adenine, thymine, guanine, and cytosine, respectively. In base pairing, adenine always pairs with thymine, and guanine always pairs with cytosine.[2]

base sequence: The order of nucleotide bases in a DNA molecule; determines structure of proteins encoded by that DNA.[1]

behavioral genetics: The study of genes that may influence behavior.[1]

bioinformatics: The merger of biotechnology and information technology with the goal of revealing new insights and principles in biology.[3]

birth defect: Any harmful trait, physical or biochemical, present at birth, whether a result of a genetic mutation or some other nongenetic factor.[1]

candidate gene: A gene located in a chromosome region suspected of being involved in a disease.[1]

carrier: An individual who possesses an unexpressed, recessive trait.[1]

cell: The basic unit of any living organism that carries on the biochemical processes of life.[1]

centimorgan (cM): A unit of measure of recombination frequency. One centimorgan is equal to a 1% chance that a marker at one genetic locus will be separated from a marker at a second locus due to crossing over in a single generation. In human beings, one centimorgan is equivalent, on average, to one million base pairs.[1]

centromere: A specialized chromosome region to which spindle fibers attach during cell division.[1]

chromosomal deletion: The loss of part of a chromosome's DNA.[1]

chromosomal inversion: Chromosome segments that have been turned 180 degrees. The gene sequence for the segment is reversed with respect to the rest of the chromosome.[1]

chromosome: The self-replicating genetic structure of cells containing the cellular DNA that bears in its nucleotide sequence the linear array of genes.[1]

chromosome region p: A designation for the short arm of a chromosome.[1]

chromosome region q: A designation for the long arm of a chromosome.[1]

clone: An exact copy made of biological material such as a DNA segment (for example, a gene or other region), a whole cell, or a complete organism.[1]

cloning: Using specialized DNA technology to produce multiple, exact copies of a single gene or other segment of DNA to obtain enough material for further study. This process, used by researchers in the Human Genome Project, is referred to as cloning DNA. The resulting cloned (copied) collections of DNA molecules are called clone libraries.

A second type of cloning exploits the natural process of cell division to make many copies of an entire cell. The genetic makeup of these cloned cells, called a cell line, is identical to the original cell. A third type of cloning produces complete, genetically identical animals such as the famous Scottish sheep, Dolly.[1]

codominance: Situation in which two different alleles for a genetic trait are both expressed.[1]

codon: Three bases in a DNA or RNA sequence which specify a single amino acid.[2]

complementary sequence: Nucleic acid base sequence that can form a double-stranded structure with another DNA fragment by following base-pairing rules (A pairs with T and C with G). The complementary sequence to GTAC for example, is CATG.[1]

complex trait: Trait that has a genetic component that does not follow strict Mendelian inheritance. May involve the interaction of two or more genes or gene-environment interactions.[1]

congenital: Any trait present at birth, whether the result of a genetic or nongenetic factor.[1]

craniosynostosis: A birth defect whereby an infant's skull bones are already fused at birth. Because this defect may interfere with the ability of the brain to grow normally, it is often necessary to operate on affected children.[2]

crossing over: The breaking during meiosis of one maternal and one paternal chromosome, the exchange of corresponding sections of DNA, and the rejoining of the chromosomes. This process can result in an exchange of alleles between chromosomes.[1]

cytogenetics: The study of the physical appearance of chromosomes.[1]

cytoplasmic trait: A genetic characteristic in which the genes are found outside the nucleus, in chloroplasts or mitochondria. Results in offspring inheriting genetic material from only one parent.[1]

cytosine (C): A nitrogenous base, one member of the base pair GC (guanine and cytosine) in DNA.[1]

deletion: A loss of part of the DNA from a chromosome; can lead to a disease or abnormality.[1]

deoxyribose: A type of sugar that is one component of DNA (deoxyribonucleic acid).[1]

diploid: A full set of genetic material consisting of paired chromosomes, one from each parental set. Most animal cells except the gametes have a diploid set of chromosomes. The diploid human genome has 46 chromosomes.[1]

DNA (deoxyribonucleic acid): The molecule that encodes genetic information. DNA is a double-stranded molecule held together by weak bonds between base pairs of nucleotides. The four nucleotides in DNA contain the bases adenine (A), guanine (G), cytosine (C), and thymine (T). In nature, base pairs form only between A and T and between G and C; thus the base sequence of each single strand can be deduced from that of its partner.[1]

DNA repair genes: Genes encoding proteins that correct errors in DNA sequencing.[1]

DNA replication: The use of existing DNA as a template for the synthesis of new DNA strands. In humans and other eukaryotes, replication occurs in the cell nucleus.[1]

DNA sequence: The relative order of base pairs, whether in a DNA fragment, gene, chromosome, or an entire genome.[1]

domain: A discrete portion of a protein assumed to fold independently of the rest of the protein and possessing its own function.[3]

dominant: An allele that is almost always expressed, even if only one copy is present.[1]

double helix: The structural arrangement of DNA, which looks something like an immensely long ladder twisted into a helix, or coil. The sides of the "ladder" are formed by a backbone of sugar and phosphate molecules, and the "rungs" consist of nucleotide bases joined weakly in the middle by hydrogen bonds.[2]

electrophoresis: A method of separating large molecules (such as DNA fragments or proteins) from a mixture of similar molecules. An electric current is passed through a medium containing the mixture, and each kind of molecule travels through the medium at a different rate, depending on its electrical charge and size. Agarose and acrylamide gels are the media commonly used for electrophoresis of proteins and nucleic acids.[1]

embryonic stem (ES) cells: An embryonic cell that can replicate indefinitely, transform into other types of cells, and serve as a continuous source of new cells.[1]

enzyme: A protein that acts as a catalyst, speeding the rate at which a biochemical reaction proceeds but not altering the direction or nature of the reaction.[1]

epistasis: One gene interferes with or prevents the expression of another gene located at a different locus.[1]

eukaryote: Cell or organism with membrane-bound, structurally discrete nucleus and other well-developed subcellular compartments. Eukaryotes include all organisms except viruses, bacteria, and blue-green algae.[1]

exon: The region of a gene that contains the code for producing the gene's protein. Each exon codes for a specific portion of the complete protein. In some species (including humans), a gene's exons are separated by long regions of DNA (called introns or sometimes "junk DNA") that have no apparent function.[2]

fingerprinting: In genetics, the identification of multiple specific alleles on a person's DNA to produce a unique identifier for that person.[1]

forensics: The use of DNA for identification. Some examples of DNA use are to establish paternity in child support cases; establish the presence of a suspect at a crime scene, and identify accident victims.[1]

fraternal twin: Siblings born at the same time as the result of fertilization of two ova by two sperm. They share the same genetic relationship to each other as any other siblings.[1]

full gene sequence: The complete order of bases in a gene. This order determines which protein a gene will produce.[1]

functional genomics: The study of genes, their resulting proteins, and the role played by the proteins the body's biochemical processes.[1]

gamete: Mature male or female reproductive cell (sperm or ovum) with a haploid set of chromosomes (23 for humans).[1]

GC-rich area: Many DNA sequences carry long stretches of repeated G (guanine) and C (cytosine) which often indicate a gene-rich region.[1]

gene: The fundamental physical and functional unit of heredity. A gene is an ordered sequence of nucleotides located in a particular position on a particular chromosome that encodes a specific functional product (a protein or RNA molecule).[1]

gene amplification: Repeated copying of a piece of DNA; a characteristic of tumor cells.[1]

gene expression: The process by which a gene's coded information is converted into the structures present and operating in the cell. Expressed genes include those that are transcribed into mRNA and then translated into protein and those that are transcribed into RNA but not translated into protein (for example, transfer and ribosomal RNAs).[1]

gene family: Group of closely related genes that make similar products.[1]

gene mapping: Determination of the relative positions of genes on a DNA molecule (chromosome or plasmid) and of the distance, in linkage units or physical units, between them.[1]

gene pool: All the variations of genes in a species.[1]

gene product: The biochemical material, either RNA or protein, resulting from expression of a gene. The amount of gene product is used to measure how active a gene is; abnormal amounts can be correlated with disease-causing alleles.[1]

gene therapy: An experimental procedure aimed at replacing, manipulating, or supplementing nonfunctional or misfunctioning genes with healthy genes.[1]

gene transfer: Incorporation of new DNA into and organism's cells, usually by a vector such as a modified virus. Used in gene therapy.[1]

genetic code: The sequence of nucleotides, coded in triplets (codons) along the mRNA, that determines the sequence of amino acids in protein synthesis. A gene's DNA sequence can be used to predict the mRNA sequence, and the genetic code can in turn be used to predict the amino acid sequence.[1]

genetic counseling: Provides patients and their families with education and information about genetic-related conditions and helps them make informed decisions.[1]

genetic discrimination: Prejudice against those who have or are likely to develop an inherited disorder.[1]

genetic engineering: Altering the genetic material of cells or organisms to enable them to make new substances or perform new functions.[1]

genetic illness: Sickness, physical disability, or other disorder resulting from the inheritance of one or more deleterious alleles.[1]

genetic marker: A gene or other identifiable portion of DNA whose inheritance can be followed.[1]

genetic mosaic: An organism in which different cells contain different genetic sequence. This can be the result of a mutation during development or fusion of embryos at an early developmental stage.[1]

genetic polymorphism: Difference in DNA sequence among individuals, groups, or populations (for example, genes for blue eyes versus brown eyes).[1]

genetic predisposition: Susceptibility to a genetic disease. May or may not result in actual development of the disease.[1]

genetic screening: Testing a group of people to identify individuals at high risk of having or passing on a specific genetic disorder.[1]

genetic testing: Analyzing an individual's genetic material to determine predisposition to a particular health condition or to confirm a diagnosis of genetic disease.[1]

genetics: The study of inheritance patterns of specific traits.[1]

genome: All the genetic material in the chromosomes of a particular organism; its size is generally given as its total number of base pairs.[1]

genomics: The study of genes and their function.[1]

genotype: The genetic constitution of an organism, as distinguished from its physical appearance (its phenotype).[1]

germ cell: Sperm and egg cells and their precursors. Germ cells are haploid and have only one set of chromosomes (23 in all), while all other cells have two copies (46 in all).[1]

germ line: The continuation of a set of genetic information from one generation to the next.[1]

germ line gene therapy: An experimental process of inserting genes into germ cells or fertilized eggs to cause a genetic change that can be passed on to offspring. May be used to alleviate effects associated with a genetic disease.[1]

guanine (G): A nitrogenous base, one member of the base pair GC (guanine and cytosine) in DNA.[1]

haploid: A single set of chromosomes (half the full set of genetic material) present in the egg and sperm cells of animals and in the egg and pollen cells of plants. Human beings have 23 chromosomes in their reproductive cells.[1]

hemizygous: Having only one copy of a particular gene. For example, in humans, males are hemizygous for genes found on the Y chromosome.[1]

hereditary cancer: Cancer that occurs due to the inheritance of an altered gene within a family.[1]

heterozygosity: The presence of different alleles at one or more loci on homologous chromosomes.[1]

homologous recombination: Swapping of DNA fragments between paired chromosomes.[1]

homology: Similarity in DNA or protein sequences between individuals of the same species or among different species.[1]

homozygote: An organism that has two identical alleles of a gene.[1]

Human Genome Initiative: Collective name for several projects begun in 1986 by the U.S. Department of Energy (DOE) to create an ordered set of DNA segments from known chromosomal locations, develop new computational methods for analyzing genetic map and DNA sequence data, and develop new techniques and instruments for detecting and analyzing DNA. This DOE initiative is now known as the Human Genome Program. The joint national effort, led by DOE and the National Institutes of Health (NIH), is known as the Human Genome Project.[1]

identical twin: Twins produced by the division of a single zygote; both have identical genotypes.[1]

imprinting: A phenomenon in which the disease phenotype depends on which parent passed on the disease gene. For instance, both Prader-Willi and Angelman syndromes are inherited when the same part of chromosome 15 is missing. When the father's complement of 15 is missing, the child has Prader-Willi, but when the mother's complement of 15 is missing, the child has Angelman syndrome.[1]

independent assortment: During meiosis each of the two copies of a gene is distributed to the germ cells independently of the distribution of other genes.[1]

informed consent: An individual willingly agrees to participate in an activity after first being advised of the risks and benefits.[1]

inherit: In genetics, to receive genetic material from parents through biological processes.[1]

insertion: A chromosome abnormality in which a piece of DNA is incorporated into a gene and thereby disrupts the gene's normal function.[1]

interphase: The period in the cell cycle when DNA is replicated in the nucleus; followed by mitosis.[1]

intron: A noncoding sequence of DNA that is initially copied into RNA but is cut out of the final RNA transcript.[2]

junk DNA: Stretches of DNA that do not code for genes; most of the genome consists of so-called junk DNA which may have regulatory and other functions. Also called non-coding DNA.[1]

karyotype: A photomicrograph of an individual's chromosomes arranged in a standard format showing the number, size, and shape of each chromosome type; used in low-resolution physical mapping to correlate gross chromosomal abnormalities with the characteristics of specific diseases.[1]

kilobase (kb): Unit of length for DNA fragments equal to 1000 nucleotides.[1]

knockout: Deactivation of specific genes; used in laboratory organisms to study gene function.[1]

linkage: The proximity of two or more markers (for example, genes, RFLP [restriction fragment length polymorphism] markers) on a chromosome; the closer the markers, the lower the probability that they will be separated during DNA repair or replication processes, and hence the greater the probability that they will be inherited together.[1]

linkage disequilibrium: Where alleles occur together more often than can be accounted for by chance. Indicates that the two alleles are physically close on the DNA strand.[1]

linkage map: A map of the relative positions of genetic loci on a chromosome, determined on the basis of how often the loci are inherited together. Distance is measured in centimorgans (cM).[1]

localize: Determination of the original position (locus) of a gene or other marker on a chromosome.[1]

locus (plural, loci): The position on a chromosome of a gene or other chromosome marker; also, the DNA at that position. The use of locus is sometimes restricted to mean expressed DNA regions.[1]

long-range restriction mapping: Restriction enzymes are proteins that cut DNA at precise locations. Restriction maps depict the chromosomal positions of restriction-enzyme cutting sites. These are used as biochemical "signposts," or markers of specific areas along the chromosomes. The map will detail the positions where the DNA molecule is cut by particular restriction enzymes.[1]

malformation: A structural defect inherited in an organ or part of an organ that results from abnormal fetal development.[2]

mass spectrometry: An instrument used to identify chemicals in a substance by their mass and charge.[1]

megabase (Mb): Unit of length for DNA fragments equal to 1 million nucleotides and roughly equal to 1 cM (centimorgan).[1]

meiosis: The process of two consecutive cell divisions in the diploid progenitors of sex cells. Meiosis results in four rather than two daughter cells, each with a haploid set of chromosomes.[1]

Mendelian inheritance: One method in which genetic traits are passed from parents to offspring. Named for Gregor Mendel, who first studied and recognized the existence of genes and this method of inheritance.[1]

messenger RNA (mRNA): RNA (ribonucleic acid) that serves as a template for protein synthesis.[1]

metaphase: A stage in mitosis or meiosis during which the chromosomes are aligned along the equatorial plane of the cell.[1]

microarray: Sets of miniaturized chemical reaction areas that may also be used to test DNA fragments, antibodies, or proteins.[1]

mitochondrial DNA: The genetic material found in mitochondria, the organelles that generate energy for the cell. Not inherited in the same fashion as nucleic DNA.[1]

mitosis: The process of nuclear division in cells that produces daughter cells that are genetically identical to each other and to the parent cell.[1]

molecular medicine: The treatment of injury or disease at the molecular level. Examples include the use of DNA-based diagnostic tests or medicine derived from DNA sequence information.[1]

monogenic disorder: A disorder caused by mutation of a single gene.[1]

monosomy: Possessing only one copy of a particular chromosome instead of the normal two copies.[1]

motif: A short conserved region in a protein sequence. Motifs are frequently highly conserved parts of domains.[3]

mutagen: An agent that causes a permanent genetic change in a cell. Does not include changes occurring during normal genetic recombination.[1]

mutation: Any heritable change in DNA sequence.[1]

nitrogenous base: A nitrogen-containing molecule having the chemical properties of a base. DNA contains the nitrogenous bases adenine (A), guanine (G), cytosine (C), and thymine (T).[1]

nucleic acid: A large molecule composed of nucleotide subunits.[1]

nucleolar organizing region: A part of the chromosome containing rRNA genes.[1]

nucleotide: A subunit of DNA or RNA consisting of a nitrogenous base (adenine, guanine, thymine, or cytosine in DNA; adenine, guanine, uracil, or cytosine in RNA), a phosphate molecule, and a sugar molecule (deoxyribose in DNA and ribose in RNA). Thousands of nucleotides are linked to form a DNA or RNA molecule.[1]

nucleus: The cellular organelle in eukaryotes that contains most of the genetic material.[1]

oligogenic: A phenotypic trait produced by two or more genes working together.[1]

oncogene: A gene, one or more forms of which is associated with cancer. Many oncogenes are involved, directly or indirectly, in controlling the rate of cell growth.[1]

orthologous: Homologous sequences in different species that arose from a common ancestral gene during speciation; may or may not be responsible for a similar function.[3]

p53: A gene which normally regulates the cell cycle and protects the cell from damage to its genome. Mutations in this gene cause cells to develop cancerous abnormalities.[2]

pedigree: A family tree diagram that shows how a particular genetic trait or disease has been inherited.[1]

penetrance: The probability of a gene or genetic trait being expressed. "Complete" penetrance means the gene or genes for a trait are expressed in all the population who have the genes. "Incomplete" penetrance means the genetic trait is expressed in only part of the population. The percent penetrance also may change with the age range of the population.[1]

peptide: Two or more amino acids joined by a bond called a "peptide bond."[1]

pharmacogenomics: The study of the interaction of an individual's genetic makeup and response to a drug.[1]

phenocopy: A trait not caused by inheritance of a gene but appears to be identical to a genetic trait.[1]

phenotype: The physical characteristics of an organism or the presence of a disease that may or may not be genetic.[1]

physical map: A map of the locations of identifiable landmarks on DNA (for example, restriction-enzyme cutting sites, genes), regardless of inheritance. Distance is measured in base pairs. For the human genome, the lowest-resolution physical map is the banding patterns on the 24 different chromosomes; the highest-resolution map is the complete nucleotide sequence of the chromosomes.[1]

pleiotropy: One gene that causes many different physical traits such as multiple disease symptoms.[1]

pluripotency: The potential of a cell to develop into more than one type of mature cell, depending on environment.[1]

polydactyly: An abnormality in which a person is born with more than the normal number of fingers or toes.[2]

polygenic disorder: Genetic disorder resulting from the combined action of alleles of more than one gene (for example, heart disease, diabetes, and some cancers). Although such disorders are inherited, they depend on the simultaneous presence of several alleles; thus the hereditary patterns usually are more complex than those of single-gene disorders.[1]

polymerase chain reaction (PCR): A method for amplifying a DNA base sequence using a heat-stable polymerase and two 20-base primers, one complementary to the (+) strand at one end of the sequence to be amplified and one complementary to the (-) strand at the other end. Because the newly synthesized DNA strands can subsequently serve as additional templates for the same primer sequences, successive rounds of primer annealing, strand elongation, and dissociation produce rapid and highly specific amplification of the desired sequence. PCR also can be used to detect the existence of the defined sequence in a DNA sample.[1]

polymerase, DNA or RNA: Enzyme that catalyzes the synthesis of nucleic acids on preexisting nucleic acid templates, assembling RNA from ribonucleotides or DNA from deoxyribonucleotides.[1]

polymorphism: Difference in DNA sequence among individuals that may underlie differences in health. Genetic variations occurring in more than 1% of a population would be considered useful polymorphisms for genetic linkage analysis.[1]

polypeptide: A protein or part of a protein made of a chain of amino acids joined by a peptide bond.[1]

population genetics: The study of variation in genes among a group of individuals.[1]

positional cloning: A technique used to identify genes, usually those that are associated with diseases, based on their location on a chromosome.[1]

premature chromosome condensation (PCC): A method of studying chromosomes in the interphase stage of the cell cycle.[1]

privacy: In genetics, the right of people to restrict access to their genetic information.[1]

pronucleus: The nucleus of a sperm or egg prior to fertilization.[1]

protein: A large molecule composed of one or more chains of amino acids in a specific order; the order is determined by the base sequence of nucleotides in the gene that codes for the protein. Proteins are required for the structure, function, and regulation of the body's cells, tissues, and organs; and each protein has unique functions. Examples are hormones, enzymes, and antibodies.[1]

proteomics: The study of the full set of proteins encoded by a genome.[1]

pseudogene: A sequence of DNA similar to a gene but nonfunctional; probably the remnant of a once-functional gene that accumulated mutations.[1]

purine: A nitrogen-containing, double-ring, basic compound that occurs in nucleic acids. The purines in DNA and RNA are adenine and guanine.[1]

pyrimidine: A nitrogen-containing, single-ring, basic compound that occurs in nucleic acids. The pyrimidines in DNA are cytosine and thymine; in RNA, cytosine and uracil.[1]

recessive gene: A gene which will be expressed only if there are 2 identical copies or, for a male, if one copy is present on the X chromosome.[1]

reciprocal translocation: When a pair of chromosomes exchange exactly the same length and area of DNA. Results in a shuffling of genes.[1]

recombinant DNA technology: Procedure used to join together DNA segments in a cell-free system (an environment outside a cell or organism). Under appropriate conditions, a recombinant DNA molecule can enter a cell and replicate there, either autonomously or after it has become integrated into a cellular chromosome.[1]

recombination: The process by which progeny derive a combination of genes different from that of either parent. In higher organisms, this can occur by crossing over.[1]

regulatory region or sequence: A DNA base sequence that controls gene expression.[1]

repetitive DNA: Sequences of varying lengths that occur in multiple copies in the genome; it represents much of the human genome.[1]

restriction fragment length polymorphism (RFLP): Variation between individuals in DNA fragment sizes cut by specific restriction enzymes; polymorphic sequences that result in RFLPs are used as markers on both physical maps and genetic linkage maps. RFLPs usually are caused by mutation at a cutting site.[1]

restriction-enzyme cutting site: A specific nucleotide sequence of DNA at which a particular restriction enzyme cuts the DNA. Some sites occur frequently in DNA (for example, every several hundred base pairs); others much less frequently (rare-cutter; for example, every 10,000 base pairs).[1]

ribose: The five-carbon sugar that serves as a component of RNA.[1]

ribosomal RNA (rRNA): A class of RNA found in the ribosomes of cells.[1]

ribosomes: Small cellular components composed of specialized ribosomal RNA and protein; site of protein synthesis.[1]

risk communication: In genetics, a process in which a genetic counselor or other medical professional interprets genetic test results and advises patients of the consequences for them and their offspring.[1]

RNA (ribonucleic acid): A chemical found in the nucleus and cytoplasm of cells; it plays an important role in protein synthesis and other chemical activities of the cell. The structure of RNA is similar to that of DNA. There are several classes of RNA molecules, including messenger RNA, transfer RNA, ribosomal RNA, and other small RNAs, each serving a different purpose.[1]

segregation: The normal biological process whereby the two pieces of a chromosome pair are separated during meiosis and randomly distributed to the germ cells.[1]

sequencing: Determination of the order of nucleotides (base sequences) in a DNA or RNA molecule or the order of amino acids in a protein.[1]

sex chromosome: The X or Y chromosome in human beings that determines the sex of an individual. Females have two X chromosomes in diploid cells; males have an X and a Y chromosome. The sex chromosomes comprise the 23rd chromosome pair in a karyotype.[1]

sex-linked: Traits or diseases associated with the X or Y chromosome; generally seen in males.[1]

single nucleotide polymorphism (SNP): DNA sequence variations that occur when a single nucleotide (A, T, C, or G) in the genome sequence is altered.[1]

single-gene disorder: Hereditary disorder caused by a mutant allele of a single gene (for example, Duchenne muscular dystrophy, retinoblastoma, sickle cell disease).[1]

somatic cell: Any cell in the body except gametes and their precursors.[1]

somatic cell genetic mutation: A change in the genetic structure that is neither inherited nor passed to offspring. Also called acquired mutations.[1]

spectral karyotype (SKY): A graphic of all an organism's chromosomes, each labeled with a different color. Useful for identifying chromosomal abnormalities.[1]

sporadic cancer: Cancer that occurs randomly and is not inherited from parents. Caused by DNA changes in one cell that grows and divides, spreading throughout the body.[1]

stem cell: Undifferentiated, primitive cells in the bone marrow that have the ability both to multiply and to differentiate into specific blood cells.[1]

substitution: In genetics, a type of mutation due to replacement of one nucleotide in a DNA sequence by another nucleotide or replacement of one amino acid in a protein by another amino acid.[1]

suppressor gene: A gene that can suppress the action of another gene.[1]

syndrome: The group or recognizable pattern of symptoms or abnormalities that indicate a particular trait or disease.[1]

tandem repeat sequences: Multiple copies of the same base sequence on a chromosome; used as markers in physical mapping.[1]

telomerase: The enzyme that directs the replication of telomeres.[1]

telomere: The end of a chromosome. This specialized structure is involved in the replication and stability of linear DNA molecules.[1]

teratogenic: Substances such as chemicals or radiation that cause abnormal development of a embryo.[1]

thymine (T): A nitrogenous base, one member of the base pair AT (adenine-thymine).[1]

toxicogenomics: The study of how genomes respond to environmental stressors or toxicants. Combines genome-wide mRNA expression profiling with protein expression patterns using bioinformatics to understand the role of gene-environment interactions in disease and dysfunction.[1]

transcription: The synthesis of an RNA copy from a sequence of DNA (a gene); the first step in gene expression.[1]

transcription factor: A protein that binds to regulatory regions and helps control gene expression.[1]

transcriptome: The full complement of activated genes, mRNAs, or transcripts in a particular tissue at a particular time[1]

transfer RNA (tRNA): A class of RNA having structures with triplet nucleotide sequences that are complementary to the triplet nucleotide coding sequences of mRNA. The role of tRNAs in protein synthesis is to bond with amino acids and transfer them to the ribosomes, where proteins are assembled according to the genetic code carried by mRNA.[1]

transgenic: An experimentally produced organism in which DNA has been artificially introduced and incorporated into the organism's germ line.[1]

translation: The process in which the genetic code carried by mRNA directs the synthesis of proteins from amino acids.[1]

translocation: A mutation in which a large segment of one chromosome breaks off and attaches to another chromosome.[1]

transposable element: A class of DNA sequences that can move from one chromosomal site to another.[1]

trisomy: Possessing three copies of a particular chromosome instead of the normal two copies.[1]

tumor suppressor gene: A protective gene that normally limits the growth of tumors. When a tumor suppressor is mutated, it may fail to keep a cancer from growing. *BRCA1* and *p53* are well-known tumor suppressor genes.[2]

uracil: A nitrogenous base normally found in RNA but not DNA; uracil is capable of forming a base pair with adenine.[1]

X chromosome: One of the two sex chromosomes, X and Y. Females have two X chromosomes.[1]

Y chromosome: One of the two sex chromosomes, X and Y. Males have one X chromosome and one Y chromosome.[1]

zinc-finger protein: A secondary feature of some proteins containing a zinc atom; a DNA-binding protein.[1]

Chapter 70

Newborn Screening Programs in the United States

Newborn screening programs exist in all 50 states and the District of Columbia. Each of these 51 programs has identified a contact whose responsibility is laboratory protocol and another knowledgeable about program and follow-up issues. A few states prefer follow-up issues and laboratory issues to be handled by the same contact and those are so noted. Several states use regional or other out-of-state laboratories; these are noted.

Alabama Laboratory

Bureau of Clinical Laboratories
8140 AUM Drive
Montgomery, AL 36130-0001
Phone: 334-260-3400
Fax: 334-274-9800

Alabama Follow-up

Newborn Screening Metabolic
Coordinator
8140 AUM Drive
Montgomery, AL 36130-0001
Phone: 334-260-3400
Fax: 334-260-3439

This chapter includes "New Born Screening Programs in the U.S." with tables from "U.S. National Screening Status Report," reprinted with permission from the National Newborn Screening and Genetics Resource Center (NNSGRC). For additional information, contact the NNSGRC at 1912 W. Anderson Lane, Suite 210, Austin, TX 78757, 512-454-6419, or visit their website at http://genes-r-us.uthscsa.edu. Contact information in this chapter was updated and verified in July 2004.

Alaska Laboratory

Newborn Screening Section
Oregon Public Health
Laboratory
1717 SW 10th Avenue
Portland, OR 97207-0275
Phone: 503-229-6576
Fax: 503-229-6989
Website: http://
www.ohd.hr.state.or.us/nbs

Alaska Follow-up

Newborn Metabolic Screening
Coordinator
Alaska Department of Health
3601 C Street, Suite 934
Anchorage, AK 99524
Phone: 907-269-3499
Fax: 907-269-3465
Website: http://
www.hss.state.ak.us/dhcs/
metabolic/default.htm

Arizona Laboratory

Arizona State Health
Laboratory
250 North 17th Avenue
Phoenix, AZ 85007
Phone: 602-542-1188
Fax: 602-542-0760
Website: http://
www.hs.state.az.us/lab

Arizona Follow-up

Newborn Screening Program
Manager
Office of Women's and Children's
Health
150 North 18th Avenue, Suite 320
Phoenix, AZ 85007
Toll-Free: 800-548-8381
Phone: 602-364-1409
Fax: 602-364-1495
TDD: 602-256-7577
Website: http://
www.hs.state.az.us/phs/owch/
newbrnscrn.htm

Arkansas Laboratory

Division of Public Laboratories
Arkansas Department of Health
4815 W. Markham Street, Slot 47
Little Rock, AR 72205-3867
Phone: 501-661-2000
Fax: 501-661-2310
Website: http://
www.healthyarkansas.com

Arkansas Follow-up

Newborn Screening Coordinator
Arkansas Department of Health
4815 W. Markham Street, Slot 17
Little Rock, AR 72205-3867
Phone: 501-661-2000
Fax: 501-661-2310
Website: http://
www.healthyarkansas.com

California Laboratory

Genetic Disease Laboratory
California Department of
Health Services
P.O. Box 997413
Sacramento, CA 95899-7413
Phone: 510-231-1502
Fax: 510-540-2228
Website: http://www.dhs.ca.gov/
pcfh/gdb/gdbindex.htm

California Follow-up

Clinical Chemistry Laboratory
California Department of
Health Services
P.O. Box 997413
Sacramento, CA 95899-7413
Phone: 510-412-5846
Fax: 510-412-1560

Colorado Laboratory

Colorado Department of Public
Health and Environment
8100 Lowry Boulevard
Denver, CO 80230-6928
Phone: 303-692-3090
Fax: 303-344-9989
Website: http://
www.cdphe.state.co.us/lr/
lrhom.htm

Colorado Follow-up

Colorado Department of Public
Health and Environment
Children and Youth with Special
Health Care Needs
300 Cherry Creek Drive South
Denver, CO 80246-1530
Phone: 303-692-2370
Fax: 303-782-5576
Website: http://
www.cdphe.state.co.us/ps/hcp/
newbornmetabolic/
newbornhom.asp
E-mail:
cdphe.psdrequests@state.co.us

Connecticut Laboratory

Connecticut Department of
Public Health
P.O. Box 1689
Hartford, CT 06144
Phone: 860-509-8513
Fax: 860-509-8697
Website: http://
www.dph.state.ct.us

Connecticut Follow-up

Connecticut Department of
Public Health
410 Capitol Ave., M.S. #11 MAT
P.O. Box 340308
Hartford, CT 06134-0308
Phone: 860-509-8081
Fax: 860-509-7720
Website: http://
www.dph.state.ct.us/BCH/NBS/
NBS.htm

Delaware Laboratory

Delaware Public Health
Laboratory
30 Sunnyside Road
P.O. Box 1047
Smyrna, DE 19977-1047
Phone: 302-653-2870
Fax: 302-653-2877
Website: http://www.state.de.us/
dhss/main/maps/labs/
dphlab.htm

Delaware Follow-up

Newborn Screening Coordinator
Delaware Division of Public
Health
417 Federal Street
Dover, DE 19901
Toll-Free: 888-459-2943
Phone: 302-459-2943
Fax: 302-739-3008
Website: http://www.state.de.us/
dhss/dph/chca/dphnsp1.html

District of Columbia Laboratory

Pediatrix Screening
90 Emerson Lane
Bridgeville, PA 15017
Toll-Free: 866-463-6436
Phone: 412-220-2300
Fax: 412-220-0784
Website: http://
www.pediatrixscreening.com

District of Columbia Follow-up

D.C. Department of Health
825 N. Capital Street NE
Washington, DC 20002
Phone: 202-442-5999
Fax: 202-727-7754
Website: http://dchealth.dc.gov

Florida Laboratory

Clinical Chemistry and Infant
Screening
Department of Health and
Rehabilitation Services
P.O. Box 210
Jacksonville, FL 32231
Phone: 904-791-1641
Fax: 904-791-1671
Website: http://
www.doh.state.fl.us/lab/
index.html

Florida Follow-up

Children's Medical Services
Florida Department of Health
4052 Bald Cypress Way
Tallahassee, FL 32399-1707
Phone: 850-245-4444, ext. 2254
Fax: 850-921-5385
Website: http://
www.doh.state.fl.us/cms

Georgia Laboratory

Manager of Laboratory
Georgia Department of Human
Resources
1749 Clairmont Road
Decatur, GA 30033
Phone: 404-327-7900
Fax: 404-327-7919
Website: http://
health.state.ga.us/programs/lab

Georgia Follow-up

Genetics Program Manager
Office of Infant and Child Health
Family Health Branch 11th Floor
2 Peachtree Street, NW
Atlanta, GA 30303-3142
Phone: 404-657-6357
Fax: 404-463-6729
Website: http://
health.state.ga.us/programs/
child/index.shtml

Hawaii Laboratory

Newborn Screening Section
Oregon Public Health
Laboratory
1717 SW 10th Avenue
Portland, OR 97207-0275
Phone: 503-229-6576
Fax: 503-229-6989
Website: http://
www.ohd.hr.state.or.us/nbs

Hawaii Follow-up

Newborn Screening Program
Coordinator
Children with Special Health
Needs Branch
741 Sunset Avenue
Honolulu, HI 96816
Phone: 808-733-9058
Fax: 808-733-9068
Website: http://www.hawaii.gov/
health/family-child-health/
cshcn/index.html

Idaho Laboratory

Newborn Screening Section
Oregon Public Health
Laboratory
1717 SW 10th Avenue
Portland, OR 97207-0275
Phone: 503-229-6576
Fax: 503-229-6989
Website: http://
www.ohd.hr.state.or.us/nbs

Idaho Follow-up

Children's Special Health/NBS/
Genetics Programs
Idaho Department of Health
and Welfare
Bureau of Clinical and
Prevention Services
450 West State Street
Boise, ID 83720
Phone: 208-334-5962
Fax: 208-334-7307
Website: http://
www2.state.id.us/dhw/health/
bocaps/cshp.htm

Illinois Laboratory

Division of Laboratories
Illinois Department of Public
Health
P.O. Box 12279
Chicago, IL 60612
Phone: 312-793-1053
Fax: 312-793-1322
Website: http://
www.idph.state.il.us

Illinois Follow-up

Illinois Department of Public
Health
Division of Health Assessment
and Screening
Genetics/Newborn Screening/
SIDS Program
P.O. Box 12279
Chicago, IL 60612
Phone: 312-793-1053
Fax: 312-793-1322
Website: http://
www.idph.state.il.us

Indiana Laboratory

Indiana Newborn Screening
Riley Children's Hospital
702 Barnhill Drive, Room 0940
Indianapolis, IN 46202
Phone: 317-278-2502
Fax: 317-274-6678

Indiana Follow-up

Director, Newborn Screening
Program
Indiana State Department of
Health
2 North Meridian Street, 7F
Indianapolis, IN 46204
Phone: 317-233-1231
Fax: 317-233-1281
Website: http://www.in.gov/isdh/
programs/mch/nsp.htm

Iowa Laboratory

Newborn Screening Laboratory
University Hygienic Laboratory
1521 2nd Avenue
Des Moines, IA 50319
Phone: 515-243-0141
Fax: 515-243-3071

Iowa Follow-up

State Coordinator for Genetic
Services
Iowa Department of Public
Health
Lucas State Office Building
Des Moines, IA 50319
Phone: 515-281-5593
Fax: 515-242-6384
Website: http://
www.idph.state.ia.us/genetics/
genetic_services.asp

Kansas Laboratory

Neonatal Chemistry Laboratory
Forbes Field, Building 740
Topeka, KS 66620-0001
Phone: 785-296-1650
Fax: 785-296-1641
Website: http://
www.kdhe.state.ks.us/labs/
neonatal.html

Kansas Follow-up

Bureau for Children Youth and
Families
Kansas Department of Health
and Environment
1000 SW Jackson, Suite 220
Topeka, KS 66612
Toll-Free: 800-332-6262
Phone: 785-291-3363
Fax: 785-296-6553
Website: http://
www.kdhe.state.ks.us/bcyf

Kentucky Laboratory

Division of Laboratory Services
Kentucky Department of Public
Health
100 Sower Boulevard
Frankfort, KY 40601
Phone: 502-564-4446
Fax: 502-564-7019
Website: http://chs.ky.gov/
publichealth/laboratory-
services.htm

Kentucky Follow-up

Newborn Screening Follow-Up
Section
Kentucky Department of Public
Health
100 Sower Boulevard
Frankfort, KY 40601
Phone: 502-564-4446
Fax: 502-564-7019
Website: http://chs.ky.gov/
publichealth/laboratory-
services.htm

Louisiana Laboratory

Newborn Screening Laboratory
Louisiana Department of Health
and Hospitals
325 Loyola Avenue, Room 308
New Orleans, LA 70112
Phone: 504-568-5070
Fax: 504-568-7722
Website: http://
www.oph.dhh.state.la.us/
geneticdisease/newbornscreen/
index.html

Louisiana Follow-up

Louisiana Department of Health
and Hospitals
325 Loyola Avenue, Room 308
New Orleans, LA 70112
Phone: 504-568-5070
Fax: 504-568-7722
Website: http://
www.oph.dhh.state.la.us/
geneticdisease/newbornscreen/
index.html

Maine Laboratory

New England Regional Newborn
Screening Program
University of Massachusetts
Medical School
305 South Street
Jamaica Plain, MA 02130-3597
Phone: 617-983-6300
Fax: 617-522-2846
Website: http://
www.umassmed.edu/nbs

Maine Follow-up

Maine Newborn Screening
Program Coordinator
Maine Bureau of Health
11 State House Station
286 Water Street
Augusta, ME 04333
Phone: 207-287-5351
Fax: 207-287-4743
Website: http://www.state.me.us/
dhs/bohdcfh/gen/index2.htm

Maryland Laboratory

Newborn Screening Laboratory
Maryland Department of Health
and Mental Hygiene
201 W. Preston Street
Baltimore, MD 21201
Phone: 410-767-6170
Fax: 410-333-7112
Website: http://
www.fha.state.md.us/genetics/
html/nbs_ndx.html

Maryland Follow-up

Division of Hereditary Disease
Maryland Department of Health
and Mental Hygiene
201 W. Preston Street
Baltimore, MD 21201
Phone: 410-767-6170
Fax: 410-333-7112
Website: http://
www.fha.state.md.us/genetics/
html/nbs_ndx.html

Massachusetts Laboratory

University of Massachusetts
Medical School
New England Regional Newborn
Screening Program
University of Massachusetts
Medical School
305 South Street
Jamaica Plain, MA 02130-3597
Phone: 617-983-6300
Fax: 617-522-2846
Website: http://
www.umassmed.edu/nbs

Massachusetts Follow-up

University of Massachusetts
Medical School
New England Regional Newborn
Screening Program
University of Massachusetts
Medical School
305 South Street
Jamaica Plain, MA 02130-3597
Phone: 617-983-6300
Fax: 617-522-2846
Website: http://
www.umassmed.edu/nbs

Michigan Laboratory

Newborn Screening Laboratory
Michigan Department of Health
3500 N. Martin Luther King Jr.
Boulevard
P.O. Box 30195
Lansing, MI 48909
Phone: 517-335-8095
Fax: 517-335-9419
Website: http://mi.gov/
newbornscreening

Michigan Follow-up

Community Living, Children
and Families
Michigan Department Health
3423 N. Martin Luther King, Jr.
Boulevard
P.O. Box 30195
Lansing, MI 48909
Phone: 517-335-9205
Fax: 517-335-9419
Website: http://mi.gov/
newbornscreening

Minnesota Laboratory

Minnesota Department of
Health
Public Health Laboratory
717 SE Delaware
P.O. Box 9441
Minneapolis, MN 55440-9441
Phone: 612-676-5260
Fax: 612-676-5514
Website: http://
www.health.state.mn.us/divs/
phl/index.html

Minnesota Follow-up

Newborn Screening Follow-up
Specialist
Minnesota Department of
Health
Golden Rule Building, Suite 400
P.O. Box 64882
St. Paul, MN 55164-0882
Phone: 651-215-8960
Website: http://
www.health.state.mn.us/divs/fh/
mcshn/nbsfaq.htm

Mississippi Laboratory

Pediatrix Screening
90 Emerson Lane
Bridgeville, PA 15017
Toll-Free: 866-463-6436
Phone: 412-220-2300
Fax: 412-220-0784
Website: http://
www.pediatrixscreening.com

Mississipi Follow-up

Mississippi State Department of
Health
Newborn Screening Program
P.O. Box 1700
Jackson, MS 39215-1700
Toll-Free: 800-489-7670
Phone: 601-576-7619
Fax: 601-354-6032
Website: http://
www2.state.tn.us/health/MCH/
genetics.htm

Table 70.1. U.S. National Screening Status Report, updated July 1, 2004 (MS/MS details are show in Table 70.2).

The U.S. National Screening Status Report lists the status of newborn screening in the United States. The condition must be required by the state in order for a dot "•" to be added. A circle in brackets [•] indicates that MS/MS is used for detecting the analyte of interest.

State	PKU	CH	GAL	MSUD	HCY	BIO	SCD	CAH	CF	MS/MS Testing	OTHER
Alabama	•	•	•			•	•	•			
Alaska	[•]	•	•	[•]	[•]	•	•	•		•	
Arizona	•	•	•	•	•	•	•	•			
Arkansas	•	•	•				•				
California	•	•	•				•				
Colorado	•	•	•			•	•	•	•		
Connecticut	[•]	•	•	[•]	[•]	•	•	•	A	•	HIV
D.C.	[•]	•	•	[•]	[•]		•				G6PD(C)
Delaware	[•]	•	•	[•]	[•]		•	•		•	
Florida	•	•	•				•	•			
Georgia	•	•	•	•	•	•	•	•		C	TYR
Hawaii	[•]	•	•	[•]	[•]	•	•	•		•	
Idaho	[•]	•	•	[•]	[•]	•	•	•		•	
Illinois	[•]	•	•	[•]	[•]	•	•	•		•	
Indiana	[•]	•	•	[•]	[•]	•	•	•		•	
Iowa	[•]	•	•	[•]	[•]	•	•	•		•	
Kansas	•	•	•				•				
Kentucky	•	•	•				•				
Louisiana	•	•	•			•	•	•			
Maine	[•]	•	•	[•]	[•]	•	•	•		•	
Maryland	[•]	•	•	[•]	[•]	•	•	•		•	
Massachusetts	[•]	•	•	[•]		•	•	•	B	•	TOXO
Michigan	[•]	•	•	[•]		•	•	•		•	
Minnesota	[•]	•	•	[•]	[•]		•	•		•	
Mississippi	[•]	•	•	[•]	[•]	•	•	•	•	•	

State														G6PD(C)
Missouri	●	●	●	C	C	C	●	●	C			●		
Montana	●	●	●	[A]	[A]	A	●	●	A	A	A	C		
Nebraska	[●]	●	●	[A]	[A]	●	●	●	●		●			
Nevada	[●]	●	●	[●]	[●]	●	●	A	●					TOXO
New Hampshire	[●]	●	●	[●]	[●]		●	●	●		●			
New Jersey	●	●	●	[●]		●	●	●	●		●			
New Mexico		●	●				●	●	●					
New York	[●]	●	●	[●]	[●]	●	●	●	●		●	●		HIV
North Carolina	[●]	●	●	[●]	[●]		●	●	●		●			
North Dakota	[●]	●	●	[●]	[●]	●	●	●	●		●			
Ohio	[●]	●	●	[●]	[●]		●	●	●		●			
Oklahoma	●	●	●				●		C	C	C	C		
Oregon	[●]	●	●	[●]	[●]	A	●	●	●	A	●	●		G6PD (A)
Pennsylvania	[●]	●	●	[A]	[A]	●	●	●	●		A	A		
Rhode Island	[●]	●	●	[●]	[●]	●	●	●	●		●	●		
South Carolina	[●]	●	●	C	C	C	●	●	●	C	●			
South Dakota	[●]	●	●	[A]	[A]		●	A	A		A	A		
Tennessee	●	●	●	[●]	[●]	●	●	●	●		●	●		
Texas	●	●	●				●		●					
Utah	●	●	●				●		●					
Vermont	[●]	●	●	[●]	[●]	●	●	●	●		●			
Virginia	[●]	●	●	[●]	[●]	●	●	●	●		●	●		
Washington	[●]	●	●			●	●	●	●		●	●		
West Virginia		●	●				●	●	●			●		
Wisconsin	[●]	●	●	[●]		●	●	●	●	●	●	●		
Wyoming	●	●	●			C	C	●	●	●		●		

PKU- Phenylketonuria, **CH**- Congenital Hypothyroidism, **GAL**- Galactosemia, **MSUD**-Maple Syrup Urine disease, **HCY** - Homocystinuria, **BIO** - Biotinidase, **SCD** - Sickle Cell Disease, **CAH** - Congenital Adrenal Hyperplasia, **CF** - Cystic Fibrosis, **MS/MS** -Tandem Mass Spectrometry, **HIV** - Human Immunodeficiency Virus, **G6PD** - Glucose 6 Phosphate Dehydrogenase Disease, **TYR** - Tyrosinemia, **TOXO** - Toxoplasmosis

A = selected populations, limited pilot programs, or by request (not mandated), **B** = universal testing on all babies (not mandated), **C** = testing mandated but not yet implemented

Table 70.2. MS/MS conditions Screened (by State), updated July 1, 2004.

Disorder	CPT-1	CPT-2	CAT	LCHAD	GA-II	SCAD	SCHAD	MCAD	MCKAT	TFP	L/VLCAD	2,4 Di.	GA-1	HMG	IBCD	IVA	MA	3-MCC	MMA	BKT	PA	2MBCD	MCD	3MGA	MHBD	ARG	ASA	CPS	CIT I&II	HHH	NKH	5-OXO	TYR-I	TYR-II
	Fatty Acids												**Organic Acids**													**Amino/Urea**								
Alabama	●	●	●	●	●	●		●			●		●	●	●	●	●	●	●	●	●	●	●	●	●	●	●		●				●	●
Alaska																																		
Arizona																																		
Arkansas				●				●																										
California																																		
Colorado																																		
Connecticut				●				C																										
D. of Columbia																																		
Delaware		●	●	●	●	●		●			●		●	●	●	●		●	●	●	●	●	●			●	●		●				●	●
Florida		●	●	●	●	●		●			●		●	●	●	●	●	●	●	●	●	●	●	●	●	●	●		●				●	●
Georgia		●	●	●	●	●		●			●		●	●	●	●	●	●	●	●	●	●	●	●	●	●	●		●				●	●
Hawaii		●		●	●	●		●		●	●		●	●	●	●	●	●	●	●	●	●	●	●		●	●		●				●	●
Idaho	●	●	●	●	●	●		●		●	●		●	●	●	●	●	●	●	●	●	●	●	●		●	●		●				●	●
Illinois	●						●	●	●	●																								
Indiana	●	●	●	●	●	●	●	●		●	●	●	●	●	●	●	●	●	●	●	●	●	●	●		●	●	●	●	●	●		●	●
Iowa *							●	●		●																								
Kansas																																		
Kentucky																																		
Louisiana																																		
Maine																																		
Maryland		B		B	B	B		●		●	B		B	B	●	B		B	B	B	B	●	●	●	●	B	B		B	B			B	B
Massachusetts		●	●	●	●	●	●	●		●	●		●	●	●	●		●	●	●	●	●	●	●		●	●		●	●			●	●
Michigan		B		B	B	B		●			B		B	B		B		B	B	B	B					B	B		B	B			B	B
Minnesota		●	●	●	●	●	●	●		●	●		●	●	●	●		●	●	●	●	●	●	●	●	●	●		●			●	●	●
Mississippi	●	●	●	●	●	●	●	●		●	●		●	●	●	●	●	●	●	●	●	●	●	●	●	●	●	●	●	●			●	●
Missouri	●	●		●	●	●		●			●		●	●		●	●	●	●	●	●					●	●		●				●	●
Montana		A		A	A	A		C			A	A	C	A		C	C	A	A	A	A					A	A		A				A	A
Nebraska		A	A	A	A	A		●		A	A	A	A	A	A	A	A	A	A	A	A	A				A	A		A	A	A	A	A	A

The abbreviations used in the table:

Carnitine / Acyl-CoA disorders:

CPT-1 — Carnitine Palmitoyl Transferase Def. I
CPT-II — Carnitine Palmitoyl Transferase Def. I
CAT — Carnitine /Acylcarnitine Translocase Def.
CUD — Carnitine Uptake Defect
LCHAD — Long-Chain Hydroxy Acyl-CoA Dehydrog.
GA-II — Multiple Acyl-CoA Dehydrogenase Deficiency
SCAD — Short-Chain Acyl-CoADehydrogenase Def.
SCHAD — Short-Chain Hydroxy Acyl -CoA Dehydr. Def.
MCAD — Medium-Chain Acyl-CoA Dehydrogenase Def.
MCKAT — Medium-Chain 3-Ketoacyl-CoA Thiolase Def.
TFP — Trifunctional Protein Def.
L/VLCAD — Long/Very Long-Chain Acyl-CoA Dehy.

Organic acid disorders:

2,4,Di — 2,4 Dienoyl-CoA Reductase Def.
GA-I — Glutaric Aciduria Type I
HMG — 3-Hydroxy-3-Methylglutaryl CoA Lyase
IBCD — Isobutyryl-CoA Dehydrogenase Def.
IVA — Isovaleric Acidemia
MA — Malonic Aciduria
3MCC — 3-Methylcrotonyl-CoA Carboxyl Def.
MMA — Methylmalonic Acidemia
BKT — Mitochondrial Acetoacetyl-CoA Thiolase
PA — Propionic Acidemia
2MBCD — 2-Methylbutyryl-CoA Dehydrogenase
MCD — Multiple CoA Carboxylase

Amino acid / urea cycle disorders:

3MGA — 3-methylglutaconyl-CoA hydratase def.
MHBD — 2-Methyl-3-hydroxybutyryl CoA dehydrogenase
ARG — Argininemia
ASA — Argininosuccinate Lyase Deficiency
CPS — Carbamoylphosphate Synthetase Deficiency
CIT — Citrullinemia Type 1 or II-
HHH — Hyperammonemia/ornithinemia/ citrullinuria
NKH — Nonketotic hyperglycinemia
5-OXO — 5-oxoprolinuria-
TYR-I — Tyrosinemia type I
TYR-II — Tyrosinemia type II

* Full screening with MS/MS mandated, with disorders to be delineated as they are identified. List includes disorders routinely screened, and disorders that can be detected with current markers.
The test has to be a requirement of the state (mandated) in order for a (●) to be added
A = (not mandated) select populations, limited pilot programs or by request,   B = (not mandated) universal pilot on all babies,   C = testing mandated but not yet implemented

States listed in the table: Nevada, New Hampshire, New Jersey, New Mexico, New York, North Carolina*, North Dakota, Ohio, Oklahoma, Oregon, Pennsylvania, Rhode Island, South Carolina, South Dakota, Tennessee, Texas, Utah, Vermont, Virginia, Washington, West Virginia, Wisconsin, Wyoming

Missouri Laboratory

State Public Health Laboratory
307 W. McCarty
Jefferson City, MO 65102
Phone: 573-751-5284
Fax: 573-522-8155
Website: http://
www.health.state.mo.us/Lab

Missouri Follow-up

Bureau of Children with Special
Health Care Needs
930 Wildwood Drive
Jefferson City, MO 65102-0570
Toll-Free: 800-451-0669
Phone: 573-751-6246
Fax: 573-573-6237
Website: http://
www.health.state.mo.us/SHCN

Montana Laboratory

Montana Public Health
Laboratory
1400 Broadway
Helena, MT 59604
Toll-Fee: 800-821-7284
Phone: 406-444-3444
Fax: 406-444-1802
Website: http://
www.dphhs.state.mt.us/hpsd/
index.htm

Montana Follow-up

Montana Department of Public
Health and Human Services
1400 Broadway
C-314 Cogswell Building
Helena, MT 59620-2951
Phone: 406-444-6858
Fax: 406-444-2606
Website: http://
www.dphhs.state.mt.us

Nebraska Laboratory

Nebraska Newborn Screening
Program
Nebraska State Health
Department
P.O. Box 95044
Lincoln, NE 68509-5044
Phone: 402-471-9731
Fax: 402-471-7049
TDD: 402-471-9570
Website: http://
www.hhs.state.ne.us/hew/fah/
nsp/stateplan.htm

Nebraska Follow-up

Nebraska Newborn Screening
Program
Nebraska State Health
Department
P.O. Box 95044
Lincoln, NE 68509-5044
Phone: 402-471-9731
Fax: 402-471-7049
TDD: 402-471-9570
Website: http://
www.hhs.state.ne.us/hew/fah/
nsp/stateplan.htm

Nevada Laboratory

Newborn Screening Section
Oregon Public Health
Laboratory
1717 SW 10th Avenue
Portland, OR 97207-0275
Phone: 503-229-6576
Fax: 503-229-6989
Website: http://
www.ohd.hr.state.or.us/nbs

Nevada Follow-up

Maternal and Child Health
Nurse Consultant
3427 Goni Road, Suite 108
Carson City, NV 89706
Phone: 775-684-3460
Fax: 775-687-1383
Website: http://
health2k.state.nv.us/BEIS

New Hampshire Laboratory

New England Regional Newborn
Screening Program
University of Massachusetts
Medical School
305 South Street
Jamaica Plain, MA 02130-3597
Phone: 617-983-6300
Fax: 617-522-2846
Website: http://
www.umassmed.edu/nbs

New Hampshire Follow-up

Newborn Screening Program
Bureau of Maternal Child
Health
29 Hazen Drive
Concord NH 03301
Phone: 603-271-4225
Fax: 603-271-4519
Website: http://
www.umassmed.edu/nbs/nh.cfm

New Jersey Laboratory

Inborn Errors of Metabolism
Laboratory
New Jersey State Department of
Health
Public Health and
Environmental Laboratories
CN 361
Trenton, NJ 08625
Phone: 609-292-5605
Fax: 609-530-3347

New Jersey Follow-up

Newborn Biochemical Screening
Program
New Jersey State Department of
Health
P.O. Box 360
Trenton, NJ 08625
Phone: 609-292-1582
Fax: 609-292-3580
Website: http://www.state.nj.us/
health/fhs/nbs2000/index.html

New Mexico Laboratory

New Mexico Department of
Health
Scientific Laboratory
700 NE Camino de Salud
Albuquerque, NM 87196
Phone: 505-841-2500
Fax: 505-841-2543
Website: http://sld.state.nm.us/
lab/default.htm

New Mexico Follow-up

New Mexico Department of
Health
Scientific Laboratory
Newborn Metabolic Screening
P.O. Box 4700
Albuquerque, NM 87196
Phone: 505-841-2581
Fax: 505-841-2560
Website: http://sld.state.nm.us/
lab/default.htm

New York Laboratory

Wadsworth Center
New York State Department of
Health
P.O. Box 509
Albany, NY 12201-0509
Phone: 518-473-1993
Fax: 518-486-2095
Website: http://
health.state.ny.us

New York Follow-up

Wadsworth Center
New York State Department of
Health
P.O. Box 509
Albany, NY 12201-0509
Phone: 518-473-7552
Fax: 518-474-0405
Website: http://
health.state.ny.us

North Carolina Laboratory

State Laboratory of Public
Health
Newborn Screening Branch
P.O. Box 28047
Raleigh, NC 27611-8047
Phone: 919-733-3937
Fax: 919-715-8610
http://www.dhhs.state.nc.us/dph

North Carolina Follow-up

State Laboratory of Public
Health
Newborn Screening Branch
P.O. Box 28047
Raleigh, NC 27611-8047
Phone: 919-733-3937
Fax: 919-715-8610
http://www.dhhs.state.nc.us/dph

North Dakota Laboratory

Newborn Screening Laboratory
University Hygienic Laboratory
1521 2nd Avenue
Des Moines, IA 50319
Phone: 515-243-0141
Fax: 515-243-3071

North Dakota Follow-up

Division of Maternal and Child
Health
North Dakota Department of
Health
600 East Boulevard
Bismarck, ND 58505-0200
Toll-Free: 800-472-2286
Phone: 701-328-2493
Fax: 701-328-1412
Website: http://www.ndmch.com

Ohio Laboratory

Newborn Screening Laboratory
Ohio Department of Health
Laboratory
P.O. Box 2568
Columbus, OH 43216-2568
Toll-Free: 888-634-5227
Phone: 614-644-4590
Fax: 614-644-4677
Website: http://
www.odh.state.oh.us/
ODHPrograms/NEWBRN/
nbrn1.htm

Ohio Follow-up

Supervisor, Newborn Screening
Section
Ohio Bureau of Public Health Labs
P.O. Box 2568
Columbus OH 43216-2568
Toll-Free: 888-634-5227
Phone: 614-644-4590
Fax: 614-644-4677
Website: http://
www.odh.state.oh.us/
ODHPrograms/NEWBRN/
nbrn1.htm

Oklahoma Laboratory

Metabolic Disease Screening
Oklahoma Health Laboratory
P.O. Box 24106
Oklahoma City, OK 73124
Phone: 405-271-5070
Fax: 405-271-4850
Website: http://
www.health.state.ok.us/
PROGRAM/phl

Oklahoma Follow-up

Newborn Screening Nurse
Coordinator
Oklahoma State Department of
Health
1000 NE 10th Street #709
Oklahoma City, OK 73117-1299
Phone: 405-271-9444 ext 56735
Fax: 405-271-4892
Website: http://
www.health.state.ok.us

671

Oregon Laboratory

Newborn Screening Section
Oregon Public Health
Laboratory
1717 SW 10th Avenue
Portland, OR 97207-0275
Phone: 503-229-6576
Fax: 503-229-6989
Website: http://
www.dhs.state.or.us/
publichealth/phl

Oregon Follow-up

Pacific NW Regional Screening
Program
Oregon Public Health
Laboratory
1717 SW 10th Avenue
Portland, OR 97207-0275
Phone: 503-229-6576
Fax: 503-229-6989
Website: http://
www.ohd.hr.state.or.us/nbs

Pennsylvania Laboratory

Division of Newborn Disease
Prevention and Identification
Bureau of Family Health,
Pennsylvania Department of
Health
7th Floor Health and Welfare Bldg.
Harrisburg, PA 17108
Phone: 717-783-8143
Fax: 717-705-9386
Website: http://
www.dsf.health.state.pa.us/
health/site/default.asp

Pennsylvania Follow-up

Division of Newborn Disease
Prevention and Identification
Bureau of Family Health,
Pennsylvania Department of
Health
7th Floor Health and Welfare Bldg.
Harrisburg, PA 17108
Phone: 717-783-8143
Fax: 717-705-9386
Website: http://
www.dsf.health.state.pa.us/
health/site/default.asp

Rhode Island Laboratory

New England Regional Newborn
Screening Program
University of Massachusetts
Medical School
305 South Street
Jamaica Plain, MA 02130-3597
Phone: 617-983-6300
Fax: 617-522-2846
Website: http://
www.umassmed.edu/nbs

Rhode Island Follow-up

Newborn Screening Coordinator
Rhode Island Department of
Health
3 Capitol Hill, Room 305
Providence, RI 02908
Phone: 401-222-4601
Fax: 401-222-6985
Website: http://
www.health.ri.gov/genetics/
newborn.htm

South Carolina Laboratory

Division of Analytical Chemistry
South Carolina Department of
Health and Environmental
Control
8231 Parklane Road
Columbia, SC 29202
Phone: 803-896-0963
Fax: 803-935-7357
Website: http://www.scdhec.net/
hs/lab/AnalytChemDiv.htm

South Carolina Follow-up

Division of Women and
Children's Health
South Carolina Department of
Health and Environmental
Control
P.O. Box 101106
Columbia, SC 29211
Phone: 803-898-0777
Fax: 803-898-0337
Website: http://www.scdhec.gov/
hs/mch/wcs/index.htm

South Dakota Laboratory

South Dakota Department of
Health
600 East Capitol Avenue
Pierre, SD 57501-2536
Phone: 605-773-3361
Fax: 605-773-5509
Website: http://www.state.sd.us/
doh

South Dakota Follow-up

South Dakota Department of
Health
600 East Capitol Avenue
Pierre, SD 57501-2536
Phone: 605-773-3361
Fax: 605-773-5509
Website: http://www.state.sd.us/
doh

Tennessee Laboratory

Microbiology Division
Laboratory Services
Tennessee Department of
Health and Environment
630 Hart Lane
Nashville, TN 37247-0801
Phone: 615-262-6300
Fax: 615-262-6393
Website: http://
www2.state.tn.us/Lab/index.htm

Tennessee Follow-up

Maternal and Child Health
Division
Cordell Hall Building, Floor 5
425 N. 5th Avenue
Nashville, TN 37247-4701
Phone: 615-262-6304
Fax: 615-262-6458
Website: http://
www2.state.tn.us/health/MCH/
genetics.htm

Texas Laboratory

Bureau of Laboratories
Texas Department of Health
1100 W. 49th Street
Austin, TX 78756
Phone: 512-458-7318
Fax: 512-458-7294
Website: http://
www.tdh.state.tx.us/lab

Texas Follow-up

Bureau of Child Health
Texas Department of Health
1100 W. 49th Street
Austin, TX 78756
Toll-Free: 800-422-2956
Fax: 512-458-7421
Website: http://
www.tdh.state.tx.us/newborn/
newborn.htm

Utah Laboratory

Bureau of Microbiology
Division of Laboratory Services
44 Medical Drive
Salt Lake City, UT 84113
Phone: 801-584-8469
Fax: 801-584-8501
Website: http://health.utah.gov/
els/microbiology

Utah Follow-up

Genetic Nurse Consultant
Newborn Metabolic Screening
Program
Utah Department of Health,
F.H.S. Division
44 N. Medical Drive
P.O. Box 144710
Salt Lake City, UT 84114-4710
Phone: 801-584-8256
Fax: 801-536-0962
Website: http://health.utah.gov/
newbornscreening

Vermont Laboratory

New England Regional Newborn
Screening Program
University of Massachusetts
Medical School
305 South Street
Jamaica Plain, MA 02130-3597
Phone: 617-983-6300
Fax: 617-522-2846
Website: http://
www.umassmed.edu/nbs

Vermont Follow-up

Vermont Department of Health
Division of Health Improvement
Newborn Screening Program
108 Cherry Street
Burlington, VT 05402
Phone: 802-863-7338
Fax: 802-651-1634
Website: http://
www.healthyvermonters.info/hi/
hi.shtml

Virginia Laboratory

Newborn Screening Laboratory
Division of Consolidated
Laboratories
600 North 5ᵗʰ Street
Richmond, VA 23219
Phone: 804-648-4480
Fax: 804-371-7973
Website: http://
dcls.dgs.state.va.us

Virginia Follow-up

Virginia Department of Health
Division of Women and Infant
Health
109 Governer Street
Richmond, VA 23219
Phone: 804-225-7751
Fax: 804-786-3442
Website: http://
www.vahealth.org/genetics/
index.htm

Washington Laboratory

Office of Newborn Screening
Washington State Department
of Health
1610 NE 150ᵗʰ Street
Shoreline, WA 98155
Phone: 206-361-2902
Fax: 206-361-4996
Website: http://www.doh.wa.gov/
ehsphl/phl/newborn

Washington Follow-up

Genetics Services Section
Office of Maternal and Child
Health
Washington State Department
of Health
Community and Family Health
NewMarket Industrial Campus,
Building 10
Olympia, WA 98504
Phone: 253-395-6741
Website: http://www.doh.wa.gov/
cfh/mch/Genetics/default.htm

West Virginia Laboratory

Office of Laboratory Services
West Virginia Department of
Health and Human Resources
167 11ᵗʰ Avenue
South Charleston, WV 25303
Phone: 304-558-3530
Fax: 304-558-2006
Website: http://www.wvdhhr.org/
labservices/index.cfm

West Virginia Follow-up

Office of Maternal and Child
Health
West Virginia Department of
Health and Human Resources
350 Capital Street #427
Charleston, WV 25301-3714
Phone: 304-558-5388
Fax: 304-558-7164
Website: http://www.wvdhhr.org/
mcfh

Wisconsin Laboratory

Newborn Screening Laboratory
Wisconsin State Laboratory of
Hygiene
465 Henry Mall
Madison, WI 53706
Phone: 608-262-6547
Fax: 608-262-5494
Website: http://
www.slh.wisc.edu/newborn/
index.php

Wisconsin Follow-up

Newborn Screening Laboratory
Wisconsin State Laboratory of
Hygiene
465 Henry Mall
Madison, WI 53706
Phone: 608-262-6547
Fax: 608-262-5494
Website: http://
www.slh.wisc.edu/newborn/
index.php

Wyoming Laboratory

Colorado Department of Public
Health and Environment
8100 Lowry Boulevard
Denver, CO 80230-6928
Phone: 303-692-3090
Fax: 303-344-9989
Website: http://
www.cdphe.state.co.us/lr/
lrhom.htm

Wyoming Follow-up

Department of Health
Hathaway Building, Floor 4
Cheyenne, WY 82002
Phone: 307-777-7166
Fax: 307-777-5580
Website: http://
wdhfs.state.wy.us/WDH/
Programs.htm

Chapter 71

Resources for Information about Genetics and Genetic Research

American Society of Human Genetics
9650 Rockville Pike
Bethesda, MD 20814
Toll-Free: 866-HUM-GENE
Phone: 301-571-7300
Website: http://www.ashg.org
E-mail: society@ashg.org

Association of Birth Defect Children, Inc.
930 Woodcock Road, Suite 225
Orlando, FL 32803
Toll-Free: 800-313-2232
Phone: 407-895-0802
Fax: 407-895-0824
Website: http://www.birthdefects.org
E-mail: staff@birthdefects.org

Canadian Genetic Diseases Network
2150 Western Parkway, Suite 201
Vancouver, BC V6T 1V6
Phone: 604-221-7300
Fax: 604-221-0778
Website: http://ww.cgdn.ca
E-mail: info@cgdn.ca

Center for Human and Molecular Genetics
Genetic Service Outreach Program
150 Bergen Street
Newark, NJ 07103
Phone: 201-982-3300
Fax: 201-982-3310
Website: http://www.theuniversityhospital.com/physservdirectory/html/genetics.htm

---

Resources listed in this chapter were compiled from various sources deemed accurate. All contact information was verified and updated in July 2004. Inclusion does not constitute endorsement.

Center for Jewish Genetic Diseases
Mount Sinai School of Medicine
Box 1497
One Gustave L. Levy Place
New York, NY 10029
Phone: 212-659-6774
Consultations/Screening:
212-241-6947
Website: http://www.mssm.edu/
Jewish_genetics

Center for the Study and Treatment of Jewish Genetic Diseases
University of Pittsburgh
Dept. of Human Genetics
E1651 BST
Pittsburgh, PA 15213
Toll-Free: 800-334-7980
Website: http://www.pitt.edu/
~geneorb/ctr-jewish.html

Children's Medical Center
The Genetics Center
One Children's Plaza
Dayton, OH 45404-1815
Phone: 937-226-8300
Website: http://www.cmc-dayton
.org/index.cfm

Cincinnati Children's Hospital Medical Center
3333 Burnet Avenue
Cincinnati, OH 45339-3039
Toll-Free: 800-344-2462
Phone: 513-636-4200
TTY: 513-636-4900
Website: http://
www.cincinnatichildrens.org

Council for Responsible Genetics
5 Upland Road, Suite 3
Cambridge, MA 02140
Phone: 617-868-0870
Fax: 617-491-5344
Website: http://www.gene-watch.org
E-mail: crg@gene-watch.org

Emory Genetics Laboratory
Emory University School of Medicine
Whitehead Biomedical Research Building
615 Michael Street, Suite 301
Atlanta, GA 30322
Phone: 404-727-5624
Fax: 404-727-3949
Website: http://
server2k.genetics.emory.edu/lab/
user
E-mail: info@genetics.emory.edu

GeneCare Medical Genetics Center
201 Sage Rd., Suite 300
Chapel Hill, NC 27514
Toll-Free: 800-277-4363
Phone: 919-942-0021
Fax: 919-967-9519
Website: http://
www.genecare.com
E-mail: info@genecare.com

GeneTests
9725 Third Avenue NE, Suite 602
Seattle, WA 98115-8735
Phone: 206-221-4674
Fax: 206-221-4679
Website: http://www.genetests.org
E-mail: genetests@genetests.org

Genetic Alliance
4301 Connecticut Avenue NW
Suite 404
Washington, DC 20008-2369
Toll-Free: 800-336-GENE (4363)
Phone: 202-966-5557
Fax: 202-966-8553
http://www.geneticalliance.org
E-mail:
information@geneticalliance.org

Genetics Education and Counseling Program
University of Pittsburgh
Department of Human Genetics
E1651 Biomedical Science Tower
Pittsburgh, PA 15213
Toll-Free: 800-640-GENE (640-4363)
Fax: 412-624-3020
Website: http://www.pitt.edu/
~edugene
E-mail: edugene@pitt.edu

Genetics Education Center
University of Kansas Medical
Center
Department of Neurology
3901 Rainbow Boulevard
Kansas City, Kansas 66160-7314
Phone: 913-588-6022
Website: http://kumc.edu/gec

Genetics Home Reference
National Library of Medicine
8600 Rockville Pike
Bethesda, MD 20894
Phone: 301-594-5983
Fax: 301-402-1384
Toll-Free: 888-FIND-NLM
Website: http://
www.ghr.nlm.nih.gov

Hereditary Disease Foundation
1303 Pico Boulevard
Santa Monica, CA 90405
Phone: 310-450-9913
Fax: 310-450-9532
Website: http://
www.hdfoundation.org
E-mail: cures@
hdfoundation.org

Howard Hughes Medical Institute
Office of Communications
4000 Jones Bridge Road
Chevy Chase, MD 20815-6789
Phone: 301-215-8500
Website: http://www.hhmi.org

MAGIC Foundation
6645 W. North Avenue
Oak Park, IL 60302
Phone: 708-383-0808
Fax: 708-383-0899
Website: http://
www.magicfoundation.org

March of Dimes Birth Defects Foundation
1275 Mamaroneck Avenue
White Plains, NY 10605
Toll-Free: 888-663-4637
Website: http://
www.modimes.org

Mayo Foundation for Medical Education and Research and Mayo Clinic

200 First Street SW
Rochester, MN 55905
Toll-Free: 800-297-1185
Phone: 507-284-2511
Fax: 507-284-0161
Website: http://
www.mayohealth.org
Website: http://mayoclinic.org

Medical College of Virginia

Department of Human Genetics
P.O. 980033
Richmond, VA 23298-0033
Phone: 804-828-9632
Fax: 804-828-3760
Website: http://
www.vipbg.vcu.edu/hg

Mountain States Genetic Network

8129 West Fremont Avenue
Littleton, CO 80128
Phone: 303-978-0125
Fax: 303-948-1890
Website: http://www.mostgene.org
E-mail: mostgenes@msn.com

National Center for Biotechnology Information

U.S. National Library of Medicine
8600 Rockville Pike
Building 38A
Bethesda, MD 20894
Phone: 301-496-2475
Fax: 301-480-9241
Website: http://
www.ncbi.nlm.nih.gov
E-mail: info@ncbi.nlm.nih.gov

National Center for Education in Maternal and Child Health

2115 Wisconsin Ave. NW, Suite 601
Washington, DC 20007-2292
Phone: 202-784-9770
Fax: 202-784-9777
Website: http://www.ncemch.org
E-mail: nchlibrary@ncemch.org

National Center on Birth Defects and Developmental Disabilities

Centers for Disease Control and Prevention
1600 Clifton Rd., Mailstop E-86
Atlanta, GA 30333
Phone: 404-498-3890
Website: http://www.cdc.gov/ncbddd

National Human Genome Research Institute

Office of Policy and Public Affairs
Building 31, Room 4B09
31 Center Drive, MSC 2152
Bethesda, MD 20892-2152
Phone: 301-402-0911
Fax: 301-402-2218
Website: http://www.genome.gov

National Institute of Child Health and Human Development

NICHD Clearinghouse
P.O. Box 3006
Rockville, MD 20847
Toll-Free: 800-370-2943
Fax: 301-984-1473
Website: http://www.nichd.nih.gov
E-mail: NICHDClearinghouse
@iqsolutions.com

National Institute of Neurological Disorders and Stroke

P.O. Box 5801
Bethesda, MD 20824
Toll-Free: 800-352-9424
Phone: 301-496-5751
TTY: 301-468-5981
Website: http://
www.ninds.nih.gov

National Newborn Screening and Genetics Resource Center

1912 W. Anderson Lane, Suite 210
Austin, TX 78757
Phone: 512-454-6419
Fax: 512-454-6509
Website: http://genes-r-us.uthscsa.edu

National Organization for Rare Disorders, Inc.

55 Kenosia Avenue
P.O. Box 1968
Danbury, CT 06813-1968
Toll-Free: 800-999-6673
Phone: 203-744-0100
Fax: 203-798-2291
TDD: 203-797-9590
Internet: http://
www.rarediseases.org
E-mail: orphan@rarediseases.org

National Society of Genetic Counselors

233 Canterbury Drive
Wallingford, PA 19086
Phone: 610-872-7608
Website: http://www.nsgc.org
E-mail: FYI@nsgc.org

Oak Ridge National Laboratory

P.O. Box 2008
Oak Ridge, TN 37831
Phone: 865-574-7199
Fax: 865-574-9998
Website: http://www.ornl.gov

Office of Rare Diseases

National Institutes of Health
6100 Executive Boulevard
Room 3B01, MSC 7518
Bethesda, MD 20892-7518
Phone: 301-402-4336
Fax: 301-480-9655
Website: http://
rarediseases.info.nih.gov
E-mail: ord@od.nih.gov

Online Mendelian Inheritance in Man (OMIM)

Johns Hopkins University
Website: http://
www.ncbi.nlm.nih.gov/omim

University of Maryland School of Medicine

Human Genetics Programs
655 W. Baltimore
Bressler Building 11-037
Baltimore, MD 21201
Phone: 410-328-8919
Website: http://
medschool.umaryland.edu

***University of Rochester
Medical Center***
Division of Genetics
601 Elmwood Avenue/Box 641
Rochester, NY 14642
Phone: 582-275-4602
Website: http://
www.urmc.rochester.edu/
Genetics

Chapter 72

Genetic Disorders:
A Directory of Information
and Support Resources

Resources in this chapter are arranged alphabetically by key word. Key words within organization names are shown in boldface type. For organization's whose focus may not be apparent from the organization name, key words are added in brackets.

Billy Barty Foundation, Inc.
[Achondroplasia]
929 W. Olive Avenue, Suite L
Burbank, CA 91506
Toll-Free: 800-891-4022
Phone: 818-953-5410
Fax: 818-953-7129 fax

Human Growth Foundation
National Office
[Achondroplasia]
997 Glen Cove Avenue, Suite 5
Glen Head, NY 11545
Toll-Free: 800-451-6434
Fax: 516-671-4055
Website: http://www.hgfound.org
E-mail: hgf1@hgfound.org

Little People of America
[Achondroplasia]
5289 NE Elam Young Parkway,
Suite F-700
Hillsboro, OR 97124
Toll-Free: 888-572-2001
Phone: 503-846-1562
Fax: 503-846-1590
Website: http://
www.lpaonline.org
E-mail: info@lpaonline.org

The resources listed in this chapter provide a starting point for further research. They were compiled from various sources deemed accurate. All contact information was verified and updated in July 2004. Inclusion does not constitute endorsement.

Short Stature Foundation
[Achondroplasia]
17200 Jamboree Road, Suite J
Irvine, CA 92714-5828
Toll-Free: 800-243-9273
Phone: 714-474-4554
Fax: 714-261-9035

Acoustic Neuroma Association
600 Peachtree Parkway, Suite 108
Cumming, GA 30041-6899
Phone: 770-205-8211
Fax: 770-205-0239
Website: http://anausa.org
E-mail: ANAUSA@aol.com

National **Adrenal Diseases**
Foundation
505 Northern Boulevard
Great Neck, NY 11021
Phone: 516-487-4992
Website: http://
www.medhelp.org/nadf
E-mail: nadfmail@aol.com

Aicardi Syndrome Newsletter,
Inc.
1510 Polo Fields Court
Louisville, KY 40245
Phone: 502-244-9152
Website://
www.aicardisyndrome.org
E-mail: AICNews@aol.com

International **Albinism** Center
University of Minnesota
P.O. Box 485 Mayo
420 Delaware Street SE
Minneapolis, MN 55455
Phone: 612-624-0144
Website: http://
www.cbc.umn.edu/iac

NOAH (National Organization
for **Albinism** and Hypo-
pigmentation)
P.O. Box 959
East Hampstead, NH 03826-0959
Toll-Free: 800-473-2310
Phone: 603-887-2310
Website: http://
www.albinism.org
E-mail:
webmaster@albinism.org

Network for 9p- Support **[Alfi's
Syndrome]**
393 N. Grass Valley Road
Pine Valley, UT 84781
Phone: 435-574-1121
Website: http://
www.9pminus.org

Asthma and **Allergy**
Foundation of America
1233 20th Street, NW
Suite 402
Washington, DC 20036
Toll-Free: 800-727-8462
Phone: 202-466-7643
Fax: 202-466-8940
Website: http://www.aafa.org
E-mail: info@aafa.org

National Institute of **Allergy**
and Infectious Diseases
Building 31, Room 7A-50
31 Center Drive MSC 2520
Bethesda, MD 20892-2520
Phone: 301-496-5598
Website: http://
www.niaid.nih.gov

684

National **Alopecia Areata**
Foundation
P.O. Box 150760
San Rafael, CA 94915-0760
Phone: 415-472-3780
Fax: 415-472-5343
Website: http://www.naaf.org

Alpha-1 Association **[Alpha-1
Antitrypsin Deficiency]**
275 West Street
Suite 210
Annapolis, MD 21401
Toll-Free: 800-521-3025
Phone: 202-887-1900
Fax: 202-887-1964
Website: http://www.alpha1.org
E-mail: info@alpha1.org

Alzheimer's Association
225 N. Michigan Avenue
Floor 17
Chicago, IL 60601
Toll-Free 800-272-3900
Phone: 312-335-8700
Fax: 312-335-1110
TDD: 312-335-8882
Website: http://www.alz.org
E-mail: info@alz.org

Alzheimer's Disease
Education and Referral Center
ADEAR Center
P.O. Box 8250
Silver Spring, MD 20907-8250
Toll-Free: 800-438-4380
Fax: 301-495-3334
Website: http://
www.alzheimers.org
E-mail: adear@alzheimers.org

**Amyotrophic Lateral
Sclerosis** Association
27001 Agoura Road
Suite 150
Calabasas Hills, CA 91301-5104
Toll-Free: 800-782-4747
Phone: 818-880-9007
Fax: 818-880-9006
Website: http://www.alsa.org
E-mail: alsinfo@alsa-
national.org

Iron Disorders Institute
[Anemia]
P.O. Box 2031
Greenville, SC 29602
Toll-Free: 888-565-4766
Phone: 864-292-1175
Fax: 864-292-1878
Website: http://
www.irondisorders.org
E-mail:
patientservices@irondisorders.org

Angelman Syndrome
Foundation
3015 E. New York Street
Suite A2265
Aurora, IL 60504
Toll-Free: 800-432-6435
Phone: 630-978-4245
Fax: 630-978-7408
Website: http://
www.angelman.org
E-mail: info@angelman.org

Angelman Syndrome
Information for Families and
Professionals
Website: http://
www.asclepius.com/angel

Arnold-Chiari Family Network
647 Spring Street
Weymouth, MA 02188-3528
Phone: 617-337-2368

American Juvenile **Arthritis**
Organization
1314 Spring Street, NW
Atlanta, GA 30309
Toll-Free: 800-283-7800
Phone: 404-872-7100
Fax: 404-872-0457

National **Ataxia** Foundation
2600 Fernbrook Lane
Suite 119
Minneapolis, MN 55447-4752
Phone: 763-553-0020
Fax: 763-553-0167
Website: http://www.ataxia.org
E-mail: naf@ataxia.org

Autism Society of America
7910 Woodmont Avenue
Suite 300
Bethesda, MD 20814-3015
Toll-Free: 800-328-8476
Phone: 301-657-0881
Website: http://www
.autism-society.org
E-mail: info@autism-society.org

Purine Research Society
[Autism]
5424 Beech Avenue
Bethesda, MD 20814-1730
Phone: 301-530-0354
Fax: 301-564-9597
Website: http://www2.dgsys.com/
~purine
E-mail: purine@erols.com

Barth Syndrome Foundation,
Inc.
P.O. Box 974
Perry, FL 32348
Phone: 850-223-1128
Fax: 402-421-1926
Website: http://
www.barthsyndrome.org
E-mail:
inquiries.rd@barthsyndrome.org

Batten Disease Support and
Research Association
120 Humphries Dr.
Suite 2
Reynoldsburg, OH 43068
Toll-Free: 800-448-4570
Phone: 740-927-4298
Website: http://bdsra.org
E-mail: bdsra1@bdsra.org

Children's Brain Disease
Foundation **[Batten Disease]**
Parnassus Heights Medical
Building, Suite 900
350 Parnassus Avenue
San Francisco, CA 94117
Phone: 415-565-6259
Fax: 415-863-3452

Institute for Basic Research
[Batten Disease]
1050 Forest Hill Road
Staten Island, NY 10314
Phone: 718-494-0600
Fax: 718-698-3803

JNCL (Juvenile Neuronal Ceroid Lipofuscinoses) Research Fund **[Batten Disease]**
P.O. Box 766
Mundelein, IL 60060
Website: http://www.jnclresearch.org
E-mail: Contactus@jnclresearch.org

Nathan's Battle Foundation
[Batten Disease]
459 South State Road 135
Greenwood, IN 46142
Phone: 317-888-7396
Fax: 317-888-0504
Website: http://www.nathansbattle.com

Beckwith-Wiedemann Support Network
2711 Colony Road
Ann Arbor, MI 48104
Toll-Free: 800-837-2976
Phone: 734-973-0263
Fax: 734-973-9721
Website: http://www.Beckwith-wiedemann.org
E-mail: bwsn@Beckwith-wiedemann.org

American **Behçet's** Disease Association
P.O. Box 19952
Amarillo, TX 79114
Toll-Free: 800-7BEHCETS
Website: http://www.behcets.com

American Council of the **Blind**
1155 15th Street NW, Suite 1004
Washington, DC 20005
Toll-Free: 800-424-8666
Phone: 202-467-5081
Fax: 202-467-5085
Website: http://www.acb.org
E-mail: info@acb.org

American Foundation for the **Blind**
11 Penn Plaza, Suite 300
New York, NY 10001
Toll-Free: 800-232-5463
Phone: 212-502-7600
Fax: 212-502-7777
Website: http://www.afb.org
E-mail: afbinfo@afb.net

National Association for Parents of Children with Visual Impairments (NAPVI)
[Blindness/Visual Impairment]
P.O. Box 317
Watertown, MA 02471
Toll-Free: 800-562-6265
Phone: 617-972-7441
Fax: 617-972-7444
Website: http://www.napvi.org
E-mail: napvi@perkins.org

Canavan Disease Research
P.O. Box 8194
Rolling Meadows, IL 60008-8194
Phone: 800-833-2194
Website: http://www.canavanresearch.org
E-mail: canavan@canavanresearch.org

Canavan Foundation
450 West End Avenue, #10C
New York, NY 10024
Toll-Free: 877-4-CANAVAN
(422-6282)
Phone: 212-873-4640
Fax: 212-873-7892
Website: http://
www.canavanfoundation.org
E-mail:
info@canavanfoundation.org

Canavan Research Foundation
Fairwood Professional Building
New Fairfield, CT 06812
Phone: 203-746-2436
Fax: 203-746-3205
Website: http://www.canavan.org
E-mail:
canavanresearch@aol.com

National Tay-Sachs and Allied
Diseases Association [**Canavan**
Disease]
2001 Beacon Street, Suite 204
Brighton, MA 02135
Toll-Free: 800-90-NTSAD
Phone: 617-277-4463
Fax: 617-277-0134
Website: http://www.ntsad.org
E-mail: info@ntsad.org

American **Cancer** Society
599 Clifton Road, NE
Atlanta, GA 30329-4251
Phone: 404-329-7622
Fax: 404-636-5567
Toll-Free: 800-227-2345
Website: http://www.cancer.org

Candlelighters Childhood
Cancer Foundation
P.O. Box 498
Kensington, MD 20895-0498
Toll-Free: 800-366-2223
Phone: 301-962-3520
Fax: 301-962-3521
Website: http://
www.candlelighters.org
E-mail: staff@candlelighters.org

National **Cancer** Institute
Building 31, Room 10A24
Bethesda, MD 20892
Toll-Free: 800-4-CANCER
Phone: 301-496-5583
TTY: 800-332-8615
Website: http://www.cancer.gov

American **Celiac** Society
59 Crystal Avenue
West Orange, NJ 07052
Phone: 504-737-3293
Fax: 504-973-8808
E-mail:
americeliacsoc@netscape.net

Celiac Disease Foundation
13251 Ventura Boulevard, #1
Studio City, CA 91604
Phone: 818-990-2354
Fax: 818-990-2379
Website: http://www.celiac.org
E-mail: cdf@celiac.org

Celiac Sprue Association/USA Inc.
P.O. Box 31700
Omaha, NE 68131-0700
Toll-Free: 877-CSA-4CSA
Phone: 402-558-0600
Fax: 402-558-1347
Website: http://www.csaceliacs.org
E-mail: celiacs@celiacs.org

Gluten-Free Living [**Celiac Disease**]
19A Broadway
Hawthorne, NY 10532
Phone: 914-741-5420
Website: http://www.glutenfreeliving.com
E-mail: info@glutenfreeliving.com

United **Cerebral Palsy** Associations, Inc.
1660 L Street, NW, Suite 700
Washington, DC 20036
Toll-Free: 800-872-5827
Phone: 202-776-0406
TTY: 202-973-7197
Fax: 202-776-0414
Website: http://www.ucp.org
E-mail: national@ucp.org

Charcot-Marie-Tooth Association
2700 Chestnut Parkway
Chester, PA 19013-4867
Toll-Free: 800-606-CMTA (2682)
Phone: 610-499-9264
Fax: 610-499-9267
Website: http://www.charcot-marie-tooth.org
E-mail: CMTAssoc@aol.com

CMT International [**Charcot-Marie-Tooth Disorder**]
1852 Lockhill-Selma
Suite 108
San Antonio, TX 78213
Phone: 210-348-6939
Fax: 210-348-6938
Website: http://www.cmt-int.com
E-mail: cmtsales@cmt-int.com

Chromosome Deletion Outreach
P.O. Box 724
Boca Raton, FL 33429-0724
Phone: 516-395-4252
Website: http://www.chromodisorder.org

Unique: Rare **Chromosome Disorder** Support Group
P.O. Box 2189
Caterham, Surrey, CR3 5GN
England
Phone: 011 44 1883 330766
Website: http://www.rarechromo.org
info@rarechromo.org

Chronic Granulomatous Disease Association, Inc.
2616 Monterey Road
San Marino, CA 91108-1646
Phone: 626-441-4118
Website: http://home.socal.rr.com/cgda
E-mail: cgda@socal.rr.com

Cleft Palate Foundation
1504 East Franklin Street
Suite 102
Chapel Hill, NC 27514-2820
Toll-Free: 800-24-CLEFT (242-5338)
Phone: 919-933-9044
Fax: 919-933-9604
Website: http://www.cleftline.org
E-mail: info@cleftline.org

Coffin-Lowry Syndrome
Foundation
3045 255th Avenue, SE
Sammamish, WA 98075
Phone: 425-842-1523
Website: http://clsfoundation.tripod.com
E-mail: CLSFoundation@yahoo.com

Cornelia de Lange Syndrome
Foundation
302 West Main Street, #100
Avon, CT 06001
Toll-Free: 800-223-8355
Phone: 860-676-8166
Fax: 860-676-8337
Website: http://www.cdlsusa.org
E-mail: info@cdlsusa.org

Children's **Craniofacial**
Association
13140 Coit Road, Suite 307
Dallas, TX 75240
Toll-Free: 800-535-3643
Phone: 214-570-9099
Website: http://www.ccakids.com
E-mail: contactCCA@ccakids.com

Craniofacial Foundation of
America
975 East Third Street, Box 269
Chattanooga, TN 37403
Toll-Free: 800-418-3223
Phone: 423-778-9192
Fax: 423-778-8172
Website: http://www.erlanger.org/craniofacial/found1.html

FACES: The National
Craniofacial Association
P.O. Box 11082
Chattanooga, TN 37401
Toll-Free: 800-332-2372
Phone: 423-266-1632
Website: http://www.faces-cranio.org
E-mail: faces@faces-cranio.org

Forward Face **[Craniofacial Conditions]**
317 East 34th Street
Suite 901A
New York, NY 10016
Phone: 212-684-5860
Fax: 212-684-5864
Website: http://www.forwardface.org

Foundation for Nager and Miller
Syndromes **[Craniofacial Conditions]**
13210 SE 342nd Street
Auburn, WA 98092
Toll-Free: 800-507-FNMS
Phone: 253-288-7679
Website: http://www.nagerormillersynd.com

Let's Face It USA
[Craniofacial Conditions]
P.O. Box 29972
Bellingham, WA 98228-1972
Phone: 360-676-7325
Website: http://www.faceit.org
E-mail: letsfaceit@faceit.org

5P- Society **[Cri Du Chat]**
P.O. Box 268
Lakewood, CA 90714-0268
Toll-Free: 888-970-0777
Phone: 714-901-1544
Website: http://www.fivepminus.org

Cri Du Chat Support Group of Australia
104 Yarralumla Drive
Langwarin, VIC 3910, Australia
Phone: 011 61 3 9561 8134
Fax: 011 61 3 9791 8577
Website: http://
www.criduchat.asn.au
E-mail: info@criduchat.asn.au

Crouzon Support Network
P.O. Box 1272
Edmonds, WA 98020
Phone: 425-672-1697
Fax: 425-778-9089
Website: http://www.crouzon.org
E-mail: crouzons-owner
@yahoogroups.com

Cystic Fibrosis Foundation
6931 Arlington Road, Suite 200
Bethesda, MD 20814
Toll-Free: 800-344-4823
Phone: 301-951-4422
Fax: 301-951-6378
Website: http://www.cff.org
E-mail: info@cff.org

Cystinosis Foundation, Inc.
604 Veronon Street
Oakland, CA 94610
Toll-Free: 800-392-8458
Phone: 599-222-7997
Website: http://
www.cystinosisfoundation.org
E-mail: email@cyctinosis.com

Alexander Graham Bell
Association for the **Deaf**, Inc.
3417 Volta Place, NW
Washington, DC 20007-2778
Phone: 202-337-5220
Fax: 202-337-8314
TTY: 202-337-5221
Website: http://www.agbell.org

American Society for **Deaf**
Children
P.O. Box 3355
Gettysburg, PA 17325
Toll-Free: 800-942-ASDC (2732)
Phone: 717-334-7922 (Business
Voice and TTY)
Fax: 717-334-8808
Website: http://
www.deafchildren.org
E-mail: ASDC1@aol.com

Better Hearing Institute
[Deafness]
515 King Street, Suite 420
Alexandria, VA 22314
Phone: 703-684-3391
Website: http://
www.betterhearing.org
E-mail: mail@betterhearing.org

Deafness Research Foundation
1050 17th Street, NW
Suite 701
Washington, DC 20036
Phone: 202-289-5850
Website: http://www.drf.org
E-mail: webmaster@drf.org

Gallaudet Research Institute
[Deafness]
Gallaudet University
800 Florida Avenue, NE
Washington, DC 20002
Phone: 202-651-5575
Website: http://gri.gallaudet.edu

Harvard Medical School Center
for Hereditary **Deafness**
65 Landsdowne Street
Cambridge, MA 02139
Phone: 617-768-8291
Fax: 617-768-8510
Website: http://
hearing.harvard.edu
E-mail:
hearing@hms.harvard.edu

National Association of the **Deaf**
814 Thayer
Silver Spring, MD 20910
Phone: 301-587-1788
TTY: 301-587-1789
Fax: 301-587-1791
Website: http://www.nad.org
E-mail: NADinfo@nad.org

National Institute on **Deafness**
and Other Communication
Disorders Clearinghouse
31 Center Drive, MCS 2320
Bethesda, MD 20892-3456
Toll-Free: 800-241-1044 (Voice)
Toll-Free: 800-241-1055 (TTY)
Phone: 301-496-7243
Fax: 301-402-0018
TTY: 301-402-0252
Website: http://
www.nidcd.nih.gov
E-mail: nidcdinfo@nidcd.nih.gov

Self Help for Hard of Hearing
People, Inc. (SHHH) **[Deafness]**
7910 Woodmont Ave., Suite 1200
Bethesda, MD 20814
Phone: 301-657-2248
TTY: 301-657-2249
Fax: 301-913-9413
Website: http://
www.hearingloss.org
E-mail:
information@hearingloss.org

National **Diabetes** Information
Clearinghouse
One Information Way
Bethesda, MD 20892
Toll-Free: 800-860-8747
Phone: 301-654-3327
Website: http://
diabetes.niddk.nih.gov

American **Diabetes** Association
1701 North Beauregard St.
Alexandria, VA 22311
Toll-Free: 800-342-2383
Website: http://www.diabetes.org
E-mail: AskADA@diabetes.org

Juvenile **Diabetes** Research Foundation International
120 Wall Street
New York, NY 10005-4001
Toll-Free: 800-533-2873
Fax: 212-785-9595
Website: http://www.jdf.org
E-mail: info@jdrf.org

American **Digestive** Health Foundation
4930 Del Ray Avenue
Bethesda, MD 20814
Phone: 301-654-2055
Fax: 301-654-5920
Website: http://www.gastro.org
E-mail: member@gastro.org

National **Digestive Diseases** Information Clearinghouse
2 Information Way
Bethesda, MD 20892-3570
Website: http://www.niddk.nih.gov
E-mail: nddic@info.niddk.nih.gov

Association of University Centers on **Disabilities**
1010 Wayne Avenue, Suite 920
Silver Spring, MD 20910
Phone: 301-588-8252
Fax: 301-588-2842
Website: http://www.aucd.org

Federation for Children with Special Needs **[Disabilities]**
1135 Tremont St., Suite 420
Boston, MA 02120
Toll-Free: 800-331-0688
Phone: 617-236-7210
Fax: 617-572-2094
Website: http://www.fcsn.org
E-mail: fcsninfo@fcsn.org

Institute for Basic Research in Developmental **Disabilities**
1050 Forest Hill Road
Staten Island, NY 10314
Phone: 718-494-0600
Fax: 718-698-3803

National Dissemination Center for Children with **Disabilities** (NICHCY)
P.O. Box 1492
Washington, DC 20013-1492
Toll-Free: 800-695-0285
Phone: 202-884-8200
Fax: 202-884-8441
Website: http://www.nichcy.org
E-mail: nichcy@aed.org

TASH: The Association for Persons with Severe Handicaps **[Disabilities]**
29 West Susquehanna Avenue
Suite 210
Baltimore, MD 21204
Phone: 410-828-8274
Fax: 410-828-6706
Website: http://tash.org
E-mail: infotash.org

Family Village: A Global Community of **Disability-Related Resources**
Waisman Center
University of Wisconsin-Madison
1500 Highland Avenue
Madison, WI 53705-2280
Website: http://www.familyvillage.wisc.edu
E-mail: familyvillage@waisman.wisc.edu

International Resource Center
for **Down Syndrome**
Keith Building
1621 Euclid Avenue
Suite 514
Cleveland, OH 44115
Toll-Free: 800-899-3039 (in Ohio
only)
Phone: 216-621-8806
Fax: 216-621-4504

National Association for **Down Syndrome**
P.O. Box 4542
Oak Brook, IL 60522
Phone: 630-325-9112
Website: http://www.nads.org
E-mail: info@nads.org

National **Down Syndrome** Congress
1370 Center Drive
Suite 102
Atlanta, GA 30338
Toll-Free: 800-232-6372
Phone: 770-604-9500
Website: http://www.ndsccenter.org
E-mail: info@ndsccenter.org

National **Down Syndrome** Society
666 Broadway
New York, NY 10012
Toll-Free: 800-221-4602
Phone: 212-460-9330
Website: http://www.ndss.org
E-mail: info@ndss.org

Dysautonomia Foundation, Inc.
633 Third Avenue
12th Floor
New York, NY 10017
Phone: 212-949-6644
Website: http://www.familialdysautonomia.org
E-mail: info@familialdysautonomia.org

National Foundation for **Ectodermal Dysplasias**
410 East Main Street
Mascoutah, IL 62258
Phone: 618-566-2020
Fax: 618-566-4718
Website: http://www.nfed.org
E-mail: info@nfed.org

Ehlers-Danlos National Foundation
6399 Wilshire Blvd.
Suite 200
Los Angeles, CA 90048
Phone: 323-651-3038
Fax: 323-651-1366
Website: http://www.ednf.org
E-mail: staff@ednf.org

Dystrophic **Epidermolysis Bullosa** Research Association of America, Inc.
5 West 36th Street
Suite 404
New York, NY 10018
Phone: 212-868-1573
Website: http://www.debra.org
E-mail: staff@debra.org

Epilepsy Foundation of
America
4351 Garden City Dr. #406
Landover, MD 20785
Toll-Free: 800-332-1000;
800-332-4050
Phone: 301-459-3700
Fax: 301-577-2684
Website: http://
www.epilepsyfoundation.org
E-mail:
info@epilepsyfoundation.org

Fabry Support Information
Group
108 NE 2nd Street
Suite C
P.O. Box 510
Concordia, MO 64020-0510
Phone: 660-463-1355
Fax: 660-463-1356
Website: http://www.fabry.org
E-mail: info@fabry.org

International Center for **Fabry
Disease**
Department of Human Genetics
Mount Sinai School of Medicine
Box 1497
Fifth Avenue at 100th Street
New York, NY 10029
Toll-Free: 866-322-7963
Phone: 212-659-6700
Fax: 212-360-1809
Website: http://www.mssm.edu/
genetics/fabry
E-mail: fabry.disease@mssm.edu

Fanconi Amenia Research
Fund, Inc.
1801 Willamette Street
Suite 200
Eugene, OR 97401
Phone: 541-687-4658
Fax: 541-687-0548
Website: http://www.fanconi.org
E-mail: info@fanconi.org

Conquer **Fragile X** Foundation
189 Bradley Place, Suite 1
Palm Beach, FL 33480
Phone: 561-833-3457
Fax: 877-275-1192
Website: http://www.cfxf.org
E-mail: mail@cfxf.org

FRAXA Research Foundation
[Fragile X]
45 Pleasant Street
Newburyport, MA 01950
Phone: 978-462-1866
Fax: 978-463-9985
Website: http://www.fraxa.org
E-mail: info@frax.org

National **Fragile X** Foundation
P.O. Box 190488
San Francisco, CA 94119
Toll-Free: 800-688-8765
Phone: 925-938-9300
Fax: 925-938-9315
Website: http://www.nfxf.org
E-mail: NATLFX@FragileX.org

Freeman-Sheldon Parent
Support Group
509 East Northmont Way
Salt Lake City, UT 87103
Phone: 801-364-7060
Website: http://www.fspsg.org

Friedreich's Ataxia Research Alliance
2001 Jefferson Davis Hwy.
Suite 209
Arlington, VA 22202
Phone: 703-413-4468
Fax: 703-413-4467
Website: http://www.frda.org
E-mail: fara@frda.org

Adult Metabolic Transition Project **[Galactosemia]**
Website: http://
depts.washington.edu/transmet
E-mail:
transmet@u.washington.edu

American Liver Foundation
[Galactosemia]
75 Maiden Lane
Suite 603
New York, NY 10038
Toll-Free: 800-GO LIVER (465-4837)
Phone: 212-668-1000
Fax: 212-483-8179
Website: http://
liverfoundation.org
E-mail: info@liverfoundation.org

Parents of **Galactosemic** Children
885 Del Sol Street
Sparks, NV 89436
Phone: 775-626-0885
Website: http://
www.galactosemia.org

Save Babies Through Screening Foundation, Inc.
[Galactosemia]
4 Manor View Circle
Malvern, PA 19355-1622
Toll-Free: 888-454-3383
Fax: 610-993-0545
Website: http://
www.savebabies.org
E-mail: email@savebabies.org

National **Gaucher** Foundation
5410 Edson Lane, Suite 260
Rockville, MD 20852-3130
Toll-Free: 800-428-2437
Phone: 301-816-1515
Fax: 301-816-1516
Website: http://
www.gaucherdisease.org
E-mail: ngf@gaucherdisease.org

American Liver Foundation
[Gilbert Syndrome]
75 Maiden Lane, Suite 603
New York, NY 10038
Toll-Free: 800-GO LIVER (465-4837)
Phone: 212-668-1000
Fax: 212-483-8179
Website: http://liverfoundation.org
E-mail: info@liverfoundation.org

Congenital Lactic Acidosis Support Group **[Glutaric Acidemia]**
P.O. Box 480282
1620 Maple Avenue
Denver, CO 80248-0282
Phone: 303-287-4953
Website: http://www.kumc.edu/
gec/support/lactic_a.html

National Urea Cycle Disorders
Foundation **[Glutaric
Acidemia]**
4841 Hill Street
La Canada, CA 91011
Toll-Free: 800-38-NUCDF
Website: http://www.nucdf.org
E-mail: info@nucdf.org

Association for **Glycogen
Storage Disease**
P.O. Box 896
Durant, IA 52747
Phone: 563-785-6038
Website: http://www.agsdus.org

American **Heart** Association
7272 Greenville Avenue
Dallas, TX 75231
Toll-Free: 800-242-8721
Phone: 214-373-6300
Website: http://
www.americanheart.org
E-mail: inquire@amhrt.org

American **Hemochromatosis**
Society Inc.
4044 West Lake Mary Boulevard
Unit #104, PMB 416
Lake Mary, FL 32746-2012
Toll-Free: 888-655-IRON (4766)
Phone: 407-829-4488
Fax: 407-333-1284
Website: http://
www.americanhs.org
E-mail: mail@americanhs.org

Iron Disorders Institute, Inc.
[Hemochromatosis]
P.O. Box 2031
Greenville, SC 29602
Toll-Free: 888-565-IRON (4766)
Phone: 864-292-1175
Fax: 864-292-1878
Website: http://
www.irondisorders.org
E-mail:
publications@irondisorders.org

National **Hemophilia**
Foundation
116 West 32nd Street, 11th Floor
New York, NY 10001
Toll-free: 800-42-HANDI
Phone: 212-328-3700
Fax: 212-328-3777
Website: http://www.hemophilia.org
E-mail: info@hemophilia.org

World Federation of
Hemophilia
1425 René Lévesque Blvd. West
Suite 1010
Montréal, Québec H3G 1T7
Canada
Phone: 514-875-7944
Fax: 514-875-8916
Website: http://www.wfh.org
E-mail: wfh@wfh.org

HHT Foundation International
**[Hereditary Hemorrhagic
Telangiectasia]**
P.O. Box 329
Monkton, MD 21111
Toll-Free: 800-448-6389
Phone: 410-357-9932
Fax: 410-357-9931
Website: http://www.hht.org
E-mail: hhtinfo@hht.org

Hermansky-Pudlak Syndrome Network Inc.
One South Road
Oyster Bay, NY 11771-1905
Toll-Free: 800-789-9HPS (9477)
Phone: 516-992-3440
Fax: 516-922-4022

Histiocytosis Association of America
72 East Holly Avenue
Suite 101
Pitman, NJ 08071
Phone: 856-589-6606
Fax: 856-589-6614
Website: http://www.histio.org
E-mail: association@histio.org

Hereditary Disease Foundation **[Huntington's Disease]**
1303 Pico Boulevard
Santa Monica, CA 90405
Phone: 310-450-9913
Fax: 310-450-9532
Website: http://www.hdfoundation.org
E-mail: cures@hdfoundation.org

Huntington's Disease Society of America
158 West 29th Street
7th Floor
New York, NY 10001-5300
Toll-Free: 800-345-HDSA (4372)
Phone: 212-242-1968
Fax: 212-239-3430
Website: http://www.hdsa.org
E-mail: hdsainfo@hdsa.org

National MPS Society **[Hurler's Syndrome]**
P.O. Box 736
Bangor, ME 04402-0736
Phone: 207-947-1445
Fax: 207-990-3074
Website: http://mpssociety.org
E-mail: info@mpssociety.org

Foundation for **Ichthyosis** and Related Skin Types, Inc.
1601 Valley Forge Road
Lansdale, PA 19446
Phone: 215-631-1411
Fax: 215-631-1413
Website: http://www.scalyskin.org
E-mail: info@scalyskin.org

Metabolic Information Network **[Inborn Errors of Metabolism]**
P.O. Box 670847
Dallas, TX 75367-0847
Toll-Free: 800-945-2188
Phone: 214-696-2188
Fax: 214-696-3258

Society for Inherited Metabolic Disorders **[Inborn Errors of Metabolism]**
Oregon Health Sciences University/L473
3181 Southwest Sam Jackson Park Road
Portland, OR 97201
Phone: 503-449-2795
Website: http://www.simd.org

International **Joseph Diseases** Foundation, Inc.
P.O. Box 994268
Redding, CA 96099
Phone: 510-246-4722
Website: http://www.ijdf.net
E-mail: mjd@ijdf.net

Joubert Syndrome Foundation
6931 South Carlinda Ave.
Columbia, MD 21046
Phone: 410-997-8084
Fax: 410-992-9184
Website: http://www.joubertsyndrome.org

Kennedy's Disease Association
P.O. Box 1105
Coarsegold, CA 93614-1105
Phone: 559-658-5950
Website: http://www.kennedysdisease.org
E-mail: info@kennedysdisease.org

Klinefelter Syndrome and Associates
P.O. Box 119
Roseville, CA 95678-0119
Toll-Free: 888-XXY-WHAT (888-999-9428)
Phone: 916-773-2999
Website: http://www.genetic.org/ks
E-mail: ksinfo@genetic.org

Klippel-Trenaunay Support Group
4610 Wooddale Avenue
Edina, MN 55424
Phone: 952-925-2596
Website: http://www.k-t.org

Krabbe's Family Network
P.O. Box 563
East Aurora, NY 14052
Website: http://www.krabbes.net

Hunter's Hope Foundation
[Leukodystrophy]
P.O. Box 643
Orchard Park, NY 14127
Toll-Free: 877-984-HOPE (4673)
Phone: 716-667-1200
Fax: 716-667-1212
Website: http://www.huntershope.org
E-mail: info@huntershope.org

Myelin Project
[Leukodystrophy]
2136 Gallows Road, Suite E
Dunn Loring, VA 22027
Toll-Free: 800-869-3546
Phone: 703-560-5400
Fax: 703-560-0706
Website: http://www.myelin.org
E-mail: mp@myelin.org

United **Leukodystrophy** Foundation
2304 Highland Drive
Sycamore, IL 60178
Toll-Free: 800-728-5483
Phone: 815-895-3211
Fax: 815-895-2432
Website: http://www.ulf.org
E-mail: ulf@tbcnet.com

National Tay-Sachs and Allied
Diseases Association [**Lipid
Storage Disorders**]
2001 Beacon Street, Suite 204
Brighton, MA 02135
Toll-Free: 800-90-NTSAD (906-
8723)
Phone: 617-277-4463
Fax: 617-277-0134
Website: http://www.ntsad.org
E-mail: info@ntsad.org

American **Liver** Foundation
75 Maiden Lane, Suite 603
New York, NY 10038-4810
Toll-Free: 800-465-4837
Phone: 212-668-1000
Fax: 212-483-8179
Website: http://
www.liverfoundation.org
E-mail: info@liverfoundation.org

Lowe's Syndrome Association,
Inc.
222 Lincoln Street
West Lafayette, IN 47906
Phone: 765-743-3634
Website: http://
www.lowesyndrome.org
E-mail: info@lowesyndrome.org

Maple Syrup Urine Disease
Family Support Group
24806 SR 119
Goshen, IN 46526
Phone: 574-862-2992
Fax: 574-862-2012
Website: http://www
.msud-support.org

National **Marfan** Foundation
22 Manhasset Avenue
Port Washington, NY 11050
Toll-Free: 800-862-7326
(8-MARFAN)
Phone: 516-883-8712
Fax: 516-883-8040
Website: http://www.marfan.org
E-mail: staff@marfan.org

American Association on
Mental Retardation
444 North Capitol Street, NW
Suite 846
Washington, DC 20001
Toll-Free: 800-424-3688
Phone: 202-387-1968
Fax: 202-387-2193
Website: http://www.aamr.org

The Arc [**Mental Retardation**]
1010 Wayne Ave., Suite 650
Silver Spring, MD 20910
Toll-Free: 800-433-5255
Phone: 301-565-3842
Fax: 301-565-5342
Website: http://thearc.org
E-mail: info@Thearc.org

Mental Retardation and
Developmental Disabilities
Branch
National Institute of Child
Health and Human
Development
Executive Building, Room 4B09G
6100 Executive Blvd., MSC 7510
Bethesda, MD 20892-7510
Phone: 301-496-1383
Website: http://
www.nichd.nih.gov/about/crmc/
mrdd/mrdd.htm

Muscular Dystrophy Association
[**Mitochondrial Disease**]
3300 E. Sunrise Drive
Tucson, AZ 85718
Toll-Free: 800-572-1717
Website: http://www.mdausa.org
E-mail: mda@mdausa.org

United **Mitochondrial Disease** Foundation
8085 Saltsburg Road
Suite 201
Pittsburgh, PA 15239
Phone: 412-793-8077
Fax: 412-793-6477
Website: http://www.umdf.org
E-mail: info@umdf.org

Mucolipidosis IV Foundation
719 East 17th Street
Brooklyn, NY 11230
Website: http://www.ml4.org
Phone: 718-434-5067
Fax: 718-859-7371
Website: http://www.ml4.org

National MPS Society, Inc.
[**Mucopolysaccharidoses**]
P.O. Box 736
Bangor, ME 04402-0736
Phone: 207-947-1445
Fax: 207-990-3074
Website: http://
www.mpssociety.org
E-mail: info@mpssociety.org

Myelin Project [**Multiple Sclerosis**]
2136 Gallows Road, Suite E
Dunn Loring, VA 22027
Toll-Free: 800-869-3546
Phone: 703-560-5400
Fax: 703-560-0706
Website: http://www.myelin.org
E-mail: mp@myelin.org

National **Multiple Sclerosis** Society
733 Third Avenue, 6th Floor
New York, NY 10017-3288
Toll-Free: 800-FIGHT-MS (344-4867)
Phone: 212-986-3240
Fax: 212-986-7981
Website: http://www.nmss.org
E-mail: nat@nmss.org

Duchenne **Muscular Dystrophy** Research Center
621 Charles Young Drive South
Life Science Building
University of California
Los Angeles, CA 90095
Phone: 310-206-8390
Fax: 310-825-8489
Website: http://
www.lifesci.ucla.edu/physci/DMD
E-mail: dmdrc@physci.ucla.edu

Muscular Dystrophy Association
3300 East Sunrise Drive
Tucson, AZ 85718-3208
Toll-Free: 800-572-1717
Phone: 520-529-2000
Fax: 520-529-5300
Website: http://www.mdausa.org
E-mail: mda@mdausa.org

Parent Project Duchenne's
Muscular Dystrophy
4785 Emerald Way
Middletown, OH 45044
Toll-Free: 800-714-5437
Phone: 513-424-0696
Fax: 513-425-9907
Website: http://
www.parentdmd.org

Myasthenia Gravis
Foundation
1821 University Avenue W
Suite S256
St. Paul, MN 55104
Toll-Free: 800-541-5454
Phone: 651-917-6256
Fax: 651-917-1835
Website: http://
www.myaasthenia.org
E-mail: mgfa@myasthenia.org

National **Neurofibromatosis**
Foundation
95 Pine St., 16th Floor
New York, NY 10005
Toll-Free: 800-323-7938
Phone: 212-344-6633
Fax: 212-747-0004
Website: http://www.nf.org
E-mail: nnff@nf.org

Neurofibromatosis, Inc.
8855 Annapolis Road
Suite 110
Lanham, MD 20706-2924
Toll-Free: 800-942-6825
Phone: 301-918-4600
Website: http://www.nfinc.org
E-mail: nfinfo@nfinc.org

Neuropathy Association
60 East 42nd Street, Suite 942
New York, NY 10165-0999
Toll-Free: 800-247-6968
Phone: 212-692-0662
Fax: 212-692-0668
Website: http://
www.neuropathy.org
E-mail: info@neuropathy.org

Jim Lambright **Niemann-Pick**
Foundation
22831 61st Ave. SE, Suite B
Woodinville, WA 98072-8674
Phone: 425-486-5303
Fax: 425-486-5373
Website: http://
www.lambrightfoundation.org
E-mail:
help@lambrightfoundation.org

National **Niemann-Pick**
Disease Foundation
P.O. Box 49
415 Madison Ave.
Ft. Atkinson, WI 53538
Toll-Free: 877-287-3672
Phone: 920-563-0930
Fax: 920-563-0931
Website: http://www.nnpdf.org
E-mail: nnpdf@idcnet.com

Ara Parseghian Medical
Research Foundation
[Niemann-Pick Type C]
3530 East Campo Abierto Rd.
Suite 105
Tucson, AZ 85718-3327
Phone: 520-577-5106
Fax: 520-577-5212
Website: http://www.parseghian.org
E-mail: victory@parseghian.org

Organic Acidemia Association
13210 35th Avenue North
Plymouth, MN 55441
Phone: 763-559-1797
Fax: 763-694-0017
Website: http://www.oaanews.org
E-mail: ooaanews@aol.com

Osteogenesis Imperfecta
Foundation, Inc.
804 Diamond Ave.
Suite 210
Gaithersburg, MD 20878
Toll-Free: 800-981-2663
Phone: 301-947-0083
Fax: 301-947-0456
Website: http://www.oif.org
E-mail: bonelink@oif.org

Oxalosis and Hyperoxaluria
Foundation
201 E. 19th Street, #12E
New York, NY 10003
Toll-Free: 800-OHF-8699
Phone: 212-777-0470
Fax: 212-777-0471
Website: http://www.ohf.org
E-mail: execdriector@ohf.org

Paget Foundation for **Paget's
Disease** of Bone
120 Wall Street
Suite 1602
New York, NY 10005-4001
Toll-Free: 800-23-PAGET
Phone: 212-509-5335
Fax: 212-509-8492
Website: http://www.paget.org
E-mail: PagetFdn@aol.com

Pallister-Killian Family
Support Group
3700 Wyndale Court
Fort Worth, TX 76109
Phone: 817-927-8854
Fax: 817-927-2073

National **Parkinson**
Foundation, Inc.
Bob Hope Parkinson Research
Center
1501 N.W. 9th Avenue
Bob Hope Road
Miami, FL 33136-1494
Toll-Free: 800-327-4545
Phone: 305-547-6666
Fax: 305-243-5595
Website: http://
www.parkinson.org
E-mail: contact@parkinson.org

Parkinson's Disease and
Movement Disorder Center
University of Kansas Medical
Center
Department of Neurology
3599 Rainbow Blvd.
Kansas City, KS 66160-7314
Phone: 913-588-6782
Fax: 913-588-6920
Website: http://www.kumc.edu/
parkinson

**Pelizaeus-Merzbacher
Disease** Foundation
333 Homestead Avenue
Haddonfield, NJ 08033
Phone: 856-795-1539
Website: http://
www.pmdfoundation.org

Children's PKU Network
[Phenylketonuria]
3790 Via de la Valle, Suite 120
Del Mar, CA 92014
Toll-Free: 800-377-6677
Phone: 858-509-0767
Fax: 858-509-0768
Website: http://
www.pkunetwork.org
E-mail: pkunetwork@aol.com

National PKU News
[Phenylketonuria]
6869 Woodlawn Ave. NE, #116
Seattle, WA 98115-5469
Phone: 206-525-8140
Fax: 206-525-5023
Website: http://pkunews.org

American Association of Kidney
Patients **[Polycystic Kidney
Disease]**
3505 E. Frontage Road, Suite 315
Tampa, FL 33607
Toll-Free: 800-749-2257
Phone: 813-636-8100
Fax: 813-636-8122
Website: http://www.aakp.org
E-mail: info@aakp.org

National Kidney and Urologic
Diseases Information
Clearinghouse **[Polycystic
Kidney Disease]**
3 Information Way
Bethesda, MD 20892-3580
Toll-Free: 800-891-5390
Phone: 301-654-4415
Fax: 301-907-8906
Website: http://www.niddk.nih.gov/
health/kidney/nkudic.htm
E-mail: nkudic@info.niddk.nih.gov

Polycystic Kidney Research
Foundation
9221 Ward Parkway
Suite 400
Kansas City, MO 64114-3367
Toll-Free: 800-PKD-CURE (753-
2873)
Phone: 816-931-2600
Fax: 816-931-8655
Website: http://www.pkdcure.org
E-mail:
pkdcure@pkrfoundation.org

Intestinal Multiple **Polyposis**
and Colorectal Cancer
P.O. Box 11
Conyngham, PA 18219
Phone: 570-788-1818
Fax: 570-788-4046
E-mail: impacc@epix.net

Acid Maltase Deficiency
Association **[Pompe Disease]**
P.O. Box 700248
San Antonio, TX 78270
Phone: 210-494-6144
Fax: 210-490-7161
Website: http://www.amda-
pompe.org

American **Porphyria**
Foundation
P.O. Box 22712
Houston, TX 77227
Phone: 713-266-9617
Website: http://
www.porphyriafoundation.com
E-mail: porphyrus@aol.com

Prader-Willi Syndrome
Association
5700 Midnight Pass Road
Sarasota, FL 34242
Toll-Free: 800-926-4797
Phone: 941-312-0400
Fax: 941-312-0142
Website: http://
www.pwsausa.org

Immune Deficiency Foundation
[Primary Immunodeficiency]
40 West Chesapeake Avenue
Suite 308
Towson, MD 21204
Toll-Free: 800-296-4433
Phone: 410-461-3127
Fax: 410-321-9165
Website: http://
www.primaryimmune.org
E-mail: idf@primaryimmune.org

Primary Immunodeficiency
Association
Alliance House
12 Caxton Street
London SW1H 0QS England
Phone: 011 44 20 7 976 7640
Fax: 011 44 20 7 976 7641
Website: http://www.pia.org.uk
E-mail: info@pia.org.uk

International **Progeria** Registry
Progeria Research Foundation
P.O. Box 3453
Peabody, MA 01961-3453
Phone: 978-535-2594
Fax: 978-535-5849
Website: http://
www.progeriaresearch.org
E-mail:
info@progeriaresearch.org

Hutchinson-Gilford **Progeria**
Syndrome Network
P.O. Box 650113
Sterling, VA 20165-0113
Website: http://www.laze.net/
progeria

National **Prune Belly**
Syndrome Network
P.O. Box 2125
Evansville, IN 47728-0125
Phone: 310-826-6865
Fax: 310-794-9962

National Organization for **Rare**
Disorders, Inc.
55 Kenosia Avenue
P.O. Box 1968
Danbury, CT 06813-1968
Toll-Free: 800-999-6673
Phone: 203-744-0100
Fax: 203-798-2291
TDD: 203-797-9590
Internet: http://
www.rarediseases.org
E-mail:
orphan@rarediseases.org

Retinitis Pigmentosa (RP)
International
P.O. Box 900
Woodland Hills, CA 91365
Toll-Free: 800-344-4877
Phone: 818-992-0500
Fax: 818-992-3265
Website: http://
rpinternatinal.org
E-mail: info@rpinternatinal.org

RP Foundation Fighting Blindness **[Retinitis Pigmentosa]**
11435 Cronhill Drive
Owings Mills, MD 21117-2220
Toll-Free: 800-683-5555
Phone: 410-225-9400
TDD: 410-225-9409
Fax: 410-255-3936
Website: http://www.blindness.org

International **Rett Syndrome** Association
9121 Piscataway Road
Clinton, MD 20735
Toll-Free: 800-818-RETT (8388)
Phone: 301-856-3334
Fax: 301-856-3336
Website: http://www.rettsyndrome.org
E-mail: irsa@rettsyndrome.org

Association for Children with **Russell-Silver Syndrome**
22 Hoyt Street
Madison, NJ 07940-1604
Phone: 201-377-4531
Fax: 201-822-2715

National Tay-Sachs and Allied Diseases Association **[Sandhoff Disease]**
2001 Beacon Street
Suite 204
Brighton, MA 02135
Toll-Free: 800-906-8723
Fax: 617-277-0134
Website: http://ntsad.org
E-mail: info@ntsad.org

Scleroderma Foundation
12 Kent Way
Suite 101
Byfield, MA 01922
Toll-Free: 800-722-4673
Phone: 978-463-5843
Fax: 978-463-5819
Website: http://www.scleroderma.org
E-mail: sfinfo@scleroderma.org

National **Scoliosis** Foundation
5 Cabot Place
Stoughton, MA 02072
Toll-Free: 800-673-6922
Phone: 781-341-6333
Website: http://www.scoliosis.org
E-mail: NSF@scoliosis.org

Shwachman-Diamond Syndrome Foundation
710 Brassie Drive
Grand Junction, CO 81506
Toll-Free: 877-SDS-INTL (737-4685)
Phone: 614-939-2324
Fax: 970-255-8293
Website: http://www.Shwachman-diamond.org
E-mail: 4sskids@Shwachman-diamond.org

American **Sickle Cell** Anemia Association
10300 Carnegie Avenue
Cleveland Clinic
Cleveland, OH 44106
Phone: 216-229-8600
Fax: 216-229-4500
Website: http://www.ascaa.org

Sickle Cell Disease Association of America, Inc.
200 Corporate Point
Suite 495
Culver City, CA 90230-7633
Toll-Free: 800-421-8453
Phone: 310-216-6363
Fax: 310-215-3722
Website: http://www.sicklecelldisease.org
E-mail: scdaa@sicklecelldisease.org

Sickle Cell Information Center
Emory University School of Medicine Department of Pediatrics
P.O. Box 109
Grady Memorial Hospital
80 Jessie Hill Jr. Drive SE
Atlanta, GA 30303
Phone: 404-616-3572
Fax: 404-616-5998
Website: http://scinfo.org

National **Sjögren's Syndrome** Association
3201 W. Evans Drive
Phoenix, AZ 85023
Toll-Free: 800-395-6772
Phone: 602-993-7227

Sjögren's Syndrome Foundation, Inc.
8120 Woodmont Avenue
Bethesda, MD 20814
Toll-Free: 800-475-6473
Fax: 301-718-0322
Website: http://www.sjogrens.org

Sotos Syndrome Support Association
23614 Airosa Place
Moreno Valley, CA 92387
Toll-Free: 888-246-7772
Website: http://www.well.com/user/sssa
E-mail: sssa@well.com

Spastic Paraplegia Foundation, Inc.
209 Park Road
Chelmsford, MA 01824
Phone: 703-495-9261
Website: http://sp-foundation.org
E-mail: info@sp-foundation.org

Spina Bifida Association of America
4590 MacArthur Boulevard
Suite 250
Washington, DC 20007-4226
Toll-Free: 800-621-3141
Phone: 202-944-6385
Website: http://www.sbaa.org
E-mail: sbaa@sbaa.org

Families of SMA **[Spinal Muscular Atrophy]**
National Headquarters
P.O. Box 196
Libertyville, Illinois 60048-0196
Toll-Free: 800-886-1762
Phone: 847-367-7620
Fax: 847-367-7623
Website: http://www.fsma.org
E-mail: info@fsma.org

Spondylitis Association of
America
P.O. Box 5872
Sherman Oaks, CA 91413
Toll-Free: 800-777- 8189
Website: http://
www.spondylitis.org
E-mail: info@spondylitis.org

Stickler [Syndrome] Involved
People
15 Angelina Drive
Augusta, KS 67010
Phone: 316-775-2993
Website: http://www.sticklers.org
E-mail: sip@sticklers.org

Stickler Syndrome Support
Group
P.O. Box 371
Walton-on-Thames
Surrey, KT12 2YS England
Phone: 011 44 1932 267635
Website: http://
www.stickler.org.uk
E-mail: info@stickler.org.uk

National **Tay-Sachs** and Allied
Diseases Association
2001 Beacon Street
Suite 204
Brighton, MA 02135
Toll-Free: 800-90-NTSAD (906-
8723)
Phone: 617-277-4463
Fax: 617-277-0134
Website: http://www.ntsad.org
E-mail: info@ntsad.org

Chromosome 18 Registry and
Research Society **[Tetrasomy
18p]**
6302 Fox Head
San Antonio, TX 78247
Phone: 210-657-4968
Website: http://
www.chromosome18.org
E-mail:
office@chromosome18.org

Cooley's Anemia Foundation,
Inc. **[Thalassemia]**
129-09 26th Avenue, #203
Flushing, NY 11354
Toll-Free: 800-522-7222
Phone: 718-321-2873
Fax: 718-321-3340
Website: http://
www.thalassemia.org

TAR Syndrome Association
**[Thrombocytopenia-Absent
Radius Syndrome]**
212 Sherwood Drive, RD 1
Linwood, NJ 08221-9745
Phone: 609-927-0418
E-mail: tarsa@aol.com

Tourette Syndrome
Association, Inc.
42-40 Bell Boulevard
Bayside, NY 11361-2820
Toll-Free: 800-237-0717
Phone: 718-224-2999
Fax: 718-279-9596
Website: http://www.tsa-usa.org
E-mail: ts@tsa-usa.org

Cleft Palate Foundation
[Treacher Collins Syndrome]
1504 East Franklin Street
Suite 102
Chapel Hill, NC 27514-2820
Toll-Free: 800-24-CLEFT (242-5338)
Phone: 919-933-9044
Fax: 919-933-9604
Website: http://www.cleftline.org
E-mail: info@cleftline.org

Treacher Collins Foundation
P.O. Box 683
Norwich, VT 05055-0683
Toll-Free: 800-823-2055
Phone: 802-649-3050
Website: http://
www.treachercollinsfnd.org

Tuberous Sclerosis Alliance
801 Roeder Road, Suite 750
Silver Spring, MD 20910
Toll-Free: 800-225-6872
Fax: 301-562-9870
Website: http://
www.tsalliance.org
E-mail: info@tsalliance.org

Turner Syndrome Society of
the United States
14450 T.C. Jester, Suite 260
Houston, TX 77014
Toll-Free: 800-365-9944
Phone: 832-249-9988
Fax: 832-249-9987
Website: http://www
.turner-syndrome-us.org
E-mail: tssus@
turner-syndrome-us.org

National Urea Cycle
Disorders Foundation
4841 Hill Street
La Canada, CA 91011
Toll-Free: 800-38-NUCDF
Website: http://www.nucdf.org
E-mail: info@nucdf.org

National Kidney and Urologic
Diseases Information
Clearinghouse
3 Information Way
Bethesda, MD 20892-3580
Toll-Free: 800-891-5390
Website: http://
kidney.niddk.nih.gov

National Vitiligo Foundation
700 Olympic Plaza Circle
Suite 404
Tyler, TX 75701
Phone: 903-534-2737
Fax: 903-534-1545
Website: http://www.nvfi.org
E-mail:
vitiligo@vitiligofoundation.org

Von Hippel-Lindau Family
Alliance
171 Clinton Road
Brookline, MA 02445
Toll-Free: 800-767-4VHL (4845)
Phone: 617-277-5667
Fax: 858-712-8712
Website: http://www.vhl.org
E-mail: info@vhl.org

National Hemophilia
Foundation **[Von Willebrand
Disease]**
116 West 32nd Street, 11th Floor
New York, NY 10001
Toll-Free: 800-42-HANDI
Phone: 212-328-3700
Fax: 212-328-3777
Website: http://
www.hemophilia.org
E-mail: HANDI@hemophilia.org

World Federation of Hemophilia
[Von Willebrand Disease]
1425 René Lévesque Boulevard
West, Suite 1010
Montréal, Québec H3G 1T7
Canada
Phone: 514-875-7944
Fax: 514-785-8916
Website: http:///www.wfh.org
E-mail: wfh@wfh.org

Williams Syndrome
Association
P.O. Box 297
Clawson, MI 48017-0297
Toll-Free: 800-806-1817
Phone: 248-244-2229
Fax: 248-244-2230
Website: http://www
.williams-syndrome.org
E-mail:
info@williams-syndrome.org

Williams Syndrome
Foundation
University of California
Irvine, CA 92697-2310
Phone: 949-824-7259
Website: http://www.wsf.org

National Center for the Study of
Wilson's Disease
432 West 58th Street, Suite 614
New York, NY 10019
Phone: 212-523-8717
Fax: 212-523-8708

Wilson's Disease Association
1802 Brookside Drive
Wooster, OH 44691
Toll-Free: 800-399-0266
Phone: 330-264-1450
Fax: 509-757-6418
Website: http://
www.wilsonsdisease.org
E-mail: wda@sssnet.com

Primary Immunodeficiency
Association **[Wiskott-Aldrich
Syndrome]**
Alliance House
12 Caxton Street
London SW1H 0QS England
Phone: 011 44 20 7 976 7640
Fax: 011 44 20 7 976 7641
Website: http://www.pia.org.uk
E-mail: info@pia.org.uk

4P- Support Group **[Wolf-
Hirschhorn Syndrome]**
1123 16th Avenue, 351
Longview, WA 98632
Website: www.4p-supportgroup.org

Xeroderma Pigmentosum
Society
437 Snydertown Road
Craryville, NY 12521
Toll-Free: 877-977-2873
Phone: 518-851-2612
Website: http://www.xps.org
E-mail: xps@xps.org

Index

Index

Page numbers followed by 'n' indicate a footnote. Page numbers in *italics* indicate a table or illustration.

A

ABCD symptoms (skin cancer), described 412
acetaldehyde 487
acetyl-CoA alpha-glucosaminide acetyltransferase 221
achondroplasia
 information resources 683–84
 prenatal testing 519
Acid Maltase Deficiency Association, contact information 704
acid sphingomyelinase (ASM) 226–27, 230
Acoustic Neuroma Foundation, contact information 684
acquired mutations, described 38–39
acute myelogenous leukemia (AML) 92
ADA *see* Americans with Disabilities Act
A.D.A.M., Inc., publications
 Edwards syndrome 339n
 Fanconi anemia 92n
 Patau syndrome 369n

A.D.A.M., Inc., publications, continued
 trisomy 13 369n
 trisomy 18 339n
Adams, Kenneth 466
Adderall (dexamethamphetamine) *355*
addictions, genetic factors 486–98
additive genetic effects, defined 635
ADEAR *see* Alzheimer's Disease Education and Referral Center
adenine (A)
 defined 635
 described 4, *5*, 595
 human genome *16*, 16–17
adenoma sebaceum 292
adenosine triphosphate (ATP), organelle DNA 17
ADHD *see* attention deficit hyperactivity disorder
adolescents
 Angelman syndrome 309
 chronic conditions 538
 fragile X syndrome 352, 356
 hemochromatosis 97
 Klinefelter syndrome 361–62, 363–64
 Turner syndrome 380
adrenoleukodystrophy (ALD) 190–92
Adult Metabolic Transition Project, Web site address 696

713

adults
  adrenoleukodystrophy 191
  Gaucher disease 211–12
  Klinefelter syndrome 362, 366–67
  myotonic muscular dystrophy 267–68
  neuronal ceroid lipofuscinoses 201
  spinal muscular atrophy 275
  urea cycle disorders 185
adverse drug reactions (ADR) 623
affected relative pair, defined 635
afibrinogenemia 85–86
African Americans
  Brown oculocutaneous albinism 64
  oculocutaneous albinism 61
  sickle cell disease 104
agalsidase beta 207
age factor
  Angelman syndrome 303
  Huntington disease 161–62
  mitochondrial myopathies 257
  pregnancy 301–2
  prostate cancer 414
  Refsum disease 196
  Rett syndrome 285
  special education services 550–51
Aicardi Syndrome Newsletter, Inc., contact information 684
Alabama, newborn screening programs 655, *664*, *666*
Alaska, newborn screening programs 656, *664*, *666*
albinism
  alleles 34
  overview 57–66
Albright, Fuller 359
Alcohol Alert (NIAAA) 486n
alcohol dehydrogenase 487
alcoholism, genetic factors 486–92
ALD *see* adrenoleukodystrophy
aldehyde dehydrogenase 487
Aldurazyme (laronidase) 225
Alexander disease 192
alleles
  defined 635
  described 6
  genetic variation 29, 31–34
  nicotine addiction 496–97

allergies
  diesel fumes 466–68
  genetic factors 464–66
allogeneic, defined 635
alpha-1 antitrypsin deficiency, overview 67–76
Alpha-1 Association, contact information 685
alpha-1 emphysema 69
alpha-galactosidase A 206, 207
alpha-L-iduronidase 218
alpha-N-acetylglucosaminidase 221
Alport syndrome *157*
ALS *see* amyotrophic lateral sclerosis
alternative splicing, described 25
Alzheimer's Association, contact information 685
Alzheimer's disease
  genetic basis *615*
  genetic factors 471–76
Alzheimer's Disease Education and Referral Center (ADEAR)
  contact information 475, 685
  genetics publication 471n
"Alzheimer's Disease Genetics Fact Sheet" (ADEAR) 471n
amantadine *355*
ambiguous genitals 421–22
American Association of Kidney Patients, contact information 704
American Association on Mental Retardation, contact information 700
American Behçet's Disease, contact information 687
American Cancer Society, contact information 688
American Celiac Society, contact information 688
American Council of the Blind, contact information 687
American Diabetes Association, contact information 692
American Digestive Health Foundation, contact information 693
American Foundation for the Blind, contact information 687
American Heart Association
  contact information 697
  Web site address 455

American Hemochromatosis Society, Inc., contact information 697
American Juvenile Arthritis Organization, contact information 686
American Liver Foundation, contact information 296, 696, 700
American Porphyria Foundation, contact information 704
American Sickle Cell Anemia Association, contact information 706
American Society for Deaf Children, contact information 691
American Society of Human Genetics, contact information 677
Americans with Disabilities Act (ADA) 559–60
amino acids
  defined 635
  described 9
  isoleucine 175–76
  leucine 175–76
  phenylalanine 20
  proteins 11
  serine 20
  translation chart *21*
  tyrosinemia 183
  valine 175–76
AML *see* acute myelogenous leukemia
ammonia, urea cycle disorders 184–87
amniocentesis
  albinism 65
  Down syndrome 333
  Klinefelter syndrome 361
  prenatal tests 524
  Tay-Sachs disease 240–41
  thalassemia 109
amyotrophic lateral sclerosis (ALS), research 603, 606
Amyotrophic Lateral Sclerosis Association, contact information 685
androgen insensitivity syndrome 422
androgen therapy, Fanconi anemia 95
anemia 152
  see also Cooley's anemia; Fanconi anemia; sickle cell disease
aneuploidy, described 43–44
Angelman, Harry 303
Angelman syndrome 303–9

Angelman Syndrome Foundation
  Angelman syndrome publication 303n
  contact information 685
Angelman Syndrome Information for Families and Professionals, Web site address 685
angiomyolipomas 291
anomalous trichromacy, described 113
anosmia, Refsum disease 196
anterior horn cells 273
antibodies, described *10*
anticipation, defined 636
anticoagulant medications, afibrinogenemia 86
antisense, defined 636
aortic stenosis (AS) 440–41
aplastic anemia, Fanconi anemia 92
apoptosis, described 14
Ara Parseghian Medical Research Foundation, contact information 702
Arbuckle, Margaret 495
The Arc, contact information 700
arginase 186
argininosuccinase acid lyase 186
argininosuccinic acid synthetase 186
argininosuccinic aciduria 186
Arizona, newborn screening programs 656, *664*, *666*
Arkansas, newborn screening programs 656, *664*, *666*
arylsulfatase A 194
AS *see* aortic stenosis
ASD *see* atrial septal defect
ASM *see* acid sphingomyelinase
aspartame 179
Association for Children with Russell-Silver Syndrome, contact information 706
Association for Glycogen Storage Disease, contact information 697
Association of Birth Defect Children, Inc., contact information 677
Association of University Centers on Disabilities, contact information 693

715

asthma
  alpha-1 antitrypsin deficiency 70
  genetic factors 464–66
Asthma and Allergy Foundation of
  America, contact information 684
Asthmabusters, Web site address 547
ataxia, neuronal ceroid lipofuscinoses
  201
ATGC (adenine, thymine, guanine,
  cytosine) 636
  see also adenine; cytosine; guanine;
    thymine
ATP *see* adenosine triphosphate
atrial septal defect (ASD) 442–43
atrioventricular canal defect 443–44
atrioventricular septal defect 443–44
attention deficit hyperactivity disorder (ADHD) 480, *615*
audiologists, hereditary deafness 156
Autism Society of America, contact
  information 686
autism spectrum disorders, Rett syndrome 285
autoradiography, defined 636
autosomal dominant disorders
  Charcot-Marie-Tooth disease 252
  congenital spondyloepiphyseal dys-
    plasia 153
  defined 636
  depicted *453*
  described *42*, 48
  multiple epiphyseal dysplasia 152
  polycystic kidney disease 419
  pseudoachondroplastic dysplasia
    152–53
  Schwartz-Jampel syndrome 153
  statistics 41
autosomal recessive disorders
  afibrinogenemia 86
  Bloom syndrome 147
  described *42*, 48
  diastrophic dysplasia 149
  Dyggve-Melchior-Clausen syndrome
    149
  Ellis-van Creveld syndrome 149
  Fanconi anemia 92
  Gaucher disease 210
  McKusick type metaphyseal chon-
    drodysplasia 152

autosomal recessive disorders, continued
  mucopolysaccharidoses 216
  multiple epiphyseal dysplasia 152
  Niemann-Pick disease 230
  polycystic kidney disease 420
  spinal muscular dystrophy 281
  statistics 41
  tyrosinemia 182
  urea cycle disorders 186
autosomes
  defined 636
  depicted *8*
  described 7–8, 300, 320
avuncular relationship, defined 636

B

Bacon, Bruce R. 96n
balloon angioplasty 441
balloon valvuloplasty 440
Barth syndrome 250–51
Barth Syndrome Foundation, contact
  information 686
Billy Barty Foundation, Inc., contact
  information 683
basal cell carcinoma 411–12
base, defined 636
base pairs
  defined 636
  depicted *5*
base sequence, defined 636
"The Basics: Genes and How They
  Work" (NLM) 3n
Batten disease 200–205
"Batten Disease Fact Sheet" (NINDS)
  200n
Batten Disease Support and Research
  Association, contact information
  686
Beaulieu, Jean-Martin 495
Becker, Peter Emil 261
Becker muscular dystrophy 262
Beckwith-Wiedemann Support Network, contact information 687
behavioral genetics
  defined 636
  overview 613–21

Alexander Graham Bell Association for the Deaf, Inc., contact information 691
beta-galactosidase 222
beta-glucuronidase 223
Better Hearing Institute, contact information 691
"Beyond Genes: Scientists Venture Deeper into the Human Genome" (NHGRI) 583n
bicuspid aortic valve 441–42
bioinformatics, defined 636
biotin, described 172
biotinidase deficiency, overview 172–73
biphasic positive airway pressure 279
bipolar disorder 478–79
birth defects
    defined 637
    newborn screening 531–33
    prenatal screening 517–29
bladder exstrophy 420–21
bleeding disorders *see* afibrinogenemia; hemophilia; von Willebrand disease
blood disorders *see* Fanconi anemia; hemochromatosis; sickle cell disease; thalassemia
blood types, described 35
Bloom syndrome 147
BMAP *see* Brain Molecular Anatomy Project
Boerwinkle, Eric 459–62
Bogardus, Clifton 429–30
bone crises 211, 214
bone dysplasia, Schwartz-Jampel syndrome 153
bone marrow failure, Fanconi anemia 92
bone marrow transplantation
    Fanconi anemia 94–95
    Krabbe disease 194
    metachromatic leukodystrophy 195
    mucopolysaccharidoses 223
    Niemann-Pick disease 233
    thalassemia 108
    urea cycle disorders 187
Boujaoude, Lina 535n
Bourneville's disease *see* tuberous sclerosis complex

Boyse, Kyla 535n
brachycephaly
    Hallermann-Streiff syndrome 150
    Weill-Marchesani syndrome 154
brachydactyly
    diastrophic dysplasia 148
    pseudoachondroplastic dysplasia 152
    Weill-Marchesani syndrome 154
Brain and Tissue Bank for Developmental Disorders 205
Brain Molecular Anatomy Project (BMAP) 482
Branchio-oto-renal syndrome *157*
Brave Kids, Web site address 547
breast cancer, heredity 407–9
breathing ventilators 279
brittle bone disease *see* osteogenesis imperfecta
bronchitis, alpha-1 antitrypsin deficiency 70
bronchospasms, alpha-1 antitrypsin deficiency 70
Brown, W. Ted 608
Brown oculocutaneous albinism 64
bubble baby syndrome 629
Buphenyl (sodium phenylbutyrate) 186

C

café au lait spots 292
CAG repeats, Huntington disease 160, 162–63, *163*
CAH *see* congenital adrenal hyperplasia
California, newborn screening programs 657, *664*, *666*
Canadian Genetic Diseases Network, contact information 677
Canavan disease 193–94
Canavan Disease Research, contact information 687
Canavan Foundation, contact information 688
Canavan Research Foundation, contact information 688

cancer
    apoptosis 14
    Bloom syndrome 147
    Fanconi anemia 92, 96
    Gaucher disease 211
    genetics 396–416
    urea cycle disorders 187
candidate gene, defined 637
Candlelighters Childhood Cancer
    Foundation, contact information 688
carbamazepine *355*
carbamyl phosphate synthetase 186
cardiac rhabdomyomas 291
cardiomyopathies, described 450
carnitine 250, 258
Caron, Marc G. 493–95
carriers
    alleles 33
    alpha-1 antitrypsin deficiency 68
    cystic fibrosis 130
    defined 637
    DiGeorge syndrome 322–23
    Gaucher disease 210–11, 212
    hemophilia 78–79, 83–84
    inheritance 51
    mucopolysaccharidoses 216–17
    neuronal ceroid lipofuscinoses 201
    Niemann-Pick disease 230
    Pelizaeus-Merzbacher disease 195
    phenylketonuria 178
    spinal muscular atrophy 273
    spinal muscular dystrophy 281–82
    Tay-Sachs disease 237–38
    urea cycle disorders 186
Catapres TTS (clonidine) *355*
CDC *see* Centers for Disease Control
    and Prevention
Celexa (citalopram) *355*
Celiac Disease Foundation, contact
    information 688
Celiac Sprue Association/USA, Inc.,
    contact information 689
cell death *see* apoptosis
cell differentiation, translation 28
cell division
    chromosomes 7
    depicted *13*
    described 12
    see also meiosis; mitosis

cells
    defined 637
    described 3–4, 299
    proteins 39
Center for Human and Molecular
    Genetics, contact information 677
Center for Jewish Genetic Diseases,
    contact information 678
Center for the Study and Treatment
    of Jewish Genetic Diseases, contact
    information 678
Centers for Disease Control and Pre-
    vention (CDC), publications
    gene-environment interaction 393n
    newborn screening 177n
centimorgan (cM), defined 637
central dogma, described 11
central nervous system
    Alexander disease 192
    Angelman syndrome 308
    Krabbe disease 194
    neurofibromatosis type 1 244
    Pelizaeus-Merzbacher disease 195
    Sandhoff disease 234
    tuberous sclerosis complex 289
centromeres
    chromosomes *24*
    defined 637
    depicted *7*
    described 9, 299, 311, 320
    sequences 23
ceroid 64
CF *see* cystic fibrosis
CG-rich area, defined 640
Charcot, Jean-Martin 251
Charcot-Marie-Tooth Association,
    contact information 689
Charcot-Marie-Tooth disease 251–57,
    603–6
"Charcot-Marie-Tooth Disease Fact
    Sheet" (NINDS) 251
Chediak-Higashi syndrome (CHS)
    64–65
chemical reactions, enzymes *10*
Arnold Chiari Family Network, con-
    tact information 686
children
    adrenoleukodystrophy 191
    Alexander disease 192

children, continued
Angelman syndrome 303
Canavan disease 193–94
chronic conditions 535–48
cystic fibrosis 129–33
DiGeorge syndrome 319–23
Down syndrome 329–37
Duchenne muscular dystrophy 261–62
electromyography 276
fragile X syndrome 343–58
galactosemia 173–74
hemochromatosis 97
Hurler-Scheie syndrome 219
Hurler syndrome 219
Klinefelter syndrome 362
Krabbe disease 194
Maroteaux-Lamy syndrome 222
metachromatic leukodystrophy 194–95
myotonic muscular dystrophy 266–67
neurofibromatosis type 1 244
neuronal ceroid lipofuscinoses 200–201
Niemann-Pick disease 227
phenylketonuria 177–78
Refsum disease 196
Sanfilippo syndrome 221
Scheie syndrome 219
sickle cell disease 102–3
Sly syndrome 223
spinal muscular atrophy 274–75
Tay-Sachs disease 236–37
thalassemia 108
tyrosinemia 182–83
urea cycle disorders 184–85
Williams syndrome 387–90
Children's Brain Disease Foundation, contact information 686
Children's Craniofacial Association, contact information 690
Children's Medical Center, contact information 678
Children's PKU Network, contact information 704
"Children with Chronic Conditions" (Laundy; Boujaoude) 535n
chloroplast, described 17
chorea 159–60

chorionic villus sampling (CVS)
Down syndrome 333
Klinefelter syndrome 361
prenatal tests 522–23
Tay-Sachs disease 240–41
thalassemia 109
Christmas, Stephen 83
Christmas disease *see* hemophilia B
chromosomal deletion, defined 637
chromosomal disorders 43–44, 520
chromosomal inversion, defined 637
Chromosome 18 Registry and Research Society, contact information 708
chromosome 22q11 deletions 320–23
chromosome abnormalities
described 300–302
Down syndrome 329
"Chromosome Abnormalities Fact Sheet" (NHGRI) 299n
Chromosome Deletion Outreach, contact information 689
chromosome region p
defined 637
depicted 7
described 9
chromosome region q
defined 637
depicted 7
described 9
chromosomes
alcoholism 489–90
Alzheimer's disease 472
Angelman syndrome 304
Charcot-Marie-Tooth disease 603–5
cystic fibrosis 130
defined 637
depicted 24
described 6–8, 47–48, 299–300
Huntington disease 160
inheritance 31–32
neurofibromatoses 247
Parkinson disease 469–70
Prader-Willi syndrome 374
chronic conditions, coping strategies 535–48
Chronic Granulomatous Disease Association, Inc., contact information 689

chronic obstructive pulmonary disease (COPD), alpha-1 antitrypsin deficiency 70
CHS *see* Chediak-Higashi syndrome
Cincinnati Children's Hospital Medical Center
allergies publication 464n
contact information 678
cirrhosis
described 69, 73
galactosemia 173–74
cis-acting, described 26
citalopram *355*
citrullinemia 186
Civil Rights Act 561
CK *see* creatine kinase
classic tyrosinase-negative oculocutaneous albinism (OCA1A) 62
cleft palate
diastrophic dysplasia 149
Kniest syndrome 151
Patau syndrome 370
Cleft Palate Foundation, contact information 690, 709
"Clinical Features of Turner Syndrome" (NICHD) 379n
"Clinical Info: Early Intervention and Down Syndrome" (Dmitriev) 333n
clonazepam 165
clone, defined 637
clonidine *355*
cloning
defined 637–38
positional, defined 648
clotting process
afibrinogenemia 85–86
hemophilia 78, 80–81
von Willebrand disease 87
clubfeet, diastrophic dysplasia 148
cM *see* centimorgan
CMD *see* congenital muscular dystrophy
CMT International, contact information 689
coarctation of the aorta 441
cocaine 494
Cockayne syndrome 147–48
codominance, defined 638

codons
defined 638
described 11, 20, *21*
human genome 24–25
translation 22
coenzyme Q 258
Coffin-Lowry Syndrome, contact information 690
collagen
Ehlers-Danlos syndrome 117, 120
osteogenesis imperfecta 117
Collins, Francis S. 431, 583–84, 600, 603, 607–10
colon cancer, heredity 409–11
Colorado, newborn screening programs 657, *664, 666*
color blindness *see* color vision defects
"Color Blindness" (University of Illinois) 111n
color vision defects 111–13
complementary sequence, defined 638
complex trait, defined 638
Concerta (methylphenidate) *355*
congenital, defined 638
congenital adrenal hyperplasia (CAH) 421–22, 532–33
congenital cardiovascular defects 439–49
congenital heart disease 457
Congenital Lactic Acidosis Support Group, contact information 696
congenital muscular dystrophy (CMD) 269–70
congenital myotonic muscular dystrophy 269
congenital spondyloepiphyseal dysplasia 153–54
Connecticut, newborn screening programs 657, *664, 666*
connective tissue disorders, described 116–28
see also Ehlers-Danlos syndrome; Marfan syndrome
conotruncal anomaly face syndrome 320
Conquer Fragile X Foundation, contact information 695
Conquering Diabetes: Highlights of Program Efforts, Research Advances and Opportunities (NIDDK) 425n

contraction stress test, prenatal tests 527

Cooke, David A. 513n

Cooley's anemia, described 108

Cooley's Anemia Foundation, Inc., contact information 708

copper absorption 295–96

Cordero, José 182

Cornelia de Lange Syndrome Foundation, contact information 690

coronary artery spasm 457

Council for Responsible Genetics, contact information 678

coxa vara, congenital spondyloepiphyseal dysplasia 153

CPK *see* creatine phosphokinase

CPS *see* urea cycle disorders

Craniofacial Foundation of America, contact information 690

craniosynostosis, defined 638

creatine kinase (CK) 271

creatine phosphokinase (CPK) 275

Cri Du Chat Support Group of Australia, Inc.
contact information 691
cri du chat syndrome publication 311n

cri du chat syndrome 311–18

crossing over, defined 638

Crouzon Support Network, contact information 691

cryoprecipitate 80–81, 89

cryptorchidism
Edwards syndrome 339
Patau syndrome 370

CVS *see* chorionic villus sampling

Cyr, Michel 495

cystic fibrosis (CF)
CFTR gene 39
overview 129–33
prenatal testing 519

Cystic Fibrosis Foundation, contact information 547, 691

Cystinosis Foundation, Inc., contact information 691

cytogenetics, defined 638

cytoplasm
defined 3
described 3, 11

cytoplasmic trait, defined 638

cytosine (C)
defined 638
described 4, *5*, 595
human genome *16*, 16–17

D

Darwin, Charles 30

DCM *see* dilated cardiomyopathy

DDAVP *see* desmopressin acetate

Deafness Research Foundation, contact information 692

Dejerine-Sottas disease 253

Delaware, newborn screening programs 658, *664*, *666*

deletions
Angelman syndrome 304
cri du chat syndrome 312
defined 638
described 40, 300
DiGeorge syndrome 319

dementia
Batten disease 203
metachromatic leukodystrophy 195
mitochondrial myopathies 257

dental defects
Hallermann-Streiff syndrome 150
McKusick type metaphyseal chondrodysplasia 152
Williams syndrome 388

deoxyribonucleic acid (DNA)
chromosomes 6
defined 639
described 4–5, 10–11
gene mutations 39–40
human genome 16–17, 616
mitochondria 53
mitochondrial, defined 646
Tay-Sachs disease 239

deoxyribose
defined 639
described 16

Depakote (valproic acid) *355*

depression
Huntington disease 165
Klinefelter syndrome 364

desmopressin acetate (DDAVP) 80–
  81, 89
deuteranomaly 113
deuteranopia 112
dexamethamphetamine *355*
Dexedrine (dexamethamphetamine)
  355
DHA *see* docosahexanoic acid
diabetes mellitus
  genetic factors 425–32
  myotonic muscular dystrophy 268
  Turner syndrome 382
"Diagnosing Williams Syndrome"
  (Williams Syndrome Association)
  387n
diastrophic dysplasia 148–49
Diaz-Sanchez, David 467
dichromacy, described 112–13
"Dictionary of Genetic Terms" (Oak
  Ridge National Laboratory) 635n
diet and nutrition
  familial disorders 37
  maple sugar urine disease 176
  mucopolysaccharidoses 223
  phenylketonuria 179
  Prader-Willi syndrome 375
  Refsum disease 196–97
  spinal muscular dystrophy 280
DiGeorge, Angelo 319
DiGeorge syndrome 319–23
dilated cardiomyopathy (DCM) 450–
  55
diploid
  defined 639
  described 31
disability categories, described 551–
  54
distal muscular dystrophy 270
distal myopathy 270
distal spinal muscular atrophy
  (dSMA) 605
District of Columbia (Washington,
  DC), newborn screening programs
  658, *664, 666*
divalproex *355*
Dmitriev, Valentine 332n, 337
DNA chain, described 16–17
"DNA Chip Technology" (NHGRI) 587n
DNA microarray technology 592–93

"DNA Microarray Technology"
  (NHGRI) 587n
DNA microchip technology 590–92
DNA polymerase, defined 648
DNA repair genes, defined 639
DNA replication, defined 639
DNA sequence, defined 639
docosahexanoic acid (DHA) 191
domain, defined 639
dominance, law 31
dominant, defined 639
dominant disorders
  hypochondroplasia 151
  prenatal testing 518–19
dominant inheritance, depicted *453*
dopamine 488
double helix
  defined 639
  depicted *5*
  described 17
Down syndrome
  diagnosis 331
  early intervention 333–37
  health issues 332–33
  overview 326–30
"Down Syndrome" (NICHCY) 326n
"Down Syndrome Facts" (National
  Down Syndrome Society) 332n
D-penicillamine 296
"Drug Addiction, Learning Share
  Common Brain Protein" (Duke University Medical Center) 493n
dSMA *see* distal spinal muscular atrophy
Duchenne, Guillaume Benjamin
  Amand 261
Duchenne muscular dystrophy 261–
  62
Duchenne Muscular Dystrophy Research Center, contact information
  701
Duke University Medical Center,
  drug addiction publication 493n
duplications
  cri du chat syndrome 312
  described 40, 300
dwarfism, overview 147–54
Dyggve-Melchior-Clausen syndrome
  149

Dysautonomia Foundation, Inc., contact information 694
dysfibrinogenemia 85–86
dyslexia, genetic basis *615*
dysplasia, dwarfism 148–49, 151, 152–54
dysthymia 478–79
dystonia, Huntington disease 165
Dystrophic Epidermolysis Bullosa Research Association of America, Inc., contact information 694

E

Easter Seals *see* National Easter Seal Society
EB *see* epidermolysis bullosa
Ebstein's anomaly 442
ectopia lentis, Weill-Marchesani syndrome 154
EDS *see* Ehlers-Danlos syndrome
education
Down syndrome 327–28
fragile X syndrome 352–53
genetic testing 515
special education services 549–56
Turner syndrome 382–83
Edwards syndrome 339–41
Effexor (venlafaxine) *355*
Ehlers-Danlos National Foundation, contact information 694
Ehlers-Danlos syndrome (EDS)
described 116–17
overview 120–21
Eisenmenger's complex 443
electrophoresis, defined 639
Ellis-van Creveld syndrome 149
embolism 457
embryonic development, translation 28
embryonic stem (EX) cells, defined 640
Emory Genetics Laboratory, contact information 678
emotional concerns
fragile X syndrome 349–50
Huntington disease 165
Marfan syndrome 127

emphysema, alpha-1 antitrypsin deficiency 68–71
endocardial cushion defect 443–44
endocrinologists
Klinefelter syndrome 364
triple X syndrome 378
endoplasmic reticulum
defined 3
described 3
environmental factors
chromosome abnormalities 302
familial disorders 37
hearing loss 158
nicotine addiction 496
prostate cancer 414
enzymes
defined 640
described *10*
Fabry disease 206
glycogen storage disease 136
neuronal ceroid lipofuscinoses 202
neutrophil elastase 67
Niemann-Pick disease 226
Sandhoff disease 234
Tay-Sachs disease 236–37
epicanthal folds
cri du chat syndrome 314
triple X syndrome 377
epidermolysis bullosa (EB), described 117
Epilepsy Foundation of America, contact information 695
epiloia *see* tuberous sclerosis complex
epispadias 420–21
epistasis
defined 640
described 34
epithelial cells, cystic fibrosis 129–30, 131
Eriksson, Maria 609–10
erythema, sun exposure 62
erythropoietin, Fanconi anemia 94
esterification 231
ethical issues
gene therapy 631–32
genetic testing 516
Human Genome Project 580–81

ethnic factors
  Canavan disease 193–94
  cystic fibrosis 130
  genetic conditions 44
  hemochromatosis 97
  Niemann-Pick disease 228, *231*
  oculopharyngeal muscular dystro-
    phy 271
  phenylketonuria 177
  sickle cell disease 104
  Tay-Sachs disease 238
eukaryotes
  defined 640
  described 21
  transcription 22
"Evaluating Gene Tests: Some Considerations" (Oak Ridge National
  Laboratory) 513n
"Evidence Builds That Genes Influence
  Cigarette Smoking" (Zickler) 495n
evolution, recombination 21
exercise
  Huntington disease 166
  muscular dystrophy 263
exons
  defined 640
  described 21
"Extending the Successful Prevention
  of Mental Retardation through
  Newborn Screening" (CDC) 177n
"Extraordinary Research Opportunities: The Genetics of Diabetes"
  (NIDDK) 425n
eye color, somatic mosaicism 35
eye disorders
  albinism 58, 59–61
  Angelman syndrome 308
  Batten disease 202
  color vision defects 111–13
  congenital spondyloepiphyseal dys-
    plasia 154
  Hallermann-Streiff syndrome 150
  Hurler syndrome 219
  Marfan syndrome 123, 126
  mucolipidoses 215
  mucopolysaccharidoses 218
  myotonic muscular dystrophy 268
  neuronal ceroid lipofuscinoses 200–
    201

eye disorders, continued
  Patau syndrome 369–70
  tuberous sclerosis 291
  Weill-Marchesani syndrome 154
  Wilson disease 295

F

Fabrazyme (agalsidase beta) 207
Fabry disease 206–9
"Fabry Disease" (NLM) 206n
Fabry Support Information Group,
  contact information 695
FACES: The National Craniofacial
  Association, contact information
  690
facial angiofibromas 292
facioscapulohumeral muscular dys-
  trophy (FSHD) 263–66
factor VIII concentrate 80–81, 89
factor VIII deficiency *see* hemophilia A
factor IX deficiency *see* hemophilia A
"Facts About Albinism" (King, et al.)
  57n
*Facts about Angelman Syndrome: In-
  formation for Families* (Angelman
  Syndrome Foundation) 303n
"Facts about Duchenne and Becker
  Muscular Dystrophies (DMD and
  BMD)" (MDA) 258n
"Facts About Facioscapulohumeral
  Muscular Dystrophy" (MDA) 258n
"Facts About Genetic Disorders"
  (MDA) 47n
"Facts about Limb-Girdle Muscular
  Dystrophy (LGMD)" (MDA) 258n
"Facts about Myotonic Muscular Dys-
  trophy" (MDA) 258n
"Facts about Rare Muscular Dystro-
  phies: Congenital, Distal, Emery-
  Dreifuss and Oculopharyngeal Mus-
  cular Dystrophies" (MDA) 258n
familial adenomatous polyposis (FAP)
  410
familial dilated cardiomyopathy 450–
  55
"Familial Dilated Cardiomyopathy"
  (Ku, et al.) 450n

"Families and Fragile X Syndrome" (NICHD) 343n
Families of SMA
  contact information 283, 707
  spinal muscular atrophy publication 273n
family issues
  chronic conditions 535–48
  genetic disorders 37–45
  hereditary cancer 396–406
Family Village: A Global Community of Disability-Related Resources, contact information 693
Fanconi anemia, overview 92–96
Fanconi Anemia Research Fund, Inc. contact information 695
Fanconi anemia publication 92n
"Fanconi's Anemia" (A.D.A.M., Inc.) 92n
FAP *see* familial adenomatous polyposis
Fauci, Anthony S. 466
FDA *see* US Food and Drug Administration
"FDA Approves First Treatment for Genetic Metabolic Disorder Including Hurler Dystrophy" (FDA) 216n
Federation for Children with Special Needs, contact information 693
Feiger, Jennie 450n
Feingold, Elise A. 584
fertility, Klinefelter syndrome 366
fertilization, translation 28
fetal tissue implant techniques, hemophilia 81, 85
fibrillin-1 117
fibrinogen 85–86
filipin 232
financial considerations
  Down syndrome 336–37
  future planning 571–76
  genetic testing 509–10
fingerprinting, defined 640
Fischbeck, Kenneth 604, 606
FISH *see* fluorescence in situ hybridization
5P- Society, contact information 691
Florida, newborn screening programs 658, *664*, *666*

fluorescence in situ hybridization (FISH)
  Angelman syndrome 304
  described 588–89
  DiGeorge syndrome 320–21
  Williams syndrome 390
"Fluorescence in Situ Hybridization (FISH)" (NHGRI) 587n
fluoxetine 165, *355*
fluvoxamine *355*
FMRP *see* fragile X mental retardation
folic acid *355*
Food and Drug Administration (FDA) *see* US Food and Drug Administration
forehead plaques 292
forensics, defined 640
forensic testing, described 509
Forward Face, contact information 690
Foundation for Ichthyosis and Related Skin Types, Inc., contact information 698
Foundations for Nager and Miller Syndromes, contact information 690
4P- Support Group, contact information 710
foveal hypoplasia, albinism 61
fragile X mental retardation (FMRP) 344–46, 357–58
fragile X syndrome 343–58, *615*
frameshift mutation, described 40
fraternal twin, defined 640
FRAXA Research Foundation, contact information 695
Freeman-Sheldon Parent Support Group, contact information 695
Friedreich's Ataxia Research Alliance, contact information 696
FSHD *see* facioscapulohumeral muscular dystrophy
full gene sequence, defined 640
fumarylacetoacetate hydrolase 183
functional genomics, defined 640
future planning, special needs persons 571–76
"Futures and Special Needs Planning for Persons with a Disability" (National Down Syndrome Society) 571n

G

GABA *see* gamma-aminobutyric acid
gabapentin *355*
Gabitril (tiagabine) *355*
Gainetdinov, Raul 495
galactocerebrosidase 194
galactosemia
  newborn screening 532
  overview 173–74
Gallaudet Research Institute, contact information 692
gametes
  defined 640
  genetic variation 29, 31
  inheritance 31–32
  organelle DNA 17
gamma-aminobutyric acid (GABA) 489, 490
gastroenterologists, hemochromatosis 99
Gaucher, Philippe Charles Ernest 211
Gaucher disease 210–15
GC *see* glucocerebroside
GC rich area, defined 640
GCSF *see* granulocyte colony stimulating factor
G-CSF *see* granulocyte colony stimulating factor
gender factor
  Alexander disease 192
  Barth syndrome 250
  Becker muscular dystrophy 262
  color vision defects 112–13
  Duchenne muscular dystrophy 261
  Edwards syndrome 339
  Fabry disease 207
  fragile X syndrome 343, 345–46, 349
  hemochromatosis 97
  hemophilia 78–79, 83–84
  Klinefelter syndrome 359–67
  mitochondria 17–18
  Rett syndrome 285–86
  sex chromosomes 7–8, 33
  spondyloepiphyseal dysplasia tarda 154
  triple X syndrome 377
  urea cycle disorders 185
  X-linked inheritance 41–43, 48–49

gene amplification, defined 641
GeneCare Medical Genetics Center, contact information 678
gene conversion, described 599
"Gene-Environment Interaction Fact Sheet" (CDC) 393n
gene expression
  defined 641
  described 10, 12, 15, 26
  inheritance 32
  mutation 39
  see also proteins; transcription; translation
gene expressivity, described 514–15
gene family, defined 641
"Gene Hunting" (NIMH) 481n
gene mapping, defined 641
gene mutations
  described 37–40
  hemochromatosis 96
gene penetrance, described 514
gene pool, defined 641
gene product, defined 641
"General Information about Disabilities" (NICHCY) 549n
gene regulation, described 12
genes
  address 8–9
  AGPAT2 *428*
  albinism *62*
  ALMS1 *428*
  Alzheimer's disease 471–72
  apolipoprotein E 473–74
  BRCA1 407–9
  BRCA2 407–9
  BTD 172
  cancer 396–416
  CDKN2 413
  CF 130–31
  CFTR 39
  COMP 153
  connexin-32 253
  defined 641
  Delta F508 130
  described 6, *6*, 15–16
  diabetes 429–32
  environment 393–94
  FABP2 430
  Fanconi anemia 92

genes, continued
  5-HTTLPR 497
  FMR1 344–49, 357
  G4.5 251
  GARS 603–6
  GFAP 192
  GLA 206
  glucokinase *428*
  HD 160
  HE1 232
  Hex-A 237
  HFE 96–97
  hMLH1 410
  hMSH2 410
  HNF-1alpha *428*
  HNF-1beta *428*
  HNF4A 430–32
  HNF-4alpha *428*
  hPMS2 410
  hPMSI 410
  human genome 21–26
  IL-4Rα 464
  IPF-1 (PDX) *428*
  Lamin A/C *428*
  LEP (164160) *436*
  LEPR (601007) *436*
  LMNA 609–11
  MC4R (155541) *436*
  mental illness 481–83
  muscular dystrophy 259
  NF1 247
  NF2 247
  ocular albinism *58*
  P0 253
  p53 647
  Parkin 469–70
  PC1 (162150) *436*
  PiZZ 68–69, 73
  POMC1 (176830) *436*
  proteins 10–11, 22–24
  PSD-95 494–95
  PWS 304
  Rett syndrome 287
  Scurfin *428*
  Seipin *428*
  SHOX 380
  SIM1 (603128) *436*
  TAZ1 251
  thalassemia 107

genes, continued
  tRNALeu *428*
  TRP1 64
  TSC1 290, 294
  TSC2 290, 294
  tyrosinase 63
  UBE3A 304–5, *305*
  Wolframin *428*
gene switching, described 25–26
GeneTests, contact information 678
gene therapy
  Charcot-Marie-Tooth disease 256–57
  cri du chat syndrome 318
  cystic fibrosis 133
  defined 641
  fragile X syndrome 357
  hemophilia 81, 85
  mucopolysaccharidoses 224
  Niemann-Pick disease 233
  overview 627–32
  phenylketonuria 181
  sickle cell disease 106
Genetic Alliance, contact information 679
genetic code, defined 641
genetic conditions, naming conventions 44–45
genetic counseling
  Alzheimer's disease 474
  cancer 400–402
  defined 641
  dilated cardiomyopathy 455
  Down syndrome 330
  hemophilia 83
  overview 501–6
  Tay-Sachs disease 241
  triple X syndrome 378
genetic discrimination
  defined 642
  described 511, 515
  insurance coverage 567–70
  legislation 565
"Genetic Disorders" (NLM) 37n
genetic disorders, overview 37–45
genetic emphysema, alpha-1-antitrypsin deficiency 69
genetic engineering, defined 642
"Genetic Features of Turner Syndrome" (NICHD) 379n

genetic illness, defined 642
genetic marker, defined 642
genetic mosaic, defined 642
genetic mutations, transcription 25
genetic polymorphism, defined 642
genetic predisposition, defined 642
"Genetic Risk for Allergy and Asthma
  Affects 20 to 40 Percent of Population" (Cincinnati Children's Hospital Medical Center) 464n
genetics, defined 642
genetic screening, defined 642
Genetics Education and Counseling
  Program, contact information 679
Genetics Education Center, contact
  information 679
Genetics Home Reference, contact information 679
*Genetics Home Reference: Your Guide
  to Understanding Genetic Conditions* (NLM) 37n, 579n
"Genetics Linked with Sudden Cardiac Death from Heart Disease"
  (HeartCenterOnline, Inc.) 456n
"Genetics Privacy and Legislation"
  (Oak Ridge National Laboratory)
  557n
genetics professionals, heredity counseling 43
genetic testing
  defined 642
  diabetes 427
  dilated cardiomyopathy 454
  hearing loss 156
  hemochromatosis 100
  Huntington disease 162–64
  muscular dystrophy 272
  overview 507–12
  spinal muscular atrophy 275
  workplace discrimination 562
"Genetic Testing" (NLM) 507n
genetic variation, mechanisms 28–35
gene transfer, defined 641
"Gene Variants May Increase Susceptibility to Type 2 Diabetes" (NIH) 425n
genital defects 417–23
genome
  defined 642
  described 15–16

genomic imprinting, methylation 27
genomics, defined 642
*Genomics and Its Impact on
  Medicine and Society: A 2001
  Primer* (Oak Ridge National
  Laboratory) 635n
genotype, defined 642
genu valgum, pseudoachondroplastic
  dysplasia 152
genu varum, pseudoachondroplastic
  dysplasia 152
Georgia, newborn screening programs 659, *664, 666*
germ cell, defined 642
germ line, defined 642
germ line gene therapy, defined 643
germline mutations, described 38
glial fibrillary acidic protein 192
globin protein 26–27
globotriaosylceramide 206
glucocerebrosidase (GC) 212,
  213–14
glucose screening, prenatal tests
  526
Gluten-Free Living, contact information 689
glycogen storage disease (GSD), overview 135–38
glycosaminoglycans 216–17
GM-CSF *see* granulocyte-macrophage
  colony-stimulating factor
Golgi apparatus, defined 3
gonadal dysgenesis 422
gonadotropins, Klinefelter syndrome
  362
Goodman, Jesse 208
Gordon, Harold 497
Gordon, Leslie 608
gout, glycogen storage disease 138
granulocyte colony stimulating factor
  (GCSF) 94, 250
granulocyte-macrophage colony-
  stimulating factor (GM-CSF),
  Fanconi anemia 94
Green, Eric D. 585, 604
Kathryn and Alan C. Greenberg Center for Skeletal Dysplasias, Web site
  address 146
Greer, Wenda 230

growth disorders, overview 140–43
see also achondroplasia; Bloom syndrome; Cockayne syndrome; congenital spondyloepiphyseal dysplasia; diastrophic dysplasia; dwarfism; Dyggve-Melchior-Clausen syndrome; Ellis-van Creveld syndrome; Hallermann-Streiff syndrome; hypochondroplasia; Kniest syndrome; Laron syndrome; McKusick type metaphyseal chondrodysplasia; metatropic dysplasia I; multiple epiphyseal dysplasia; pseudoachondroplastic dysplasia; Schwartz-Jampel syndrome; spondyloepiphyseal dysplasia tarda; Weill-Marchesani syndrome
growth factors, Fanconi anemia 94
growth hormone, Laron syndrome 151
growth hormone deficiency 149–50
GSD *see* glycogen storage disease
guanfacine *355*
guanine (G)
  defined 643
  described 4, *5*, 595
  human genome *16*, 16–17
guanosine triphosphatase-activating protein 247
gynecomastia
  Klinefelter syndrome 363
  spinal muscular atrophy 275

H

Haefemeyer, James W. 57n, 66
Hallermann-Streiff syndrome 150
haloperidol 165
Hamer, Dean 613n
haploid
  defined 643
  described 31
Harvard Brain Tissue Resource Center, contact information 170, 205, 248
Harvard Medical School, deafness publication 155n

Harvard Medical School Center for Hereditary Deafness, contact information 692
Haussler, David 585
Hawaii, newborn screening programs 659, *664*, *666*
HD *see* Huntington disease
health insurance *see* insurance
Health Insurance Portability and Accountability Act (HIPAA) 560–61
hearing impairment
  Hunter syndrome 220
  mucopolysaccharidoses 217–18
  newborn screening 533
  Refsum disease 196
  Williams syndrome 389
hearing loss 155–58
HeartCenterOnline, Inc.
  contact information 457
  heart disease publication 456n
heart problems
  DiGeorge syndrome 319, 320, 321–22
  Edwards syndrome 340
  genetic factors 438–57
  Marfan syndrome 123, 126
  myotonic muscular dystrophy 268
  Patau syndrome 370
  Turner syndrome 380–81
  Williams syndrome 388
hematologists
  hemochromatosis 99
  sickle cell disease 103
hemizygous, defined 643
hemochromatosis, overview 96–101
hemoglobin
  described 26
  sickle cell disease 101
  thalassemia 107–8
hemophilia A, overview 78–82
hemophilia B, overview 83–85
heparan N-sulfatase 221
heparin 81
hepatologists, hemochromatosis 99
hereditary cancer
  defined 643
  overview 396–406
hereditary deafness, overview 155–58
Hereditary Disease Foundation, contact information 679, 698

hereditary motor and sensory neuropathy 251
hereditary mutations, described 38
hereditary neuropathy with predisposition to pressure palsy (HNPP) 252
hereditary nonpolyposis colorectal cancer (HNPCC) 410–11
heredity, mechanisms 28–35
heritable, described 116
Hermansky-Pudlak syndrome (HPS) 64
Hermansky-Pudlak Syndrome Network, Inc., contact information 698
Hershey, Gurjit Khurana 464–65
heterozygosity, defined 643
heterozygous, described 32
hexosaminidase A 234, 236–37
HGNC *see* HUGO Gene Nomenclature Committee
HGPS *see* Hutchinson-Gilford progeria syndrome
HHT Foundation International, contact information 697
high blood pressure *see* hypertension
HIPAA *see* Health Insurance Portability and Accountability Act
Histiocytosis Association of America, contact information 698
histone proteins, depicted 7
hitchhiker thumbs, diastrophic dysplasia 148
HLA *see* human leukocyte antigens
HNPCC *see* hereditary nonpolyposis colorectal cancer
homologous recombination, defined 643
homology, defined 643
homozygote, defined 643
homozygous, described 32
Howard Hughes Medical Institute, contact information 679
"How is NPD Diagnosed?" (National Niemann-Pick Disease Foundation) 226n
"How is NPD Transmitted?" (National Niemann-Pick Disease Foundation) 226n
HPS *see* Hermansky-Pudlak syndrome (HPS)

HUGO Gene Nomenclature Committee (HGNC), described 45
Human Brain and Spinal Fluid Resource Center, contact information 170, 205, 248
human genome
  overview 15–35
  research 583–85
Human Genome Initiative, described 643
Human Genome Project
  genes 393
  overview 579–82
"The Human Genome Project and Genomic Research" (NLM) 579n
Human Genome Project Information, genetic testing publication 513n
Human Growth Foundation
  contact information 683
  Web site address 146
human leukocyte antigens (HLA) 427
Hunter's Hope Foundation, contact information 699
Hunter syndrome 216, 220
Huntington, George 159
Huntington disease (HD)
  genetic basis *615*
  overview 159–70
  prenatal testing 519
"Huntington's Disease - Hope through Research" (NINDS) 159
Huntington's Disease Society of America, contact information 698
Hurler-Scheie syndrome 219–20
Hurler syndrome
  described 218–19
  treatment 225–26
Hutchinson-Gilford progeria syndrome (HGPS), research 607–11
Hutchinson-Gilford Progeria Syndrome Network, contact information 705
hyaluronidase deficiency 223
hydronephrosis 419
hydrops fetalis 223
hydroxyurea 103
hyperactivity
  Angelman syndrome 306
  cri du chat syndrome 317

hyperammonemia 185–87
hypercalcemia, Williams syndrome
  388
hypertelorism, cri du chat syndrome
  314
hypertension (high blood pressure),
  genetic factors 459–62
hypertrophic cardiomyopathy 456
hypochondroplasia 150–51
hypofibrinogenemia 85–86
hypoglycemia, tyrosinemia 183
hypomelanotic macules 292
hypopigmentation
  albinism 62
  Angelman syndrome 308
  Hermansky-Pudlak syndrome 62
hypoplastic left heart syndrome 448–
  49
hypospadias 421
hypostasis, described 34
hypothyroidism, newborn screening
  532
hypotonia
  congenital spondyloepiphyseal dys-
    plasia 153
  metachromatic leukodystrophy 195
  Patau syndrome 370
  urea cycle disorders 185
hypotrichosis, Hallermann-Streiff
  syndrome 150

I

I-cell disease 214
ichthyosis, Refsum disease 196
Idaho, newborn screening programs
  659, *664, 666*
IDEA *see* Individuals with Disabilities Education Act
identical twin, defined 643
idiopathic dilated cardiomyopathy 451
Illinois, newborn screening programs
  660, *664, 666*
imaging technologies
  Batten disease 203
  Huntington disease 168–69
Immune Deficiency Foundation, contact information 705

immune system, DiGeorge syndrome
  319
imperfect albinism *see*
  oculocutaneous albinism
imprinting, defined 643–44
inborn errors of metabolism *see*
  biotinidase deficiency; galactosemia;
  Gaucher disease; maple sugar urine
  disease; phenylketonuria; tyrosinemia; urea cycle disorders
incomplete albinism *see*
  oculocutaneous albinism
independent assortment
  defined 644
  law 31
Indiana, newborn screening programs 660, *664, 666*
Indiana University Medical Center,
  contact information 169
individualized education plan (IEP)
  352–53
Individuals with Disabilities Education Act (IDEA) 352–56, 549–56
influenza vaccine, alpha-1 antitrypsin deficiency 70
informed consent, defined 644
inherit, defined 644
inheritance
  described 31–32
  genetic conditions 41
inheritance patterns
  afibrinogenemia 86
  described *42*
  Ehlers-Danlos syndrome 121
  hemophilia 78–79, 83–84
  overview 47–53
insertion
  defined 644
  described 40
Institute for Basic Research in Developmental Disabilities, contact information 686, 693
insurance
  discrimination legislation 563
  genetic discrimination 567–70
intermittent positive pressure
  breathing (IPPB) 280
International Albinism Center, contact information 66, 684

International Center for Fabry Disease, contact information 695
International Joseph Diseases Foundation, Inc., contact information 699
International Progeria Registry, contact information 705
International Resource Center for Down Syndrome, contact information 694
International Rett Syndrome Association, contact information 706
interphase, defined 644
interstitial deletion, cri du chat syndrome 312
Intestinal Multiple Polyposis and Colorectal Cancer, contact information 704
introns
defined 644
described 21
inversion, cri du chat syndrome 312
inversions, described 301
Iowa, newborn screening programs 660, *664*, *666*
IPPB *see* intermittent positive pressure breathing
iris color, albinism 60
iron chelators, thalassemia 108
Iron Disorders Institute, contact information 685, 697
iron overload disease 96–101

J

Jansky-Bielschowsky disease 201
Jervell syndrome *157*
Jewish genetic diseases
Bloom syndrome 147
Gaucher disease 210–15
Niemann-Pick disease 228, *231*
Tay-Sachs disease 236, 238
JNCL (Juvenile Neuronal Ceroid Lipofuscinoses) Research Fund, contact information 687
Johanssen, Wilhelm 15
Johns Hopkins University, achondroplasia publication 144n

Joubert Syndrome, contact information 699
junk DNA
defined 644
described 23
Juvenile Diabetes Research Foundation International, contact information 547, 693
juvenile hemochromatosis 97
juvenile spinal muscular atrophy 274

K

Kansas, newborn screening programs 661, *664*, *666*
karyotype
defined 644
described 300
Klinefelter syndrome 361, 366
triple X syndrome 378
Kawasaki disease 457
Kayser-Fleischer ring 295–96
kb *see* kilobase
Kearns-Sayre syndrome 257
Kennedy's Disease Association, contact information 699
Kentucky, newborn screening programs 661, *664*, *666*
key ages, described 33
kidney problems
tuberous sclerosis 291
Turner syndrome 380
Williams syndrome 388
see also polycystic kidney disease
kidney stones, glycogen storage disease 138
kilobase (kb), defined 644
kinesins 253
King, Richard A. 57n, 66
Klinefelter, Harry 359
Klinefelter syndrome 359–67
Klinefelter Syndrome and Associates, contact information 699
Klippel-Trenaunay Support Group, contact information 699
Kniest syndrome 151
knockout, defined 644

Krabbe disease 194
Krabbe's Family Network, contact information 699
Ku, Lisa 450n
Kufs disease 201
Kugelberg-Welander disease 273, 274
kyphoscoliosis
  congenital spondyloepiphyseal dysplasia 153
  metatropic dysplasia 151
kyphosis
  diastrophic dysplasia 148
  pseudoachondroplastic dysplasia 153

L

L-acetylcarnitine *355*
ladder *see* double helix
Jim Lambright Niemann-Pick Foundation, contact information 702
Lamictal (lamotrigine) *355*
lamotrigine *355*
Lange-Nielsen syndrome *157*
laronidase 225
Laron syndrome 151
late onset Tay-Sachs disease 241–42
Late Onset Tay-Sachs Foundation, late onset Tay-Sachs disease publication 236n
laughter, Angelman syndrome 306–7
Laundy, Jennifer 535n
law of dominance 31
law of independent assortment 31
law of segregation 31
LCR *see* locus control region
"Learning About Breast Cancer" (NHGRI) 407n
"Learning About Colon Cancer" (NHGRI) 409n
"Learning about Parkinson's Disease" (NHGRI) 469n
"Learning About Prostate Cancer" (NHGRI) 414n
"Learning About Skin Cancer" (NHGRI) 411n

"Learning about Thalassemia" (NHGRI) 107n
legal planning, special needs persons 571–76
legislation
  free appropriate public education 352–56
  genetics privacy 557–65
Lejeune, Jerome 313
Lerman, Caryn 496–97
LeRoy, Bonnie S. 57n, 66
Let's Face It, contact information 691
leukemia 92, 147
leukodystrophies, overview 189–97
LGMD *see* limb-girdle muscular dystrophy
Li, Ting-Kai 490
Lieberman, Jack 67n
life expectancy
  Charcot-Marie-Tooth disease 252
  cri du chat syndrome 316
  cystic fibrosis 132
  Edwards syndrome 341
  Ehlers-Danlos syndrome 121
  Fanconi anemia 95
  hemochromatosis 99
  Hunter syndrome 220
  Hurler-Scheie syndrome 220
  Hurler syndrome 219
  Morquio syndrome 222
  muscular dystrophy 263
  Niemann-Pick disease 227
  Patau syndrome 371
  Rett syndrome 286
  Sandhoff disease 235
  Sanfilippo syndrome 221
  Scheie syndrome 219
  Sly syndrome 223
  special needs planning 571–76
  spinal muscular atrophy 277
  Tay-Sachs disease 236
  triple X syndrome 378
limb ataxia, Pelizaeus-Merzbacher disease 196
limb-girdle muscular dystrophy (LGMD) 262–63
linkage, defined 644
linkage disequilibrium, defined 645
linkage map, defined 645

lipid storage diseases *see* Batten disease; Fabry disease; Gaucher disease; mucolipidoses; mucopolysaccharidoses; Niemann-Pick disease; Sandhoff disease; Tay-Sachs disease
lipofuscins 201–2
lipopigments 201–2, 204
Liscum, Laura 233
lithium 165
lithium carbonate *355*
Little People of America (LPA)
   contact information 683
   Web site address 146
liver disorders
   alpha-1 antitrypsin deficiency 67–68, 73–76
   cirrhosis 69
   galactosemia 173–74
   glycogen storage disease 136–37
   tyrosinemia 182–83
   urea cycle disorders 187
liver transplantation 74
localize, defined 645
locus, defined 645
locus control region (LCR), described 27
long Q-T syndrome 457
long-range restriction mapping, defined 645
Lorenzo's Oil 191
Louisiana, newborn screening programs 661, *664, 666*
Lowe's Syndrome Association, Inc., contact information 700
lumbar lordosis
   congenital spondyloepiphyseal dysplasia 153
   pseudoachondroplastic dysplasia 153
lung disorders
   alpha-1 antitrypsin deficiency 68, 69–73
   cystic fibrosis 129–33
   Marfan syndrome 124, 126
lung transplantation 72
Luvox (fluvoxamine) *355*
lymphopenia, McKusick type metaphyseal chondrodysplasia 152

lysosomal storage diseases
   mucolipidosis 218
   mucopolysaccharidoses 217
lysosomes
   defined 4
   described 4
Niemann-Pick disease 226

M

Macones, George 520–21, 528–29
macrocephaly, hypochondroplasia 150
macrophages, described 14
MAGIC Foundation, contact information 679
Maine, newborn screening programs 662, *664, 666*
maintenance therapy, hemochromatosis 99
major depressive disorder 478–79
major histocompatibility complex (MHC) 426–27
malabsorption, McKusick type metaphyseal chondrodysplasia 152
malformation, defined 645
manic depression *see* bipolar disorder
maple sugar urine disease (MSUD), overview 175–76
Maple Syrup Urine Disease Family Support Group, contact information 700
March of Dimes
   contact information 679
   publications
      phenylketonuria 177n
      sickle cell disease 101n
Marfan syndrome
   described 117
   overview 122–28
Marie, Pierre 251
Maroteaux-Lamy syndrome 222
Maryland, newborn screening programs 662, *664, 666*
Massachusetts, newborn screening programs 663, *664, 666*
mass spectrometry, defined 645
maternal blood screening, prenatal tests 523–24

maternal inheritance *42*
maternal phenylketonuria 180
maturity onset diabetes of the young (MODY) 432
Mayo Foundation for Medical Education and Research and Mayo Clinic, contact information 680
Mb *see* megabase
McClellan, Mark B. 208–9
McGuffin, Peter 613n
McKusick type metaphyseal chondrodysplasia 151–52
MDA *see* Muscular Dystrophy Association
meconium 131
MECP2 *see* methyl cytosine binding protein 2
MED *see* multiple epiphyseal dysplasia
Medical College of Virginia, contact information 680
megabase (Mb), defined 645
meiosis
    defined 645
    depicted *13*
    described 12, 301
    genetic variation 30
    inheritance 31
    Klinefelter syndrome 359–60
    segregation 650
melanin, described 57–58
melanoma 412
melatonin *355*
Mendel, Gregor 15, 30–31
Mendelian inheritance, defined 645
    see also Online Mendelian Inheritance in Man
Mendel's laws, described 30–35
menstrual cycle, Turner syndrome 384
mental illness, heredity 478–84
mental retardation
    Angelman syndrome 307–8
    congenital muscular dystrophy 270
    Dyggve-Melchior-Clausen syndrome 149
    fragile X syndrome 343
    hypochondroplasia 150
    maple sugar urine disease 175

mental retardation, continued
    mucolipidoses 214
    phenylketonuria 177
    Sly syndrome 223
Merville, Scott 462
messenger RNA (mRNA)
    defined 645
    described 11, 20
    transcription 22, 26
messengers, described *10*
Mestroni, Luisa 450n
Metabolic Information Network, contact information 698
metachromatic leukodystrophy (MLD) 194–95
metaphase, defined 645
metaphyseal chondrodysplasia 152
metatropic dysplasia I 151
methionine, translation 22
methylation, DNA structure 27
methyl cytosine binding protein 2 (MECP2) 287–88
methylphenidate *355*
MHC *see* major histocompatibility complex
Michigan, newborn screening programs 663, *664, 666*
microarray, defined 646
microcephaly
    cri du chat syndrome 313
    neuronal ceroid lipofuscinoses 200
    Patau syndrome 370
    phenylketonuria 180
microdontia, McKusick type metaphyseal chondrodysplasia 152
micrognathia
    cri du chat syndrome 313
    diastrophic dysplasia 149
    Edwards syndrome 339
    Patau syndrome 370
microphthalmia
    Hallermann-Streiff syndrome 150
    Patau syndrome 370
milestones, described 33
Minnesota, newborn screening programs 663, *664, 666*
missense mutation, described 40
Mississippi, newborn screening programs 663, *664, 666*

Missouri, newborn screening programs
665, *666*, 668
mitochondria
defined 4
described 4, 257
inheritance 52
described *42*
mutations 52–53
organelle DNA 17–18
mitochondrial DNA
defined 646
described 17
mitochondrial encephalomyopathy
257
mitochondrial myopathies 257–58
mitosis
defined 646
depicted *13*
described 12, 301
genetic variation 30
MLD *see* metachromatic leukodystrophy
MMD *see* myotonic muscular dystrophy
MODY *see* maturity onset diabetes of
the young
molecular medicine, defined 646
molluscum fibrosum 292
monochromacy, described 112
monogenic disorder, defined 646
monosomy
defined 646
described 300
Montana, newborn screening programs *665*, *666*, 668
"More Information: Glossary" (National
Center for Biotechnology Information) 635n
Morquio syndrome 222
mosaicism
cri du chat syndrome 312–13
described 301
Down syndrome 330
fragile X syndrome 345
Klinefelter syndrome 365
motif, defined 646
Mountain States Genetic Network,
contact information 680
mRNA *see* messenger RNA

MSUD *see* maple sugar urine disease
mucolipidoses 214–15, 218
mucopolysaccarides *see* glycosaminoglycans
mucopolysaccharidoses, overview
216–26
"The Mucopolysaccharidoses Fact
Sheet" (NINDS) 216n
Mucolipidosis IV Foundation, contact
information 701
Mullis, Kary B. 587
multifactorial disorders, prenatal
testing 520
multigenic, described 34
multiple epiphyseal dysplasia (MED)
152
multiple myeloma, Gaucher disease
211
muscular dystrophies 258–72
Muscular Dystrophy Association (MDA)
contact information 701
publications
genetic disorders 47n
muscular dystrophies 258n
mutagen, defined 646
mutations
cancer 396
defined 646
genetic testing 514
genetic variation 29–30
mitochondria 52–53
see also gene mutations
Myasthenia Gravis Foundation, contact information 702
myelin 189, 190, 194, 195, 196, 197,
252–53
Myelin Project, contact information
699, 701
myoclonic jerks 201
myoclonus epilepsy 257
myopia
congenital spondyloepiphyseal dysplasia 154
Weill-Marchesani syndrome 154
myotonic muscular dystrophy (MMD)
266–69
myotonic myopathy, Schwartz-Jampel
syndrome 153
Mysoline (primidone) *355*

N

N-acetylgalactosamine 4-sulfatase
222
N-acetylgalactosamine 6-sulfatase
222
N-acetylglucosamine 6-sulfatase 221
N-acetylglutamate synthetase 185
naltrexone 489
nandrolone decanoate 95
"Nanomedicine" (NHGRI) 587n
nanomedicine, described 593–94
NAPVI *see* National Association for
Parents of Children with Visual Impairments
Nathan's Battle Foundation, contact
information 687
National Adrenal Diseases Foundation, contact information 684
National Alopecia Areata Foundation,
contact information 685
National Association for Down
Syndrome, contact information 694
National Association for Parents
of Children with Visual Impairments (NAPVI), contact information 687
National Association of the Deaf, contact information 692
National Ataxia Foundation, contact
information 686
National Cancer Institute, contact information 688
National Center for Biotechnology Information (NCBI)
contact information 680
gene map 476
publications
genomes 15n
glossary 635n
pharmacogenomics 623n
signal nucleotide polymorphisms
595n
National Center for Education in Maternal and Child Health, contact information 680
National Center for the Study of
Wilson's Disease, contact information 710

National Center on Birth Defects and
Developmental Disabilities, contact
information 680
National Diabetes Information Clearinghouse, contact information 692
National Digestive Diseases Information Clearinghouse, contact information 693
National Disease Research Interchange (NDRI) 205
National Dissemination Center for
Children with Disabilities
(NICHCY)
contact information 693
publications
disabilities information 549n
Down syndrome 326n
National Down Syndrome Congress,
contact information 694
National Down Syndrome Society
contact information 694
publications
Down syndrome causes 329n
Down syndrome health issues
332n
special needs planning 571n
National Easter Seal Society, contact
information 547
National Foundation for Ectodermal
Dysplasias, contact information 694
National Fragile X Foundation, contact information 695
National Gaucher Foundation
contact information 213, 696
Gaucher disease publication 210n
National Hemophilia Foundation,
contact information 697, 710
National Human Genome Research
Institute (NHGRI)
Alzheimer's disease 476
contact information 680
publications
breast cancer 407n
chromosome abnormalities 299n
colon cancer 409n
DNA chip technology 587n
DNA microarray technology 587n
fluorescence in situ hybridization
587n

National Human Genome Research
Institute (NHGRI), continued
publications, continued
glossary 635n
human genome 583n
nanomedicine 587n
Parkinson disease 469n
polymerase chain reaction 587n
prostate cancer 414n
skin cancer 411n
spectral karyotyping 587n
thalassemia 107n
Y chromosome gene preservation
599n
National Institute on Drug Abuse
(NIDA), nicotine addiction publication 495n
National Institute of Allergy and Infectious Diseases (NIAID), contact
information 684
National Institute of Arthritis and
Musculoskeletal and Skin Diseases
(NIAMS), Marfan syndrome publication 122n
National Institute of Child Health
and Human Development (NICHD)
contact information 680
Mental Retardation and Develop-
mental Disabilities Branch, con-
tact information 700
publications
fragile X syndrome 343n
Turner syndrome 379n
National Institute of Diabetes and
Digestive and Kidney Diseases
(NIDDK), publications
diabetes mellitus 425n
Wilson disease 295n
National Institute of Mental Health
(NIMH)
gene hunting publication 481n
Web site address 480
National Institute of Neurological
Disorders and Stroke (NINDS)
contact information 681
publications
Barth syndrome 250n
Batten disease 200n
Charcot-Marie-Tooth disease 251

National Institute of Neurological
Disorders and Stroke (NINDS), continued
publications, continued
Huntington disease 159
leukodystrophies 189n
mitochondrial myopathies 257n
mucolipidoses 214n
mucopolysaccharidoses 216n
neurofibromatosis 243n
Sandhoff disease 234n
tuberous sclerosis 289n
National Institute on Alcohol Abuse
and Alcoholism (NIAAA), heredity
publication 486
National Institute on Deafness and
Other Communication Disorders Clearinghouse, contact information 692
National Institutes of Health (NIH),
diabetes mellitus publication 425n
National Kidney and Urologic Diseases Information Clearinghouse,
contact information 704, 709
National Library of Medicine (NLM),
publications
Fabry disease 206n
genes 3n
genetic disorders 37n
genetic testing 507n
Human Genome Project 579n
National Marfan Foundation, contact
information 700
National Mental Health Association
(NMHA), Web site address 480
National MPS Society, contact infor-
mation 698, 701
National Multiple Sclerosis Society,
contact information 701
National Newborn Screening and
Genetics Resource Center, contact
information 681
National Newborn Screening and Ge-
netics Resource Center (NNSGRC),
newborn screening programs publi-
cation 655n
National Niemann-Pick Disease
Foundation
contact information 234, 702
Niemann-Pick disease publication 226n

National Organization for Rare Disorders, Inc., contact information 681, 705

National Parkinson Foundation, Inc., contact information 703

National PKU News, contact information 704

National Prune Belly Syndrome Network, contact information 705

National Scoliosis Foundation, contact information 706

National Sjögren's Syndrome Association, contact information 707

National Society of Genetic Counselors
contact information 476, 681
Web site address 455

National Tay-Sachs and Allied Diseases Association
contact information 688, 700, 706, 708
Tay-Sachs disease publication 236n

National Urea Cycle Disorders Foundation (NUCDF)
contact information 697, 709
urea cycle disorders publication 184n

National Vitiligo Foundation, contact information 709

NCBI *see* National Center for Biotechnology Information

NCL *see* neuronal ceroid lipofuscinoses

NDRI *see* National Disease Research Exchange

Nebraska, newborn screening programs *665*, *666*, 668

nefazodone *355*

neonatal hemochromatosis 97

nerve signals, albinism 61

nervous system, Marfan syndrome 123, 126

Network for 9p- Support, contact information 684

neurofibromatoses 243–48

Neurofibromatosis, Inc., contact information 702

"Neurofibromatosis Fact Sheet" (NINDS) 243n

neurofibromatosis type 1 (NF1) 243–45, 246–48

neurofibromatosis type 2 (NF2) *157*, 245–48

neurofilaments 253

neurological disorders, research 603–6

neurologists
Huntington disease 165
Tay-Sachs disease 236

neuromuscular disorders *see* Barth syndrome; Charcot-Marie-Tooth disease; mitochondrial myopathies; muscular dystrophies; spinal muscular atrophy

neuronal ceroid lipofuscinoses (NCL) 200–205

Neurontin (gabapentin) *355*

Neuropathy Association, contact information 702

neuroticism, S allele 497

neutropenia
Barth syndrome 250
McKusick type metaphyseal chondrodysplasia 152

neutrophil elastase
described 67
emphysema 69

neutrophils, panniculitis 69

Nevada, newborn screening programs *665*, *667*, 669

"New Born Screening Programs in the U.S." (NNSGRC) 655n

New Hampshire, newborn screening programs *665*, *667*, 669

New Jersey, newborn screening programs *665*, *667*, 669

New Mexico, newborn screening programs *665*, *667*, 670

New York state, newborn screening programs *665*, *667*, 670

NF1 *see* neurofibromatosis type 1

NF2 *see* neurofibromatosis type 2

NHGRI *see* National Human Genome Research Institute

NHPP *see* hereditary neuropathy with predisposition to pressure palsy

NIAAA *see* National Institute on Alcohol Abuse and Alcoholism

NIAID *see* National Institute of Allergy and Infectious Diseases

NIAMS *see* National Institute of Arthritis and Musculoskeletal and Skin Diseases
NICHCY *see* National Dissemination Center for Children with Disabilities
NICHD *see* National Institute of Child Health and Human Development
Nicholson, Linda 506
NIDA *see* National Institute on Drug Abuse
NIDDK *see* National Institute of Diabetes and Digestive and Kidney Diseases
Niemann-Pick disease 226–34
NIMH *see* National Institute of Mental Health
NINDS *see* National Institute of Neurological Disorders and Stroke
"NINDS Adrenoleukodystrophy Information Page" (NINDS) 189n
"NINDS Alexander Disease Information Page" (NINDS) 189n
"NINDS Barth Syndrome Information Page" (NINDS) 250n
"NINDS Canavan Disease Information Page" (NINDS) 189n
"NINDS Krabbe Disease Information Page" (NINDS) 189n
"NINDS Leukodystrophy Information Page" (NINDS) 189n
"NINDS Metachromatic Leukodystrophy Information Page" (NINDS) 189n
"NINDS Mitochondrial Myopathies Information Page" (NINDS) 257n
"NINDS Mucolipidoses Information Page" (NINDS) 214n
"NINDS Pelizaeus-Merzbacher Disease Information Page" (NINDS) 189n
"NINDS Refsum Disease Information Page" (NINDS) 189n
"NINDS Sandhoff Disease Information Page" (NINDS) 234n
"NINDS Zellweger Syndrome Information Page" (NINDS) 189n
nitrogenous base, defined 646

NLM *see* National Library of Medicine
NMHA *see* National Mental Health Association
NNSGRC *see* National Newborn Screening and Genetics Resource Center
NOAH (National Organization for Albinism and Hypopigmentation), contact information 684
nondisjunction Down syndrome, described 329–30
nonsense mutation, described 40
nonstress test, prenatal tests 526–27
Norbottnian Gaucher disease 212
North Carolina, newborn screening programs *665, 667,* 670
North Dakota, newborn screening programs *665, 667,* 671
nortriptyline 165
NUCDF *see* National Urea Cycle Disorders Foundation
nuclear DNA, described 4, 16–17
nucleic acid
    defined 646
    described 16
nucleolar organizing region, defined 646
nucleotides
    defined 646
    described 5, 16, 624
nucleus
    defined 4, 646
    described 4
    inheritance 52
nystagmus
    albinism 59–60
    color vision defects 112
    Pelizaeus-Merzbacher disease 196
    Refsum disease 196

O

Oak Ridge National Laboratory
    contact information 681
    publications
        genetics privacy legislation 557n
        glossary 635n

obesity
  diabetes mellitus 427–28
  genetic factors 433–36
  Prader-Willi syndrome 374
"Obesity" (CDC) 433n
"Obesity and Genetics: What We
  Know, What We Don't Know and
  What It Means" (CDC) 433n
OCA *see* oculocutaneous albinism
OCA1 *see* tyrosinase related
  oculocutaneous albinism
OCA1A *see* classic tyrosinase-negative
  oculocutaneous albinism
OCA1B 62
OCA3 *see* TRP1-related
  oculocutaneous albinism
ocular albinism 65
oculocutaneous albinism (OCA), de-
  scribed 61–62
oculopharyngeal muscular dystrophy
  (OPMD) 270–71
odontoid hypoplasia 222
Office of Rare Diseases, contact infor-
  mation 681
Ohio, newborn screening programs
  665, *667*, 671
OI *see* osteogenesis imperfecta
Oklahoma, newborn screening programs *665*, *667*, 671
olanzapine *355*
oligogenic, defined 647
OMIM *see* Online Mendelian Inheritance in Man
oncogene, defined 647
one gene-one enzyme theory 25
"One Size Does Not Fit All: The
  Promise of Pharmacogenomics"
  (NCBI) 623n
Online Mendelian Inheritance in
  Man (OMIM), Web site address 476,
  681
OPMD *see* oculopharyngeal muscular
  dystrophy
Oregon, newborn screening programs
  665, *667*, 672
organelle DNA, described 17
organelles, described 3–4
Organic Academia Association, contact information 703

ornithine transcarbamylase 186
Orphan Drug Act 187, 209, 226
orthologous, defined 647
osteogenesis imperfecta (OI), described 117
Osteogenesis Imperfecta Foundation,
  Inc., contact information 703
osteoporosis, Turner syndrome 381–82
otolaryngologists, hereditary deafness 156
Our-Kids, Web site address 548
Oxalosis and Hyperoxaluria Foundation, contact information 703
oxymetholone 95

P

p53 gene, defined 647
Pacer (Parent Advocacy Coalition for
  Educational Rights), contact information 548
Padman, Raj 133
Page, David C. 599
Paget Foundation for Paget's Disease
  of Bone, contact information 703
pain episodes, sickle cell disease 103
palindromes, described 600
Pallister-Killian Family Support
  Group, contact information 703
palmitoyl-protein thioesterase 202,
  203
panniculitis
  described 69
  treatment 74
parahydroxy phenyllactic acid 183
parahydroxy phenylpyruvic acid 183
parapodium 280
parathyroid glands, DiGeorge syndrome 319
Parent Project Duchenne's Muscular
  Dystrophy, contact information 702
Parents of Galactosemic Children,
  contact information 696
Parkinson disease, genetic factors
  469–70
Parkinson's Disease and Movement
  Disorder Center, contact information 703

paroxetine *355*
Parry's disease 201
partial albinism *see* oculocutaneous albinism
partial trisomy, cri du chat syndrome 312
Patau syndrome 369–71
patent ductus arteriosus (PDA) 439–40
paternal uniparental disomy (UPD) 304, *305*
"Patient Guide to Achondroplasia" (Johns Hopkins University) 144n
Paxil (paroxetine) *355*
PCC *see* premature chromosome condensation
PCR *see* polymerase chain reaction
PDA *see* patent ductus arteriosus
pedigree, defined 647
Pelizaeus-Merzbacher disease (PMD) 195–96
Pelizaeus-Merzbacher Disease Foundation, contact information 703
Pendred syndrome *157*
penetrance, defined 647
Pennsylvania, newborn screening programs *665*, *667*, 672
peptide, defined 647
percutaneous umbilical blood sampling (PUBS), Down syndrome 333
percutaneous umbilical vein sampling (PUVS), prenatal tests 527–28
peripheral neurofibromatosis *see* neurofibromatosis type 1
peripheral neuropathies, described 251–52
peripheral neuropathy, Refsum disease 196
peroneal muscular atrophy 251
peroxisomes
  defined 4
  described 4
  Zellweger syndrome 197
PGD *see* preimplantation genetic diagnosis
P-gene related oculocutaneous albinism (OCA2) 63
phakomas 291

pharmacogenomics
  defined 647
  described 582
  overview 623–26
phenobarbital *355*
phenocopy, defined 647
phenotypes
  alpha-1 antitrypsin deficiency 68, *71*
  defined 647
phenotypic traits, genetic variation 28–29
phenylalanine 177, 179, 180, 183
phenylketonuria (PKU)
  newborn screening 532
  overview 177–82
phosphate molecules, nuclear DNA 16
photophobia, albinism 60
photoreceptors, described 111
photosensitivity
  Bloom syndrome 147
  Cockayne syndrome 147
physical map, defined 647
phytanic acid 196–97
pigmentation, albinism 57, 61–62, 63
"The Pima Indians: Genetic Research" (NIDDK) 425n
The Pima Indians: Pathfinders for Health (NIDDK) 425n
pinnae, diastrophic dysplasia 148, 149
pituitary gland, growth hormone deficiency 149
PKD *see* polycystic kidney disease
PKU *see* phenylketonuria
"PKU" (March of Dimes) 177n
plasma membrane
  defined 4
  described 4
pleiotropism, described 34
pleiotropy, defined 647
Plomin, Robert 613n
pluripotency, defined 647
PMD *see* Pelizaeus-Merzbacher disease
pneumonia vaccine, alpha-1 antitrypsin deficiency 70
poliosis 292
polycystic kidney disease (PKD) 419–20

Polycystic Kidney Research Foundation, contact information 704
polydactyly
  defined 647
  Ellis-van Creveld syndrome 149
  Patau syndrome 370
polygenic disorder, defined 648
polymerase, DNA or RNA, defined 648
polymerase binding, DNA structure 27
polymerase chain reaction (PCR)
  defined 648
  described 587–88
"Polymerase Chain Reaction (PCR)" (NHGRI) 587n
polymorphisms
  asthma 464–65
  defined 648
  genetic variation 29, 619
polypeptide, defined 648
population genetics, defined 648
Port-A-Lung 279
positional cloning, defined 648
Prader-Willi syndrome 373–76
Prader-Willi Syndrome Association
  contact information 376, 705
  Prader-Willi syndrome publication 373n
pregnancy
  genetic counseling 501–6
  genetic testing 508
  phenylketonuria 180, 181–82
  sickle cell disease 104–5
preimplantation genetic diagnosis (PGD) 241
premature chromosome condensation (PCC), defined 648
premutation, described 345
Primary Immunodeficiency Association, contact information 705, 710
primidone *355*
privacy, defined 649
progeria, research 607–11
prokaryotes, transcription 22
promoter region, described 344
promoter sequence, described 26
pronucleus, defined 649
prostate cancer, heredity 414–16
protanomaly 113

protanopia 112
protease inhibitors, Pi 68
protein replacement, fragile X syndrome 357–58
proteins
  alpha-1 antitrypsin 67
  CFTR 129
  collagen 117, 120
  defined 649
  described 6, 9–11, 16, 19–20
  fragile X syndrome 344
  GAP 247
  neutrophil elastase 67, 69
  PMP-22 252
proteomics, defined 649
Prozac (fluoxetine) *355*
PS *see* pulmonary stenosis
pseudoachondroplastic dysplasia 152–53
pseudogene
  defined 649
  described 23–24
pseudo-Hurler polydystrophy 214
PUBS *see* percutaneous umbilical blood sampling
pulmonary atresia 446–47
pulmonary function tests, cystic fibrosis 132
pulmonary stenosis (PS) 440
Purine Research Society, contact information 686
purines
  defined 649
  described 16
  human genome 16–17
  see also adenine; guanine
PUVS *see* percutaneous umbilical vein sampling
pyrimidines
  defined 649
  described 16
  human genome 16–17
  see also cytosine; thymine

Q

"Questions and Answers about Fabry Disease" (NLM) 206n

"Questions and Answers about
Marfan Syndrome" (NIAMS) 122n
"Questions and Answers about
Mucopolysaccharidoses" (NINDS)
216n
"Questions and Answers about PKU"
(March of Dimes) 177n
"Questions and Answers on Prader-
Willi Syndrome" (Prader-Willi Syn-
drome Association) 373n
quetiapine *355*

R

racial factor
hypertension 460
sickle cell disease 104
recessive disorders, prenatal testing 519
recessive gene, defined 649
recessive inheritance
described 47–51
Fanconi anemia 92
hemophilia 78–79
reciprocal translocation, defined 649
reciprocating gait orthosis (RGO) 280
recombinant DNA technology
defined 649
Fabry disease 207
recombination, defined 649
red OCA *see* TRP1-related
oculocutaneous albinism (OCA3)
Refsum disease 196–97
regulatory sequences
defined 650
described 23
renal agenesis 418
repeat expansion, described 40
repetitive DNA, defined 650
repressor proteins, translation 28
"Researchers Discover Use of Novel
Mechanism Preserves Y Chromosome Genes" (NHGRI) 599n
Resta, Robert 503
restriction-enzyme cutting site, defined 650
restriction fragment length polymorphism (RFLP), defined 650
restriction points, described 14

"Rethinking Behavior Genetics"
(Hamer) 613n
retinitis pigmentosa, Refsum disease 196
Retinitis Pigmentosa (RP) International, contact information 705
Rett syndrome 285–88
RFLP *see* restriction fragment length
polymorphism
RGO *see* reciprocating gait orthosis
Rhode Island, newborn screening programs *665, 667,* 672
riboflavin 258
ribonucleic acid (RNA)
defined 650
described 10–11, 19
see also messenger RNA; ribosomal
RNA; small nuclear RNA; transfer RNA
ribose, defined 650
ribosomal RNA (rRNA)
defined 650
described 19
ribosomes
defined 4, 650
described 4, 11
Riley, Brien 613n
ring chromosome, cri du chat syndrome 312
rings, described 301
risk communication, defined 650
Risperdal (risperidone) *355*
risperidone *355*
Ritalin (methylphenidate) *355*
RNA *see* ribonucleic acid
RNA polymerase
defined 648
described 22, 26
translation 28
RP Foundation Fighting Blindness,
contact information 706
rRNA *see* ribosomal RNA
Rufous OCA *see* TRP1-related
oculocutaneous albinism (OCA3)

S

Sabril (vigabatrin) *355*
Sachs, Bernard 236

Sandhoff disease 234–35
Sanfilippo syndrome 221–22
Santavuori-Haltia disease 200–201
satellite DNA, described 23
Save Babies Through Screening
 Foundation, Inc., contact informa-
 tion 696
Scheie syndrome 219
schizophrenia 479, *615*
Schwann cells 253
Schwartz-Jampel syndrome (SJS) 153
*A Science Primer: A Basic Introduc-
 tion to the Science Underlying
 NCBI Resources* (NCBI) 15n
*A Science Primer: Just the Facts: A Ba-
 sic Introduction to the Science Underlying NCBI Resources* (NCBI) 595n
Scleroderma Foundation, contact information 706
scoliosis
 diastrophic dysplasia 148
 Kniest syndrome 151
 spinal muscular atrophy 280
SDS *see* Shwachman-Diamond syndrome
SEDT *see* spondyloepiphyseal dysplasia tarda
segregation
 defined 650
 law 31
seizures
 Angelman syndrome 305–6
 Patau syndrome 369
 tuberous sclerosis 292
Self Help for Hard of Hearing People,
 Inc. (SHHH), contact information 692
sequencing
 defined 650
 described 4–5, 595–96
 Y chromosome 599–601
Seroquel (quetiapine) *355*
serotonin 489, 497, 619
sertraline 165, *355*
Serzone (nefazodone) *355*
severe aortic stenosis 457
sex chromosomes
 defined 651
 described 7–8, 300, 320
 inheritance 33

sex-linked, defined 651
sexual behavior, Klinefelter syndrome
 365
shagreen patches 292
SHHH *see* Self Help for Hard of
 Hearing People, Inc.
Shine-Dalgarno sequence, described
 22
Short Stature Foundation, contact information 684
Shwachman-Diamond syndrome
 (SDS) 131
Shwachman-Diamond Syndrome
 Foundation, contact information
 706
sialidosis 214
sickle cell disease
 newborn screening 532
 overview 101–6
 prenatal testing 519
"Sickle Cell Disease" (March of
 Dimes) 101n
Sickle Cell Disease Association of
 America, Inc., contact information
 707
Sickle Cell Information Center, contact information 707
single-gene disorder, defined 651
single nucleotide polymorphism
 (SNP)
 defined 651
 described 616, 624–25
 overview 595–98
Sjögren's Syndrome Foundation, Inc.,
 contact information 707
SJS *see* Schwartz-Jampel syndrome
skin cancer, heredity 411–13
skin disorders, Marfan syndrome 123
skin tags 292
SKY *see* spectral karyotype
sleep disorders
 Angelman syndrome 308
 mucopolysaccharidoses 223
Sly syndrome 223
SMA *see* spinal muscular atrophy
small nuclear RNA (snRNA), described 19
Smith-McCort dwarfism 149
SMN *see* survival motor neuron

smoking cessation, alpha-1 antitrypsin deficiency 70
SNP *see* single nucleotide polymorphism
"SNPs: Variations on a Theme" (NCBI) 595n
snRNA *see* small nuclear RNA
Society for Inherited Metabolic Disorders, contact information 698
sodium benzoate 186
sodium phenylbutyrate 186
SOFT *see* Support Organization for Trisomy 18, 13 and Related Disorders
Solomon, Richard 535n
somatic cell, defined 651
somatic cell genetic mutation, defined 651
somatic mosaicism, eye color 35
Sotnikova, Tatyana 495
Sotos Syndrome Support Association, contact information 707
South Carolina, newborn screening programs *665*, *667*, 673
South Dakota, newborn screening programs *665*, *667*, 673
spastic paraplegia 195–96
Spastic Paraplegia Foundation, Inc., contact information 707
spectral karyotype (SKY)
defined 651
described 589–90
"Spectral Karyotyping" (NHGRI) 587n
spherophakia, Weill-Marchesani syndrome 154
sphingomyelinase 226
Spielmeyer-Vogt-Sjögren-Batten disease 200
Spina Bifida Association of America, contact information 707
spina bifida occulta, diastrophic dysplasia 148
spinal cord injury, diastrophic dysplasia 148–49
spinal muscular atrophy (SMA) 273–83, 605
Spondylitis Association of America, contact information 708

spondyloepiphyseal dysplasia tarda (SEDT) 154
sporadic cancer, defined 651
sporadic mutations, described 38
Sprintzen, Robert 319
squamous cell carcinoma 412
Starbright Foundation, contact information 548
statistics
alpha-1 antitrypsin deficiency 68
Angelman syndrome 303
Barth syndrome 250
breast cancer 407
chronic conditions 536
colon cancer 409
cystic fibrosis 130, 131
Down syndrome 326
Edwards syndrome 339
Fabry disease 206
Gaucher disease 210, 211
glycogen storage disease 136
hemophilia A 78
hemophilia B 83
Marfan syndrome 122
mucopolysaccharidoses 216, 220, 222
neuronal ceroid lipofuscinoses 201
Niemann-Pick disease *231*
phenylketonuria 177
polycystic kidney disease 420
Prader-Willi syndrome 373
prostate cancer 414
skin cancer 411
triple X syndrome 377
tuberous sclerosis complex 289
Turner syndrome 379
stem cells, defined 651
Stevens, Barton Y. 576
Stickler Involved People, contact information 708
Stickler syndrome *157*
Stickler Syndrome Support Group, contact information 708
Stimate nasal spray 81
storage molecules, described *10*
strabismus
albinism 60
Angelman syndrome 308
stroke, sickle cell disease 103

structural components, described *10*
structural genes, described 23
subaortic stenosis 442
subluxation, diastrophic dysplasia 148
substance abuse
    genetic factors 493–98
    heredity 480
substitution, defined 651
subungual fibromas 292
succinylacetoacetate 183
succinylacetone 183
sudden cardiac death, genetic factors 456–57
sugar molecules, nuclear DNA 16
sugar-phosphate backbone, depicted *5*
Summers, C. Gail 57n, 66
Support Organization for Trisomy 18, 13 and Related Disorders (SOFT), contact information 341, 371
suppressor gene, defined 651
surgical procedures
    liver transplantation 74
    lung transplantation 72
    lung volume reduction 75
    tuberous sclerosis 293
survival motor neuron (SMN) 275
Symmetrel (amantadine) *355*
symphalangism, diastrophic dysplasia 148
syndrome, defined 651

T

Takao, Atsuyoshi 320
talipes, diastrophic dysplasia 148
"Talking Glossary of Genetic Terms" (NHGRI) 635n
tandem repeat sequences, defined 652
TAR Syndrome Association, contact information 708
TASH: The Association for Persons with Severe Handicaps, contact information 693
Tay, Warren 236
Taylor, Matthew 450n
Tay-Sachs disease
    overview 236–42
    prenatal testing 519

"Tay-Sachs Disease (Classical Infantile Form)" (National Tay-Sachs and Allied Diseases Association, Inc.) 236n
T cells, McKusick type metaphyseal chondrodysplasia 152
teenagers *see* adolescents
Tegretol (carbamazepine) *355*
telangiectasia 147
telomerase, defined 652
telomeres
    chromosomes *24*
    sequences 23
Tenex (guanfacine) *355*
Tennessee, newborn screening programs *665, 667*, 673
teratogenic, defined 652
terminus, described 9
testosterone, Klinefelter syndrome 363–66
tests
    albinism 65
    alpha-1 antitrypsin deficiency 71
    ambiguous genitals 422
    Batten disease 202–3
    breast cancer 408
    Canavan disease 193
    Charcot-Marie-Tooth disease 255
    color vision defects 113
    connective tissue disorders 119
    cystic fibrosis 132
    dilated cardiomyopathy 450–51
    Down syndrome 332–33
    Edwards syndrome 340
    Fanconi anemia 93–94
    FEV1 (forced expiratory volume) 75
    fragile X syndrome 356–57
    Gaucher disease 210, 212
    glycogen storage disease 137
    growth hormone deficiency 150
    hemochromatosis 98, 100
    Huntington disease 163–64
    Klinefelter syndrome 361
    liver disease 73–74
    maple sugar urine disease 175–76
    Marfan syndrome 124–25
    mucopolysaccharidoses 223
    muscular dystrophy 271–72
    neurofibromatoses 246

tests, continued
  newborn screening 531–33
  Niemann-Pick disease 230–32
  Patau syndrome 370
  phenylketonuria 178–79
  prenatal 517–29
  prostate cancer 415
  pulmonary function 132
  sickle cell disease 105
  skin cancer 413
  spinal muscular atrophy 275–76
  Tay-Sachs disease 238–40
  thalassemia 108–9
  transferrin saturation 100
  triple X syndrome 378
  tuberous sclerosis 293
  tyrosinemia 183
  urinary tract defects 418
  Williams syndrome 389–90
tetralogy of Fallot 445
Texas, newborn screening programs
  665, *667*, 674
thalassemia
  overview 107–9
  prenatal testing 519
  sickle cell disease 102
  treatment 27
thrombosis, treatment 86
thymine (T)
  defined 652
  described 4, *5*, 595
  human genome *16*, 16–17
thymus gland, DiGeorge syndrome
  319
thyroid, Turner syndrome 382
tiagabine *355*
tobacco use, alpha-1 antitrypsin deficiency 70, 71, 75
Tooth, Henry 251
Topamax (topiramate) *355*
topiramate *355*
Torres, Gonzalo 495
total anomalous pulmonary venous
  connection 448
Tourette Syndrome Association, Inc.,
  contact information 708
"Toward Behavioral Genomics"
  (McGuffin, et al.) 613n
toxicogenomics, defined 652

trans-acting, describe 26
transaminases, tyrosinemia 183
transcription
  control 26–28
  defined 652
  depicted *11*
  described 10–11, 20, 22
  introns 21
transcription factor, defined 652
transcriptome, defined 652
transferrin saturation test 100
transfer RNA (tRNA)
  defined 652
  described 11, 19
transgenic, defined 652
translation
  control 28
  defined 652
  depicted *11*
  described 10–11, 22
translocation
  cri du chat syndrome 312
  defined 652
  described 300–301
  Down syndrome 330
transport molecules, described *10*
transposable element, defined 653
transposition of great arteries 445–
  46
trazodone *355*
Treacher Collins Foundation, contact
  information 709
tricuspid atresia 446
trientine hydrochloride 296
triple X syndrome 377–78
trisomy
  defined 653
  described 300
trisomy 13 *see* Patau syndrome
"Trisomy 13" (A.D.A.M., Inc.) 369n
trisomy 18 *see* Edwards syndrome
"Trisomy 18" (A.D.A.M., Inc.) 339n
trisomy 21 *see* Down syndrome
tritanomaly 113
tritanopia 112–13
tRNA *see* transfer RNA
TRP1-related oculocutaneous albinism (OCA3) 64
True, William 496

truncus arteriosus 447
TSC *see* tuberous sclerosis complex
Tuberous Sclerosis Alliance, contact information 709
tuberous sclerosis complex (TSC) 289–94
"Tuberous Sclerosis Fact Sheet" (NINDS) 289n
tumor suppressing gene, defined 653
Turkkan, Jaylan 496
Turner syndrome 379–85
Turner Syndrome Society of the United States, contact information 709
22q11 deletions 320–23
twins
  behavior genetics 617
  identical, defined 643
  nicotine addiction 495–96
tyrosinase gene 63
tyrosinase related oculocutaneous albinism (OCA1) 62
tyrosinemia, overview 182–83

U

UCBT *see* umbilical cord blood transplantation
ultrasound, prenatal tests 525–26
ultraviolet radiation, skin cancer 412–13
umbilical cord blood transplantation (UCBT), mucopolysaccharidoses 224
Understanding Spinal Muscular Atrophy: A Comprehensive Guide (Families of SMA) 273n
"Understanding the Basics" (NUCDF) 184n
Understanding the Genetics of Deafness: A Guide for Patients and Families (Harvard Medical School) 155n
ungual fibromas 292
unipolar disorder 478–79
Unique: Rare Chromosome Disorder Support Group, contact information 689

United Cerebral Palsy Associations, Inc., contact information 689
United Leukodystrophy Foundation, contact information 699
United Mitochondrial Disease Foundation, Muscular Dystrophy Association 701
University of Colorado Cardiovascular Institute, Web site address 455
University of Illinois, color blindness publication 111n
University of Maryland School of Medicine, contact information 681
University of Michigan Health System, publications
  pediatric chronic conditions 535n
  XXX syndrome 377n
University of Rochester Medical Center, contact information 682
UPD *see* paternal uniparental disomy
uracil, defined 653
urea cycle disorders (CPS), overview 184–87
uric acid, glycogen storage disease 138
urinary tract defects 417–23
"U.S. National Screening Status Report" (NNSGRC) 655n
US Food and Drug Administration (FDA), genetic metabolic disorders publication 216n
Usher syndrome *157*
Utah, newborn screening programs *665, 667*, 674

V

vaccines
  Haemophilus influenzae type b 102
  meningitis 102
  pneumonia 102
valproic acid *355*
velocardiofacial syndrome (VCFS) 319–21
venlafaxine *355*
ventricular septal defect (VSD) 443
Vermont, newborn screening programs *665, 667*, 674

vertical supranuclear gaze palsy (VSGP) 229
vigabatrin *355*
Virginia, newborn screening programs *665, 667*, 675
visual acuity, albinism 59
Von-Hippel-Lindau Family Alliance, contact information 709
von Recklinghausen's neurofibromatosis *see* neurofibromatosis type 1
von Willebrand disease (vWD) 87–89
VSD *see* ventricular septal defect
VSGP *see* vertical supranuclear gaze palsy
vWD *see* von Willebrand disease

W

Waardenburg syndrome *157*
warfarin 81
Washington, DC *see* District of Columbia
Washington state, newborn screening programs *665, 667*, 675
Waterston, Robert H. 599
Weill-Marchesani syndrome 154
Werdnig-Hoffman disease 273, 274
West Virginia, newborn screening programs *665, 667*, 675
"What are the Signs and Symptoms of NPD?" (National Niemann-Pick Disease Foundation) 226n
"What Causes Down Syndrome" (National Down Syndrome Society) 329n
What Every Family Should Know, 6th Edition (National Tay-Sachs and Allied Diseases Association) 236n
"What is a Genome?" (NCBI) 15n
"What is Cri du Chat Syndrome?" (Cri Du Chat Support Group of Australia, Inc.) 311n
"What Is Fanconi Anemia?" (Fanconi Anemia Research Fund, Inc.) 92n
"What Is Gaucher Disease" (National Gaucher Foundation) 210n

"What is Late Onset Tay-Sachs" (Late Onset Tay-Sachs Foundation) 236n
"What Is Niemann-Pick Disease?" (National Niemann-Pick Disease Foundation) 226n
"What is Williams Syndrome?" (Williams Syndrome Association) 387n
"What Treatment Is Available for NPD?" (National Niemann-Pick Disease Foundation) 226n
Williams, Roger 462
Williams syndrome 387–90
Williams Syndrome Association contact information 710
Williams syndrome publication 387n
Williams Syndrome Foundation, contact information 710
Wilson, Richard K. 599
Wilson disease 295–96
"Wilson's Disease" (NIDDK) 295n
Wilson's Disease Association, contact information 296, 710
Wisconsin, newborn screening programs *665, 667*, 676
Wolff-Parkinson-White syndrome 456–57
workplace discrimination legislation 561–63
World Federation of Hemophilia, contact information 697, 710
Wyoming, newborn screening programs *655, 667*, 676

X

X chromosome
adrenoleukodystrophy 191
Barth syndrome 250
Charcot-Marie-Tooth disease 254
defined 653
described 8–9, 300
Fabry disease 207
fragile X syndrome 344, 346–47
Rett syndrome 288
Turner syndrome 383–84
see also sex chromosomes

X chromosome monosomy 383
X chromosome mosaicism 383–84
xeroderma pigmentosa-Cockayne
syndrome 148
Xeroderma Pigmentosum Society,
contact information 710
Xian, Hong 496
X-inactivation
described 23
X-linked disorders
prenatal testing 519
X-linked dominant conditions
described *42*, 48–49
statistics 41
X-linked ocular albinism 65
X-linked recessive conditions
described *42*, 48–49
Pelizaeus-Merzbacher disease
195
statistics 43
"XXX Syndrome (Trisomy X)" (University of Michigan) 377n
XXY males *see* Klinefelter syndrome

Y

Yao, Wei-Dong 494
Y chromosome
analysis 599–601
defined 653
described 8–9, 300
see also sex chromosomes
Young, Richard A. 431
*Your Child: Development and Behavior
Resources* (University of Michigan)
377n, 535n

Z

Zavesca 233
Zellweger syndrome 197
Zickler, Patrick 495n
zinc acetate 296
zinc-finger protein, defined 653
Zoloft (sertraline) *355*
Zyprexa (olanzapine) *355*

Health Reference Series
COMPLETE CATALOG

Adolescent Health Sourcebook

Basic Consumer Health Information about Common Medical, Mental, and Emotional Concerns in Adolescents, Including Facts about Acne, Body Piercing, Mononucleosis, Nutrition, Eating Disorders, Stress, Depression, Behavior Problems, Peer Pressure, Violence, Gangs, Drug Use, Puberty, Sexuality, Pregnancy, Learning Disabilities, and More

Along with a Glossary of Terms and Other Resources for Further Help and Information

Edited by Chad T. Kimball. 658 pages. 2002. 0-7808-0248-9. $78.

"It is written in clear, nontechnical language aimed at general readers. . . . Recommended for public libraries, community colleges, and other agencies serving health care consumers."
—*American Reference Books Annual, 2003*

"Recommended for school and public libraries. Parents and professionals dealing with teens will appreciate the easy-to-follow format and the clearly written text. This could become a 'must have' for every high school teacher." —*E-Streams, Jan '03*

"A good starting point for information related to common medical, mental, and emotional concerns of adolescents." —*School Library Journal, Nov '02*

"This book provides accurate information in an easy to access format. It addresses topics that parents and caregivers might not be aware of and provides practical, useable information." —*Doody's Health Sciences Book Review Journal, Sep-Oct '02*

"Recommended reference source."
—*Booklist, American Library Association, Sep '02*

■

AIDS Sourcebook, 3rd Edition

Basic Consumer Health Information about Acquired Immune Deficiency Syndrome (AIDS) and Human Immunodeficiency Virus (HIV) Infection, Including Facts about Transmission, Prevention, Diagnosis, Treatment, Opportunistic Infections, and Other Complications, with a Section for Women and Children, Including Details about Associated Gynecological Concerns, Pregnancy, and Pediatric Care

Along with Updated Statistical Information, Reports on Current Research Initiatives, a Glossary, and Directories of Internet, Hotline, and Other Resources

Edited by Dawn D. Matthews. 664 pages. 2003. 0-7808-0631-X. $78.

ALSO AVAILABLE: AIDS Sourcebook, 1st Edition. Edited by Karen Bellenir and Peter D. Dresser. 831 pages. 1995. 0-7808-0031-1. $78.

AIDS Sourcebook, 2nd Edition. Edited by Karen Bellenir. 751 pages. 1999. 0-7808-0225-X. $78.

"The 3rd edition of the *AIDS Sourcebook*, part of Omnigraphics' *Health Reference Series*, is a welcome update. . . . This resource is highly recommended for academic and public libraries."
—*American Reference Books Annual, 2004*

"Excellent sourcebook. This continues to be a highly recommended book. There is no other book that provides as much information as this book provides."
—*AIDS Book Review Journal, Dec-Jan 2000*

"Recommended reference source."
—*Booklist, American Library Association, Dec '99*

"A solid text for college-level health libraries."
—*The Bookwatch, Aug '99*

Cited in *Reference Sources for Small and Medium-Sized Libraries, American Library Association, 1999*

■

Alcoholism Sourcebook

Basic Consumer Health Information about the Physical and Mental Consequences of Alcohol Abuse, Including Liver Disease, Pancreatitis, Wernicke-Korsakoff Syndrome (Alcoholic Dementia), Fetal Alcohol Syndrome, Heart Disease, Kidney Disorders, Gastrointestinal Problems, and Immune System Compromise and Featuring Facts about Addiction, Detoxification, Alcohol Withdrawal, Recovery, and the Maintenance of Sobriety

Along with a Glossary and Directories of Resources for Further Help and Information

Edited by Karen Bellenir. 613 pages. 2000. 0-7808-0325-6. $78.

"This title is one of the few reference works on alcoholism for general readers. For some readers this will be a welcome complement to the many self-help books on the market. Recommended for collections serving general readers and consumer health collections."
—*E-Streams, Mar '01*

"This book is an excellent choice for public and academic libraries."
—*American Reference Books Annual, 2001*

"Recommended reference source."
—*Booklist, American Library Association, Dec '00*

"Presents a wealth of information on alcohol use and abuse and its effects on the body and mind, treatment, and prevention." —*SciTech Book News, Dec '00*

"Important new health guide which packs in the latest consumer information about the problems of alcoholism." —*Reviewer's Bookwatch, Nov '00*

SEE ALSO Drug Abuse Sourcebook, Substance Abuse Sourcebook

753

Allergies Sourcebook, 2nd Edition

Basic Consumer Health Information about Allergic Disorders, Triggers, Reactions, and Related Symptoms, Including Anaphylaxis, Rhinitis, Sinusitis, Asthma, Dermatitis, Conjunctivitis, and Multiple Chemical Sensitivity

Along with Tips on Diagnosis, Prevention, and Treatment, Statistical Data, a Glossary, and a Directory of Sources for Further Help and Information

Edited by Annemarie S. Muth. 598 pages. 2002. 0-7808-0376-0. $78.

ALSO AVAILABLE: Allergies Sourcebook, 1st Edition. Edited by Allan R. Cook. 611 pages. 1997. 0-7808-0036-2. $78.

"This book brings a great deal of useful material together. . . . This is an excellent addition to public and consumer health library collections."
—American Reference Books Annual, 2003

"This second edition would be useful to laypersons with little or advanced knowledge of the subject matter. This book would also serve as a resource for nursing and other health care professions students. It would be useful in public, academic, and hospital libraries with consumer health collections."   —E-Streams, Jul '02

■

Alternative Medicine Sourcebook, 2nd Edition

Basic Consumer Health Information about Alternative and Complementary Medical Practices, Including Acupuncture, Chiropractic, Herbal Medicine, Homeopathy, Naturopathic Medicine, Mind-Body Interventions, Ayurveda, and Other Non-Western Medical Traditions

Along with Facts about such Specific Therapies as Massage Therapy, Aromatherapy, Qigong, Hypnosis, Prayer, Dance, and Art Therapies, a Glossary, and Resources for Further Information

Edited by Dawn D. Matthews. 618 pages. 2002. 0-7808-0605-0. $78.

ALSO AVAILABLE: Alternative Medicine Sourcebook, 1st Edition. Edited by Allan R. Cook. 737 pages. 1999. 0-7808-0200-4. $78.

"Recommended for public, high school, and academic libraries that have consumer health collections. Hospital libraries that also serve the public will find this to be a useful resource."   —E-Streams, Feb '03

"Recommended reference source."
—Booklist, American Library Association, Jan '03

"An important alternate health reference."
—MBR Bookwatch, Oct '02

"A great addition to the reference collection of every type of library." —American Reference Books Annual, 2000

Alzheimer's Disease Sourcebook, 3rd Edition

Basic Consumer Health Information about Alzheimer's Disease, Other Dementias, and Related Disorders, Including Multi-Infarct Dementia, AIDS Dementia Complex, Dementia with Lewy Bodies, Huntington's Disease, Wernicke-Korsakoff Syndrome (Alcohol-Reated Dementia), Delirium, and Confusional States

Along with Information for People Newly Diagnosed with Alzheimer's Disease and Caregivers, Reports Detailing Current Research Efforts in Prevention, Diagnosis, and Treatment, Facts about Long-Term Care Issues, and Listings of Sources for Additional Information

Edited by Karen Bellenir. 645 pages. 2003. 0-7808-0666-2. $78.

ALSO AVAILABLE: Alzheimer's, Stroke & 29 Other Neurological Disorders Sourcebook, 1st Edition. Edited by Frank E. Bair. 579 pages. 1993. 1-55888-748-2. $78.

ALSO AVAILABLE: Alzheimer's Disease Sourcebook, 2nd Edition. Edited by Karen Bellenir. 524 pages. 1999. 0-7808-0223-3. $78.

"This very informative and valuable tool will be a great addition to any library serving consumers, students and health care workers."
—American Reference Books Annual, 2004

"This is a valuable resource for people affected by dementias such as Alzheimer's. It is easy to navigate and includes important information and resources."
—Doody's Review Service, Feb. 2004

"Recommended reference source."
—Booklist, American Library Association, Oct '99

SEE ALSO Brain Disorders Sourcebook

■

Arthritis Sourcebook, 2nd Edition

Basic Consumer Health Information about Osteoarthritis, Rheumatoid Arthritis, Other Rheumatic Disorders, Infectious Forms of Arthritis, and Diseases with Symptoms Linked to Arthritis, Featuring Facts about Diagnosis, Pain Management, and Surgical Therapies

Along with Coping Strategies, Research Updates, a Glossary, and Resources for Additional Help and Information

Edited by Amy L. Sutton. 593 pages. 2004. 0-7808-0667-0. $78.

ALSO AVAILABLE: Arthritis Sourcebook, 1st Edition. Edited by Allan R. Cook. 550 pages. 1998. 0-7808-0201-2. $78.

". . . accessible to the layperson."
—Reference and Research Book News, Feb '99

Asthma Sourcebook

Basic Consumer Health Information about Asthma, Including Symptoms, Traditional and Nontraditional Remedies, Treatment Advances, Quality-of-Life Aids, Medical Research Updates, and the Role of Allergies, Exercise, Age, the Environment, and Genetics in the Development of Asthma

Along with Statistical Data, a Glossary, and Directories of Support Groups, and Other Resources for Further Information

Edited by Annemarie S. Muth. 628 pages. 2000. 0-7808-0381-7. $78.

"A worthwhile reference acquisition for public libraries and academic medical libraries whose readers desire a quick introduction to the wide range of asthma information." — *Choice, Association of College & Research Libraries, Jun '01*

"Recommended reference source." — *Booklist, American Library Association, Feb '01*

"Highly recommended." — *The Bookwatch, Jan '01*

"There is much good information for patients and their families who deal with asthma daily." — *American Medical Writers Association Journal, Winter '01*

"This informative text is recommended for consumer health collections in public, secondary school, and community college libraries and the libraries of universities with a large undergraduate population." — *American Reference Books Annual, 2001*

Attention Deficit Disorder Sourcebook

Basic Consumer Health Information about Attention Deficit/Hyperactivity Disorder in Children and Adults, Including Facts about Causes, Symptoms, Diagnostic Criteria, and Treatment Options Such as Medications, Behavior Therapy, Coaching, and Homeopathy

Along with Reports on Current Research Initiatives, Legal Issues, and Government Regulations, and Featuring a Glossary of Related Terms, Internet Resources, and a List of Additional Reading Material

Edited by Dawn D. Matthews. 470 pages. 2002. 0-7808-0624-7. $78.

"Recommended reference source." — *Booklist, American Library Association, Jan '03*

"This book is recommended for all school libraries and the reference or consumer health sections of public libraries." — *American Reference Books Annual, 2003*

Back & Neck Sourcebook, 2nd Edition

Basic Consumer Health Information about Spinal Pain, Spinal Cord Injuries, and Related Disorders, Such as Degenerative Disk Disease, Osteoarthritis, Scoliosis,

Sciatica, Spina Bifida, and Spinal Stenosis, and Featuring Facts about Maintaining Spinal Health, Self-Care, Pain Management, Rehabilitative Care, Chiropractic Care, Spinal Surgeries, and Complementary Therapies

Along with Suggestions for Preventing Back and Neck Pain, a Glossary of Related Terms, and a Directory of Resources

Edited by Amy L. Sutton. 600 pages. 2004. 0-7808-0738-3 $78.

ALSO AVAILABLE: *Back & Neck Disorders Sourcebook, 1st Edition.* Edited by Karen Bellenir. 548 pages. 1997. 0-7808-0202-0. $78.

"The strength of this work is its basic, easy-to-read format. Recommended." — *Reference and User Services Quarterly, American Library Association, Winter '97*

Blood & Circulatory Disorders Sourcebook

Basic Information about Blood and Its Components, Anemias, Leukemias, Bleeding Disorders, and Circulatory Disorders, Including Aplastic Anemia, Thalassemia, Sickle-Cell Disease, Hemochromatosis, Hemophilia, Von Willebrand Disease, and Vascular Diseases

Along with a Special Section on Blood Transfusions and Blood Supply Safety, a Glossary, and Source Listings for Further Help and Information

Edited by Karen Bellenir and Linda M. Shin. 554 pages. 1998. 0-7808-0203-9. $78.

"Recommended reference source." — *Booklist, American Library Association, Feb '99*

"An important reference sourcebook written in simple language for everyday, non-technical users. " — *Reviewer's Bookwatch, Jan '99*

Brain Disorders Sourcebook

Basic Consumer Health Information about Strokes, Epilepsy, Amyotrophic Lateral Sclerosis (ALS/Lou Gehrig's Disease), Parkinson's Disease, Brain Tumors, Cerebral Palsy, Headache, Tourette Syndrome, and More

Along with Statistical Data, Treatment and Rehabilitation Options, Coping Strategies, Reports on Current Research Initiatives, a Glossary, and Resource Listings for Additional Help and Information

Edited by Karen Bellenir. 481 pages. 1999. 0-7808-0229-2. $78.

"Belongs on the shelves of any library with a consumer health collection." — *E-Streams, Mar '00*

"Recommended reference source." — *Booklist, American Library Association, Oct '99*

SEE ALSO *Alzheimer's Disease Sourcebook*

Breast Cancer Sourcebook, 2nd Edition

Basic Consumer Health Information about Breast Cancer, Including Facts about Risk Factors, Prevention, Screening and Diagnostic Methods, Treatment Options, Complementary and Alternative Therapies, Post-Treatment Concerns, Clinical Trials, Special Risk Populations, and New Developments in Breast Cancer Research

Along with Breast Cancer Statistics, a Glossary of Related Terms, and a Directory of Resources for Additional Help and Information

Edited by Sandra J. Judd. 600 pages. 2004. 0-7808-0668-9. $78.

ALSO AVAILABLE: Breast Cancer Sourcebook, 1st Edition. Edited by Edward J. Prucha and Karen Bellenir. 580 pages. 2001. 0-7808-0244-6. $78.

"It would be a useful reference book in a library or on loan to women in a support group."
— *Cancer Forum, Mar '03*

"Recommended reference source."
— *Booklist, American Library Association, Jan '02*

"This reference source is highly recommended. It is quite informative, comprehensive and detailed in nature, and yet it offers practical advice in easy-to-read language. It could be thought of as the 'bible' of breast cancer for the consumer." — *E-Streams, Jan '02*

"The broad range of topics covered in lay language make the *Breast Cancer Sourcebook* an excellent addition to public and consumer health library collections."
— *American Reference Books Annual 2002*

"From the pros and cons of different screening methods and results to treatment options, *Breast Cancer Sourcebook* provides the latest information on the subject."
— *Library Bookwatch, Dec '01*

"This thoroughgoing, very readable reference covers all aspects of breast health and cancer.... Readers will find much to consider here. Recommended for all public and patient health collections."
— *Library Journal, Sep '01*

SEE ALSO Cancer Sourcebook for Women, Women's Health Concerns Sourcebook

Breastfeeding Sourcebook

Basic Consumer Health Information about the Benefits of Breastmilk, Preparing to Breastfeed, Breastfeeding as a Baby Grows, Nutrition, and More, Including Information on Special Situations and Concerns Such as Mastitis, Illness, Medications, Allergies, Multiple Births, Prematurity, Special Needs, and Adoption

Along with a Glossary and Resources for Additional Help and Information

Edited by Jenni Lynn Colson. 388 pages. 2002. 0-7808-0332-9. $78.

SEE ALSO Pregnancy & Birth Sourcebook

"Particularly useful is the information about professional lactation services and chapters on breastfeeding

when returning to work.... *Breastfeeding Sourcebook* will be useful for public libraries, consumer health libraries, and technical schools offering nurse assistant training, especially in areas where Internet access is problematic."
— *American Reference Books Annual, 2003*

Burns Sourcebook

Basic Consumer Health Information about Various Types of Burns and Scalds, Including Flame, Heat, Cold, Electrical, Chemical, and Sun Burns

Along with Information on Short-Term and Long-Term Treatments, Tissue Reconstruction, Plastic Surgery, Prevention Suggestions, and First Aid

Edited by Allan R. Cook. 604 pages. 1999. 0-7808-0204-7. $78.

"This is an exceptional addition to the series and is highly recommended for all consumer health collections, hospital libraries, and academic medical centers."
— *E-Streams, Mar '00*

"This key reference guide is an invaluable addition to all health care and public libraries in confronting this ongoing health issue."
— *American Reference Books Annual, 2000*

"Recommended reference source."
— *Booklist, American Library Association, Dec '99*

SEE ALSO Skin Disorders Sourcebook

Cancer Sourcebook, 4th Edition

Basic Consumer Health Information about Major Forms and Stages of Cancer, Featuring Facts about Head and Neck Cancers, Lung Cancers, Gastrointestinal Cancers, Genitourinary Cancers, Lymphomas, Blood Cell Cancers, Endocrine Cancers, Skin Cancers, Bone Cancers, Sarcomas, and Others, and Including Information about Cancer Treatments and Therapies, Identifying and Reducing Cancer Risks, and Strategies for Coping with Cancer and the Side Effects of Treatment

Along with a Cancer Glossary, Statistical and Demographic Data, and a Directory of Sources for Additional Help and Information

Edited by Karen Bellenir. 1,119 pages. 2003. 0-7808-0633-6. $78.

ALSO AVAILABLE: Cancer Sourcebook, 1st Edition. Edited by Frank E. Bair. 932 pages. 1990. 1-55888-888-8. $78.

New Cancer Sourcebook, 2nd Edition. Edited by Allan R. Cook. 1,313 pages. 1996. 0-7808-0041-9. $78.

Cancer Sourcebook, 3rd Edition. Edited by Edward J. Prucha. 1,069 pages. 2000. 0-7808-0227-6. $78.

"With cancer being the second leading cause of death for Americans, a prodigious work such as this one, which locates centrally so much cancer-related information, is clearly an asset to this nation's citizens and others." — *Journal of the National Medical Association, 2004*

"This title is recommended for health sciences and public libraries with consumer health collections."
— *E-Streams, Feb '01*

"... can be effectively used by cancer patients and their families who are looking for answers in a language they can understand. Public and hospital libraries should have it on their shelves."
— *American Reference Books Annual, 2001*

"Recommended reference source."
— *Booklist, American Library Association, Dec '00*

Cited in *Reference Sources for Small and Medium-Sized Libraries, American Library Association, 1999*

"The amount of factual and useful information is extensive. The writing is very clear, geared to general readers. Recommended for all levels." — *Choice, Association of College & Research Libraries, Jan '97*

SEE ALSO Breast Cancer Sourcebook, Cancer Sourcebook for Women, Pediatric Cancer Sourcebook, Prostate Cancer Sourcebook

Cancer Sourcebook for Women, 2nd Edition

Basic Consumer Health Information about Gynecologic Cancers and Related Concerns, Including Cervical Cancer, Endometrial Cancer, Gestational Trophoblastic Tumor, Ovarian Cancer, Uterine Cancer, Vaginal Cancer, Vulvar Cancer, Breast Cancer, and Common Non-Cancerous Uterine Conditions, with Facts about Cancer Risk Factors, Screening and Prevention, Treatment Options, and Reports on Current Research Initiatives

Along with a Glossary of Cancer Terms and a Directory of Resources for Additional Help and Information

Edited by Karen Bellenir. 604 pages. 2002. 0-7808-0226-8. $78.

ALSO AVAILABLE: Cancer Sourcebook for Women, 1st Edition. Edited by Allan R. Cook and Peter D. Dresser. 524 pages. 1996. 0-7808-0076-1. $78.

"An excellent addition to collections in public, consumer health, and women's health libraries."
— *American Reference Books Annual, 2003*

"Overall, the information is excellent, and complex topics are clearly explained. As a reference book for the consumer it is a valuable resource to assist them to make informed decisions about cancer and its treatments." — *Cancer Forum, Nov '02*

"Highly recommended for academic and medical reference collections." — *Library Bookwatch, Sep '02*

"This is a highly recommended book for any public or consumer library, being reader friendly and containing accurate and helpful information."
— *E-Streams, Aug '02*

"Recommended reference source."
— *Booklist, American Library Association, Jul '02*

SEE ALSO Breast Cancer Sourcebook, Women's Health Concerns Sourcebook

Cardiovascular Diseases & Disorders Sourcebook, 1st Edition

SEE Heart Diseases & Disorders Sourcebook, 2nd Edition

Caregiving Sourcebook

Basic Consumer Health Information for Caregivers, Including a Profile of Caregivers, Caregiving Responsibilities and Concerns, Tips for Specific Conditions, Care Environments, and the Effects of Caregiving

Along with Facts about Legal Issues, Financial Information, and Future Planning, a Glossary, and a Listing of Additional Resources

Edited by Joyce Brennfleck Shannon. 600 pages. 2001. 0-7808-0331-0. $78.

"Essential for most collections."
— *Library Journal, Apr 1, 2002*

"An ideal addition to the reference collection of any public library. Health sciences information professionals may also want to acquire the *Caregiving Sourcebook* for their hospital or academic library for use as a ready reference tool by health care workers interested in aging and caregiving." — *E-Streams, Jan '02*

"Recommended reference source."
— *Booklist, American Library Association, Oct '01*

Child Abuse Sourcebook

Basic Consumer Health Information about the Physical, Sexual, and Emotional Abuse of Children, with Additional Facts about Neglect, Munchausen Syndrome by Proxy (MSBP), Shaken Baby Syndrome, and Controversial Issues Related to Child Abuse, Such as Withholding Medical Care, Corporal Punishment, and Child Maltreatment in Youth Sports, and Featuring Facts about Child Protective Services, Foster Care, Adoption, Parenting Challenges, and Other Abuse Prevention Efforts

Along with a Glossary of Related Terms and Resources for Additional Help and Information

Edited by Dawn D. Matthews. 620 pages. 2004. 0-7808-0705-7. $78.

Childhood Diseases & Disorders Sourcebook

Basic Consumer Health Information about Medical Problems Often Encountered in Pre-Adolescent Children, Including Respiratory Tract Ailments, Ear Infections, Sore Throats, Disorders of the Skin and Scalp, Digestive and Genitourinary Diseases, Infectious Diseases, Inflammatory Disorders, Chronic Physical and Developmental Disorders, Allergies, and More

Along with Information about Diagnostic Tests, Common Childhood Surgeries, and Frequently Used Medications, with a Glossary of Important Terms and Resource Directory

Edited by Chad T. Kimball. 662 pages. 2003. 0-7808-0458-9. $78.

"This is an excellent book for new parents and should be included in all health care and public libraries."
—*American Reference Books Annual, 2004*

Colds, Flu & Other Common Ailments Sourcebook

Basic Consumer Health Information about Common Ailments and Injuries, Including Colds, Coughs, the Flu, Sinus Problems, Headaches, Fever, Nausea and Vomiting, Menstrual Cramps, Diarrhea, Constipation, Hemorrhoids, Back Pain, Dandruff, Dry and Itchy Skin, Cuts, Scrapes, Sprains, Bruises, and More

Along with Information about Prevention, Self-Care, Choosing a Doctor, Over-the-Counter Medications, Folk Remedies, and Alternative Therapies, and Including a Glossary of Important Terms and a Directory of Resources for Further Help and Information

Edited by Chad T. Kimball. 638 pages. 2001. 0-7808-0435-X. $78.

"A good starting point for research on common illnesses. It will be a useful addition to public and consumer health library collections."
—*American Reference Books Annual 2002*

"Will prove valuable to any library seeking to maintain a current, comprehensive reference collection of health resources. . . . Excellent reference."
—*The Bookwatch, Aug '01*

"Recommended reference source."
—*Booklist, American Library Association, July '01*

Communication Disorders Sourcebook

Basic Information about Deafness and Hearing Loss, Speech and Language Disorders, Voice Disorders, Balance and Vestibular Disorders, and Disorders of Smell, Taste, and Touch

Edited by Linda M. Ross. 533 pages. 1996. 0-7808-0077-X. $78.

"This is skillfully edited and is a welcome resource for the layperson. It should be found in every public and medical library."
—*Booklist Health Sciences Supplement, American Library Association, Oct '97*

Congenital Disorders Sourcebook

Basic Information about Disorders Acquired during Gestation, Including Spina Bifida, Hydrocephalus, Cerebral Palsy, Heart Defects, Craniofacial Abnormalities, Fetal Alcohol Syndrome, and More

Along with Current Treatment Options and Statistical Data

Edited by Karen Bellenir. 607 pages. 1997. 0-7808-0205-5. $78.

"Recommended reference source."
—*Booklist, American Library Association, Oct '97*

SEE ALSO *Pregnancy & Birth Sourcebook*

Consumer Issues in Health Care Sourcebook

Basic Information about Health Care Fundamentals and Related Consumer Issues, Including Exams and Screening Tests, Physician Specialties, Choosing a Doctor, Using Prescription and Over-the-Counter Medications Safely, Avoiding Health Scams, Managing Common Health Risks in the Home, Care Options for Chronically or Terminally Ill Patients, and a List of Resources for Obtaining Help and Further Information

Edited by Karen Bellenir. 618 pages. 1998. 0-7808-0221-7. $78.

"Both public and academic libraries will want to have a copy in their collection for readers who are interested in self-education on health issues."
—*American Reference Books Annual, 2000*

"The editor has researched the literature from government agencies and others, saving readers the time and effort of having to do the research themselves. Recommended for public libraries."
—*Reference and User Services Quarterly, American Library Association, Spring '99*

"Recommended reference source."
—*Booklist, American Library Association, Dec '98*

Contagious Diseases Sourcebook

Basic Consumer Health Information about Infectious Diseases Spread by Person-to-Person Contact through Direct Touch, Airborne Transmission, Sexual Contact, or Contact with Blood or Other Body Fluids, Including Hepatitis, Herpes, Influenza, Lice, Measles, Mumps, Pinworm, Ringworm, Severe Acute Respiratory Syndrome (SARS), Streptococcal Infections, Tuberculosis, and Others

Along with Facts about Disease Transmission, Antimicrobial Resistance, and Vaccines, with a Glossary and Directories of Resources for More Information

Edited by Karen Bellenir. 643 pages. 2004. 0-7808-0736-7. $78.

Contagious & Non-Contagious Infectious Diseases Sourcebook

Basic Information about Contagious Diseases like Measles, Polio, Hepatitis B, and Infectious Mononucleosis, and Non-Contagious Infectious Diseases like Tetanus and Toxic Shock Syndrome, and Diseases Occurring as Secondary Infections Such as Shingles and Reye Syndrome

Along with Vaccination, Prevention, and Treatment Information, and a Section Describing Emerging Infectious Disease Threats

Edited by Karen Bellenir and Peter D. Dresser. 566 pages. 1996. 0-7808-0075-3. $78.

Death & Dying Sourcebook

Basic Consumer Health Information for the Layperson about End-of-Life Care and Related Ethical and Legal Issues, Including Chief Causes of Death, Autopsies, Pain Management for the Terminally Ill, Life Support Systems, Insurance, Euthanasia, Assisted Suicide, Hospice Programs, Living Wills, Funeral Planning, Counseling, Mourning, Organ Donation, and Physician Training

Along with Statistical Data, a Glossary, and Listings of Sources for Further Help and Information

Edited by Annemarie S. Muth. 641 pages. 1999. 0-7808-0230-6. $78.

"Public libraries, medical libraries, and academic libraries will all find this sourcebook a useful addition to their collections."
— *American Reference Books Annual, 2001*

"An extremely useful resource for those concerned with death and dying in the United States."
— *Respiratory Care, Nov '00*

"Recommended reference source."
— *Booklist, American Library Association, Aug '00*

"This book is a definite must for all those involved in end-of-life care." — *Doody's Review Service, 2000*

■

Dental Care & Oral Health Sourcebook, 2nd Edition

Basic Consumer Health Information about Dental Care, Including Oral Hygiene, Dental Visits, Pain Management, Cavities, Crowns, Bridges, Dental Implants, and Fillings, and Other Oral Health Concerns, Such as Gum Disease, Bad Breath, Dry Mouth, Genetic and Developmental Abnormalities, Oral Cancers, Orthodontics, and Temporomandibular Disorders

Along with Updates on Current Research in Oral Health, a Glossary, a Directory of Dental and Oral Health Organizations, and Resources for People with Dental and Oral Health Disorders

Edited by Amy L. Sutton. 609 pages. 2003. 0-7808-0634-4. $78.

ALSO AVAILABLE: *Oral Health Sourcebook, 1st Edition.* Edited by Allan R. Cook. 558 pages. 1997. 0-7808-0082-6. $78.

"This book could serve as a turning point in the battle to educate consumers in issues concerning oral health."
— *American Reference Books Annual, 2004*

"Unique source which will fill a gap in dental sources for patients and the lay public. A valuable reference tool even in a library with thousands of books on dentistry. Comprehensive, clear, inexpensive, and easy to read and use. It fills an enormous gap in the health care literature." — *Reference and User Services Quarterly, American Library Association, Summer '98*

"Recommended reference source."
— *Booklist, American Library Association, Dec '97*

Depression Sourcebook

Basic Consumer Health Information about Unipolar Depression, Bipolar Disorder, Postpartum Depression, Seasonal Affective Disorder, and Other Types of Depression in Children, Adolescents, Women, Men, the Elderly, and Other Selected Populations

Along with Facts about Causes, Risk Factors, Diagnostic Criteria, Treatment Options, Coping Strategies, Suicide Prevention, a Glossary, and a Directory of Sources for Additional Help and Information

Edited by Karen Belleni. 602 pages. 2002. 0-7808-0611-5. $78.

"*Depression Sourcebook* is of a very high standard. Its purpose, which is to serve as a reference source to the lay reader, is very well served."
— *Journal of the National Medical Association, 2004*

"Invaluable reference for public and school library collections alike." — *Library Bookwatch, Apr '03*

"Recommended for purchase."
— *American Reference Books Annual, 2003*

■

Diabetes Sourcebook, 3rd Edition

Basic Consumer Health Information about Type 1 Diabetes (Insulin-Dependent or Juvenile-Onset Diabetes), Type 2 Diabetes (Noninsulin-Dependent or Adult-Onset Diabetes), Gestational Diabetes, Impaired Glucose Tolerance (IGT), and Related Complications, Such as Amputation, Eye Disease, Gum Disease, Nerve Damage, and End-Stage Renal Disease, Including Facts about Insulin, Oral Diabetes Medications, Blood Sugar Testing, and the Role of Exercise and Nutrition in the Control of Diabetes

Along with a Glossary and Resources for Further Help and Information

Edited by Dawn D. Matthews. 622 pages. 2003. 0-7808-0629-8. $78.

ALSO AVAILABLE: *Diabetes Sourcebook, 1st Edition.* Edited by Karen Bellenir and Peter D. Dresser. 827 pages. 1994. 1-55888-751-2. $78.

Diabetes Sourcebook, 2nd Edition. Edited by Karen Bellenir. 688 pages. 1998. 0-7808-0224-1. $78.

"This edition is even more helpful than earlier versions. . . . It is a truly valuable tool for anyone seeking readable and authoritative information on diabetes."
— *American Reference Books Annual, 2004*

"An invaluable reference." — *Library Journal, May '00*

Selected as one of the 250 "Best Health Sciences Books of 1999." — *Doody's Rating Service, Mar-Apr 2000*

"Provides useful information for the general public."
— *Healthlines, University of Michigan Health Management Research Center, Sep/Oct '99*

". . . provides reliable mainstream medical information . . . belongs on the shelves of any library with a consumer health collection." — *E-Streams, Sep '99*

"Recommended reference source."
— *Booklist, American Library Association, Feb '99*

Diet & Nutrition Sourcebook, 2nd Edition

Basic Consumer Health Information about Dietary Guidelines, Recommended Daily Intake Values, Vitamins, Minerals, Fiber, Fat, Weight Control, Dietary Supplements, and Food Additives

Along with Special Sections on Nutrition Needs throughout Life and Nutrition for People with Such Specific Medical Concerns as Allergies, High Blood Cholesterol, Hypertension, Diabetes, Celiac Disease, Seizure Disorders, Phenylketonuria (PKU), Cancer, and Eating Disorders, and Including Reports on Current Nutrition Research and Source Listings for Additional Help and Information

Edited by Karen Bellenir. 650 pages. 1999. 0-7808-0228-4. $78.

ALSO AVAILABLE: Diet & Nutrition Sourcebook, 1st Edition. Edited by Dan R. Harris. 662 pages. 1996. 0-7808-0084-2. $78.

"This book is an excellent source of basic diet and nutrition information." *— Booklist Health Sciences Supplement, American Library Association, Dec '00*

"This reference document should be in any public library, but it would be a very good guide for beginning students in the health sciences. If the other books in this publisher's series are as good as this, they should all be in the health sciences collections."
—American Reference Books Annual, 2000

"This book is an excellent general nutrition reference for consumers who desire to take an active role in their health care for prevention. Consumers of all ages who select this book can feel confident they are receiving current and accurate information." *—Journal of Nutrition for the Elderly, Vol. 19, No. 4, '00*

"Recommended reference source."
—Booklist, American Library Association, Dec '99

SEE ALSO Digestive Diseases & Disorders Sourcebook, Eating Disorders Sourcebook, Gastrointestinal Diseases & Disorders Sourcebook, Vegetarian Sourcebook

■

Digestive Diseases & Disorders Sourcebook

Basic Consumer Health Information about Diseases and Disorders that Impact the Upper and Lower Digestive System, Including Celiac Disease, Constipation, Crohn's Disease, Cyclic Vomiting Syndrome, Diarrhea, Diverticulosis and Diverticulitis, Gallstones, Heartburn, Hemorrhoids, Hernias, Indigestion (Dyspepsia), Irritable Bowel Syndrome, Lactose Intolerance, Ulcers, and More

Along with Information about Medications and Other Treatments, Tips for Maintaining a Healthy Digestive Tract, a Glossary, and Directory of Digestive Diseases Organizations

Edited by Karen Bellenir. 335 pages. 2000. 0-7808-0327-2. $78.

"This title would be an excellent addition to all public or patient-research libraries."
—American Reference Books Annual, 2001

"This title is recommended for public, hospital, and health sciences libraries with consumer health collections." *—E-Streams, Jul-Aug '00*

"Recommended reference source."
—Booklist, American Library Association, May '00

SEE ALSO Diet & Nutrition Sourcebook, Eating Disorders Sourcebook, Gastrointestinal Diseases & Disorders Sourcebook

■

Disabilities Sourcebook

Basic Consumer Health Information about Physical and Psychiatric Disabilities, Including Descriptions of Major Causes of Disability, Assistive and Adaptive Aids, Workplace Issues, and Accessibility Concerns

Along with Information about the Americans with Disabilities Act, a Glossary, and Resources for Additional Help and Information

Edited by Dawn D. Matthews. 616 pages. 2000. 0-7808-0389-2. $78.

"It is a must for libraries with a consumer health section." *— American Reference Books Annual 2002*

"A much needed addition to the Omnigraphics *Health Reference Series.* A current reference work to provide people with disabilities, their families, caregivers or those who work with them, a broad range of information in one volume, has not been available until now. . . . It is recommended for all public and academic library reference collections." *— E-Streams, May '01*

"An excellent source book in easy-to-read format covering many current topics; highly recommended for all libraries." *— Choice, Association of College and Research Libraries, Jan '01*

"Recommended reference source."
—Booklist, American Library Association, Jul '00

■

Domestic Violence Sourcebook, 2nd Edition

Basic Consumer Health Information about the Causes and Consequences of Abusive Relationships, Including Physical Violence, Sexual Assault, Battery, Stalking, and Emotional Abuse, and Facts about the Effects of Violence on Women, Men, Young Adults, and the Elderly, with Reports about Domestic Violence in Selected Populations, and Featuring Facts about Medical Care, Victim Assistance and Protection, Prevention Strategies, Mental Health Services, and Legal Issues

Along with a Glossary of Related Terms and Resources for Additional Help and Information

Edited by Dawn D. Matthews. 628 pages. 2004. 0-7808-0669-7. $78.

ALSO AVAILABLE: Domestic Violence & Child Abuse Sourcebook, 1st Edition. Edited by Helene Henderson. 1,064 pages. 2001. 0-7808-0235-7. $78.

"Interested lay persons should find the book extremely beneficial. . . . A copy of *Domestic Violence and Child Abuse Sourcebook* should be in every public library in the United States."
— *Social Science & Medicine, No. 56, 2003*

"This is important information. The Web has many resources but this sourcebook fills an important societal need. I am not aware of any other resources of this type." — *Doody's Review Service, Sep '01*

"Recommended for all libraries, scholars, and practitioners." — *Choice, Association of College & Research Libraries, Jul '01*

"Recommended reference source."
— *Booklist, American Library Association, Apr '01*

"Important pick for college-level health reference libraries." — *The Bookwatch, Mar '01*

"Because this problem is so widespread and because this book includes a lot of issues within one volume, this work is recommended for all public libraries."
— *American Reference Books Annual, 2001*

■

Drug Abuse Sourcebook, 2nd Edition

Basic Consumer Health Information about Illicit Substances of Abuse and the Misuse of Prescription and Over-the-Counter Medications, Including Depressants, Hallucinogens, Inhalants, Marijuana, Stimulants, and Anabolic Steroids

Along with Facts about Related Health Risks, Treatment Programs, Prevention Programs, a Glossary of Abuse and Addiction Terms, a Glossary of Drug-Related Street Terms, and a Directory Resources for More Information

Edited by Catherine Ginther. 600 pages. 2004. 0-7808-0740-5. $78.

ALSO AVAILABLE: Drug Abuse Sourcebook, 1st Edition. Edited by Karen Bellenir. 629 pages. 2000. 0-7808-0242-X. $78.

"Containing a wealth of information . . . . This resource belongs in libraries that serve a lower-division under-graduate or community college clientele as well as the general public." — *Choice, Association of College and Research Libraries, Jun '01*

"Recommended reference source."
— *Booklist, American Library Association, Feb '01*

"Highly recommended." — *The Bookwatch, Jan '01*

"Even though there is a plethora of books on drug abuse, this volume is recommended for school, public, and college libraries."
— *American Reference Books Annual, 2001*

SEE ALSO Alcoholism Sourcebook, Substance Abuse Sourcebook

Ear, Nose & Throat Disorders Sourcebook

Basic Information about Disorders of the Ears, Nose, Sinus Cavities, Pharynx, and Larynx, Including Ear Infections, Tinnitus, Vestibular Disorders, Allergic and Non-Allergic Rhinitis, Sore Throats, Tonsillitis, and Cancers That Affect the Ears, Nose, Sinuses, and Throat

Along with Reports on Current Research Initiatives, a Glossary of Related Medical Terms, and a Directory of Sources for Further Help and Information

Edited by Karen Bellenir and Linda M. Shin. 576 pages. 1998. 0-7808-0206-3. $78.

"Overall, this sourcebook is helpful for the consumer seeking information on ENT issues. It is recommended for public libraries."
— *American Reference Books Annual, 1999*

"Recommended reference source."
— *Booklist, American Library Association, Dec '98*

■

Eating Disorders Sourcebook

Basic Consumer Health Information about Eating Disorders, Including Information about Anorexia Nervosa, Bulimia Nervosa, Binge Eating, Body Dysmorphic Disorder, Pica, Laxative Abuse, and Night Eating Syndrome

Along with Information about Causes, Adverse Effects, and Treatment and Prevention Issues, and Featuring a Section on Concerns Specific to Children and Adolescents, a Glossary, and Resources for Further Help and Information

Edited by Dawn D. Matthews. 322 pages. 2001. 0-7808-0335-3. $78.

"Recommended for health science libraries that are open to the public, as well as hospital libraries. This book is a good resource for the consumer who is concerned about eating disorders." — *E-Streams, Mar '02*

"This volume is another convenient collection of excerpted articles. Recommended for school and public library patrons; lower-division undergraduates; and two-year technical program students." — *Choice, Association of College & Research Libraries, Jan '02*

"Recommended reference source." — *Booklist, American Library Association, Oct '01*

SEE ALSO Diet & Nutrition Sourcebook, Digestive Diseases & Disorders Sourcebook, Gastrointestinal Diseases & Disorders Sourcebook

■

Emergency Medical Services Sourcebook

Basic Consumer Health Information about Preventing, Preparing for, and Managing Emergency Situations, When and Who to Call for Help, What to Expect in the Emergency Room, the Emergency Medical Team, Patient Issues, and Current Topics in Emergency Medicine

Along with Statistical Data, a Glossary, and Sources of Additional Help and Information

Edited by Jenni Lynn Colson. 494 pages. 2002. 0-7808-0420-1. $78.

"Handy and convenient for home, public, school, and college libraries. Recommended."
— *Choice, Association of College and Research Libraries, Apr '03*

"This reference can provide the consumer with answers to most questions about emergency care in the United States, or it will direct them to a resource where the answer can be found."
— *American Reference Books Annual, 2003*

"Recommended reference source."
— *Booklist, American Library Association, Feb '03*

Endocrine & Metabolic Disorders Sourcebook

Basic Information for the Layperson about Pancreatic and Insulin-Related Disorders Such as Pancreatitis, Diabetes, and Hypoglycemia; Adrenal Gland Disorders Such as Cushing's Syndrome, Addison's Disease, and Congenital Adrenal Hyperplasia; Pituitary Gland Disorders Such as Growth Hormone Deficiency, Acromegaly, and Pituitary Tumors; Thyroid Disorders Such as Hypothyroidism, Graves' Disease, Hashimoto's Disease, and Goiter; Hyperparathyroidism; and Other Diseases and Syndromes of Hormone Imbalance or Metabolic Dysfunction

Along with Reports on Current Research Initiatives

Edited by Linda M. Shin. 574 pages. 1998. 0-7808-0207-1. $78.

"Omnigraphics has produced another needed resource for health information consumers."
— *American Reference Books Annual, 2000*

"Recommended reference source."
— *Booklist, American Library Association, Dec '98*

Environmental Health Sourcebook, 2nd Edition

Basic Consumer Health Information about the Environment and Its Effect on Human Health, Including the Effects of Air Pollution, Water Pollution, Hazardous Chemicals, Food Hazards, Radiation Hazards, Biological Agents, Household Hazards, Such as Radon, Asbestos, Carbon Monoxide, and Mold, and Information about Associated Diseases and Disorders, Including Cancer, Allergies, Respiratory Problems, and Skin Disorders

Along with Information about Environmental Concerns for Specific Populations, a Glossary of Related Terms, and Resources for Further Help and Information

Edited by Dawn D. Matthews. 673 pages. 2003. 0-7808-0632-8. $78.

ALSO AVAILABLE: Environmentally Induced Disorders Sourcebook, 1st Edition. Edited by Allan R. Cook. 620 pages. 1997. 0-7808-0083-4. $78.

"This recently updated edition continues the level of quality and the reputation of the numerous other volumes in Omnigraphics' *Health Reference Series*."
— *American Reference Books Annual, 2004*

"Recommended reference source."
— *Booklist, American Library Association, Sep '98*

"This book will be a useful addition to anyone's library."
— *Choice Health Sciences Supplement, Association of College and Research Libraries, May '98*

". . . a good survey of numerous environmentally induced physical disorders . . . a useful addition to anyone's library."
— *Doody's Health Sciences Book Reviews, Jan '98*

". . . provide[s] introductory information from the best authorities around. Since this volume covers topics that potentially affect everyone, it will surely be one of the most frequently consulted volumes in the *Health Reference Series*." — *Rettig on Reference, Nov '97*

Environmentally Induced Disorders Sourcebook, 1st Edition

SEE Environmental Health Sourcebook, 2nd Edition

Ethnic Diseases Sourcebook

Basic Consumer Health Information for Ethnic and Racial Minority Groups in the United States, Including General Health Indicators and Behaviors, Ethnic Diseases, Genetic Testing, the Impact of Chronic Diseases, Women's Health, Mental Health Issues, and Preventive Health Care Services

Along with a Glossary and a Listing of Additional Resources

Edited by Joyce Brennfleck Shannon. 664 pages. 2001. 0-7808-0336-1. $78.

"Recommended for health sciences libraries where public health programs are a priority."
— *E-Streams, Jan '02*

"Not many books have been written on this topic to date, and the *Ethnic Diseases Sourcebook* is a strong addition to the list. It will be an important introductory resource for health consumers, students, health care personnel, and social scientists. It is recommended for public, academic, and large hospital libraries."
— *American Reference Books Annual 2002*

"Recommended reference source."
— *Booklist, American Library Association, Oct '01*

"Will prove valuable to any library seeking to maintain a current, comprehensive reference collection of health resources. . . . An excellent source of health information about genetic disorders which affect particular ethnic and racial minorities in the U.S."
— *The Bookwatch, Aug '01*

Eye Care Sourcebook, 2nd Edition

Basic Consumer Health Information about Eye Care and Eye Disorders, Including Facts about the Diagnosis, Prevention, and Treatment of Common Refractive Problems Such as Myopia, Hyperopia, Astigmatism, and Presbyopia, and Eye Diseases, Including Glaucoma, Cataract, Age-Related Macular Degeneration, and Diabetic Retinopathy

Along with a Section on Vision Correction and Refractive Surgeries, Including LASIK and LASEK, a Glossary, and Directories of Resources for Additional Help and Information

Edited by Amy L. Sutton. 543 pages. 2003. 0-7808-0635-2. $78.

ALSO AVAILABLE: Ophthalmic Disorders Sourcebook, 1st Edition. Edited by Linda M. Ross. 631 pages. 1996. 0-7808-0081-8. $78.

". . . a solid reference tool for eye care and a valuable addition to a collection."
— *American Reference Books Annual, 2004*

■

Family Planning Sourcebook

Basic Consumer Health Information about Planning for Pregnancy and Contraception, Including Traditional Methods, Barrier Methods, Hormonal Methods, Permanent Methods, Future Methods, Emergency Contraception, and Birth Control Choices for Women at Each Stage of Life

Along with Statistics, a Glossary, and Sources of Additional Information

Edited by Amy Marcaccio Keyzer. 520 pages. 2001. 0-7808-0379-5. $78.

"Recommended for public, health, and undergraduate libraries as part of the circulating collection."
— *E-Streams, Mar '02*

"Information is presented in an unbiased, readable manner, and the sourcebook will certainly be a necessary addition to those public and high school libraries where Internet access is restricted or otherwise problematic." — *American Reference Books Annual 2002*

"Recommended reference source."
— *Booklist, American Library Association, Oct '01*

"Will prove valuable to any library seeking to maintain a current, comprehensive reference collection of health resources. . . . Excellent reference."
— *The Bookwatch, Aug '01*

SEE ALSO Pregnancy & Birth Sourcebook

■

Fitness & Exercise Sourcebook, 2nd Edition

Basic Consumer Health Information about the Fundamentals of Fitness and Exercise, Including How to Begin and Maintain a Fitness Program, Fitness as a Lifestyle, the Link between Fitness and Diet, Advice for Specific Groups of People, Exercise as It Relates to Specific Medical Conditions, and Recent Research in Fitness and Exercise

Along with a Glossary of Important Terms and Resources for Additional Help and Information

Edited by Kristen M. Gledhill. 646 pages. 2001. 0-7808-0334-5. $78.

ALSO AVAILABLE: Fitness & Exercise Sourcebook, 1st Edition. Edited by Dan R. Harris. 663 pages. 1996. 0-7808-0186-5. $78.

"This work is recommended for all general reference collections."
— *American Reference Books Annual 2002*

"Highly recommended for public, consumer, and school grades fourth through college."
— *E-Streams, Nov '01*

"Recommended reference source." — *Booklist, American Library Association, Oct '01*

"The information appears quite comprehensive and is considered reliable. . . . This second edition is a welcomed addition to the series."
— *Doody's Review Service, Sep '01*

"This reference is a valuable choice for those who desire a broad source of information on exercise, fitness, and chronic-disease prevention through a healthy lifestyle." — *American Medical Writers Association Journal, Fall '01*

"Will prove valuable to any library seeking to maintain a current, comprehensive reference collection of health resources. . . . Excellent reference."
— *The Bookwatch, Aug '01*

■

Food & Animal Borne Diseases Sourcebook

Basic Information about Diseases That Can Be Spread to Humans through the Ingestion of Contaminated Food or Water or by Contact with Infected Animals and Insects, Such as Botulism, E. Coli, Hepatitis A, Trichinosis, Lyme Disease, and Rabies

Along with Information Regarding Prevention and Treatment Methods, and Including a Special Section for International Travelers Describing Diseases Such as Cholera, Malaria, Travelers' Diarrhea, and Yellow Fever, and Offering Recommendations for Avoiding Illness

Edited by Karen Bellenir and Peter D. Dresser. 535 pages. 1995. 0-7808-0033-8. $78.

"Targeting general readers and providing them with a single, comprehensive source of information on selected topics, this book continues, with the excellent caliber of its predecessors, to catalog topical information on health matters of general interest. Readable and thorough, this valuable resource is highly recommended for all libraries."
— *Academic Library Book Review, Summer '96*

"A comprehensive collection of authoritative information." — *Emergency Medical Services, Oct '95*

Food Safety Sourcebook

Basic Consumer Health Information about the Safe Handling of Meat, Poultry, Seafood, Eggs, Fruit Juices, and Other Food Items, and Facts about Pesticides, Drinking Water, Food Safety Overseas, and the Onset, Duration, and Symptoms of Foodborne Illnesses, Including Types of Pathogenic Bacteria, Parasitic Protozoa, Worms, Viruses, and Natural Toxins

Along with the Role of the Consumer, the Food Handler, and the Government in Food Safety; a Glossary, and Resources for Additional Help and Information

Edited by Dawn D. Matthews. 339 pages. 1999. 0-7808-0326-4. $78.

"This book is recommended for public libraries and universities with home economic and food science programs." *—E-Streams, Nov '00*

"Recommended reference source." *—Booklist, American Library Association, May '00*

"This book takes the complex issues of food safety and foodborne pathogens and presents them in an easily understood manner. [It does] an excellent job of covering a large and often confusing topic." *—American Reference Books Annual, 2000*

Forensic Medicine Sourcebook

Basic Consumer Information for the Layperson about Forensic Medicine, Including Crime Scene Investigation, Evidence Collection and Analysis, Expert Testimony, Computer-Aided Criminal Identification, Digital Imaging in the Courtroom, DNA Profiling, Accident Reconstruction, Autopsies, Ballistics, Drugs and Explosives Detection, Latent Fingerprints, Product Tampering, and Questioned Document Examination

Along with Statistical Data, a Glossary of Forensics Terminology, and Listings of Sources for Further Help and Information

Edited by Annemarie S. Muth. 574 pages. 1999. 0-7808-0232-2. $78.

"Given the expected widespread interest in its content and its easy to read style, this book is recommended for most public and all college and university libraries." *—E-Streams, Feb '01*

"Recommended for public libraries." *—Reference & User Services Quarterly, American Library Association, Spring 2000*

"Recommended reference source." *—Booklist, American Library Association, Feb '00*

"A wealth of information, useful statistics, references are up-to-date and extremely complete. This wonderful collection of data will help students who are interested in a career in any type of forensic field. It is a great resource for attorneys who need information about types of expert witnesses needed in a particular case. It also offers useful information for fiction and nonfiction writers whose work involves a crime. A fascinating compilation. All levels." *—Choice, Association of College and Research Libraries, Jan 2000*

"There are several items that make this book attractive to consumers who are seeking certain forensic data.... This is a useful current source for those seeking general forensic medical answers." *—American Reference Books Annual, 2000*

Gastrointestinal Diseases & Disorders Sourcebook

Basic Information about Gastroesophageal Reflux Disease (Heartburn), Ulcers, Diverticulosis, Irritable Bowel Syndrome, Crohn's Disease, Ulcerative Colitis, Diarrhea, Constipation, Lactose Intolerance, Hemorrhoids, Hepatitis, Cirrhosis, and Other Digestive Problems, Featuring Statistics, Descriptions of Symptoms, and Current Treatment Methods of Interest for Persons Living with Upper and Lower Gastrointestinal Maladies

Edited by Linda M. Ross. 413 pages. 1996. 0-7808-0078-8. $78.

". . . very readable form. The successful editorial work that brought this material together into a useful and understandable reference makes accessible to all readers information that can help them more effectively understand and obtain help for digestive tract problems." *—Choice, Association of College & Research Libraries, Feb '97*

SEE ALSO *Diet & Nutrition Sourcebook, Digestive Diseases & Disorders, Eating Disorders Sourcebook*

Genetic Disorders Sourcebook, 3rd Edition

Basic Consumer Health Information about Hereditary Diseases and Disorders, Including Facts about the Human Genome, Genetic Inheritance Patterns, Disorders Associated with Specific Genes, such as Sickle Cell Disease, Hemophilia, and Cystic Fibrosis, Chromosome Disorders, such as Down Syndrome, Fragile X Syndrome, and Turner Syndrome, and Complex Diseases and Disorders Resulting from the Interaction of Environmental and Genetic Factors, such as Allergies, Cancer, and Obesity

Along with Facts about Genetic Testing, Suggestions for Parents of Children with Special Needs, Reports on Current Research Initiatives, a Glossary of Genetic Terminology, and Resources for Additional Help and Information

Edited by Karen Bellenir. 777 pages. 2004. 0-7808-0742-1. $78.

ALSO AVAILABLE: *Genetic Disorders Sourcebook, 1st Edition.* Edited by Karen Bellenir. 642 pages. 1996. 0-7808-0034-6. $78.

Genetic Disorders Sourcebook, 2nd Edition. Edited by Kathy Massimini. 768 pages. 2001. 0-7808-0241-1. $78.

"Recommended for public libraries and medical and hospital libraries with consumer health collections." *—E-Streams, May '01*

"Important pick for college-level health reference libraries." —*The Bookwatch, Mar '01*

"Provides essential medical information to both the general public and those diagnosed with a serious or fatal genetic disease or disorder." —*Choice, Association of College and Research Libraries, Jan '97*

■

Head Trauma Sourcebook

Basic Information for the Layperson about Open-Head and Closed-Head Injuries, Treatment Advances, Recovery, and Rehabilitation

Along with Reports on Current Research Initiatives

Edited by Karen Bellenir. 414 pages. 1997. 0-7808-0208-X. $78.

■

Headache Sourcebook

Basic Consumer Health Information about Migraine, Tension, Cluster, Rebound and Other Types of Headaches, with Facts about the Cause and Prevention of Headaches, the Effects of Stress and the Environment, Headaches during Pregnancy and Menopause, and Childhood Headaches

Along with a Glossary and Other Resources for Additional Help and Information

Edited by Dawn D. Matthews. 362 pages. 2002. 0-7808-0337-X. $78.

"Highly recommended for academic and medical reference collections." —*Library Bookwatch, Sep '02*

■

Health Insurance Sourcebook

Basic Information about Managed Care Organizations, Traditional Fee-for-Service Insurance, Insurance Portability and Pre-Existing Conditions Clauses, Medicare, Medicaid, Social Security, and Military Health Care

Along with Information about Insurance Fraud

Edited by Wendy Wilcox. 530 pages. 1997. 0-7808-0222-5. $78.

"Particularly useful because it brings much of this information together in one volume. This book will be a handy reference source in the health sciences library, hospital library, college and university library, and medium to large public library."
—*Medical Reference Services Quarterly, Fall '98*

Awarded "Books of the Year Award"
—*American Journal of Nursing, 1997*

"The layout of the book is particularly helpful as it provides easy access to reference material. A most useful addition to the vast amount of information about health insurance. The use of data from U.S. government agencies is most commendable. Useful in a library or learning center for healthcare professional students."
—*Doody's Health Sciences Book Reviews, Nov '97*

Health Reference Series Cumulative Index 1999

A Comprehensive Index to the Individual Volumes of the Health Reference Series, Including a Subject Index, Name Index, Organization Index, and Publication Index

Along with a Master List of Acronyms and Abbreviations

Edited by Edward J. Prucha, Anne Holmes, and Robert Rudnick. 990 pages. 2000. 0-7808-0382-5. $78.

"This volume will be most helpful in libraries that have a relatively complete collection of the Health Reference Series." —*American Reference Books Annual, 2001*

"Essential for collections that hold any of the numerous *Health Reference Series* titles."
—*Choice, Association of College and Research Libraries, Nov '00*

■

Healthy Aging Sourcebook

Basic Consumer Health Information about Maintaining Health through the Aging Process, Including Advice on Nutrition, Exercise, and Sleep, Help in Making Decisions about Midlife Issues and Retirement, and Guidance Concerning Practical and Informed Choices in Health Consumerism

Along with Data Concerning the Theories of Aging, Different Experiences in Aging by Minority Groups, and Facts about Aging Now and Aging in the Future; and Featuring a Glossary, a Guide to Consumer Help, Additional Suggested Reading, and Practical Resource Directory

Edited by Jenifer Swanson. 536 pages. 1999. 0-7808-0390-6. $78.

"Recommended reference source."
—*Booklist, American Library Association, Feb '00*

SEE ALSO *Physical & Mental Issues in Aging Sourcebook*

■

Healthy Children Sourcebook

Basic Consumer Health Information about the Physical and Mental Development of Children between the Ages of 3 and 12, Including Routine Health Care, Preventative Health Services, Safety and First Aid, Healthy Sleep, Dental Care, Nutrition, and Fitness, and Featuring Parenting Tips on Such Topics as Bedwetting, Choosing Day Care, Monitoring TV and Other Media, and Establishing a Foundation for Substance Abuse Prevention

Along with a Glossary of Commonly Used Pediatric Terms and Resources for Additional Help and Information.

Edited by Chad T. Kimball. 647 pages. 2003. 0-7808-0247-0. $78.

"It is hard to imagine that any other single resource exists that would provide such a comprehensive guide

of timely information on health promotion and disease prevention for children aged 3 to 12."
— *American Reference Books Annual, 2004*

"The strengths of this book are many. It is clearly written, presented and structured."
— *Journal of the National Medical Association, 2004*

■

Healthy Heart Sourcebook for Women

Basic Consumer Health Information about Cardiac Issues Specific to Women, Including Facts about Major Risk Factors and Prevention, Treatment and Control Strategies, and Important Dietary Issues

Along with a Special Section Regarding the Pros and Cons of Hormone Replacement Therapy and Its Impact on Heart Health, and Additional Help, Including Recipes, a Glossary, and a Directory of Resources

Edited by Dawn D. Matthews. 336 pages. 2000. 0-7808-0329-9. $78.

"A good reference source and recommended for all public, academic, medical, and hospital libraries."
— *Medical Reference Services Quarterly, Summer '01*

"Because of the lack of information specific to women on this topic, this book is recommended for public libraries and consumer libraries."
— *American Reference Books Annual, 2001*

"Contains very important information about coronary artery disease that all women should know. The information is current and presented in an easy-to-read format. The book will make a good addition to any library."
— *American Medical Writers Association Journal, Summer '00*

"Important, basic reference."
— *Reviewer's Bookwatch, Jul '00*

SEE ALSO *Heart Diseases & Disorders Sourcebook, Women's Health Concerns Sourcebook*

■

Heart Diseases & Disorders Sourcebook, 2nd Edition

Basic Consumer Health Information about Heart Attacks, Angina, Rhythm Disorders, Heart Failure, Valve Disease, Congenital Heart Disorders, and More, Including Descriptions of Surgical Procedures and Other Interventions, Medications, Cardiac Rehabilitation, Risk Identification, and Prevention Tips

Along with Statistical Data, Reports on Current Research Initiatives, a Glossary of Cardiovascular Terms, and Resource Directory

Edited by Karen Bellenir. 612 pages. 2000. 0-7808-0238-1. $78.

ALSO AVAILABLE: *Cardiovascular Diseases & Disorders Sourcebook, 1st Edition.* Edited by Karen Bellenir and Peter D. Dresser. 683 pages. 1995. 0-7808-0032-X. $78.

"This work stands out as an imminently accessible resource for the general public. It is recommended for the reference and circulating shelves of school, public, and academic libraries."
— *American Reference Books Annual, 2001*

"Recommended reference source."
— *Booklist, American Library Association, Dec '00*

"Provides comprehensive coverage of matters related to the heart. This title is recommended for health sciences and public libraries with consumer health collections."
— *E-Streams, Oct '00*

SEE ALSO *Healthy Heart Sourcebook for Women*

Household Safety Sourcebook

Basic Consumer Health Information about Household Safety, Including Information about Poisons, Chemicals, Fire, and Water Hazards in the Home

Along with Advice about the Safe Use of Home Maintenance Equipment, Choosing Toys and Nursery Furniture, Holiday and Recreation Safety, a Glossary, and Resources for Further Help and Information

Edited by Dawn D. Matthews. 606 pages. 2002. 0-7808-0338-8. $78.

"This work will be useful in public libraries with large consumer health and wellness departments."
— *American Reference Books Annual, 2003*

"As a sourcebook on household safety this book meets its mark. It is encyclopedic in scope and covers a wide range of safety issues that are commonly seen in the home."
— *E-Streams, Jul '02*

■

Hypertension Sourcebook

Basic Consumer Health Information about the Causes, Diagnosis, and Treatment of High Blood Pressure, with Facts about Consequences, Complications, and Co-Occurring Disorders, Such as Coronary Heart Disease, Diabetes, Stroke, Kidney Disease, and Hypertensive Retinopathy, and Issues in Blood Pressure Control, Including Dietary Choices, Stress Management, and Medications

Along with Reports on Current Research Initiatives and Clinical Trials, a Glossary, and Resources for Additional Help and Information

Edited by Dawn D. Matthews and Karen Bellenir. 600 pages. 2004. 0-7808-0674-3. $78.

■

Immune System Disorders Sourcebook

Basic Information about Lupus, Multiple Sclerosis, Guillain-Barré Syndrome, Chronic Granulomatous Disease, and More

Along with Statistical and Demographic Data and Reports on Current Research Initiatives

Edited by Allan R. Cook. 608 pages. 1997. 0-7808-0209-8. $78.

Infant & Toddler Health Sourcebook

Basic Consumer Health Information about the Physical and Mental Development of Newborns, Infants, and Toddlers, Including Neonatal Concerns, Nutrition Recommendations, Immunization Schedules, Common Pediatric Disorders, Assessments and Milestones, Safety Tips, and Advice for Parents and Other Caregivers

Along with a Glossary of Terms and Resource Listings for Additional Help

Edited by Jenifer Swanson. 585 pages. 2000. 0-7808-0246-2. $78.

"As a reference for the general public, this would be useful in any library." — *E-Streams, May '01*

"Recommended reference source."
— *Booklist, American Library Association, Feb '01*

"This is a good source for general use."
— *American Reference Books Annual, 2001*

∎

Infectious Diseases Sourcebook

Basic Consumer Health Information about Non-Contagious Bacterial, Viral, Prion, Fungal, and Parasitic Diseases Spread by Food and Water, Insects and Animals, or Environmental Contact, Including Botulism, E. Coli, Encephalitis, Legionnaires' Disease, Lyme Disease, Malaria, Plague, Rabies, Salmonella, Tetanus, and Others, and Facts about Newly Emerging Diseases, Such as Hantavirus, Mad Cow Disease, Monkeypox, and West Nile Virus

Along with Information about Preventing Disease Transmission, the Threat of Bioterrorism, and Current Research Initiatives, with a Glossary and Directory of Resources for More Information

Edited by Karen Bellenir. 634 pages. 2004. 0-7808-0675-1. $78.

∎

Injury & Trauma Sourcebook

Basic Consumer Health Information about the Impact of Injury, the Diagnosis and Treatment of Common and Traumatic Injuries, Emergency Care, and Specific Injuries Related to Home, Community, Workplace, Transportation, and Recreation

Along with Guidelines for Injury Prevention, a Glossary, and a Directory of Additional Resources

Edited by Joyce Brennfleck Shannon. 696 pages. 2002. 0-7808-0421-X. $78.

"This publication is the most comprehensive work of its kind about injury and trauma."
— *American Reference Books Annual, 2003*

"This sourcebook provides concise, easily readable, basic health information about injuries. . . . This book is well organized and an easy to use reference resource suitable for hospital, health sciences and public libraries with consumer health collections."
— *E-Streams, Nov '02*

"Practitioners should be aware of guides such as this in order to facilitate their use by patients and their families." — *Doody's Health Sciences Book Review Journal, Sep-Oct '02*

"Recommended reference source."
— *Booklist, American Library Association, Sep '02*

"Highly recommended for academic and medical reference collections." — *Library Bookwatch, Sep '02*

∎

Kidney & Urinary Tract Diseases & Disorders Sourcebook

Basic Information about Kidney Stones, Urinary Incontinence, Bladder Disease, End Stage Renal Disease, Dialysis, and More

Along with Statistical and Demographic Data and Reports on Current Research Initiatives

Edited by Linda M. Ross. 602 pages. 1997. 0-7808-0079-6. $78.

∎

Learning Disabilities Sourcebook, 2nd Edition

Basic Consumer Health Information about Learning Disabilities, Including Dyslexia, Developmental Speech and Language Disabilities, Non-Verbal Learning Disorders, Developmental Arithmetic Disorder, Developmental Writing Disorder, and Other Conditions That Impede Learning Such as Attention Deficit/ Hyperactivity Disorder, Brain Injury, Hearing Impairment, Klinefelter Syndrome, Dyspraxia, and Tourette Syndrome

Along with Facts about Educational Issues and Assistive Technology, Coping Strategies, a Glossary of Related Terms, and Resources for Further Help and Information

Edited by Dawn D. Matthews. 621 pages. 2003. 0-7808-0626-3. $78.

ALSO AVAILABLE: Learning Disabilities Sourcebook, 1st Edition. Edited by Linda M. Shin. 579 pages. 1998. 0-7808-0210-1. $78.

"The second edition of *Learning Disabilities Sourcebook* far surpasses the earlier edition in that it is more focused on information that will be useful as a consumer health resource."
— *American Reference Books Annual, 2004*

"Teachers as well as consumers will find this an essential guide to understanding various syndromes and their latest treatments. [An] invaluable reference for public and school library collections alike."
— *Library Bookwatch, Apr '03*

Named "Outstanding Reference Book of 1999."
— *New York Public Library, Feb 2000*

"An excellent candidate for inclusion in a public library reference section. It's a great source of information. Teachers will also find the book useful. Definitely worth reading."
— *Journal of Adolescent & Adult Literacy, Feb 2000*

"Readable . . . provides a solid base of information regarding successful techniques used with individuals who have learning disabilities, as well as practical suggestions for educators and family members. Clear language, concise descriptions, and pertinent information for contacting multiple resources add to the strength of this book as a useful tool." — *Choice, Association of College and Research Libraries, Feb '99*

"Recommended reference source."
— *Booklist, American Library Association, Sep '98*

"A useful resource for libraries and for those who don't have the time to identify and locate the individual publications." — *Disability Resources Monthly, Sep '98*

■

Leukemia Sourcebook

Basic Consumer Health Information about Adult and Childhood Leukemias, Including Acute Lymphocytic Leukemia (ALL), Chronic Lymphocytic Leukemia (CLL), Acute Myelogenous Leukemia (AML), Chronic Myelogenous Leukemia (CML), and Hairy Cell Leukemia, and Treatments Such as Chemotherapy, Radiation Therapy, Peripheral Blood Stem Cell and Marrow Transplantation, and Immunotherapy

Along with Tips for Life During and After Treatment, a Glossary, and Directories of Additional Resources

Edited by Joyce Brennfleck Shannon. 587 pages. 2003. 0-7808-0627-1. $78.

"Unlike other medical books for the layperson, . . . the language does not talk down to the reader. . . . This volume is highly recommended for all libraries."
— *American Reference Books Annual, 2004*

■

Liver Disorders Sourcebook

Basic Consumer Health Information about the Liver and How It Works; Liver Diseases, Including Cancer, Cirrhosis, Hepatitis, and Toxic and Drug Related Diseases; Tips for Maintaining a Healthy Liver; Laboratory Tests, Radiology Tests, and Facts about Liver Transplantation

Along with a Section on Support Groups, a Glossary, and Resource Listings

Edited by Joyce Brennfleck Shannon. 591 pages. 2000. 0-7808-0383-3. $78.

"A valuable resource."
— *American Reference Books Annual, 2001*

"This title is recommended for health sciences and public libraries with consumer health collections."
— *E-Streams, Oct '00*

"Recommended reference source."
— *Booklist, American Library Association, Jun '00*

■

Lung Disorders Sourcebook

Basic Consumer Health Information about Emphysema, Pneumonia, Tuberculosis, Asthma, Cystic Fibrosis, and Other Lung Disorders, Including Facts about

Diagnostic Procedures, Treatment Strategies, Disease Prevention Efforts, and Such Risk Factors as Smoking, Air Pollution, and Exposure to Asbestos, Radon, and Other Agents

Along with a Glossary and Resources for Additional Help and Information

Edited by Dawn D. Matthews. 678 pages. 2002. 0-7808-0339-6. $78.

"This title is a great addition for public and school libraries because it provides concise health information on the lungs."
— *American Reference Books Annual, 2003*

"Highly recommended for academic and medical reference collections." — *Library Bookwatch, Sep '02*

■

Medical Tests Sourcebook, 2nd Edition

Basic Consumer Health Information about Medical Tests, Including Age-Specific Health Tests, Important Health Screenings and Exams, Home-Use Tests, Blood and Specimen Tests, Electrical Tests, Scope Tests, Genetic Testing, and Imaging Tests, Such as X-Rays, Ultrasound, Computed Tomography, Magnetic Resonance Imaging, Angiography, and Nuclear Medicine

Along with a Glossary and Directory of Additional Resources

Edited by Joyce Brennfleck Shannon. 654 pages. 2004. 0-7808-0670-0. $78.

ALSO AVAILABLE: Medical Tests, 1st Edition. Edited by Joyce Brennfleck Shannon. 691 pages. 1999. 0-7808-0243-8. $78.

"Recommended for hospital and health sciences libraries with consumer health collections."
— *E-Streams, Mar '00*

"This is an overall excellent reference with a wealth of general knowledge that may aid those who are reluctant to get vital tests performed."
— *Today's Librarian, Jan 2000*

"A valuable reference guide."
— *American Reference Books Annual, 2000*

■

Men's Health Concerns Sourcebook, 2nd Edition

Basic Consumer Health Information about the Medical and Mental Concerns of Men, Including Theories about the Shorter Male Lifespan, the Leading Causes of Death and Disability, Physical Concerns of Special Significance to Men, Reproductive and Sexual Concerns, Sexually Transmitted Diseases, Men's Mental and Emotional Health, and Lifestyle Choices That Affect Wellness, Such as Nutrition, Fitness, and Substance Use

Along with a Glossary of Related Terms and a Directory of Organizational Resources in Men's Health

Edited by Robert Aquinas McNally. 644 pages. 2004. 0-7808-0671-9. $78.

▪

Mental Health Disorders Sourcebook, 2nd Edition

Basic Consumer Health Information about Anxiety Disorders, Depression and Other Mood Disorders, Eating Disorders, Personality Disorders, Schizophrenia, and More, Including Disease Descriptions, Treatment Options, and Reports on Current Research Initiatives

Along with Statistical Data, Tips for Maintaining Mental Health, a Glossary, and Directory of Sources for Additional Help and Information

Edited by Karen Bellenir. 605 pages. 2000. 0-7808-0240-3. $78.

ALSO AVAILABLE: Mental Health Disorders Sourcebook, 1st Edition. Edited by Karen Bellenir. 548 pages. 1995. 0-7808-0040-0. $78.

"Well organized and well written."
—*American Reference Books Annual, 2001*

"Recommended reference source."
—*Booklist, American Library Association, Jun '00*

▪

Mental Retardation Sourcebook

Basic Consumer Health Information about Mental Retardation and Its Causes, Including Down Syndrome, Fetal Alcohol Syndrome, Fragile X Syndrome, Genetic Conditions, Injury, and Environmental Sources

Along with Preventive Strategies, Parenting Issues, Educational Implications, Health Care Needs, Employment and Economic Matters, Legal Issues, a Glossary, and a Resource Listing for Additional Help and Information

Edited by Joyce Brennfleck Shannon. 642 pages. 2000. 0-7808-0377-9. $78.

"Public libraries will find the book useful for reference and as a beginning research point for students, parents, and caregivers."
—*American Reference Books Annual, 2001*

"The strength of this work is that it compiles many basic fact sheets and addresses for further information in one volume. It is intended and suitable for the general public. This sourcebook is relevant to any collection providing health information for the general public."
—*E-Streams, Nov '00*

"From preventing retardation to parenting and family challenges, this covers health, social and legal issues and will prove an invaluable overview."
—*Reviewer's Bookwatch, Jul '00*

Movement Disorders Sourcebook

Basic Consumer Health Information about Neurological Movement Disorders, Including Essential Tremor, Parkinson's Disease, Dystonia, Cerebral Palsy, Huntington's Disease, Myasthenia Gravis, Multiple Sclerosis, and Other Early-Onset and Adult-Onset Movement Disorders, Their Symptoms and Causes, Diagnostic Tests, and Treatments

Along with Mobility and Assistive Technology Information, a Glossary, and a Directory of Additional Resources

Edited by Joyce Brennfleck Shannon. 655 pages. 2003. 0-7808-0628-X. $78.

". . . a good resource for consumers and recommended for public, community college and undergraduate libraries."
—*American Reference Books Annual, 2004*

▪

Muscular Dystrophy Sourcebook

Basic Consumer Health Information about Congenital, Childhood-Onset, and Adult-Onset Forms of Muscular Dystrophy, Such as Duchenne, Becker, Emery-Dreifuss, Distal, Limb-Girdle, Facioscapulohumeral (FSHD), Myotonic, and Ophthalmoplegic Muscular Dystrophies, Including Facts about Diagnostic Tests, Medical and Physical Therapies, Management of Co-Occurring Conditions, and Parenting Guidelines

Along with Practical Tips for Home Care, a Glossary, and Directories of Additional Resources

Edited by Joyce Brennfleck Shannon. 577 pages. 2004. 0-7808-0676-X. $78.

▪

Obesity Sourcebook

Basic Consumer Health Information about Diseases and Other Problems Associated with Obesity, and Including Facts about Risk Factors, Prevention Issues, and Management Approaches

Along with Statistical and Demographic Data, Information about Special Populations, Research Updates, a Glossary, and Source Listings for Further Help and Information

Edited by Wilma Caldwell and Chad T. Kimball. 376 pages. 2001. 0-7808-0333-7. $78.

"The book synthesizes the reliable medical literature on obesity into one easy-to-read and useful resource for the general public."
— *American Reference Books Annual 2002*

"This is a very useful resource book for the lay public."
—*Doody's Review Service, Nov '01*

"Well suited for the health reference collection of a public library or an academic health science library that serves the general population." —*E-Streams, Sep '01*

"Recommended reference source."
—*Booklist, American Library Association, Apr '01*

" Recommended pick both for specialty health library collections and any general consumer health reference collection." — *The Bookwatch, Apr '01*

Ophthalmic Disorders Sourcebook, 1st Edition

SEE *Eye Care Sourcebook, 2nd Edition*

■

Oral Health Sourcebook

SEE *Dental Care & Oral Health Sourcebook, 2nd Ed.*

■

Osteoporosis Sourcebook

Basic Consumer Health Information about Primary and Secondary Osteoporosis and Juvenile Osteoporosis and Related Conditions, Including Fibrous Dysplasia, Gaucher Disease, Hyperthyroidism, Hypophosphatasia, Myeloma, Osteopetrosis, Osteogenesis Imperfecta, and Paget's Disease

Along with Information about Risk Factors, Treatments, Traditional and Non-Traditional Pain Management, a Glossary of Related Terms, and a Directory of Resources

Edited by Allan R. Cook. 584 pages. 2001. 0-7808-0239-X. $78.

"This would be a book to be kept in a staff or patient library. The targeted audience is the layperson, but the therapist who needs a quick bit of information on a particular topic will also find this book useful."
— *Physical Therapy, Jan '02*

"This resource is recommended as a great reference source for public, health, and academic libraries, and is another triumph for the editors of Omnigraphics."
— *American Reference Books Annual 2002*

"Recommended for all public libraries and general health collections, especially those supporting patient education or consumer health programs."
— *E-Streams, Nov '01*

"Will prove valuable to any library seeking to maintain a current, comprehensive reference collection of health resources. . . . From prevention to treatment and associated conditions, this provides an excellent survey."
— *The Bookwatch, Aug '01*

"Recommended reference source."
— *Booklist, American Library Association, July '01*

SEE ALSO *Women's Health Concerns Sourcebook*

■

Pain Sourcebook, 2nd Edition

Basic Consumer Health Information about Specific Forms of Acute and Chronic Pain, Including Muscle and Skeletal Pain, Nerve Pain, Cancer Pain, and Disorders Characterized by Pain, Such as Fibromyalgia, Shingles, Angina, Arthritis, and Headaches

Along with Information about Pain Medications and Management Techniques, Complementary and Alternative Pain Relief Options, Tips for People Living with Chronic Pain, a Glossary, and a Directory of Sources for Further Information

Edited by Karen Bellenir. 670 pages. 2002. 0-7808-0612-3. $78.

ALSO AVAILABLE: Pain Sourcebook, 1st Edition. Edited by Allan R. Cook. 667 pages. 1997. 0-7808-0213-6. $78.

"A source of valuable information. . . . This book offers help to nonmedical people who need information about pain and pain management. It is also an excellent reference for those who participate in patient education."
— *Doody's Review Service, Sep '02*

"The text is readable, easily understood, and well indexed. This excellent volume belongs in all patient education libraries, consumer health sections of public libraries, and many personal collections."
— *American Reference Books Annual, 1999*

"A beneficial reference." — *Booklist Health Sciences Supplement, American Library Association, Oct '98*

"The information is basic in terms of scholarship and is appropriate for general readers. Written in journalistic style . . . intended for non-professionals. Quite thorough in its coverage of different pain conditions and summarizes the latest clinical information regarding pain treatment." — *Choice, Association of College and Research Libraries, Jun '98*

"Recommended reference source."
— *Booklist, American Library Association, Mar '98*

■

Pediatric Cancer Sourcebook

Basic Consumer Health Information about Leukemias, Brain Tumors, Sarcomas, Lymphomas, and Other Cancers in Infants, Children, and Adolescents, Including Descriptions of Cancers, Treatments, and Coping Strategies

Along with Suggestions for Parents, Caregivers, and Concerned Relatives, a Glossary of Cancer Terms, and Resource Listings

Edited by Edward J. Prucha. 587 pages. 1999. 0-7808-0245-4. $78.

"An excellent source of information. Recommended for public, hospital, and health science libraries with consumer health collections." — *E-Streams, Jun '00*

"Recommended reference source."
— *Booklist, American Library Association, Feb '00*

"A valuable addition to all libraries specializing in health services and many public libraries."
— *American Reference Books Annual, 2000*

■

Physical & Mental Issues in Aging Sourcebook

Basic Consumer Health Information on Physical and Mental Disorders Associated with the Aging Process, Including Concerns about Cardiovascular Disease, Pulmonary Disease, Oral Health, Digestive Disorders, Musculoskeletal and Skin Disorders, Metabolic Changes, Sexual and Reproductive Issues, and Changes in Vision, Hearing, and Other Senses

Along with Data about Longevity and Causes of Death, Information on Acute and Chronic Pain, Descriptions of Mental Concerns, a Glossary of Terms, and Resource Listings for Additional Help

Edited by Jenifer Swanson. 660 pages. 1999. 0-7808-0233-0. $78.

"This is a treasure of health information for the layperson." — *Choice Health Sciences Supplement, Association of College & Research Libraries, May 2000*

"Recommended for public libraries."
—*American Reference Books Annual, 2000*

"Recommended reference source."
— *Booklist, American Library Association, Oct '99*

SEE ALSO *Healthy Aging Sourcebook*

■

Podiatry Sourcebook

Basic Consumer Health Information about Foot Conditions, Diseases, and Injuries, Including Bunions, Corns, Calluses, Athlete's Foot, Plantar Warts, Hammertoes and Clawtoes, Clubfoot, Heel Pain, Gout, and More

Along with Facts about Foot Care, Disease Prevention, Foot Safety, Choosing a Foot Care Specialist, a Glossary of Terms, and Resource Listings for Additional Information

Edited by M. Lisa Weatherford. 380 pages. 2001. 0-7808-0215-2. $78.

"Recommended reference source."
— *Booklist, American Library Association, Feb '02*

"There is a lot of information presented here on a topic that is usually only covered sparingly in most larger comprehensive medical encyclopedias."
— *American Reference Books Annual 2002*

■

Pregnancy & Birth Sourcebook, 2nd Edition

Basic Consumer Health Information about Conception and Pregnancy, Including Facts about Fertility, Infertility, Pregnancy Symptoms and Complications, Fetal Growth and Development, Labor, Delivery, and the Postpartum Period, as Well as Information about Maintaining Health and Wellness during Pregnancy and Caring for a Newborn

Along with Information about Public Health Assistance for Low-Income Pregnant Women, a Glossary, and Directories of Agencies and Organizations Providing Help and Support

Edited by Amy L. Sutton. 626 pages. 2004. 0-7808-0672-7. $78.

ALSO AVAILABLE: *Pregnancy & Birth Sourcebook, 1st Edition.* Edited by Heather E. Aldred. 737 pages. 1997. 0-7808-0216-0. $78.

"A well-organized handbook. Recommended."
— *Choice, Association of College and Research Libraries, Apr '98*

"Recommended reference source."
— *Booklist, American Library Association, Mar '98*

"Recommended for public libraries."
— *American Reference Books Annual, 1998*

SEE ALSO *Congenital Disorders Sourcebook, Family Planning Sourcebook*

■

Prostate Cancer Sourcebook

Basic Consumer Health Information about Prostate Cancer, Including Information about the Associated Risk Factors, Detection, Diagnosis, and Treatment of Prostate Cancer

Along with Information on Non-Malignant Prostate Conditions, and Featuring a Section Listing Support and Treatment Centers and a Glossary of Related Terms

Edited by Dawn D. Matthews. 358 pages. 2001. 0-7808-0324-8. $78.

"Recommended reference source."
— *Booklist, American Library Association, Jan '02*

"A valuable resource for health care consumers seeking information on the subject. . . .All text is written in a clear, easy-to-understand language that avoids technical jargon. Any library that collects consumer health resources would strengthen their collection with the addition of the *Prostate Cancer Sourcebook*."
— *American Reference Books Annual 2002*

■

Public Health Sourcebook

Basic Information about Government Health Agencies, Including National Health Statistics and Trends, Healthy People 2000 Program Goals and Objectives, the Centers for Disease Control and Prevention, the Food and Drug Administration, and the National Institutes of Health

Along with Full Contact Information for Each Agency

Edited by Wendy Wilcox. 698 pages. 1998. 0-7808-0220-9. $78.

"Recommended reference source."
— *Booklist, American Library Association, Sep '98*

"This consumer guide provides welcome assistance in navigating the maze of federal health agencies and their data on public health concerns."
— *SciTech Book News, Sep '98*

■

Reconstructive & Cosmetic Surgery Sourcebook

Basic Consumer Health Information on Cosmetic and Reconstructive Plastic Surgery, Including Statistical Information about Different Surgical Procedures, Things to Consider Prior to Surgery, Plastic Surgery Techniques and Tools, Emotional and Psychological Considerations, and Procedure-Specific Information

Along with a Glossary of Terms and a Listing of Resources for Additional Help and Information

Edited by M. Lisa Weatherford. 374 pages. 2001. 0-7808-0214-4. $78.

"An excellent reference that addresses cosmetic and medically necessary reconstructive surgeries. . . . The

style of the prose is calm and reassuring, discussing the many positive outcomes now available due to advances in surgical techniques."
— *American Reference Books Annual 2002*

"Recommended for health science libraries that are open to the public, as well as hospital libraries that are open to the patients. This book is a good resource for the consumer interested in plastic surgery."
— *E-Streams, Dec '01*

"Recommended reference source."
— *Booklist, American Library Association, July '01*

■

Rehabilitation Sourcebook

Basic Consumer Health Information about Rehabilitation for People Recovering from Heart Surgery, Spinal Cord Injury, Stroke, Orthopedic Impairments, Amputation, Pulmonary Impairments, Traumatic Injury, and More, Including Physical Therapy, Occupational Therapy, Speech/ Language Therapy, Massage Therapy, Dance Therapy, Art Therapy, and Recreational Therapy

Along with Information on Assistive and Adaptive Devices, a Glossary, and Resources for Additional Help and Information

Edited by Dawn D. Matthews. 531 pages. 1999. 0-7808-0236-5. $78.

"This is an excellent resource for public library reference and health collections."
— *American Reference Books Annual, 2001*

"Recommended reference source."
— *Booklist, American Library Association, May '00*

■

Respiratory Diseases & Disorders Sourcebook

Basic Information about Respiratory Diseases and Disorders, Including Asthma, Cystic Fibrosis, Pneumonia, the Common Cold, Influenza, and Others, Featuring Facts about the Respiratory System, Statistical and Demographic Data, Treatments, Self-Help Management Suggestions, and Current Research Initiatives

Edited by Allan R. Cook and Peter D. Dresser. 771 pages. 1995. 0-7808-0037-0. $78.

"Designed for the layperson and for patients and their families coping with respiratory illness. . . . an extensive array of information on diagnosis, treatment, management, and prevention of respiratory illnesses for the general reader."
— *Choice, Association of College and Research Libraries, Jun '96*

"A highly recommended text for all collections. It is a comforting reminder of the power of knowledge that good books carry between their covers."
— *Academic Library Book Review, Spring '96*

"A comprehensive collection of authoritative information presented in a nontechnical, humanitarian style for patients, families, and caregivers."
— *Association of Operating Room Nurses, Sep/Oct '95*

SEE ALSO Lung Disorders Sourcebook

Sexually Transmitted Diseases Sourcebook, 2nd Edition

Basic Consumer Health Information about Sexually Transmitted Diseases, Including Information on the Diagnosis and Treatment of Chlamydia, Gonorrhea, Hepatitis, Herpes, HIV, Mononucleosis, Syphilis, and Others

Along with Information on Prevention, Such as Condom Use, Vaccines, and STD Education; And Featuring a Section on Issues Related to Youth and Adolescents, a Glossary, and Resources for Additional Help and Information

Edited by Dawn D. Matthews. 538 pages. 2001. 0-7808-0249-7. $78.

ALSO AVAILABLE: Sexually Transmitted Diseases Sourcebook, 1st Edition. Edited by Linda M. Ross. 550 pages. 1997. 0-7808-0217-9. $78.

"Recommended for consumer health collections in public libraries, and secondary school and community college libraries."
— *American Reference Books Annual 2002*

"Every school and public library should have a copy of this comprehensive and user-friendly reference book."
— *Choice, Association of College & Research Libraries, Sep '01*

"This is a highly recommended book. This is an especially important book for all school and public libraries."
— *AIDS Book Review Journal, Jul-Aug '01*

"Recommended reference source."
— *Booklist, American Library Association, Apr '01*

"Recommended pick both for specialty health library collections and any general consumer health reference collection."
— *The Bookwatch, Apr '01*

■

Skin Disorders Sourcebook

Basic Information about Common Skin and Scalp Conditions Caused by Aging, Allergies, Immune Reactions, Sun Exposure, Infectious Organisms, Parasites, Cosmetics, and Skin Traumas, Including Abrasions, Cuts, and Pressure Sores

Along with Information on Prevention and Treatment

Edited by Allan R. Cook. 647 pages. 1997. 0-7808-0080-X. $78.

". . . comprehensive, easily read reference book."
— *Doody's Health Sciences Book Reviews, Oct '97*

SEE ALSO Burns Sourcebook

■

Sleep Disorders Sourcebook

Basic Consumer Health Information about Sleep and Its Disorders, Including Insomnia, Sleepwalking, Sleep Apnea, Restless Leg Syndrome, and Narcolepsy

Along with Data about Shiftwork and Its Effects, Information on the Societal Costs of Sleep Deprivation, Descriptions of Treatment Options, a Glossary of Terms, and Resource Listings for Additional Help

Edited by Jenifer Swanson. 439 pages. 1998. 0-7808-0234-9. $78.

"This text will complement any home or medical library. It is user-friendly and ideal for the adult reader."
—*American Reference Books Annual, 2000*

"A useful resource that provides accurate, relevant, and accessible information on sleep to the general public. Health care providers who deal with sleep disorders patients may also find it helpful in being prepared to answer some of the questions patients ask."
—*Respiratory Care, Jul '99*

"Recommended reference source."
—*Booklist, American Library Association, Feb '99*

Smoking Concerns Sourcebook

Basic Consumer Health Information about Nicotine Addiction and Smoking Cessation, Featuring Facts about the Health Effects of Tobacco Use, Including Lung and Other Cancers, Heart Disease, Stroke, and Respiratory Disorders, Such as Emphysema and Chronic Bronchitis

Along with Information about Smoking Prevention Programs, Suggestions for Achieving and Maintaining a Smoke-Free Lifestyle, Statistics about Tobacco Use, Reports on Current Research Initiatives, a Glossary of Related Terms, and Directories of Resources for Additional Help and Information

Edited by Karen Bellenir. 625 pages. 2004. 0-7808-0323-X. $78.

Sports Injuries Sourcebook, 2nd Edition

Basic Consumer Health Information about the Diagnosis, Treatment, and Rehabilitation of Common Sports-Related Injuries in Children and Adults

Along with Suggestions for Conditioning and Training, Information and Prevention Tips for Injuries Frequently Associated with Specific Sports and Special Populations, a Glossary, and a Directory of Additional Resources

Edited by Joyce Brennfleck Shannon. 614 pages. 2002. 0-7808-0604-2. $78.

ALSO AVAILABLE: *Sports Injuries Sourcebook, 1st Edition.* Edited by Heather E. Aldred. 624 pages. 1999. 0-7808-0218-7. $78.

"This is an excellent reference for consumers and it is recommended for public, community college, and undergraduate libraries."
—*American Reference Books Annual, 2003*

"Recommended reference source."
—*Booklist, American Library Association, Feb '03*

Stress-Related Disorders Sourcebook

Basic Consumer Health Information about Stress and Stress-Related Disorders, Including Stress Origins and Signals, Environmental Stress at Work and Home, Mental and Emotional Stress Associated with Depression, Post-Traumatic Stress Disorder, Panic Disorder, Suicide, and the Physical Effects of Stress on the Cardiovascular, Immune, and Nervous Systems

Along with Stress Management Techniques, a Glossary, and a Listing of Additional Resources

Edited by Joyce Brennfleck Shannon. 610 pages. 2002. 0-7808-0560-7. $78.

"Well written for a general readership, the *Stress-Related Disorders Sourcebook* is a useful addition to the health reference literature."
—*American Reference Books Annual, 2003*

"I am impressed by the amount of information. It offers a thorough overview of the causes and consequences of stress for the layperson. . . . A well-done and thorough reference guide for professionals and nonprofessionals alike."
—*Doody's Review Service, Dec '02*

Stroke Sourcebook

Basic Consumer Health Information about Stroke, Including Ischemic, Hemorrhagic, Transient Ischemic Attack (TIA), and Pediatric Stroke, Stroke Triggers and Risks, Diagnostic Tests, Treatments, and Rehabilitation Information

Along with Stroke Prevention Guidelines, Legal and Financial Information, a Glossary, and a Directory of Additional Resources

Edited by Joyce Brennfleck Shannon. 606 pages. 2003. 0-7808-0630-1. $78.

"This volume is highly recommended and should be in every medical, hospital, and public library."
—*American Reference Books Annual, 2004*

Substance Abuse Sourcebook

Basic Health-Related Information about the Abuse of Legal and Illegal Substances Such as Alcohol, Tobacco, Prescription Drugs, Marijuana, Cocaine, and Heroin; and Including Facts about Substance Abuse Prevention Strategies, Intervention Methods, Treatment and Recovery Programs, and a Section Addressing the Special Problems Related to Substance Abuse during Pregnancy

Edited by Karen Bellenir. 573 pages. 1996. 0-7808-0038-9. $78.

"A valuable addition to any health reference section. Highly recommended."
—*The Book Report, Mar/Apr '97*

". . . a comprehensive collection of substance abuse information that's both highly readable and compact. Families and caregivers of substance abusers will find

the information enlightening and helpful, while teachers, social workers and journalists should benefit from the concise format. Recommended."
— *Drug Abuse Update, Winter '96/'97*

SEE ALSO Alcoholism Sourcebook, Drug Abuse Sourcebook

Surgery Sourcebook

Basic Consumer Health Information about Inpatient and Outpatient Surgeries, Including Cardiac, Vascular, Orthopedic, Ocular, Reconstructive, Cosmetic, Gynecologic, and Ear, Nose, and Throat Procedures and More

Along with Information about Operating Room Policies and Instruments, Laser Surgery Techniques, Hospital Errors, Statistical Data, a Glossary, and Listings of Sources for Further Help and Information

Edited by Annemarie S. Muth and Karen Bellenir. 596 pages. 2002. 0-7808-0380-9. $78.

"Large public libraries and medical libraries would benefit from this material in their reference collections."
— *American Reference Books Annual, 2004*

"Invaluable reference for public and school library collections alike." — *Library Bookwatch, Apr '03*

Transplantation Sourcebook

Basic Consumer Health Information about Organ and Tissue Transplantation, Including Physical and Financial Preparations, Procedures and Issues Relating to Specific Solid Organ and Tissue Transplants, Rehabilitation, Pediatric Transplant Information, the Future of Transplantation, and Organ and Tissue Donation

Along with a Glossary and Listings of Additional Resources

Edited by Joyce Brennfleck Shannon. 628 pages. 2002. 0-7808-0322-1. $78.

"Along with these advances [in transplantation technology] have come a number of daunting questions for potential transplant patients, their families, and their health care providers. This reference text is the best single tool to address many of these questions. . . . It will be a much-needed addition to the reference collections in health care, academic, and large public libraries."
— *American Reference Books Annual, 2003*

"Recommended for libraries with an interest in offering consumer health information." — *E-Streams, Jul '02*

"This is a unique and valuable resource for patients facing transplantation and their families."
— *Doody's Review Service, Jun '02*

Traveler's Health Sourcebook

Basic Consumer Health Information for Travelers, Including Physical and Medical Preparations, Transportation Health and Safety, Essential Information about Food and Water, Sun Exposure, Insect and Snake Bites, Camping and Wilderness Medicine, and Travel with Physical or Medical Disabilities

Along with International Travel Tips, Vaccination Recommendations, Geographical Health Issues, Disease Risks, a Glossary, and a Listing of Additional Resources

Edited by Joyce Brennfleck Shannon. 613 pages. 2000. 0-7808-0384-1. $78.

"Recommended reference source."
— *Booklist, American Library Association, Feb '01*

"This book is recommended for any public library, any travel collection, and especially any collection for the physically disabled."
— *American Reference Books Annual, 2001*

Vegetarian Sourcebook

Basic Consumer Health Information about Vegetarian Diets, Lifestyle, and Philosophy, Including Definitions of Vegetarianism and Veganism, Tips about Adopting Vegetarianism, Creating a Vegetarian Pantry, and Meeting Nutritional Needs of Vegetarians, with Facts Regarding Vegetarianism's Effect on Pregnant and Lactating Women, Children, Athletes, and Senior Citizens

Along with a Glossary of Commonly Used Vegetarian Terms and Resources for Additional Help and Information

Edited by Chad T. Kimball. 360 pages. 2002. 0-7808-0439-2. $78.

"Organizes into one concise volume the answers to the most common questions concerning vegetarian diets and lifestyles. This title is recommended for public and secondary school libraries." — *E-Streams, Apr '03*

"Invaluable reference for public and school library collections alike." — *Library Bookwatch, Apr '03*

"The articles in this volume are easy to read and come from authoritative sources. The book does not necessarily support the vegetarian diet but instead provides the pros and cons of this important decision. The *Vegetarian Sourcebook* is recommended for public libraries and consumer health libraries."
— *American Reference Books Annual, 2003*

Women's Health Concerns Sourcebook, 2nd Edition

Basic Consumer Health Information about the Medical and Mental Concerns of Women, Including Maintaining Health and Wellness, Gynecological Concerns, Breast Health, Sexuality and Reproductive Issues, Menopause, Cancer in Women, the Leading Causes of Death and Disability among Women, Physical Concerns of Special Significance to Women, and Women's Mental and Emotional Health

Along with a Glossary of Related Terms and Directories of Resources for Additional Help and Information

Edited by Amy L. Sutton. 748 pages. 2004. 0-7808-0673-5. $78.

ALSO AVAILABLE: Women's Health Concerns Sourcebook, 1st Edition. Edited by Heather E. Aldred. 567 pages. 1997. 0-7808-0219-5. $78.

"Handy compilation. There is an impressive range of diseases, devices, disorders, procedures, and other physical and emotional issues covered . . . well organized, illustrated, and indexed." —*Choice, Association of College and Research Libraries, Jan '98*

SEE ALSO Breast Cancer Sourcebook, Cancer Sourcebook for Women, Healthy Heart Sourcebook for Women, Osteoporosis Sourcebook

Workplace Health & Safety Sourcebook

Basic Consumer Health Information about Workplace Health and Safety, Including the Effect of Workplace Hazards on the Lungs, Skin, Heart, Ears, Eyes, Brain, Reproductive Organs, Musculoskeletal System, and Other Organs and Body Parts

Along with Information about Occupational Cancer, Personal Protective Equipment, Toxic and Hazardous Chemicals, Child Labor, Stress, and Workplace Violence

Edited by Chad T. Kimball. 626 pages. 2000. 0-7808-0231-4. $78.

"As a reference for the general public, this would be useful in any library." —*E-Streams, Jun '01*

"Provides helpful information for primary care physicians and other caregivers interested in occupational medicine. . . . General readers; professionals." —*Choice, Association of College & Research Libraries, May '01*

"Recommended reference source." —*Booklist, American Library Association, Feb '01*

"Highly recommended." —*The Bookwatch, Jan '01*

Worldwide Health Sourcebook

Basic Information about Global Health Issues, Including Malnutrition, Reproductive Health, Disease Dispersion and Prevention, Emerging Diseases, Risky Health Behaviors, and the Leading Causes of Death

Along with Global Health Concerns for Children, Women, and the Elderly, Mental Health Issues, Research and Technology Advancements, and Economic, Environmental, and Political Health Implications, a Glossary, and a Resource Listing for Additional Help and Information

Edited by Joyce Brennfleck Shannon. 614 pages. 2001. 0-7808-0330-2. $78.

"Named an Outstanding Academic Title." —*Choice, Association of College & Research Libraries, Jan '02*

"Yet another handy but also unique compilation in the extensive Health Reference Series, this is a useful work because many of the international publications reprinted or excerpted are not readily available. Highly recommended." —*Choice, Association of College & Research Libraries, Nov '01*

"Recommended reference source." —*Booklist, American Library Association, Oct '01*

Teen Health Series

Helping Young Adults Understand, Manage, and Avoid Serious Illness

Cancer Information for Teens

Health Tips about Cancer Awareness, Prevention, Diagnosis, and Treatment

Including Facts about Frequently Occurring Cancers, Cancer Risk Factors, and Coping Strategies for Teens Fighting Cancer or Dealing with Cancer in Friends or Family Members

Edited by Wilma R. Caldwell. 428 pages. 2004. 0-7808-0678-6. $58.

◼

Diet Information for Teens

Health Tips about Diet and Nutrition

Including Facts about Nutrients, Dietary Guidelines, Breakfasts, School Lunches, Snacks, Party Food, Weight Control, Eating Disorders, and More

Edited by Karen Bellenir. 399 pages. 2001. 0-7808-0441-4. $58.

"Full of helpful insights and facts throughout the book. ... An excellent resource to be placed in public libraries or even in personal collections."
— *American Reference Books Annual 2002*

"Recommended for middle and high school libraries and media centers as well as academic libraries that educate future teachers of teenagers. It is also a suitable addition to health science libraries that serve patrons who are interested in teen health promotion and education." — *E-Streams, Oct '01*

"This comprehensive book would be beneficial to collections that need information about nutrition, dietary guidelines, meal planning, and weight control. ... This reference is so easy to use that its purchase is recommended." — *The Book Report, Sep-Oct '01*

"This book is written in an easy to understand format describing issues that many teens face every day, and then provides thoughtful explanations so that teens can make informed decisions. This is an interesting book that provides important facts and information for today's teens." — *Doody's Health Sciences Book Review Journal, Jul-Aug '01*

"A comprehensive compendium of diet and nutrition. The information is presented in a straightforward, plain-spoken manner. This title will be useful to those working on reports on a variety of topics, as well as to general readers concerned about their dietary health." — *School Library Journal, Jun '01*

Drug Information for Teens

Health Tips about the Physical and Mental Effects of Substance Abuse

Including Facts about Alcohol, Anabolic Steroids, Club Drugs, Cocaine, Depressants, Hallucinogens, Herbal Products, Inhalants, Marijuana, Narcotics, Stimulants, Tobacco, and More

Edited by Karen Bellenir. 452 pages. 2002. 0-7808-0444-9. $58.

"A clearly written resource for general readers and researchers alike." — *School Library Journal*

"The chapters are quick to make a connection to their teenage reading audience. The prose is straightforward and the book lends itself to spot reading. It should be useful both for practical information and for research, and it is suitable for public and school libraries." — *American Reference Books Annual, 2003*

"Recommended reference source." — *Booklist, American Library Association, Feb '03*

"This is an excellent resource for teens and their parents. Education about drugs and substances is key to discouraging teen drug abuse and this book provides this much needed information in a way that is interesting and factual." — *Doody's Review Service, Dec '02*

◼

Fitness Information for Teens

Health Tips about Exercise, Physical Well-Being, and Health Maintenance

Including Facts about Aerobic and Anaerobic Conditioning, Stretching, Body Shape and Body Image, Sports Training, Nutrition, and Activities for Non-Athletes

Edited by Karen Bellenir. 425 pages. 2004. 0-7808-0679-4. $58.

◼

Mental Health Information for Teens

Health Tips about Mental Health and Mental Illness

Including Facts about Anxiety, Depression, Suicide, Eating Disorders, Obsessive-Compulsive Disorders, Panic Attacks, Phobias, Schizophrenia, and More

Edited by Karen Bellenir. 406 pages. 2001. 0-7808-0442-2. $58.

"In both language and approach, this user-friendly entry in the *Teen Health Series* is on target for teens needing information on mental health concerns." — *Booklist, American Library Association, Jan '02*

"Readers will find the material accessible and informative, with the shaded notes, facts, and embedded glossary insets adding appropriately to the already interesting and succinct presentation."
—*School Library Journal, Jan '02*

"This title is highly recommended for any library that serves adolescents and parents/caregivers of adolescents." —*E-Streams, Jan '02*

"Recommended for high school libraries and young adult collections in public libraries. Both health professionals and teenagers will find this book useful."
—*American Reference Books Annual 2002*

"This is a nice book written to enlighten the society, primarily teenagers, about common teen mental health issues. It is highly recommended to teachers and parents as well as adolescents."
—*Doody's Review Service, Dec '01*

■

Sexual Health Information for Teens

Health Tips about Sexual Development, Human Reproduction, and Sexually Transmitted Diseases

Including Facts about Puberty, Reproductive Health, Chlamydia, Human Papillomavirus, Pelvic Inflammatory Disease, Herpes, AIDS, Contraception, Pregnancy, and More

Edited by Deborah A. Stanley. 391 pages. 2003. 0-7808-0445-7. $58.

"This work should be included in all high school libraries and many larger public libraries. . . . highly recommended."
—*American Reference Books Annual 2004*

"Sexual Health approaches its subject with appropriate seriousness and offers easily accessible advice and information."
—*School Library Journal, Feb. 2004*

Skin Health Information For Teens

Health Tips about Dermatological Concerns and Skin Cancer Risks

Including Facts about Acne, Warts, Hives, and Other Conditions and Lifestyle Choices, Such as Tanning, Tattooing, and Piercing, That Affect the Skin, Nails, Scalp, and Hair

Edited by Robert Aquinas McNally. 430 pages. 2003. 0-7808-0446-5. $58.

"This volume, as with others in the series, will be a useful addition to school and public library collections."
—*American Reference Books Annual 2004*

"This volume serves as a one-stop source and should be a necessity for any health collection."
—*Library Media Connection*

■

Sports Injuries Information For Teens

Health Tips about Sports Injuries and Injury Protection

Including Facts about Specific Injuries, Emergency Treatment, Rehabilitation, Sports Safety, Competition Stress, Fitness, Sports Nutrition, Steroid Risks, and More

Edited by Joyce Brennfleck Shannon. 425 pages. 2003. 0-7808-0447-3. $58.

"This work will be useful in the young adult collections of public libraries as well as high school libraries."
—*American Reference Books Annual 2004*

Health Reference Series

Adolescent Health Sourcebook

AIDS Sourcebook, 3rd Edition

Alcoholism Sourcebook

Allergies Sourcebook, 2nd Edition

Alternative Medicine Sourcebook, 2nd Edition

Alzheimer's Disease Sourcebook, 3rd Edition

Arthritis Sourcebook

Asthma Sourcebook

Attention Deficit Disorder Sourcebook

Back & Neck Disorders Sourcebook

Blood & Circulatory Disorders Sourcebook

Brain Disorders Sourcebook

Breast Cancer Sourcebook

Breastfeeding Sourcebook

Burns Sourcebook

Cancer Sourcebook, 4th Edition

Cancer Sourcebook for Women, 2nd Edition

Caregiving Sourcebook

Child Abuse Sourcebook

Childhood Diseases & Disorders Sourcebook

Colds, Flu & Other Common Ailments Sourcebook

Communication Disorders Sourcebook

Congenital Disorders Sourcebook

Consumer Issues in Health Care Sourcebook

Contagious & Non-Contagious Infectious Diseases Sourcebook

Death & Dying Sourcebook

Dental Care & Oral Health Sourcebook, 2nd Edition

Depression Sourcebook

Diabetes Sourcebook, 3rd Edition

Diet & Nutrition Sourcebook, 2nd Edition

Digestive Diseases & Disorder Sourcebook

Disabilities Sourcebook

Domestic Violence Sourcebook, 2nd Edition

Drug Abuse Sourcebook

Ear, Nose & Throat Disorders Sourcebook

Eating Disorders Sourcebook

Emergency Medical Services Sourcebook

Endocrine & Metabolic Disorders Sourcebook

Environmentally Health Sourcebook, 2nd Edition

Ethnic Diseases Sourcebook

Eye Care Sourcebook, 2nd Edition

Family Planning Sourcebook

Fitness & Exercise Sourcebook, 2nd Edition

Food & Animal Borne Diseases Sourcebook

Food Safety Sourcebook

Forensic Medicine Sourcebook

Gastrointestinal Diseases & Disorders Sourcebook

Genetic Disorders Sourcebook, 2nd Edition

Head Trauma Sourcebook

Headache Sourcebook

Health Insurance Sourcebook

Health Reference Series Cumulative Index 1999

Healthy Aging Sourcebook

Healthy Children Sourcebook